Dynamic Lumbar Spine Stabilization

Ali Fahir Özer • Mario Di Silvestre
Vijay K. Goel • Deniz U. Erbulut
Editors

Dynamic Lumbar Spine Stabilization

Springer

Editors
Ali Fahir Özer
Department of Neurosurgery
Koc University School of Medicine
Istanbul, Turkey

Mario Di Silvestre
Chief of Spinal Deformity Department
Ospedale Santa Corona
Pietra Ligure, Italy

Vijay K. Goel
Department of Bioengineering &
Orthopaedic Surgery
University of Toledo
Toledo, OH, USA

Deniz U. Erbulut
Herston Biofabrication Institute
Metro North Hospital
and Health Service
Brisbane, QLD, Australia

ISBN 978-3-032-12121-9 ISBN 978-3-032-12122-6 (eBook)
https://doi.org/10.1007/978-3-032-12122-6

This Springer imprint is published by the registered company Springer Nature Switzerland AG
The registered company address is: Gewerbestrasse 11, 6330 Cham, Switzerland

"In memory of Mehdi Sasani and Vijay K. Goel"

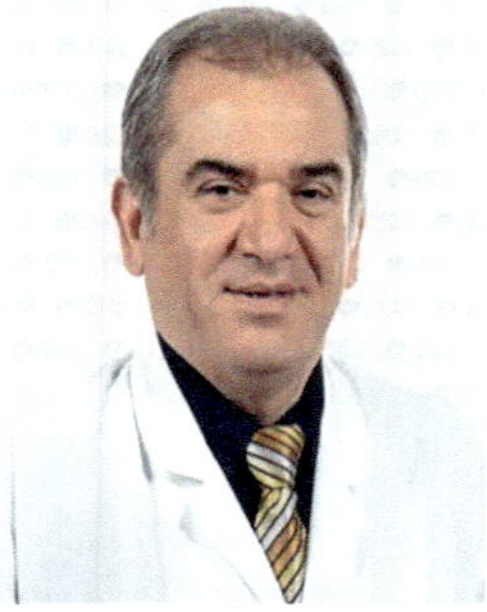

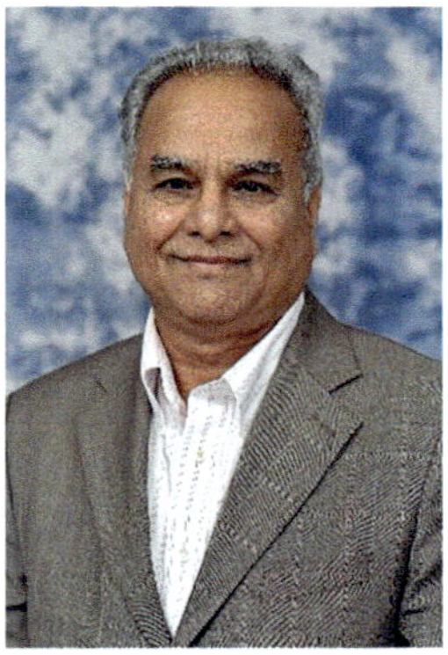

Preface

The management of spinal pathologies, recent advances in biomechanics and biomaterials, and especially the shift in understanding in surgical philosophy have led to the development of many concepts in spinal surgery from different perspectives. While spinal fusion has long represented the definitive solution for achieving spinal stability, as problems have become more apparent, problems such as adjacent segment degeneration, pseudoarthrosis, and loss of physiological mobility have become increasingly apparent through long-term clinical observation. Furthermore, disproportionately complex surgery, such as spinal fusion, is being performed to treat a simple pathology such as degenerative disc disease. The idea that "there must be a simpler solution to this disproportionate stabilization" has led surgeons to question the importance of fusion. These challenges have spurred the pursuit of motion-preserving strategies aimed at stabilizing the spine without compromising its dynamic nature.

In this context, dynamic spinal instrumentation has emerged as a significant milestone in modern spine surgery. The concept focuses on providing controlled stabilization of a functional spinal unit while preserving motion in appropriate cases. This biomechanical balance aims to preserve normal kinematics, reduce mechanical load on adjacent segments, and improve long-term patient outcomes. Various systems, such as pedicle-based structures (Dynesys®, Cosmic®, Safinaz®), interspinous devices (Coflex®, DIAM®), and hybrid stabilization designs, reflect a common goal: to restore segmental function and physiological load distribution rather than create a rigid spine.

The evidence supporting dynamic stabilization continues to expand. Short- and medium-term results demonstrate promising results in selected indications, particularly in degenerative lumbar pathologies that cause chronic instability. In this context, dynamic pedicle systems are also finding application in long-term degenerative conditions and mobile adult deformities. However, as with any emerging technology, several questions are being actively investigated. Issues such as determining optimal patient selection criteria, implant longevity, mechanical fatigue behavior, and the role of dynamic structures in multi-level or revision settings continue to define the frontiers of clinical research. The need for long-term comparative studies versus fusion remains critical to clarifying their precise role in surgical practice.

Looking ahead, the field of spinal dynamic instrumentation stands on the brink of a transformative era driven by interdisciplinary innovation. The next generation of implants will evolve beyond merely responding to physiological stresses—they will embody advanced material properties engineered to endure dynamic loading and revolutionary design architectures that sustain motion without compromising function or succumbing to fatigue. Alongside biological disc repair, these breakthroughs will converge with robotic precision, AI-guided surgical planning, and patient-specific customization, ushering in a new paradigm of truly adaptive and enduring spinal restoration. Furthermore, long-term success rates are expected to increase with advancements such as robotic guidance, AI-assisted surgical planning, and the integration of patient-specific design and precision, personalized surgery.

This book is designed to provide a comprehensive and critical review of the principles, technologies, clinical applications, and future directions of spinal dynamic instrumentation. This book reflects the collective efforts of clinicians, engineers, and scientists dedicated to preserving at least some spinal function through simple stabilization and preserving motion in appropriate cases. We hope this work serves not only as a reference for current practice but also as a foundation for continued inquiry and innovation.

We would like to express our sincere gratitude to Hınazant Talin Özkan, with whom we have worked for many years, for her unparalleled efforts and unforgettable contributions at every stage of the preparation of this book. It is impossible to forget her contribution.

As editors, we extend our gratitude to those whose expertise shaped this book, to the contributors, and to the pioneers whose vision continues to redefine the boundaries of spinal stabilization. The transition from fusion to functional preservation represents more than a technical evolution; it also signals a paradigm shift in our understanding of spinal health. This shift involves moderating stabilization, preserving motion in appropriate cases, and simplifying and improving quality of life. We will continue to work on this path until we establish our credibility.

Pietra Ligure, Italy — Mario Di Silvestre
Istanbul, Turkey — Ali Fahir Özer
Brisbane, QLD, Australia — Deniz U. Erbulut

Contents

About the Editors

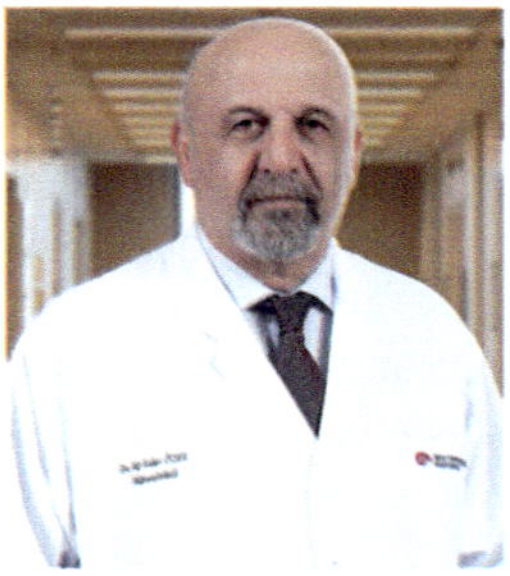

Ali Fahir Özer graduated from Atatürk University School of Medicine in 1976. He did his neurosurgery residency between 1977 and 1982 at Hacettepe University School of Medicine. He obtained his associate professorship in 1988 and full-professorship in 1994. He served as the head of neurosurgery department in Kocaeli University between 1994 and 1995. He has been working at the neurosurgery department of the American Hospital since 1995 and is currently a faculty at Koc University School of Medicine, Department of Neurosurgery. Since 2018, he is Adjunct Professor in Bioengineering and Orthopaedic Surgery Colleges of Engineering and Medicine, University of Toledo (OH, USA). He is member of Eurospine and North American Spine Society.

He also is member of the advisory board and reviewer of several journals, e.g., *The Spine Journal*, *World Neurosurgery*, *BMC Musculoskeletal Journal*, Springer, *Journal of Turkish Neurosurgery*, *Case Reports in Orthopedics*, etc. He has authored or co-authored over 230 articles and 46 book chapters, and he is also editor of 9 books. His research mainly focuses on biomechanics and dynamic stabilization of spine. He had patented Orthrus Dynamic Spinal System, Safinaz Dynamic Screw, and Cervical Disc Prosthesis.

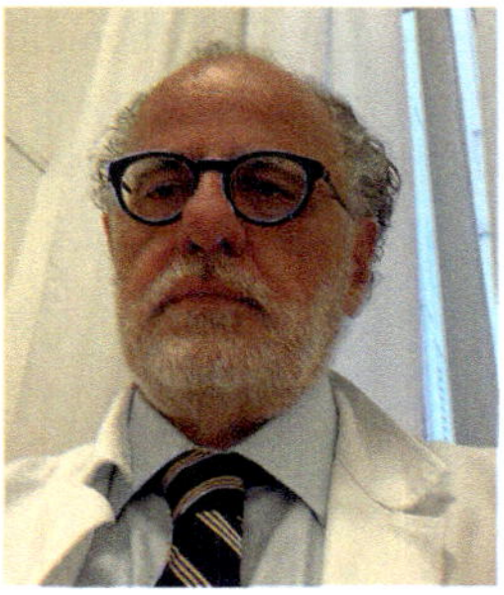

Mario Di Silvestre attended the Scoliosis Center of the Pisa University Orthopedic Clinic (Pisa, Italy) during his Orthopedics and Traumatology residency, directed by Prof. Pier Giorgio Marchetti. After his specialization, in 1984 he moved to the Scoliosis Center at the Rizzoli Orthopedic Institute in Bologna (Italy), becoming more actively involved in spine surgery under the guidance of Prof. Leonardo Gui and Prof. Romolo Savini. He was then hired back to the Rizzoli Institute in 1989, first as an orthopedics and traumatology medical assistant, then as an orthopedics and traumatology hospital assistant, and finally as a medical director of the Spine Surgery Department. Since 2017, he is responsible of the Spine Surgery at the Santa Corona Hospital in Pietra Ligure (Savona, Italy). He has many publications published in international journals and many papers presented at international meetings.

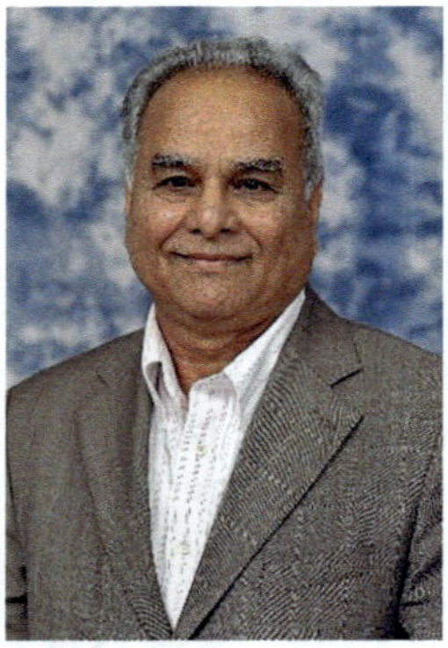

Vijay K. Goel is Professor of Orthopaedic Bioengineering and Co-Director of the Engineering Center for Orthopaedic Research Excellence (E-CORE), Department of Bioengineering and Orthopaedic Surgery, University of Toledo, Toledo (OH, USA). He has been active as professor of bioengineering over four decades, and is a globally recognized biomechanical researcher and mentor of a large number of scientists and clinicians. He is a prolific contributor to device development as an industrial advisor/entrepreneur, and a dedicated society-benefactor in developing treatments of orthopedic ailments

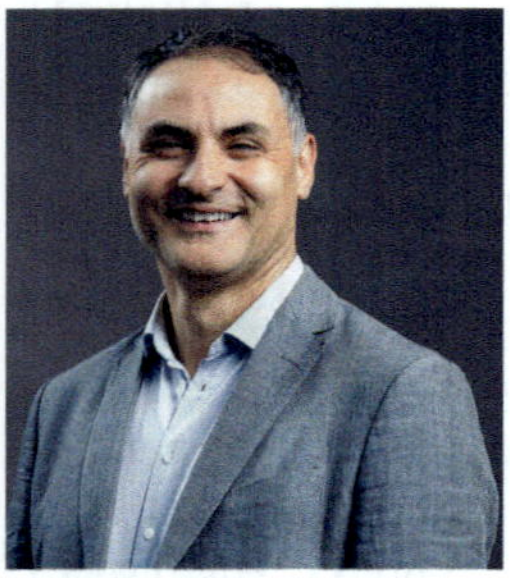

Deniz U. Erbulut received his PhD in Mechanical Engineering from the University of Melbourne in 2010. After faculty appointments in the USA and Turkey, he joined HBI as a senior research fellow in 2020. He gained about 10 years of research experience in biomechanics for understanding clinically relevant issues in medicine. Using a combination of experimental and computational tools, he performs research in in vivo/in vitro joint mechanics, human motion, musculoskeletal modeling, computational biomechanics and spinal/orthopedic implant development and testing. He holds three orthopedic implant patents for the USA and most European countries. He has been a principal investigator for several projects, teaching graduate and undergraduate level courses in the biomedical and mechanical engineering departments at various universities, and supervised several master and PhD students as a principal advisor.

Dynamic Stabilization and Philosophy

1

Mehmet Yiğit Akgün and Utku Özgen

1.1 Introduction

You may have trouble associating skills like running, taking deep breaths, and climbing with your spine. However, mammals, including humans, owe these abilities to the complex structures of their spines, which consist of five distinct regions with specialized functions. The spine, including the human spine, is one of the most important components of the system that keeps many living beings upright in nature and directly affects their vital movements [1]. The structural logic of the spine is also considered the formal logic of many design products present in human life. In terms of its organic structure and the relationship between its parts, it possesses an aesthetic appearance.

For approximately 1.9 million years, starting with Homo erectus, which is considered the evolutionary ancestor of Homo sapiens, the most defining characteristic of humans has been reflected in our spine: "Upright posture." As humans evolved to be able to walk on 2 ft, there was not much material for evolution to work with [2]. Our spine, which had a useful S-shaped curve for climbing trees, "suddenly" rotated 90 degrees. We can liken this to stacking 26 different cups and plates on top of each other and trying to maintain balance. When we think of vertebrae and discs instead of plates and cups and add the necessity of carrying an excessively heavy object like the head in balance, it becomes inevitable to experience problems related to the spine [3–5]. Jeremy DeSilva from Boston University clearly expresses this by saying, "If you were to design anatomy from scratch, the human body would definitely not be the product you would design. Unfortunately, evolution works like a bad engineer with a roll of duct tape in one hand and a stapler in the other."

Regardless of where they are in the world, human beings rush through their daily routines in order to complete their to-do lists. Due to the limited time and unfinished tasks, significant mental and physical strains occur over the years. This approach plays a significant role in the fundamental problem of spinal pain, which is one of the biggest issues of our modern age.

Pain is the primary factor that leads patients with spinal disorders to seek medical help. Along with pain, neurological deficits may also occur. However, patients' main complaints are acute-convulsive or chronic-continuous pain that interrupts their daily activities. Pain can manifest as axial pain due to rapid annular laceration or as radicular pain caused by compression on the

M. Y. Akgün (✉)
Department of Neurosurgery, Koc University Hospital, Spine Center, Istanbul, Turkey
e-mail: makgun@kuh.ku.edu.tr

U. Özgen
Department of Neurosurgery, American Hospital, Istanbul, Turkey
e-mail: utkuo@amerikanhastanesi.org

A. F. Özer et al. (eds.), *Dynamic Lumbar Spine Stabilization*,
https://doi.org/10.1007/978-3-032-12122-6_1

nerve root by a herniated disc [6]. Consequently, pain is the fundamental problem that we, as surgeons, strive to treat. The Latin phrase "primum nihil nocere" ("first, do no harm"), which we were taught in medical school, constitutes one of the fundamental ethical principles of our professional life. Therefore, treating patients with the method that poses the least potential harm becomes a "mandatory condition" for both adherence to professional ethical norms and the surgeon's recognition of success.

In modern times, lower back pain is one of the most significant issues that diminishes quality of life due to disc degeneration. While disc herniation and degeneration are often blamed as the most common causes of pain, the primary cause of lower back pain is spinal instability. The association of intervertebral disc degeneration with instability was first described by Knutsson in 1944. Knutsson identified abnormal flexion-extension displacement associated with disc degeneration on direct radiographs. Furthermore, he emphasized that sagittal displacement greater than 3 mm in dynamic radiographs should be considered a significant indication in favor of segmental instability [7].

The degenerative process of the lumbar spine and the pathology of discogenic pain were defined by Kirkaldy-Willis and Farfan in 1982 [8]. They reported that spinal stenosis and degenerative spondylolisthesis occur as a result of the degenerative process and cellular mechanisms, leading to back pain. Frymoyer and Selby introduced the concepts of primary and secondary instability and included degenerative disc disease, degenerative spondylolisthesis, and degenerative scoliotic deformities in the primary instability group [9]. Panjabi emphasized that instability leads to pathological motion, deformities, and neurological deficits [10]. Benzel classified chronic instability into two groups: glacial and dysfunctional segmental motion. According to Benzel, the most common example of glacial instability is degenerative spondylolisthesis, while degenerative disc disease is associated with dysfunctional segmental motion [11].

However, the abnormal motion used in the definition of instability does not always cause back pain. For example, although radiological abnormal motion can be observed in degenerated discs associated with spondylolisthesis, the pain is not constant. Therefore, the definition of instability has been updated to include abnormal motion at the joint surface and altered load transmission. The intervertebral disc is actually an isotropic structure filled with fluid, but it undergoes changes as it degenerates. The isotropic properties and load transmission of the intervertebral disc vary depending on disc degeneration. The "stone in the shoe" phenomenon explains the postural pain pattern in patients with lumbar disc degeneration because the loading pattern is associated with the formation of pain that shifts from one patient to another in the degenerative spine. Symptoms of back pain generally involve abnormal load distribution rather than abnormal motion as the primary source of pain. Most patients complain of postural or positional pain as the predominant symptom. Thus, the idea that achieving the most physiological load transmission will provide the most ideal surgical outcomes has emerged [12–14].

The effects of lumbar disc surgery have been debated since the procedure was introduced by Mixter and Barr in 1934 [15]. Spinal fusion, initially described by Albee and Hibbs, was first applied for the treatment of Pott's disease and spinal deformities [16, 17]. Over the years, spinal fusion has become a widely used surgical treatment for various spinal pathologies, including chronic back pain, disc herniation, spondylolisthesis, facet arthropathy, and spinal stenosis. In the past 50 years, with the advancements in technology and instrument systems, spinal fusion has become the gold standard for the treatment of various degenerative spinal disorders [18].

Despite the establishment of a common experience worldwide in fusion surgery and reported radiological success rates of up to 100%, the expected success has not been achieved when considering patient satisfaction and clinical outcomes. According to a systematic meta-analysis evaluating the results of lumbar spinal fusion, success rates range from 16% to 95% (average 70%) [19]. Additionally, increased stress formation in adjacent segments and the development of well-known adjacent segment degeneration are observed with rigid spinal implants. Furthermore, fusion surgery has some significant disadvantages, such as pain, wound issues, infections due to long operation times, pseudarthrosis, and implant fatigue insufficiency. These observations suggest that there may be successful treatments beyond fusion, considering the etiologies of back pain related to abnormal load distribution [20].

According to Wolf's law, fusion grafts should be under pressure for fusion to occur. Some researchers have believed that continuous compression on the graft is essential for the development of fusion. In rigid systems, the load is directly transmitted downward, preventing loading of the graft and creating a "stress shield" phenomenon. In dynamic pedicle systems, the load from instrumentation is shared with the anterior column, resulting in continuous load transmission on the graft and increasing the likelihood of fusion development [21].

Graf presented the concept of fusionless dynamic stabilization using his own pedicle screw at the second Eurospine Congress in Rome and later published the results. Both Graf's concept with the Graf ligament and Von Strempel's concept with the mobile screw head aim to maintain motion in the spine. They defined the dynamic pedicle screw system as a simple stabilization system that can be used only for minor instabilities [22, 23]. Alongside stabilization, the concept of motion preservation emerged with Fernstrom. Sengupta reported that larger physiological load transfers could alleviate pain and prevent adjacent segment degeneration. Additionally, it was noted that if normal motion and load transmission are restored and the degeneration is not advanced, the damaged disc can regenerate [24].

In the search for alternative spinal implants, the primary goal is to avoid the adverse effects on adjacent segments, prevent implant failure, and ultimately develop a system that allows for increased load sharing and controlled motion without compromising load transmission. Dynamic stabilization aims to maintain motion in the spinal segment and control abnormal movement while providing increased physiological load transmission between the anterior and posterior components of the spine to alleviate pain. Dynamic systems can allow for anatomical modification of the motion segment when subjected to postural changes [25].

During dynamic stabilization surgery, it is important to remember the principle we discussed earlier. As mentioned before, pain is the primary issue that needs to be addressed. Patients seek medical help to relieve their pain, so the doctor's main responsibility is to treat the patient with the least amount of risk. While alleviating the patient's pain, our second concern should be, "Can we also preserve mobility?" Surgeons should aim to accomplish both tasks without causing harm to the patient. If a surgeon can successfully achieve both objectives without causing harm, the outcome can be considered excellent [26].

Our aim was to demonstrate the biomechanical adequacy of the dynamic screw and rod system through finite element and cadaver studies. We used a rod that we developed ourselves and named it the Talin rod, as the dynamic rod. In this study, the biomechanical effects of dynamic, semi-rigid, and rigid posterior stabilization systems on the lumbar spine were reported. The resulting range of motion (ROM), facet joint loads, intradiscal pressures, and stresses in pedicle screws were observed and compared for all cases. As a result, in hybrid moment flexion, extension, and right and left lateral bending, the dynamic screw-dynamic rod combination yielded results closest to those of the intact spine. Similarly, when examining ROM values at the L4–5 segment, it was observed that the dynamic combination provided results close to those of the intact spine [27, 28].

If the aim of the pedicle dynamic system is to maintain motion, for the dynamic system to be considered ideal, it should stabilize the disrupted neutral zone in or near the normal range. Human motion segments can differ from each other due to various structural reasons. The degree of degeneration in the structures forming the motion segment is also crucial. "What is the ideal rod strain in a motion segment?" Does the ability to perform motion within normal physiological limits have any relation to age, height, or muscle volume? How much do ethnic factors affect it? Being hypermobile does not necessarily mean that the motion segments are unstable. "Do gymnasts competing in the Olympics perform their movements in pain?" In this case, it is not very likely that the expectation of achieving the characteristic of a mobile segment that varies from person to person can be fulfilled with a single rod. However, based on the satisfactory results obtained from clinically applied systems where both the rod and screw are dynamic, we have come to the conclusion that a new classification is needed [29, 30].

Fusion advocates' strongest argument is "Fusion is the natural outcome, the rest is a lie." The solution of freezing the mobility in a problematic motion segment also stems from this idea. However, it is also possible to try to restore the abnormal mobility of the problematic segment back to the normal range using a simpler procedure such as dynamic stabilization. Why burn all the bridges from the beginning? Why should we start with a more challenging option when there is a simpler alternative? Why not provide the conditions that allow the organism to make choices for itself? The answers to these questions will ultimately lead us to dynamic stability.

Throughout the history of humanity, we have witnessed that today's "truths" can become tomorrow's "errors." The process of sharpening our consciousness, questioning the unquestionable, and eliminating intellectual blindness has indeed led us to the enlightenment movement. In ancient times, Pyrrho argued that logical thinking cannot lead to infallible certainty and laid the foundations of "skepticism." In the modern era, Bacon defined skepticism as a necessary step in the pursuit of truth, stating, "If a person begins with certainties, they shall end in doubts, but if they are content to begin with doubts, they shall end in certainties." Kant also attributed a critical approach to skepticism and advocated that it is the only way to secure what we know or should know. These thinkers emphasize the importance of searching for truth and engaging in critical thinking.

Regarding the idea that nothing is fixed and everything is constantly changing, we can trace this line of thought back to philosophical doctrines that date back hundreds of years, such as those of Heraclitus, as well as to thinkers like Bergson in the twentieth century. Heraclitus, for instance, emphasized the constant flux and change in nature with his famous statement, "No man ever steps in the same river twice, for it's not the same river and he's not the same man." This notion forms the foundation of the doctrine of flux. Bergson, in his philosophy, also argued for ongoing change in everything. He described the cosmic evolution as an "élan vital," or vital impulse, characterizing change as "flux," time as the medium of flux, and "duration" as the sum total of existence. These philosophical ideas highlight the dynamic and ever-changing nature of the world and the importance of recognizing and adapting to this continuous flux. They invite us to cultivate a mindset of openness, flexibility, and an understanding that nothing remains fixed.

Absolutely, questioning dynamic systems is essential. Just like any other inquiry, it prevents us from blindly advocating for a new technology. Moreover, how can we determine what is right? The best way to do so is by actively engaging with the reality of dynamic systems.

Art increasing our knowledge of spinal anatomy, enhancing our proficiency in biomechanics, and understanding the compatibility of instrumentation systems with the spine should enable us to make informed choices by selecting what is advantageous and critiquing what is futile. Our task is to utilize these concepts to design future dynamic systems while preserving the ideal physiology of the spine. This stems from our nation's ability to utilize current technologies, accumulate knowledge, and possess confidence.

Currently, the surgical implantation of dynamic stabilization devices is invasive enough to cause disruption to muscle and ligament structures. It is well-known that these soft tissue structures play a significant role in normal spinal motion, balance, and load transmission. Over time, these devices ideally require the natural support of muscles and ligaments to function effectively. Fortunately, advancements in the surgical implantation of fusion-related devices such as interbody cages, rods, and screws have led to the emergence of minimally invasive techniques. These techniques inflict far less damage to supportive structures and are associated with faster recovery times. It appears that the optimal performance of dynamic systems may likely stem from the integration of these minimally invasive techniques with the implant itself. Indeed, when used in conjunction with motion-preserving devices, minimally invasive surgical techniques can offer more significant benefits in long-term outcomes compared to fusion procedures [31, 32].

Ultimately, the concept of dynamic stabilization presented by Graf, along with the artificial ligament he pioneered, and Strempel's articulated screw concepts lie ahead of us. Our task is to create future dynamic systems that align with the ideal spinal physiology using these concepts. This will be possible through the ability to utilize the sufficient technologies available in our country, knowledge, and self-confidence.

References

1. Jones KE, Angielczyk KD, Polly PD, Head JJ, Fernandez V, Lungmus JK, Tulga S, Pierce SE. Fossils reveal the complex evolutionary history of the mammalian regionalized spine. Science. 2018;361(6408):1249–52.
2. Oró JJ. Evolution of the brain: from behavior to consciousness in 3.4 billion years. Neurosurgery. 2004;54(6):1287–96. discussion 1296–7
3. Galbusera F, Bassani T. The spine: a strong, stable, and flexible structure with biomimetics potential. Biomimetics (Basel). 2019;4(3):60.
4. Abelin-Genevois K. Sagittal balance of the spine. Orthop Traumatol Surg Res. 2021 Feb;107(1S):102769.
5. Meyer MR, Haeusler M. Spinal cord evolution in early homo. J Hum Evol. 2015 Nov;88:43–53.
6. Schwarzer AC, Aprill CN, Derby R, Fortin J, Kine G, Bogduk N. The relative contributions of the disc and zygapophyseal joint in chronic low back pain. Spine. 1994;19(7):801–6.
7. Knutsson F. The instability associated with disc degeneration in the lumbar spine. Acta Radiol. 1944;25:593–609.
8. Kirkaldy-Willis WH, Farfan HF. Instability of the lumbar spine. Clin Orthop Relat Res. 1982;165:110–23.
9. Frymoyer JW, Selby DK. Segmental instability: rationale for treatment. Spine. 1985;10(3):280–6.
10. Panjabi MM. Clinical spinal instability and low back pain. J Electromyogr Kinesiol. 2003;13(4):371–9.
11. Benzel EC. Biomechanics of Spine Stabilization, Stability and instability of the spine. New York, NY, USA: AANS; 2001. p. 29–43.
12. McNally DS, Adams MA. Internal intervertebral disc mechanics as revealed by stress profilometry. Spine. 1992;17(1):66–73.
13. Nockels RP. Dynamic stabilization in the surgical management of painful lumbar spinal disorders. Spine. 2005;30(16):S68–72.
14. Sengupta DK. Dynamic stabilization devices in the treatment of low back pain. Neurol India. 2005;53(4):466–74.
15. Mixter WJ, Barr JS. Rupture of the intervertebral disc with involvement of the spinal canal. N Engl J Med. 1934;211:210–5.
16. Albee FH. Transplantation of a portion of the tibia into the spine for Pott's disease. JAMA. 1911;57:885.
17. Hibbs RH. An operation for progressive spinal deformities. NY J Med. 1911;93:1013.
18. Reid PC, Morr S, Kaiser MG. State of the union: a review of lumbar fusion indications and techniques for degenerative spine disease. J Neurosurg Spine. 2019;31(1):1–14.
19. Tavares WM, de França SA, Paiva WS, Teixeira MJ. A systematic review and meta-analysis of fusion rate enhancements and bone graft options for spine surgery. Sci Rep. 2022;12(1):7546.
20. Murphy RF, Mooney JF 3rd. Complications following spine fusion for adolescent idiopathic scoliosis. Curr Rev Musculoskelet Med. 2016 Dec;9(4):462–9.
21. Ahn YH, Chen WM, Lee KY, Park KW, Lee SJ. Comparison of the load-sharing characteristics between pedicle-based dynamic and rigid rod devices. Biomed Mater. 2008 Dec;3(4):044101.
22. Graf H. Evaluation of the therapeutic effect of the Graf stabilisation system. In: Proceedings of the 2nd annual meeting of the European spine society. Rome; 1991.
23. von Strempel A, Moosman D, Stoss C, Martin A. Stabilization of the degenerated lumbar spine in the non fusion technique with cosmic posterior dynamic system. World Spine J. 2006;1(1):40–7.
24. Fernström U. Arthroplasty with intercorporal endoprothesis in herniated disc and in painful disc. Acta Chir Scand Suppl. 1966;357:154–9.
25. Kaner T, Ozer AF. Dynamic stabilization for challenging lumbar degenerative diseases of the spine: a review of the literature. Adv Orthop. 2013;2013:753470.
26. Gomleksiz C, Sasani M, Oktenoglu T, Ozer AF. A short history of posterior dynamic stabilization. Adv Orthop. 2012;2012:629698.
27. Erbulut DU, Kiapour A, Oktenoglu T, Ozer AF, Goel VK. A computational biomechanical investigation of posterior dynamic instrumentation: combination of dynamic rod and hinged (dynamic) screw. J Biomech Eng. 2014;136(5):051007.
28. Oktenoglu T, Erbulut DU, Kiapour A, Ozer AF, Lazoglu I, Kaner T, Sasani M, Goel VK. Pedicle

screw-based posterior dynamic stabilisation of the lumbar spine: in vitro cadaver investigation and a finite element study. Comput Methods Biomech Biomed Engin. 2015 Aug;18(11):1252–61.
29. Beazell JR, Mullins M, Grindstaff TL. Lumbar instability: an evolving and challenging concept. J Man Manip Ther. 2010;18(1):9–14.
30. Kaner T, Sasani M, Oktenoglu T, Ozer AF. Dynamic stabilization of the spine: a new classification system. Turk Neurosurg. 2010 Apr;20(2):205–15.
31. Chang CC, Kuo CH, Chang HK, Tu TH, Fay LY, Wu JC, Cheng H, Huang WC. Minimally invasive dynamic screw stabilization using cortical bone trajectory. BMC Musculoskelet Disord. 2020;21(1):605.
32. Kuo YH, Kuo CH, Chang HK, Ko CC, Tu TH, Chang CC, Cheng H, Lirng JF, Huang WC, Wu JC. Cortical bone trajectory-based dynamic stabilization. World Neurosurg. 2022 Mar;159:e416–24.

Functional Anatomy and Load Dynamics of the Lumbar Spine

2

Shashwat Mishra, Venkata Paruchuri,
Raheel M. Dar, Nicholas Green, Yuheng Wang,
and Deniz U. Erbulut

2.1 Introduction

The lumbar spine consists of five vertebrae and five discs. These vertebrae are specialized in their function to withstand the highest loads among all spinal segments. The vertebrae within this region are the largest within the human spine [1]. The unique anatomy of the individual lumbar vertebrae and their articulations allows for the load-bearing and movement characteristics known to be associated with the lumbar spine [2]. Similarly, the lumbar intervertebral discs are the largest among their counterparts throughout the human spine. This increased size, as well as differences in their composition, results in their increased physiologic limits and load-bearing characteristics as compared to discs within other regions of the spine [3].

In vivo, these structures form a chain whose formation allows the lumbar spine to physiologically withstand loads upwards of two times one's body weight. This increase in the static and dynamic loading capabilities of the lumbar spine is not solely attributed to the anatomy and orientation of the vertebrae and intervertebral discs but also to passive and active tissues that act within this region. The elasticity of passive tissues, contractility of active tissues, and structural and compositional anatomy of the vertebrae and discs contribute to the stability of this region in an exponential, as opposed to an additive, manner [4, 5].

2.2 Lumbar Vertebral Anatomy

The ingenuity of these structures begins with the unique anatomy of the vertebral bodies. Consisting of trabecular bone and a red marrow core, surrounded by compact bone, the body of a vertebra, as seen in Fig. 2.1a, forms a kidney-like shape. This slightly umbilicated structure is the largest of its kind found throughout the human body [1, 2]. The vertebral body, as well as other structures that will be subsequently discussed in further detail below, contains perforations through which blood and lymphatic vessels traverse. Being the final site of force transfer within the spine, prior to the beginning of the

S. Mishra · R. M. Dar
University of Queensland Mayne Medical School, University in Herston, Brisbane, QLD, Australia
e-mail: shashwat.mishra@uq.net.au

V. Paruchuri
Ochsner Clinical School, University of Queensland, Brisbane, QLD, Australia
e-mail: v.paruchuri@uq.net.au

N. Green · Y. Wang
Metro North Health, Herston Biofabrication Institute, Brisbane, QLD, Australia
e-mail: nicholas.green@health.qld.gov.au

D. U. Erbulut (✉)
Herston Biofabrication Institute, Metro North Hospital and Health Service, Brisbane, QLD, Australia
e-mail: deniz.erbulut@health.qld.gov.au; erbulutdeniz@gmail.com

A. F. Özer et al. (eds.), *Dynamic Lumbar Spine Stabilization*,
https://doi.org/10.1007/978-3-032-12122-6_2

Fig. 2.1 (**a**) A transverse view of an average lumbar vertebral body. Note the umbilicated vertebral body. (**b**) A sagittal view of two lumbar vertebral bodies, demonstrating the facet or zygapophyseal joint, as well as the intervertebral disc. Note the large, broad, and slightly inferior directionality of the spinous processes. (Courtesy of Dr. Alper Yeni)

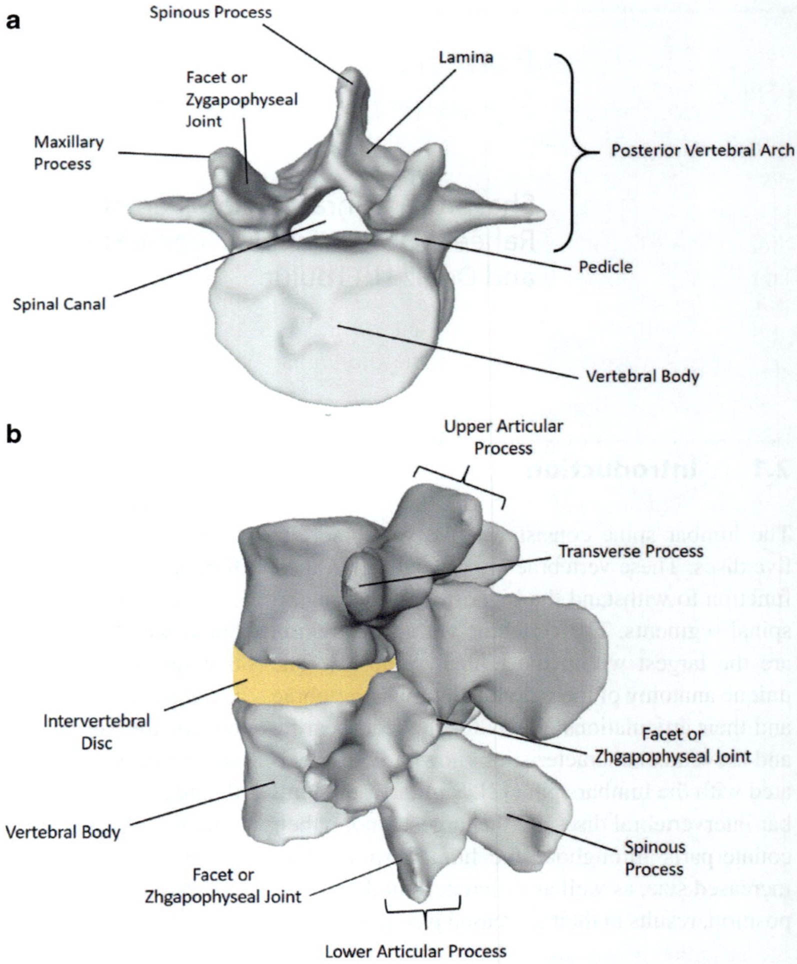

sacrum, the L5 vertebra is typically the largest of its kind within the human body [1, 2]. The L5 body is found to be taller on the anterior aspect as compared to the posterior aspect. This allows for the formation of the lumbar kyphosis, called the lumbosacral angle (LA), also known as the Cobb angle [2]. Manipulation of the LA is crucial for maintaining both static and dynamic stability [1, 2].

Protruding from the lateral aspects of the dorsal vertebral body are the pedicles, as seen in Fig. 2.1a, b [1]. Anchored to the vertebral body, they mark the beginning of the vertebral arch. The vertebral arch is defined as the structures dorsal to the vertebral body, which form the spinal canal, as per Fig. 2.1a [1]. Due to the shape of their protrusion, they form superior and inferior vertebral notches. When considered alongside an adjacent vertebra, these notches form the intervertebral foramen, allowing nerves and blood vessels to enter and exit the spinal canal [1, 2]. The transverse processes are found to be protruding laterally at the distal end of the pedicles, as seen in Fig. 2.1a, b. The L5 transverse processes are the largest of their kind in the human body [2].

As per Fig. 2.1a, the transverse processes are connected via bilateral oblique, inferior-medial projections called the lamina [1, 2]. The laminae are crucial structures, as they serve as connection points for the superior and inferior articular processes [1]. The aspect of the lamina between the superior and inferior articular processes is called the *pars interlaminaris* [1, 2]. Due to it serving as the interface between the articular processes of adjacent vertebrae, the *pars interlaminaris* faces high levels of shear forces and is a common location for fatigue- or stress-induced spondylolysis [2].

The laminae on both sides of a vertebra connect in the midline to form the spinous processes [1]. These are much larger than their cervical and thoracic counterparts, leading to their arch overlapping the vertebrae directly below them. Relative to spinous processes in the cervical and thoracic regions, those of the lumbar region are shorter and thicker [1, 2].

The specialization of the structures of the lumbar spine is not restricted to the vertebrae but also within the elastic tissues, including the discs, tendons, and ligaments [1].

2.3 Zygapophyseal Articulation of the Lumbar Spine

The articulation of the inferior articular process of a proximal vertebra and the superior articular process of a distal vertebra is called the facet joint (also known as the zygapophyseal joint). The superior articular processes of the lumbar spine extend in a somewhat vertical direction and have a curved surface within the facet joints. The mammillary process extends from the posterior side of the articular processes and serves as an attachment for the *intertransversarii* and *multifidus* muscles [1, 2]. This is unique to the lumbar spine and reflects its dual role in stabilization as well as bearing significant weight [2]. When articulating with adjacent vertebrae, this shape provides stability to the lumbar spine by allowing the joints to rotate through flexion, extension, and lateral flexion movements, while preventing axial rotation [1, 2]. The orientation of these joints changes from being within the sagittal plane in the L1–L3 region to a slight coronal rotation through L5–S1 [2]. This increase in coronal contributions at the lumbosacral joint line prevents the vertebral column from translating anteriorly and allows for a greater potential for rotational movement as compared to the other facet joints throughout this region of the spine. This rotation is, however, limited by a series of iliolumbar ligaments [1, 2]. Facet joints are innervated by the medial branches of the dorsal rami at their respective vertebral level, as well as by the medial branches of the nerve of the vertebral level above [1].

2.4 Load-Bearing Characteristics of the Lumbar Vertebrae

The anterior and middle segments of the lumbar vertebrae contribute 50%–70% of the total cross-sectional area of the functional spine unit (FSU) and thus, along with the intervertebral discs, are primarily responsible for withstanding the compressive forces placed upon the lumbar spine.

The posterior segments, on the other hand, are relatively less developed and lack the supportive bulk in the transverse plane. Therefore, their role focuses on providing dynamic stability for the lumbar spine, especially during flexion, extension, and rotation, where torsional and shear forces reign.

The articular facets in these posterior segments are found to restrict the axial rotation of the lumbar spine to ±30° in the transverse plane, after which the torque applied on the pedicle would drastically increase the likelihood of a pedicular fracture or ligamentous failure [6]. Further experiments supported this restriction with a maximum of 20° of flexion and 10° of lateral flexion when the elements of the posterior segment of the lumbar spine were isolated [7] (Fig. 2.2).

There is an inherent limitation of torsional forces tolerated by the articular facets, with lumbar mobility being adapted to incorporate these articulations with the involvement of the facet capsule and interspinous and supraspinous ligaments. The interspinous and supraspinous ligaments only provided optimal torsional resistance at 1°–2° of axial rotation [7], with their primary role being to maintain clinical stability against larger magnitudes of torsional and shear forces.

Thus, these ligaments, along with the facet capsule, are essential in allowing the lumbar spine and its associated structures to withstand axial torques for short periods of time and prevent the dynamic torsional and shear forces caused by flexion and rotational motions from directly straining the posterior vertebral segment.

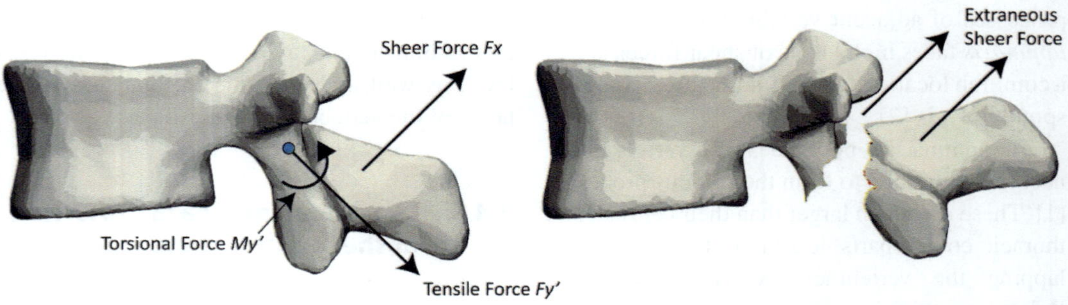

Fig. 2.2 While the vertebral body absorbs compressive forces, any torsional force caused by spinal rotation or shearing forces caused by anterior and lateral flexion of the lumbar spine results in torque on the pedicle. An excessive moment in this region makes the pedicle and surrounding structures prone to failure. (Courtesy of Prof. Özer)

2.5 Anatomy of the Lumbar Intervertebral Disc

While the vertebral bodies, facets, and processes are the primary structural components of the lumbar spine, the intervertebral discs play a critical role in mediating and propagating the various types of forces and moments exerted on the lumbar spinal column.

The dynamic nature in which forces are exerted upon the vertebrae necessitates the requirement of a viscoelastic tissue to transfer these forces to adjacent vertebrae while minimizing damage to bony structures. The intervertebral discs consist of two regions, a central mucoprotein gel, the nucleus pulposus (NP), and a fibrous periphery, the annulus fibrosus (AF) (Fig. 2.3a) [4, 5].

- The NP of the lumbar disc takes up 30%–50% of the cross-sectional area, primarily consisting of a loose mesh of fibrous filaments. It is located more posteriorly in the lumbar disc compared to its usual central position in cervical and thoracic discs. The NP is optimized for continuous compressive load bearing and shock absorption [8].
- The concentric layers of laminated fibrous tissue of the AF are helicoid and run in opposing directions for adjacent bands. The fibers are oriented at 30° to the transverse inertial plane of the disc (Fig. 2.3b). The fibers in the periphery of the AF attach directly to bony structures using Sharpey's fibers. This angle reduces to meet the inertial plane while attaching to the periosteum of the vertebral body. On the other hand, the fibers of the central zone attach to the cartilaginous end plates [9].

Interestingly, this dual composition of the intervertebral discs results in their demonstration of this very property. Under lighter loads, they remain soft and act to cushion compressive movements. However, under larger loads, the rigidity of the lumbar discs increases to prevent damage while maintaining bodily stability.

The intervertebral discs attach to their neighboring vertebral bodies via the cartilaginous end plates (CEP). The CEPs are located on the superior and inferior surfaces of the vertebral discs and serve as an articular surface of sorts between neighboring vertebrae. This hyaline cartilage serves to separate the disc from the vertebral body.

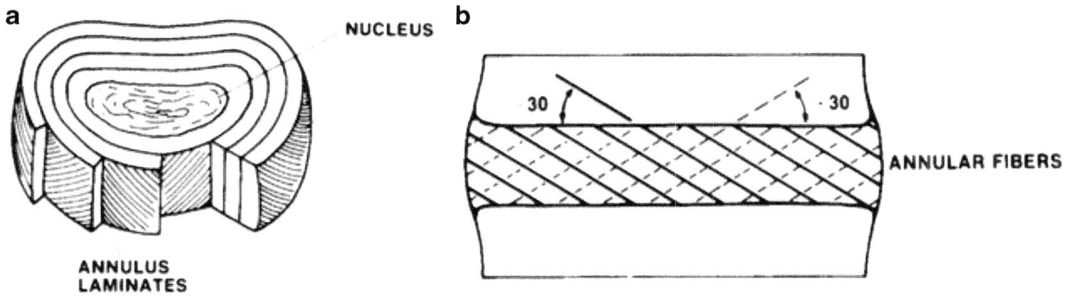

Fig. 2.3 (**a**) Cross-sectional illustration of an intervertebral disc in the transverse plane with the inner NP and outer, concentric layers of AF. (**b**) Cross-sectional illustration of an intervertebral disc in the coronal/sagittal plane depicting the alternating alignment of annular fibers to provide greater efficacy in the distribution of forces. (Reproduced with permission from Panjabi and White [3])

2.6 Load-Displacement Profile of the Lumbar Intervertebral Discs

The intervertebral discs in the lumbar spine are capable of mediating substantial loads over prolonged periods of time. Dynamic loading on the intervertebral discs at the lumbar level can exceed base static loading by over 200% [8]. The ability of the discs to bear such loads depends on their viscoelastic properties and load-rate sensitivity. The mechanical stresses on the disc are primarily tensile, with flexion, extension, and lateral flexion responsible for tensile stresses and axial rotation, exerting bending moments, resulting in shear stresses [10].

The viscoelasticity of the nucleus pulposus allows for increased load bearing but limits the load rate—the time required for a material to safely reach its maximum load without any permanent distortion [10]. This results in the NP being capable of withstanding high magnitudes of compressive loads in the upright anatomical position, with annular fibers contributing to mediating tensile stress on the periphery of the disc [9]. However, the NP is limited in mediating dynamic loads, which are characterized by higher load rates. Higher load rates result in greater elasticity in the intervertebral discs, which assists with mobility but reduces the upper limit on stability and reduces shock absorption. Therefore, dynamic loads lead to increased stress on the lumbar vertebral bodies [11].

The load-displacement profile of lumbar intervertebral discs can be determined by measuring the lateral deformation of the disc using controlled load rates (Fig. 2.4). Their load-displacement profile, with adjacent vertebral body attachments, shows a sigmoidal relationship between the load magnitude and lateral deformation of the disc [8]. This profile is indicative of the magnitude of resistive force applied by the disc being dependent on the load vector—the magnitude and direction of the load force. For load vectors with smaller magnitudes and acting along the inertial axis of the disc (primarily compressive), the intervertebral discs exhibit lesser viscoelasticity. This results in reduced resistance to movement and increased mobility and range of motion (ROM) at low loads. On the other hand, for larger load vectors with larger magnitudes and acting in a more lateral direction, the torsional components of the load vectors are emphasized. This results in greater resistance from the disc, resulting in increased rigidity and high stability at the cost of mobility [11, 12].

Larger compressive load vectors are shown to cause inelastic bending of the annular fibers,

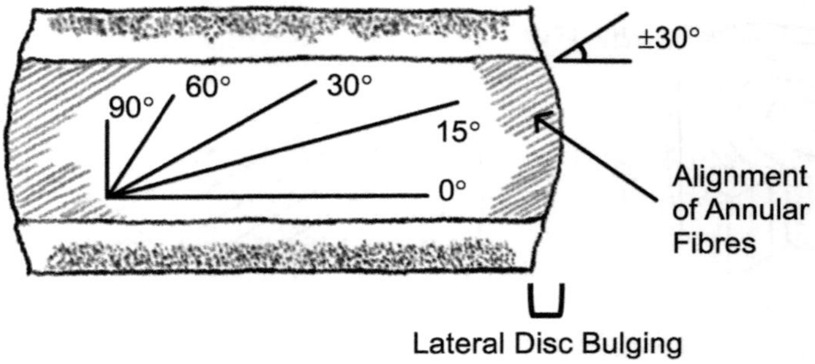

Fig. 2.4 Coronal/sagittal cross-sectional view of a lumbar intervertebral disc depicting the lateral components of varying load vectors. The AF fibers mediate any compression and torsional forces with greater efficacy if the load vector itself has a closer alignment to the annular fibers, with the fibers being most effective at handling load vectors with a 15°–30° angle to the inertial axis. However, load vectors at such angles and with significant lateral components also result in more significant lateral bulging of the AF [3]. (Illustrated by chapter authors)

resulting in permanent deformation of the disc. However, such compressive forces were unlikely to cause herniation, as the NP is specialized for such loads [13–15]. However, despite the loss of elasticity, the consequent central compression rarely causes herniation and primarily tends to result in transverse plane bulging—with a maximum disc bulge of 1.5 mm [16].

2.7 Dynamic Stress Response of the Lumbar Intervertebral Disc

Exploration of the lumbar intervertebral disc characteristics under tensile stresses demonstrated that load vectors that generate tensile stress on the disc do not occur under anatomical position or physiological lumbar movements. These stresses are mainly caused by excessive lateral flexion, where tensile stress develops on the AF when a load is applied at greater than 45° to the transverse inertial plane of the disc [6]. Tensile load vectors are normal to AF fibers, resulting in most of the load being transferred to the more pliable NP. The AF fiber orientation more closely aligns with tensile vectors in the anterior and posterior regions of the lumbar intervertebral disc compared to the lateral regions. This is theorized to provide additional compensatory support against tensile stresses to the discs since most herniations occur in the anterior and posterior directions [9] (Fig. 2.5).

2.7.1 Dynamic Response to Tensile Stresses

AF fibers provide maximum resistance against tensile stresses at approximately 15° to the transverse inertial plane of the lumbar intervertebral disc [17]. Therefore, when the lumbar spine undergoes lateral flexion of 15°, the structural stability of the intervertebral disc is shown to be optimized with the greatest burden of the load being applied to the AF fibers, ranging from 0.7 to 1.4 MPa. At different angles of lateral flexion, especially in the range of 6°–8° of lateral flexion, the NP takes on an increasing burden of the load off the AF, with a limit of 0.3 MPa. This is indicative of the disc exhibiting reduced stiffness under tension and increased stiffness under compression, with purely compressive loads being highly unlikely to cause

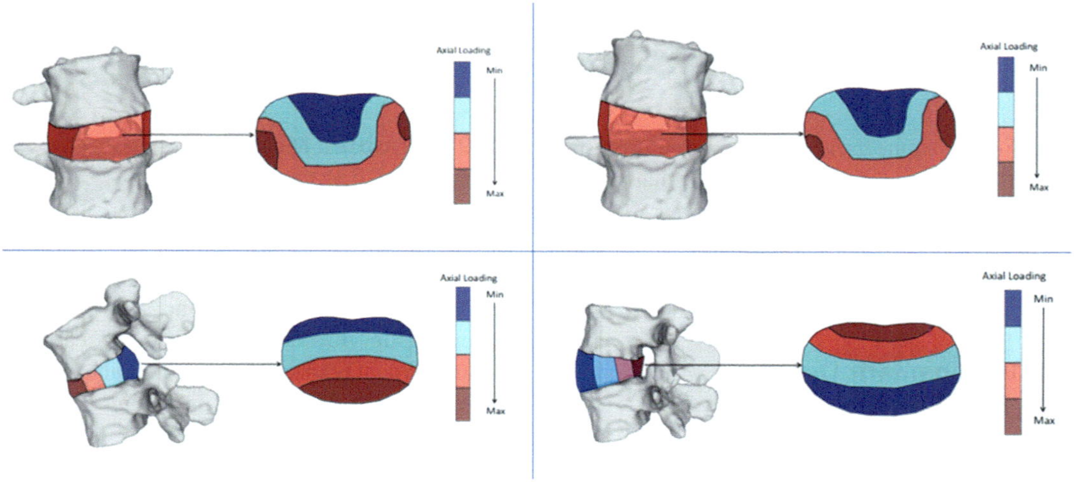

Fig. 2.5 Transverse cross-sectional illustration of a lumbar intervertebral disc depicting the distribution of the maximum tensile load capabilities in the anterior, middle, and posterior segments of the disc. The varying tensile load capabilities are according to the bending moments exerted on the disc during lumbar movements. (Courtesy of Dr. Alper Yeni)

permanent distortion to the disc. Therefore, the lumbar intervertebral disc is anisotropic—only efficient at resisting specific load vectors with varying viscoelasticity [18].

2.7.2 Inertial Displacement to Torsional Loads

The most frequent and severe lumbar intervertebral disc injuries are caused by torsional loads [6]. A torsional load profile was determined by applying a torque along the anterior-posterior inertial axis of the intervertebral disc. The torsional load profile of the lumbar intervertebral disc shows a gradual increase in torsional response at varying degrees of axial rotation, with a minimal torsional response at 1°–3°, a linear response at 3°–12°, and an increased risk of AF failure above 20° of axial rotation. Therefore, the applied torque does not uniformly distribute throughout the intervertebral disc, instead focusing along the periphery of the AF. This is likely due to the AF fibers redirecting the torsional loads away from the NP and converting the consequent torque along the anterior-posterior inertial axis into peripheral shear stresses, which measure up to 260 N/mm in the transverse inertial plane of the intervertebral disc [12].

These load profile characteristics are more prominent in the lower lumbar intervertebral discs as they tend to exhibit a greater level of hysteresis. When a small axial torque that causes 5° of lateral flexion is applied, the lower lumbar discs require over 200 cycles to show any visible signs of disc failure, with complete failure after 1000 cycles. Upper-lumbar intervertebral discs did not show this level of hysteresis [15]. Furthermore, lower lumbar discs had a slightly elevated intradiscal pressure within the NP at approximately 550 kPa in the anatomical position [19]. Both factors would be protective by contributing to reducing the rate of lumbar intervertebral disc degeneration caused by sustained dynamic loading.

2.8 Kinematics of the Lumbar Spine and Intervertebral Discs

The lumbar spine is a complex structure composed of adjacent vertebral bodies that collectively form a column with dependent mobility. Each vertebra moves in reference to its fixed adjacent vertebra.

2.8.1 Kinematic Degrees of Freedom and Axes of Rotation

The lumbar spine exhibits six degrees of freedom, which include three axes of rotation in the coronal, sagittal, and transverse planes as well as three axes of translation. The center of rotation (COR) of each vertebral body is determined by its center of mass and inertial plane and varies based on the type and degree of movement [10]. Rotational movements are often described by their instantaneous axis of rotation (IAR), which indicates the location of the COR at a specific instant during the movement of the lumbar spine (Fig. 2.6).

2.8.2 Coupled Movements and Anatomical Planes

Contrary to the simplified biomechanical models suggesting that rotation occurs strictly orthogonal or perpendicular to a plane, lumbar spine movements in vitro exhibit movement in at least two anatomical planes. Minor vertebral asymmetry leads to an off-axis COR, resulting in torque components in multiple planes [20]. This phenomenon, known as coupled movement, implies that most movements are associated with IARs that do not align with any specific anatomical plane. However, exceptions to this general observation include coupled axial rotation and lateral flexion, which tend to align with their respective anatomical axes more closely [21].

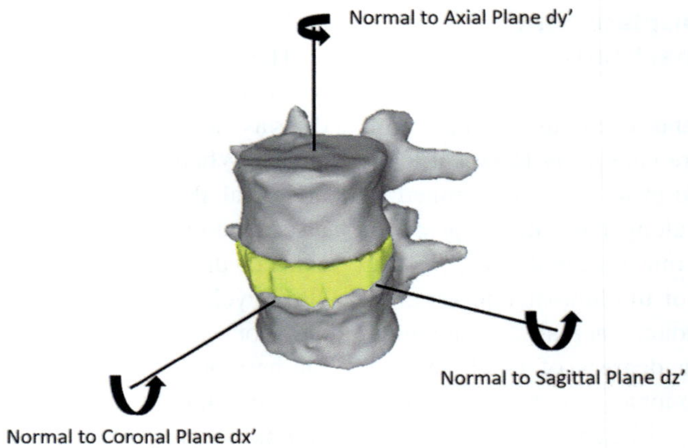

Fig. 2.6 Six degrees of freedom of the lumbar spine: three translational and three rotational axes. Movements result in a net force and/or moment in one or more of these axes, which leads to the propagation of compressive, tensile, shear, or torsional load vectors. Coupled movements of the lumbar spine have multiple axis components, and thus, any individual movement has an axis of rotation (IAR) that is a combination of the base components. (Courtesy of Dr. Alper Yeni)

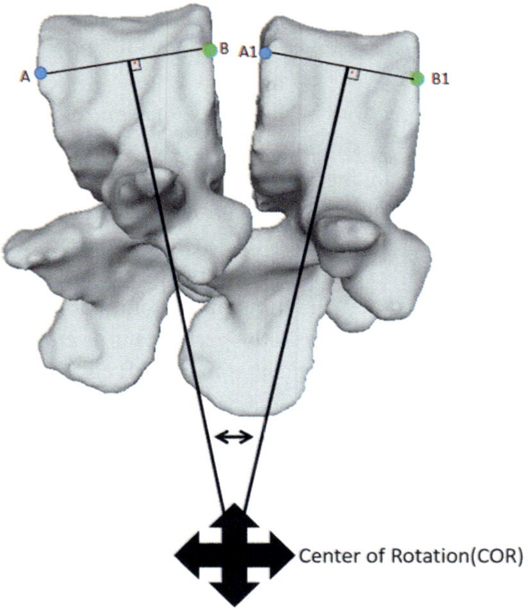

Fig. 2.7 The COR of a rotational movement of a lumbar vertebra is determined by plotting the intersection of the initial and final bisectors of the vertebral body. Therefore, the location of the COR is dependent on the angle of rotation as well as the translational distance of the movement. (Courtesy of Dr. Alper Yeni)

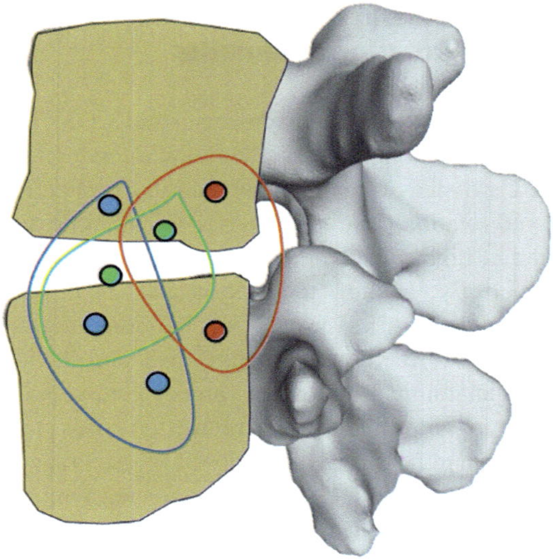

Fig. 2.8 A sagittal view of adjacent lumbar vertebrae with depictions of the primary CORs and centrode regions of flexion/extension (shown in blue), lateral flexion (shown in red), and axial rotation (shown in green) adapted from in vivo and external measurements [21, 24–26]. (Courtesy of Dr. Alper Yeni)

2.8.3 Determining the COR and Centrode

The COR of a lumbar vertebral body is determined relative to its adjacent vertebra by intersecting their bisectors, as shown in Fig. 2.7 [20].

Calculating the COR involves averaging the IARs over the full range of motion (ROM) of the lumbar spine, with smaller angular intervals providing greater accuracy [22]. The region encompassing all IARs during the complete ROM is referred to as the centrode. The centrode represents the range of possible COR positions during movement [23].

2.8.4 Flexion and Extension Kinematics

Flexion and extension movements of the lumbar spine occur primarily in the sagittal plane. The centrode for flexion and extension spans from the anterior region of the posterior third of the intervertebral disc to below the superior endplate of the inferiorly adjacent vertebra, as shown in Fig. 2.8 [21]. Consequently, the COR tends to lie within this centrode region, progressively shifting toward the posterior third of the intervertebral disc in the lower lumbar segments, particularly at L4–L5 and L5–S1 [24]. Studies have shown that the IARs cluster anteriorly during flexion and posteriorly during extension [25].

2.8.5 Lateral Flexion and Axial Rotation Kinematics

In lateral flexion movements, the COR lies toward the contralateral side of the intervertebral disc, whereas it tends to be centrally located for axial rotation [26]. With increased lateral flexion and at higher loads, the IARs shift laterally and superiorly, leading to oppositional facet joint articulation [25]. However, it is important to note that due to the coupled nature of lateral flexion and anatomical variations among individuals, isolating movements of lateral flexion poses challenges and results in relatively lower accuracy in determining the COR positions for such movements [27].

Understanding the kinematics of the lumbar spine and intervertebral discs provides valuable insights into the complex motion patterns exhibited by this region. The determination of the COR and the centrode helps characterize the position and range of possible AIR locations during different lumbar movements.

2.9 Muscular Stabilization and Dynamics of the Lumbar Spine

While the bones and ligaments of the lumbar spine are essential to stabilization and movement, so too are the lumbar spinal muscles. Expectedly, muscle mechanics can be difficult to model due to muscles being composed of numerous fascicles with a variety of attachment points. Muscles attached to the lumbar spine and auxiliary muscles have even more complicated mechanics that can be attributed to the intricate spinal curvature and diversity of attachment points in the lumbar region. This section will explore the key muscles associated with stabilization and movement of the lumbar spine and detail their relevant biomechanics.

2.9.1 Stabilization of the Lumbar Spine

The active actions of lumbar spinal muscles are necessary to promote spinal stability. It was found that an increase in the neutral zone, or range of spinal motion without resistance, can lead to spinal instability [28]. Therefore, preventing the disruption of the normal range of spinal motion is a key function of muscle stabilizers [29]. As the human body performs movements that involve the lumbar spine, such as lifting, bending, or standing, muscles such as the *multifidus* and *abdominis* (transverse and oblique) act as dynamic stabilizers [29].

The multifidus muscles are triangular muscles that are on both sides of the lumbar vertebral column. Within the lumbar region, the multifidus muscles arise from various parts of the posterior sacral region, including the sacral surface, the posterior superior iliac spine, and the sacroiliac ligament. Then the fascicles of the multifidus attach to the lateral surface of the caudal edge of the lumbar spinous processes primarily via the common tendon. Roughly, the spinous attachments of the multifidus form a 90-degree angle to the pedicular long axis. During dynamic movements of lifting and rotation, the multifidus muscles act to ensure that excess displacement of spinal structures does not occur by creating a force vector perpendicular to the long axis. In the example of lifting, an individual needs to bend to pick up the object, resulting in flexion of the lumbar spine. The multifidus muscles provide extension forces in opposition to the flexion to help control and stabilize the spine [29]. Importantly, the multifidus fascicles also attach at angles above and below 90° to the long axis in (Fig. 2.9). This variation in attachment angles allows for better stabilization since the surface of the attachment features a nonplanar curvature in reality [30].

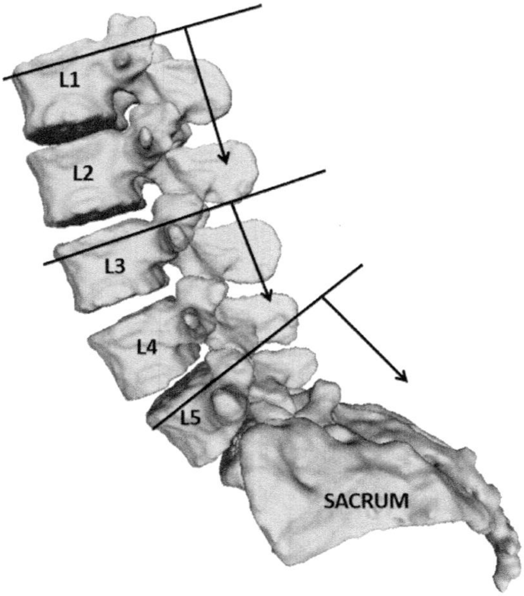

Fig. 2.9 Sagittal view of the lumbar spine with force vectors of the multifidus muscles and their respective moments applied on the vertebral bodies. (Courtesy of Dr. Alper Yeni)

While the abdominal muscles do not directly attach to the lumbar spine, the transversus abdominis and internal oblique muscles play roles in spinal stabilization [29]. The lumbar transversus abdominis is the deepest of the abdominal muscles and originates from the lateral aspect of the thoracolumbar fascia, iliac crest, and upper surface of the inguinal ligament [31]. From there, the transversus abdominis inserts into the anterior aponeurosis, linea alba, and pubic crest [31]. The internal oblique originates from the lumbar fascia, the iliac crest, and the inguinal ligament [32]. It has insertions at the inferior cartilaginous borders of ribs 10–12 and at the costal cartilage of rib 9, where the insertion fascicles merge at the linea alba [32]. Together, both the transverse and oblique abdominal muscles form a cylinder around the spine and work to increase intra-abdominal pressure [29]. This cylindrical structure, coupled with the added intra-abdominal pressure, adds to the tension of the lumbodorsal fascia [33]. From the increased tensile forces, the lumbar spine gains resistance to abnormal changes in the range of spinal motion and subsequently is more stable [29, 33].

2.9.2 Lumbar Movements and Muscle Groups

The movements of the lumbar spine can be broken down into extension, flexion, and rotation. Movements that involve lifting or power tasks involve lumbar extension and therefore involve the lumbar erector spinae and the oblique abdominal muscles [29]. Rotational movements of the lumbar spine involve those same muscles [29]. Earlier, we talked about the oblique abdominal muscles in their role as spinal stabilizers, but their primary function involves flexion and rotation [29].

The *erector spinae* are a group of muscles, as shown in Fig. 2.10 [34], that include the spinalis, longissimus, and iliocostalis muscle subgroups organized from medial to lateral [35]. The spinalis muscle group can be further subdivided into the *spinalis capitis*, *spinalis cervicis*, and *spinalis thoracis,* each of which has unique origin and insertion points [35]. However, only the *spinalis thoracis* inserts in the lumbar spine and is relevant to its movements. The *spinalis thoracis* has origin points between T1 and T4 and inserts between T11 and L2 [35]. The role of the *spinalis thoracis* itself is limited compared to the rest of the *erector spinae* group, but it does serve a small role in controlling the extension of the lumbar spine [33].

Similarly, the longissimus muscle group can be divided into capitis, cervicis, and thoracis subgroups, with the longissimus thoracis being the only muscle having lumbar attachments [35]. The *longissimus thoracis* is lateral to the *spinalis thoracis* and can be divided into a tho-

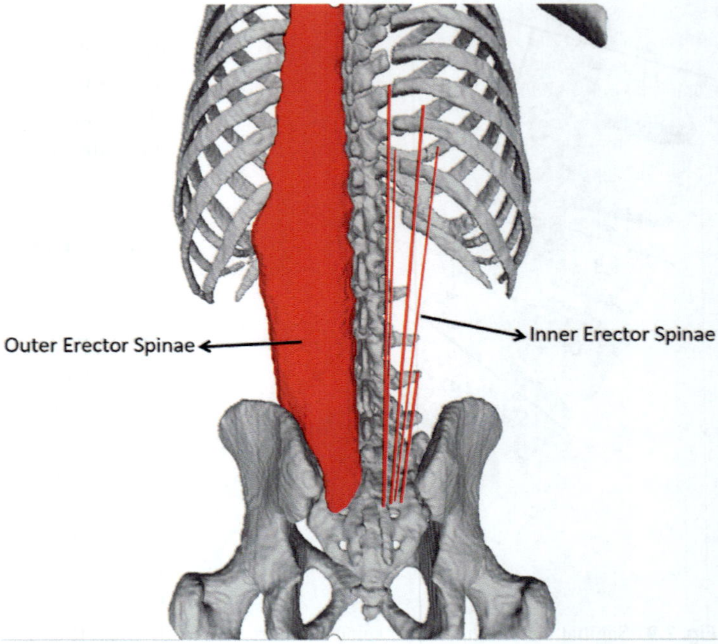

Fig. 2.10 Posterior view with varying levels of dissection of the erector spinae. (Courtesy of Dr. Alper Yeni)

racic and lumbar component based on the origin point [35]. For the thoracic component, there are multiple origin points that lie between T1 and T12, and they have insertions at L1–L5, the medial sacral crest, the posterior surface of the sacrum, and the dorsal iliac crest in Fig. 2.10 [34]. At the insertion points, the distance between the fascicles of the thoracic component and the adjacent vertebrae is minimal, and that results in a relatively reduced bending axis [36]. The shape of the fascicles themselves forms a rough arc from origin to insertion, and therefore, forces along the flexible aspect of the curvature will result in bending [33]. Since the thoracic spine has limited flexibility, the lumbar spine primarily controls the bending action of the *longissimus thoracis* pars thoracis [33]. The lumbar *longissimus thoracis* originates between L1 and L5, and the fascicles from L1 to L4 converge laterally, forming the lumbar intramuscular aponeurosis that ultimately inserts onto the ilium at its medial surface [35]. From its L5 origin point, the *longissimus thoracis* fascicles bypass integration into the aponeurosis and attach directly to the ilium and dorsal sacroiliac ligament [35]. Significantly, both the origins and insertions of the *longissimus thoracis pars lumborum* occur in or close to the lumbar region [33]. This results in short lever arms leading to a reduced bending moment [33]. Overall, the mechanical function of the lumbar component is the same as the thoracic component, and the muscle forms a curvature that allows for bending of the lumbar spine.

Finally, the iliocostalis is subdivided into the cervicis, thoracis, and lumborum components, with the *iliocostalis lumborum* being relevant to the lumbar spinal motion [35]. As with the *longissimus thoracis*, the *iliocostalis lumborum* is divided into a thoracic and lumbar component [35]. The *thoracic iliocostalis lumborum* has multiple origins at the angles of ribs 3–12, and it has insertions at the iliac crest [35]. The lumbar component originates from the thoracolumbar fascia and inserts at the iliac crest [35]. Both the thoracic and lumbar components insert at the iliac crest at the medial end and dorsal segment, but the thoracic component attaches in a linear fashion to the insertion site, while

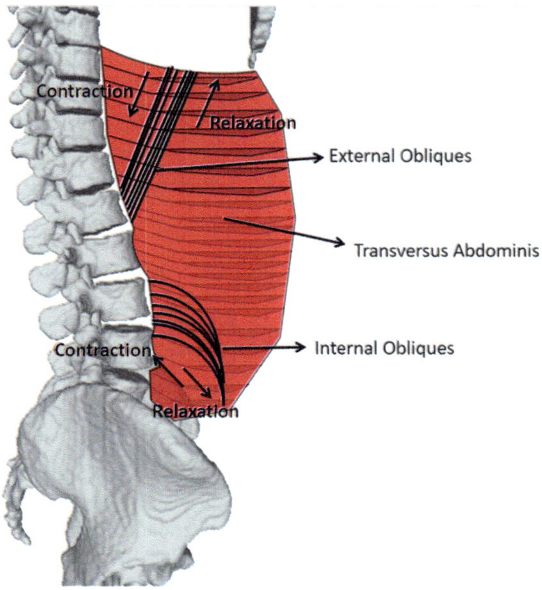

Fig. 2.11 Sagittal, dissected view of the transversus abdominis. Rotational movements using oblique muscles. Contraction of the ipsilateral internal oblique and contralateral external oblique leads to rotation in a given direction [37]. (Courtesy of Dr. Alper Yeni)

the lumbar component attaches in such a way that its insertion fascicles form a fan shape [33, 35]. The *iliocostalis lumborum* is the most posterior of the *erector spinae* muscles and therefore has the longest connection to the origin and insertion points [33]. This positioning yields a long lever arm and therefore an increased bending moment within its associated fibers [33]. Since the iliocostalis is the most lateral of the *erector spinae* muscles, it acts on the sagittal plane to control flexion and extension at angles to the plane [29, 33].

The prior discussion of the origin and insertion points for the internal oblique was discussed earlier. The external oblique originates in the shaft of ribs 5–12, as shown in Fig. 2.11 [37, 38]. Its insertion fascicles form an aponeurosis along the linea alba and also attach at the anterior iliac crest [38]. The oblique muscles act to not only form the cylindrical stabilizing apparatus of the lumbar spine but also act to rotate and flex the spine [29, 39]. Given the attachments of the obliques in the lumbar and costal regions, the contraction of muscle fibers flexes the truncal region [39]. Additionally, contraction of the obliques produces axial rotation by producing torque in the sagittal and coronal planes [40]. Specifically, the contralateral external oblique and ipsilateral internal oblique agonize lumbar rotation in a given direction as depicted in Fig. 2.11 [37]. Logically, it follows then that the ipsilateral external oblique and contralateral internal oblique act as antagonists to axial rotation. This balance is essential in providing stability to the lumbar spine during rotational movements [40].

2.10 Conclusion

The lumbar spine has a functional anatomy that maintains its stability and allows for the traditionally associated movements. From the mitigation of the shearing processes by the laminar surface to the increased tension on the lumbodorsal fascia created from the oblique muscles, the lumbar spine is stabilized through both passive and active stabilizing forces. The motion of a spinal component is determined by its center of rotation about the dimensional planes [41]. While the COR is due to the structure of the spinal component, the actual planar movements are due to the active contraction of the associated spinal muscles such as the erector spinae and oblique abdominals [41]. Considering the demands to support the rest of the body and contribute to multidimensional movement, the lumbar spine is a structure essential to human activity.

References

1. John T. Netter's clinical anatomy. Saunders/Elsevier; 2010.
2. Waxenbaum JA, Reddy V, Williams C, Futterman B. Anatomy, back, lumbar vertebrae. In: StatPearls. StatPearls Publishing; 2023.
3. Panjabi MM, White AA. Basic Biomechanics of the Spine. Neurosurgery. 1980;7:76–93.
4. Nachemson A. The load on lumbar disks in different positions of the body. Clin Orthop. 1966;45:107–22.
5. Nachemson AL, Evans JH. Some mechanical properties of the third human lumbar interlaminar ligament (ligamentum flavum). J Biomech. 1968;1:211–20.
6. Farfan HF. Muscular mechanism of the lumbar spine and the position of power and efficiency. Orthop Clin N Am. 1975;6(1):135–44. https://doi.org/10.1016/s0030-5898(20)31207-4.
7. Nagel DA, Edwards WT, Schneider E. Biomechanics of spinal fixation and fusion. Spine. 1991;16(3 Suppl):S151–4. https://doi.org/10.1097/00007632-199103001-00022.
8. Panjabi MM. Biomechanics of lumbar spine instability. In: Lumbar fusion and stabilization. Tokyo: Springer-Verlag; 1993. p. 3–9. https://doi.org/10.1007/978-4-431-68234-9_1.
9. Christophy M, Faruk Senan NA, Lotz JC, O'Reilly OM. A musculoskeletal model for the lumbar spine. Biomech Model Mechanobiol. 2011;11(1–2):19–34. https://doi.org/10.1007/s10237-011-0290-6.
10. Hirsch BE. Anatomy of the foot. In: Foot and ankle biomechanics. Elsevier; 2023. p. 3–44. https://doi.org/10.1016/b978-0-12-815449-6.00040-8.
11. Crisco JJ, Panjabi MM. Postural biomechanical stability and gross muscular architecture in the spine. In: Multiple muscle systems. New York: Springer; 1990. p. 438–50. https://doi.org/10.1007/978-1-4613-9030-5_26.
12. King AI, Yang K-H. Biomechanics of the lumbar spine. In: Frontiers in biomechanics. New York: Springer; 1986. p. 210–24. https://doi.org/10.1007/978-1-4612-4866-8_16.
13. Virgin WJ. Experimental investigations into the physical properties of the intervertebral disc. J Bone Joint Surg. 1951;33-B(4):607–11. https://doi.org/10.1302/0301-620x.33b4.607.
14. Hirsch C. The reaction of intervertebral discs to compression forces. J Bone Joint Surg Am. 1955;37(6):1188–96. https://doi.org/10.2106/00004623-195537060-00005.
15. Markolf KL, Morris JM. The structural components of the intervertebral disc. J Bone Joint Surg Am. 1974;56(4):675–87. https://doi.org/10.2106/00004623-197456040-00003.
16. Reuber M, Schultz A, Denis F, Spencer D. Bulging of lumbar intervertebral disks. J Biomech Eng. 1982;104(3):187–92. https://doi.org/10.1115/1.3138347.
17. Galante JO. Tensile properties of the human lumbar annulus fibrosus. Acta Orthop Scand. 1967;38(sup100):1–91. https://doi.org/10.3109/ort.1967.38.suppl-100.01.
18. Benzel EC. Biomechanically relevant anatomy and material properties of the spine and associated elements. In: Biomechanics of spine stabilization. New York: Thieme; 2015. https://doi.org/10.1055/b-0035-106376.
19. Nachemson AL. Disc pressure measurements. Spine. 1981;6(1):93–7. https://doi.org/10.1097/00007632-198101000-00020.
20. McCombe P, Diwan A, Wilke H-J, Patwardhan A. Biomechanics of motion preservation technologies. In: Boden SD, editor. Lumbar spine textbook [Internet]. International Society for the Study of the Lumbar Spine and Data Trace Internet Publishing, LLC. Available from: https://www.wheelessonline.com/issls/.
21. Panjabi MM, Krag MH, Goel VK. A technique for measurement and description of three-dimensional six-degree-of-freedom motion of a body joint with an application to the human spine. J Biomech. 1981;14(7):447–60. https://doi.org/10.1016/0021-9290(81)90095-6.
22. Pearcy MJ, Bogduk N. Instantaneous axes of rotation of the lumbar intervertebral joints. Spine. 1988;13(9):1033–41. https://doi.org/10.1097/00007632-198809000-00011.
23. Gertzbein SD, Holtby R, Tile M, Kapasouri A, Chan KW, Cruickshank B. Determination of a locus of instantaneous centers of rotation of the lumbar disc by moiré fringes. Spine. 1984;9(4):409–13. https://doi.org/10.1097/00007632-198405000-00015.
24. Yoshioka T, Tsuji H, Hirano N, Sainoh S. Motion characteristic of the normal lumbar spine in young adults. J Spinal Disord. 1990;3(2):103–13. https://doi.org/10.1097/00002517-199006000-00001.
25. Schmidt H, Heuer F, Claes L, Wilke H-J. The relation between the instantaneous center of rotation and facet joint forces—a finite element analysis. Clin Biomech. 2008;23(3):270–8. https://doi.org/10.1016/j.clinbiomech.2007.10.001.

26. White AA, Panjabi MM. The basic kinematics of the human spine. Spine. 1978;3(1):12–20. https://doi.org/10.1097/00007632-197803000-00003.
27. Hayes WC. Bone mechanics: from tissue mechanical properties to an assessment of structural behavior. In: Frontiers in biomechanics. New York: Springer; 1986. p. 196–209. https://doi.org/10.1007/978-1-4612-4866-8_15.
28. Panjabi MM. Clinical spinal instability and low back pain. J Electromyogr Kinesiol. 2003;13(4):371–9.
29. Izzo R, Guarnieri G, Guglielmi G, Muto M. Biomechanics of the spine. Part I: spinal stability. Eur J Radiol. 2013;82(1):118–26.
30. Macintosh JE, Bogduk N. The biomechanics of the lumbar multifidus. Clin Biomech. 1986;1(4):205–13.
31. Karunasena S, Worsley C, Hacking C, et al. Transversus abdominis muscle. Reference article, Radiopaedia.org. https://doi.org/10.53347/rID-47186. Accessed on 29 June 2023.
32. Tan S, Worsley C, Hacking C, et al. Internal oblique muscle. Reference article, Radiopaedia.org. https://doi.org/10.53347/rID-45966. Accessed on 29 June 2023.
33. Aspden RM. Review of the functional anatomy of the spinal ligaments and the lumbar erector spinae muscles. Clin Anat. 1992;5(5):372–87.
34. Kurihara Y, Yakushiji YK, Matsumoto J, Ishikawa T, Hirata K. The ribs: anatomic and radiologic considerations. Radiographics. 1999;19(1):105–19.
35. Yee J, Mellam Y, Hacking C, et al. Erector spinae group. Reference article, Radiopaedia.org. https://doi.org/10.53347/rID-45291. Accessed on 22 June 2023.
36. Macintosh JE, Bogduk NI. The attachments of the lumbar erector spinae. Spine. 1991;16(7):783–92.
37. Gordon KE, Reed O. The role of the pelvic floor in respiration: a multidisciplinary literature review. J Voice. 2020;34(2):243–9.
38. Dematawa D, Worsley C, Knipe H, et al. External oblique muscle. Reference article, Radiopaedia.org. https://doi.org/10.53347/rID-45491. Accessed on 23 June 2023.
39. McGill SM. A revised anatomical model of the abdominal musculature for torso flexion efforts. J Biomech. 1996;29(7):973–7.
40. Ng JK, Parnianpour M, Richardson CA, Kippers V. Functional roles of abdominal and back muscles during isometric axial rotation of the trunk. J Orthop Res. 2001;19(3):463–71.
41. Panjabi MM, et al. Human lumbar vertebrae: quantitative three-dimensional anatomy. Spine. 1992;17:299.

Degenerative Spine Biomechanics

3

Niloufar Shekouhi, Muzammil Mumtaz, Sudharshan Tripathi, Norihiro Nishida, Adit Padgaonkar, Thaddeus Ochs, and Vijay K. Goel

3.1 Introduction

The spine, also known as the vertebral column, is a complex structure that provides support, enables mobility, and protects the spinal cord. The interplay between the vertebrae, intervertebral discs, facet joints, ligaments, and muscles enables these critical functions, highlighting the importance of spinal biomechanics. However, degenerative changes caused by aging, injury, or genetic predisposition can disrupt the balance and lead to problems.

Degenerative spine biomechanics study the changes that happen in the spine leading to a progressive loss of function, pain, or neurologic impairment. These changes start at a microscopic level and gradually develop into noticeable, disabling symptoms. One of the critical aspects of this process is disc degeneration. The discs, which work as shock absorbers between the vertebrae, begin to deteriorate, losing their elasticity, height, and flexibility, causing spinal instability and abnormal distribution of load across the spine. This then triggers a series of events that worsen the spinal degeneration.

Back pain is a common and debilitating condition that affects nearly everyone at some point in their life. According to various studies, the prevalence of back pain ranges between 1.4% and 20%, depending on which definition of LBP is used [1]. Due to age-related degeneration only, the prevalence of back pain is extremely high in today's graying population.

Degenerative spine biomechanics can lead to conditions like spondylolysis and stenosis, which are often caused by disc degeneration. Spondylolysis can cause a vertebra to slip forward, leading to spinal instability and nerve compression. Additionally, spinal stenosis can narrow spaces in

Vijay K. Goel died before publication of this work was completed.

N. Shekouhi · S. Tripathi · N. Nishida
A. Padgaonkar · T. Ochs
Engineering Center for Orthopaedic Research Excellence (E-CORE), Departments of Bioengineering and Orthopaedics, The University of Toledo, Toledo, OH, USA
e-mail: niloufar.shekouhi@rockets.utoledo.edu; sudharshan.tripathi@utoledo.edu; nishida3@yamaguchi-u.ac.jp; adit.padgaonkar@rockets.utoledo.edu; thaddeus.ochs@rockets.utoledo.edu

M. Mumtaz (✉)
Engineering Center for Orthopaedic Research Excellence (E-CORE), Departments of Bioengineering and Orthopaedics, The University of Toledo, Toledo, OH, USA

Biomedical Engineering, West Chester University, West Chester, USA
e-mail: muzammil.mumtaz@rockets.utoledo.edu; mmumtaz626@wcupa.edu

V. K. Goel
Department of Bioengineering & Orthopaedic Surgery, University of Toledo, Toledo, OH, USA
e-mail: goelshashi1@gmail.com

A. F. Özer et al. (eds.), *Dynamic Lumbar Spine Stabilization*,
https://doi.org/10.1007/978-3-032-12122-6_3

the spinal canal, leading to numbness, pain, and weakness in the limbs. It is crucial to understand these conditions, as they can severely impact your quality of life.

Degenerative conditions affecting the spine are complex and involve changes in the mechanics of bone, disc, ligament, and muscle, alongside the effects of gravity and daily activities on the spine. Therefore, understanding degenerative spine biomechanics is crucial to understanding the biomechanics of the degenerative spine and to developing effective interventions and improving the quality of life for affected individuals. The study of these conditions is not only academically critical but also vitally relevant to public health and clinical practice.

3.2 Basics of Spinal Biomechanics

As discussed before, the spinal structure is a complex system that involves the intricate interactions between vertebrae, intervertebral discs, facet joints, ligaments, and muscles. With this foundation, we can delve deeper into the specifics of spinal biomechanics. Each of these elements—vertebrae, intervertebral discs, facet joints, ligaments, and muscles—contributes to the complex dynamics of the spine. The vertebrae provide a strong foundation to support the spine and protect the spinal cord. Intervertebral discs act as crucial shock absorbers and help to maintain spinal flexibility. Facet joints guide and control spine movement, while ligaments connect the vertebrae to muscles attached to the spine, offering stability, movement, and proper posture.

Several forces act on the spine, influencing its biomechanics. These include gravitational forces constantly exerting pressure, muscle contractions generated by various physical activities acting on the spine, and external loads arising from everyday actions like lifting or carrying objects. In response to these forces, the spine performs a range of movements, including flexion, extension, lateral bending, and rotation.

A fundamental concept in understanding and managing spinal biomechanics is the normal distribution of loads and movements in a healthy, functional spine. Within the normal spine, all loads are equally distributed on all the vertebral bodies and discs. During movements, the spine dynamically adjusts the distribution of loads to minimize stress on the spinal structures and prevent injury. The principle of load distribution is facilitated by the cervical (neck), thoracic (middle back), and lumbar (lower back) curves of the spine so that the spine is well adapted to efficiently bear the weight of the body and transmit force generated naturally during various daily movements. Any alterations in the structure or function of the spine due to degenerative changes or injury can lead to disruption of the normal loading patterns of the spinal column, resulting in increased spinal instability and the likelihood of injury that may lead to pain conditions. Therefore, this is why such basic spinal biomechanical understanding is crucial for understanding the onset and progression of degenerative spinal conditions.

3.3 Degenerative Changes in Spine Biomechanics

3.3.1 Overview of the Degenerative Process

The biomechanics of the spine are susceptible to alterations caused by degenerative processes; these changes in morphology and structure may lead to changes in the usual function of the spine and have dramatic effects on its biomechanics. As a result of such pathological shifts, abnormal load distribution, spinal instability, and consequent pain may result, underscoring the importance of studying these changes to understand the onset and progression of degenerative spinal conditions. This section will explain the nature of degenerative changes and their impact on the biomechanics of the spine, focusing on disc degeneration, spondylolysis, and spinal stenosis.

3.3.2 Changes in Disc Mechanics with Degeneration

Disc degeneration is a major component of degenerative changes in spine biomechanics. A healthy intervertebral disc, which is comprised of a lot of water and flexible fibrous rings, acts as a cushion between the vertebrae (backbones) and simplifies the mobility of the spine. However, during degeneration, the discs lose some physical properties; they are less hydrated, less flexible, and less strong. The deferring of the disc proportion and reduction of elasticity causes the unequal occlusion of the stresses on the spine and pelvis; it leads to bad consequences for the back. Also, annular fiber rupture can promote disc herniation, which is an instance of the outer, firmer part of the intervertebral disc giving way and protruding outward. As a result, the inner gel-like material pushes out and may compress nearby nerve roots and cause pain.

3.3.3 Changes in Bone and Joint Mechanics with Degeneration

Degenerative changes also have a significant impact on the mechanics of bone and joints in the spine. A common result is the formation of osteophytes, also known as bone spurs, in response to increased load and stress on the vertebral bodies caused by disc degeneration. While these growths are a way for the body to try to increase the area that bears weight and stabilize the spine, they can result in the narrowing of the spinal canal, leading to spinal stenosis. In a similar manner, the facet joints experience wear and tear, which leads to a decrease in joint space, breakdown of cartilage, and the development of osteoarthritis. The degeneration of facet joints can lead to unusual movement and contribute to instability in the spine.

3.3.4 Changes in Ligament and Muscle Mechanics with Degeneration

Degenerative changes in the spine also impact the ligaments and muscles that offer support and aid in movement. Ligaments might thicken and toughen over time as a result of chronic stress and strain, potentially resulting in a constriction of the spinal passage or the openings, known as foramina, through which nerves depart the spine. This ligamentous hypertrophy can compress nerve roots, causing pain and neurological symptoms. Muscles surrounding the spine, particularly the paraspinal muscles, can also be affected by degenerative changes. Muscle atrophy and imbalances can occur due to disuse, pain-avoidance behavior, or nerve impairment. This muscle dysfunction can reduce spinal stability, increase mechanical stress on the vertebral bodies and discs, and contribute to chronic back pain. The understanding of these changes in ligament and muscle mechanics offers valuable insights into the complex biomechanical consequences of spinal degeneration.

3.4 Disc Degeneration

3.4.1 Biological and Mechanical Changes in Disc Degeneration

The intervertebral disc (IVD) biomechanics are influenced by the extracellular matrix (ECM) properties of its two tissues: the nucleus pulposus (NP) and the annulus fibrosus (AF) [2]. Both of these tissues are composed of collagen fibers and proteoglycans (PGs); however, they differ in their amount and organization [2–4].

The nucleus pulposus (NP) contains water and negatively charged proteoglycans (PGs), creating an osmotic potential that attracts water to maintain equilibrium [2, 5]. Collagen in the nucleus forms a loose network of randomly oriented fibers. The annulus fibrosus (AF) exhibits a dense arrangement of collagen fibers in a lamellar structure with alternating angles, providing anisotropic properties that enhance the disc's resistance to bending and twisting [6, 7]. This structural feature enables the disc to maintain its stability and integrity during various movements and forces [7]. The rigid annulus structure in the circumferential direction restricts the expansion of the nucleus, resulting in an osmotic pressure that enables the intervertebral disc to withstand compressive loads [2, 8, 9].

The process of intervertebral disc degeneration in the lumbar region is characterized by a slow but steady change in the disc tissues' biological and mechanical attributes as well as tissue morphology [3, 4, 10]. As the degeneration develops, there is a noticeable increase in disc stiffness coupled with a decrease in the original hydration levels [11, 12]. Furthermore, the orientation of collagen fibers becomes more diverse as degeneration advances, creating heightened nonlinearity within the fibers [13]. This shift profoundly influences the functionality of the collagen fiber network, subsequently altering the biomechanical properties of the annular and nucleus tissues, as well as affecting the overall range of motion [13]. As a result, parameters like disc height, axial movement, facet force, and range of motion during flexion-extension experience a marked decrease [11, 12]. However, rotational instability does not invariably present in the preliminary stages of disc degeneration [14].

Computational modeling plays a crucial role in understanding the biomechanical behavior of intervertebral discs (IVDs). Several authors have predominantly focused on finite element (FE) models, which rely on observations and descriptions of disc behavior rather than detailed mechanisms [15–19].

Galbusera et al. developed four approaches to simulate the osmotic behavior of the intervertebral disc using a constant pore pressure on the boundary of the outer AF [20]. In an attempt to provide more accurate results, authors incorporated an osmotic pressure into bi-, tri-, or quadriphasic models of intervertebral disc (IVD) tissue [21–25]. However, most existing models fail to consider the content of the annulus fibrosus (AF) and the influence of vertebrae and ligaments on disc kinematics.

However, most of these studies considered AF as a fiber-reinforced ground substance and failed to incorporate the content of these tissues in their models [15–18, 26]. Moreover, only a few models of IVD were developed by considering the effect of vertebrae and ligaments on disc kinematics [26]. The multi-scale model developed by Barthelemy et al. encompasses local disc biochemical composition and spinal biomechanics and provides a promising avenue for investigating their relationship [26].

3.4.2 Causes of Disc Degeneration

Intervertebral disc degeneration is a multifactorial process that can be prompted by a variety of causes. Age is one of the primary factors, as the natural aging process often leads to a loss of disc water content, reducing its ability to handle stress and leading to wear and tear. Genetics can also play a significant role, with some individuals inheriting a predisposition to earlier and more severe disc degeneration. Lifestyle factors such as obesity, smoking, and a lack of regular exercise can exacerbate the process, contributing to faster degeneration.

Among all, the role of mechanical factors in disc degeneration, particularly excessive mechanical stress, is noteworthy [27]. One of the key factors that leads to damage to the structure and leads to decompression is an abnormal vertebral endplate [28].

Experimental evidence has shown that physical injuries to the disc or vertebral endplate can induce premature degeneration and that disruptions to the annulus or endplate almost certainly result in disc degeneration [29–33]. However, there is a reciprocal effect between endplates and the intervertebral disc [28]. Literature indicates that NP's loss of pressure can happen due to endplates bulging into the nearby vertebra or as a result of dehydration, and it could create intense stress concentrations on the endplates [28, 34, 35].

This stress could lead to microfractures, which would carry severe biomechanical implications such as implant subsidence [28, 34, 35]. This is why Liu et al. proposed that assessing the integrity of the endplates through preoperative MRI could potentially minimize the possibility of implant subsidence after interbody fusion [28].

Furthermore, in vitro studies have revealed the underlying mechanisms at play, demonstrating that physical damage to the disc leads to decompression of the disc nucleus [35, 36], alterations in disc cell metabolism [37–39], and an increased susceptibility of the annulus to nerve and blood vessel ingrowth [40].

Adding to this, research by Stefanakis et al. demonstrated an intriguing relationship between disc degeneration severity and stress gradients within the annulus [27]. They found that as disc degeneration worsens, stress gradients in the annulus escalate significantly, potentially triggering progressive annulus delamination and collapse [27]. Moreover, they suggested that despite the protective stress-shielding provided by the neural arch, these stress gradients could still contribute to the progression of the disease [27].

3.4.3 Role of Biomechanical Factors in Disc Degeneration Progression

Biomechanical factors play an important role in accelerating degeneration, particularly in the lower lumbar spine. Interestingly, research conducted by Jelec et al. highlighted compressive load and a more coronal facet orientation as the primary risk factor [41]. The authors established that coronal facet orientation facilitates rotational movements during ambulation while curtailing dorsoventral vertebral translation. This adaptation assists in managing shearing forces linked with upright posture and lumbar lordosis [41].

This particular facet orientation might play a significant role in the rapid progression of disc degeneration. In contrast, facet joint remodeling, under the influence of diverse loading conditions, could be connected to a more sagittal facet orientation and heightened facet osteoarthritis scores [41]. This sagittal orientation could align with age-related changes and altered loading circumstances, culminating in a partial loss of lumbar lordosis [41]. In essence, understanding these nuances of biomechanical causes and the subsequent adaptations within the spine can significantly inform therapeutic interventions and preventative measures for degenerative spinal disorders.

3.4.4 Segmental Instability After Disc Degeneration

The progression of disc degeneration and the onset of facet joint osteoarthritis frequently lead to a state of segmental instability. This condition manifests as an abnormal degree of movement within the spine under typical physiological load until an advanced stage is reached, wherein the intervertebral space collapses and the facet joints display severe subchondral sclerosis [41]. As this degeneration further evolves, shifts in the center of rotation lead to irregular load distribution across the disc space [42]. Studies have noted that disc degeneration undermines the spine's stabilizing mechanisms, while shear loads directed posteriorly contribute to torsional instability [43].

In a 2014 study, Melnyk et al. suggested a potential link between disc degeneration and instability in the sagittal plane [44]. This instability can promote conditions such as stenosis and neural compression, which may necessitate decompression [44]. Hutton et al., meanwhile, underscored the crucial role that the posterior elements play in maintaining spinal stability [45]. Their research suggests that preserving these structures is of vital importance in the treatment of spondylolysis and other spinal disorders [45]. In conclusion, understanding the intricate mechanics and biological alterations within the spine due to degeneration helps guide treatment strategies to mitigate the effects and preserve spinal stability.

Disc degeneration significantly impacts the muscle recruitment pattern, affecting spinal movement and stability. Kim et al. employed a computational model to analyze these changes, particularly focusing on the erect standing posture [46]. Their research indicated a shift in muscle activation: as degeneration increased, there was a rise in the activation of superficial muscles, accompanied by a decrease in deep muscle activation [46]. Such a shift, while providing temporary stability by redistributing the load, can induce muscle imbalances and overuse. Interestingly, this adjustment reduced stress on the degenerated disc, potentially slowing down the progression of degeneration [46]. This insight emphasizes the importance of tailored therapeutic interventions in managing disc degeneration.

Clinical manifestations of DDD can vary from no symptoms to mild, nonspecific symptoms to severe back pain. Disc herniation is the most seen clinical manifestation of degenerative damage. Disc bulging is caused by the nucleus pulposus pushing on the annular fibers, which can turn into disc protrusion if the nucleus escapes the annular fibers. Both of which can ultimately lead to the most dangerous, disc sequestration, where the broken disc fragments displace away from their site. The primary manifestation of such a herniation is compression of nerve structures like the spinal cord and roots, leading to radicular pain, sensory abnormalities, and weakness in the dermatomal and myotomal patterns, respectively. Lateral herniation compresses the exiting nerve root, while a central herniation affects the transversing nerve root. Patients usually present with shooting, burning pain in a dermatomal manner. On physical exam, weakness of specific muscle groups can be seen; however, most muscles receive innervation from multiple spinal roots, resulting in preserved strength in many cases. MR imaging is used conservatively for back pain, especially because most patients can improve within 6 weeks of physical therapy and pain management. However, persistent radicular pain is a major indication for MRI. Clinicians often use it for diagnosing and treatment purposes, but clinical signs are still more important because asymptomatic disc degeneration is very commonly seen on MRI. Additionally, a well-defined image of compressing structures helps clinicians administer injections as well as determine any further indication for surgery. More conservative approaches like physical therapy, lifestyle modifications, pain management, and orthotics are still first line [2].

Another age-related progressive degeneration of the spine is spondylosis, or osteoarthritis of the spine. With the number of facet joints in the spine and its dynamic motion, spondylosis is another prevalent cause of back pain in the aging population. The pathophysiology of spondylosis involves basic wear and tear, mechanical stress, and some genetic and inflammatory factors. A combination of these factors contributes to the breakdown of cartilage, bone remodeling, and the formation of osteophytes. The clinical presentation can range from mild pain to severe local or radicular pain. Other symptoms include stiffness and limited range of motion. As facet joints degenerate, osteophytes form and migrate near the joint space. They can further compress neural structures and cause radicular pain, as discussed earlier. It will present with similar shooting, burning pain in a dermatomal fashion [3].

The differential diagnosis for spondylosis always contains autoimmune inflammatory conditions like rheumatoid arthritis. Therefore, a workup including chronic inflammatory markers and autoantibodies is sometimes performed in severe cases. After such conditions have been ruled out, conservative treatment is still key since many exacerbated cases resolve on their own with pain management and physical therapy. Pain is usually managed using various nonsteroidal anti-inflammatory drugs or sometimes muscle relaxants. Opioids are not recommended. X-rays are done initially to look for obvious injuries; however, MRIs are indicated for severe or refractory cases [4].

Dynamic/functional X-rays are used to assess instability due to degeneration. Many doctors employ the use of functional imaging techniques, such as lateral flexion/extension radiographs, since they have the potential to reveal an increased translation [47].

Modic reported evidence of associated degenerative disk disease.

Modic changes classification consists of four types [48, 49]:

- Type 0: normal disc and vertebral body appearance
- Type I: presence of bone marrow edema within the vertebral body and hypervascularization
- Type II: fatty replacements of the red bone marrow within the vertebral body
- Type III: subchondral bone sclerosis

Endplate defects include Schmorl nodes, fractures, avulsions/erosions, and calcifications, which have all been considered to be clinically associated with LBP [50].

3.5 Spondylolysis and Spondylolisthesis

Spondylolysis and spondylolisthesis are two related conditions that can significantly impact spinal biomechanics. Spondylolysis, characterized as a stress fracture in a vertebra, is typically attributed to repetitive trauma, specific genetic predispositions impacting bone structure, or biomechanical factors such as anterior-posterior shear force and spinal flexure [51, 52]. To better understand the underlying factors contributing to spondylolysis, Cyron et al. experimentally induced fractures of the neural arch in 1976 [53]. Their findings revealed that such fractures are prone to propagate obliquely across the pars interarticularis [53]. In addition, their research illuminated that the force necessary to induce a fracture escalates from the first to the fifth lumbar vertebra, which can be attributed to the progressive thickening and increased robustness of the pars interarticularis in the lower lumbar region [53]. Furthermore, the prevalence of this condition in the lower lumbar regions suggests that the vertebrae in these areas are subjected to higher shear loads. This is likely due to the enhanced shear forces they endure during routine activities and the distinctive curvature associated with the lordotic nature of the lumbar spine [54].

Spondylolisthesis, on the other hand, is a condition where a vertebra, typically the one that has suffered spondylolysis, slips out of place and moves forward over the vertebra below it. This can be triggered by the initial stress fracture of spondylolysis or due to degenerative changes associated with aging, such as intervertebral disc degeneration.

During et al.'s study, it showed that postural parameters in spondylolysis patients differed significantly from those in the group of healthy volunteers, suggesting that posture may play a key role in the generation of low back pain by creating an uneven distribution of forces across the spine, leading to higher stress in certain areas [55]. Over time, this uneven stress distribution can accelerate the degeneration of intervertebral discs and other spinal structures, leading to conditions like spondylolisthesis, herniated discs, or stenosis, all of which can cause low back pain. Their observation showed that in patients with spondylolysis, an abnormal loading at the sacroiliac joint is observed, which is either due to the steeper upper sacral surface (compared to the normal group) or the deviation of the vertical line of gravity [56].

The complexity of the lumbar spine and the forces that influence its mechanics have been the subject of various studies. Skrzypiec et al., for instance, conducted a detailed investigation focusing on the distribution of shear load between intervertebral discs and apophyseal joints in the moderately degraded human lumbar spine [54]. Their findings showed that, at first, a significant portion (55%–65%) of the anterior shear load is shouldered by the apophyseal joints [54]. However, with increasing shear displacement, this proportion progressively diminishes. Conversely, the load contribution of the intervertebral disc undergoes a considerable rise, escalating from 38% to an impressive 66% [54]. This highlights the dynamic and adaptable nature of load distribution within the lumbar spine.

In a separate but equally relevant cadaver study, Green et al. illuminated the potential risks tied to specific types of physical activities to the spinal structure, specifically regarding spondylolysis [51]. Their research identified that activities incorporating alternating flexion and extension movements result in substantial stress reversals in the pars interarticularis, a region that often suffers from spondylolysis [51].

Adding to this body of knowledge, Chamoli et al. suggested a specific impact of bilateral spondylolytic defects [57]. Their research pointed to the potential for such defects to significantly overstress the posterior annulus of the affected intervertebral disc during movements such as flexion-extension and bilateral bending [57]. This insight underscores the critical role of specific anatomical defects in exacerbating the strains associated with certain movements.

Grobler et al. highlighted that isthmic spondylolisthesis lesions at L4–5 demonstrate greater instability compared to those at L5–S1 [58]. In a related study using a personalized finite element model, researchers analyzed the L5–S1 segment in patients with low-grade isthmic spondylolisthesis [59]. They identified that the pelvic morphology significantly affects the L5–S1 junction's inclination, subsequently impacting the shear forces and potentially contributing to spondylolisthesis development [59]. Collectively, these findings underline the nuanced biomechanics involved in isthmic spondylolisthesis.

In the study of spondylosis, various authors have advanced biomechanical models of spondylolisthesis [60–66]. However, these models primarily focus on general spondylolisthesis and rarely delve into the intricacies of Degenerative Lumbar Spondylolisthesis (DLS). As stated by Melnyk et al., the scarcity of literature on DLS can be attributed to its evolution over time, a result of prolonged degeneration and subsequent tissue adaptation [60, 64, 65]. Consequently, only a limited number of studies have developed models to understand this specific condition.

Among those few models, Crawford et al.'s innovative approach to spondylolisthesis modeling deserves particular attention [64]. Their method involved executing two resection procedures targeting the disc and both the anterior and posterior longitudinal ligaments. They discovered that the disc's integrity was pivotal for stability, even more so than the ligaments' attachment to the vertebral bodies [64].

Complementing the efforts of Crawford et al., Melnyk et al. have pioneered the development of an in vitro model specifically for DLS [60, 67]. Their model stands out for its intricate process of four incremental surgical destabilizations that target the facet complex and the intervertebral disc. These destabilizations resulted in a noticeable increase in shear translation. Simultaneously, the rigidity of the specimen reduced, while there was a significant increase in the range of motion [60, 67].

These contributions not only add to our understanding of spondylolisthesis and DLS but also lay the foundation for future research in the field. Further exploration and development of such models can deepen our understanding of these conditions, potentially leading to better diagnostic and treatment methods.

The biomechanical alterations due to these conditions are complex and significant. They can disrupt the balance and distribution of forces across the spinal column, causing abnormal motion and increasing the stress on the intervertebral discs and facet joints. This leads to altered spinal dynamics, contributing to the instability and potentially increasing the risk of further injury or degeneration. Collectively, these studies provide insightful perspectives into the multifaceted dynamics of the lumbar spine. They highlight the significance of continued research to deepen our understanding and develop strategies to alleviate the risks associated with conditions like spondylolysis [51, 57].

3.6 Spondylolysis

Spondylolysis is a traumatic fracture through the pars reticularis of the lumbar vertebrae that can occur at all ages and is most commonly seen at L5 and L4 [68]. L5 is the most affected vertebra due to extreme shearing forces during extension. The incidence rate in the general population is 6%–8% but increases to 63% when observing athletes only. The pathogenesis of spondylosis is a matter of debate, with many factors contributing to its development. Genetic and developmental factors, repetitive physical activity, and acute trauma are a few [5]. According to H. Saraste, the most likely mechanism involves repetitive, stressful movements on a congenitally weakened or dysplastic vertebrae [6].

X-rays have limitations in the diagnosis of spondylolysis since pars injuries can be very subtle findings [68]. For example, early stages of pars injuries with stress reactions without complete defects are radiographically occult and can only be properly evaluated on MRIs [69]. CT is useful in assessing for healing, establishing chronic spondylolysis, and ruling out another lesion [70].

Spondylolisthesis is a forward displacement of one vertebra over the other, most commonly in the lumbar region. It could be seen as a complication of a pars reticularis fracture.

Clinically, both spondylolysis and spondylolisthesis may be completely asymptomatic and show up as incidental findings on imaging. In children and adolescents, however, they represent the highest percentage of back pain [7]. Patients usually complain of back pain, and on physical exam, they present with hyperlordotic posture, pain reproduction with lumbar extension, and hamstring tightness. Spondylolisthesis can be palpated along the spinous process as a step-off through the normal curvature. The pain in both is worsened by activity and improved with rest. Some may present with radicular symptoms if neural structures are being compressed.

Normally, X-rays are the first line of imaging to check for any obvious traumatic damage to the spine. Both spondylolysis and spondylolisthesis may be appreciated on an oblique and lateral film, respectively. When clinical suspicion arises for them, a lateral 45-degree right, a collimated lateral view, and a left oblique view are performed [5]. For Spondylolysis, the classic "Scotty Dog" appearance may be seen with a lesion in the dog's neck. However, in acute injury, the gap in the pars reticularis is very narrow and may not be appreciable on a film. In some cases, CTs and MRIs can be performed for a better view. In spondylolisthesis, the forward displacement of the vertebrae is easily seen on a lateral view X-ray, which can then be graded on the Meyerding scale from I to IV [5]. Later, two more grades were added: grade 0, characterized by a normal state without displacement, and grade V, corresponding to spondyloptosis.

The Meyerding classification grade is determined by measuring the degree of slip using standing, neutral lateral radiographs of the lumbar spine. The classification system divides slip into five grades: 0%–25% is Grade I, 25%–50% is Grade II, 50%–75% is Grade III, 75%–100% is Grade IV, and >100% is Grade V. The grade percent is determined by drawing a line through the posterior wall of the superior and inferior vertebral bodies and measuring the translation of the superior vertebral body as a percentage of the distance between the two lines. This line is considered the numerator over the denominator, which is the length of the vertebral body below. Grades I and II are generally considered low-grade slip, whereas Grades III, IV, and V are considered high-grade slip. Grade V is also called spondyloptosis and is a complete slip >100%. Further assessment might include lateral flexion and extension views to evaluate segmental translation, which allows for a further assessment of mobility and slip severity.

The percentage expression of the extent of the slip is evaluated by measuring according to Taillard [71]. With the Taillard Method, the percentage of slip of the superior vertebra relative to the superior aspect of the inferior vertebra is calculated as $(A/B) \times 100$.

The trend for conservative treatment continues with spondylolysis and spondylolisthesis. Cessation of any extreme physical activity, organized physical therapy, braces and orthotics, and pain management is the first line for these injuries. For spondylolysis, bracing helps with the osseous healing of the fracture, while physical therapy aims to strengthen muscles, reduce lumbar lordosis, and loosen the hamstrings. For cases refractory to conservative treatments for more than 6 months, surgery is considered [5].

References

1. Fatoye F, Gebrye T, Odeyemi I. Real-world incidence and prevalence of low back pain using routinely collected data. Rheumatol Int. 2019;39(4):619–26.
2. Barthelemy VM, et al. A computational spinal motion segment model incorporating a matrix composition-based model of the intervertebral disc. J Mech Behav Biomed Mater. 2016;54:194–204.
3. Antoniou J, et al. The human lumbar intervertebral disc: evidence for changes in the biosynthesis and denaturation of the extracellular matrix with growth, maturation, ageing, and degeneration. J Clin Invest. 1996;98(4):996–1003.
4. Lyons G, Eisenstein SM, Sweet M. Biochemical changes in intervertebral disc degeneration. Biochim Biophys Acta (BBA) Gen Subj. 1981;673:443–53.
5. Donnan FG. The theory of membrane equilibria. Chem Rev. 1924;1(1):73–90.
6. Marchand F, Ahmed AM. Investigation of the laminate structure of lumbar disc anulus fibrosus. Spine. 1990;15(5):402–10.
7. Meakin J, Hukins D. Effect of removing the nucleus pulposus on the deformation of the annulus fibrosus during compression of the intervertebral disc. J Biomech. 2000;33(5):575–80.
8. Nachemson A, Morris JM. In vivo measurements of intradiscal pressure: discometry, a method for the determination of pressure in the lower lumbar discs. JBJS. 1964;46(5):1077–92.
9. Wilke HJ, et al. New in vivo measurements of pressures in the intervertebral disc in daily life. Spine. 1999;24(8):755–62.
10. Buckwalter JA. Aging and degeneration of the human intervertebral disc. Spine. 1995;20(11):1307–14.

11. Galbusera F, et al. The mechanical response of the lumbar spine to different combinations of disc degenerative changes investigated using randomized poroelastic finite element models. Eur Spine J. 2011;20(4):563–71.
12. Galbusera F, et al. The effect of degenerative morphological changes of the intervertebral disc on the lumbar spine biomechanics: a poroelastic finite element investigation. Comput Methods Biomech Biomed Engin. 2011;14(8):729–39.
13. Ayturk UM, et al. Modeling degenerative disk disease in the lumbar spine: a combined experimental, constitutive, and computational approach. J Biomech Eng. 2012;134(10):101003.
14. Kettler A, et al. Do early stages of lumbar intervertebral disc degeneration really cause instability? Evaluation of an in vitro database. Eur Spine J. 2011;20(4):578–84.
15. Malandrino A, Planell JA, Lacroix D. Statistical factorial analysis on the poroelastic material properties sensitivity of the lumbar intervertebral disc under compression, flexion and axial rotation. J Biomech. 2009;42(16):2780–8.
16. Noailly J, et al. How does the geometry affect the internal biomechanics of a lumbar spine bi-segment finite element model? Consequences on the validation process. J Biomech. 2007;40(11):2414–25.
17. Ruberté LM, Natarajan RN, Andersson GB. Influence of single-level lumbar degenerative disc disease on the behavior of the adjacent segments—a finite element model study. J Biomech. 2009;42(3):341–8.
18. Schmidt H, et al. Application of a new calibration method for a three-dimensional finite element model of a human lumbar annulus fibrosus. Clin Biomech. 2006;21(4):337–44.
19. Schmidt H, et al. Response analysis of the lumbar spine during regular daily activities—a finite element analysis. J Biomech. 2010;43(10):1849–56.
20. Galbusera F, et al. Comparison of four methods to simulate swelling in poroelastic finite element models of intervertebral discs. J Mech Behav Biomed Mater. 2011;4(7):1234–41.
21. Ehlers W, Karajan N, Markert B. An extended biphasic model for charged hydrated tissues with application to the intervertebral disc. Biomech Model Mechanobiol. 2009;8:233–51.
22. Schroeder Y, et al. A biochemical/biophysical 3D FE intervertebral disc model. Biomech Model Mechanobiol. 2010;9:641–50.
23. Frijns AJH, Huyghe JM, Janssen JD. A validation of the quadriphasic mixture theory for intervertebral disc tissue. Int J Eng Sci. 1997;35(15):1419–29.
24. Iatridis JC, Laible JP, Krag MH. Influence of fixed charge density magnitude and distribution on the intervertebral disc: applications of a poroelastic and chemical electric (PEACE) model. J Biomech Eng. 2003;125(1):12–24.
25. Jackson AR, Huang C-Y, Gu WY. Effect of endplate calcification and mechanical deformation on the distribution of glucose in intervertebral disc: a 3D finite element study. Comput Methods Biomech Biomed Eng. 2011;14(02):195–204.
26. Rohlmann A, et al. Analysis of the influence of disc degeneration on the mechanical behaviour of a lumbar motion segment using the finite element method. J Biomech. 2006;39(13):2484–90.
27. Stefanakis M, et al. ISSLS Prize winner: mechanical influences in progressive intervertebral disc degeneration. Spine (Phila Pa 1976). 2014;39(17):1365–72.
28. Liu J, et al. Biomechanical properties of lumbar endplates and their correlation with MRI findings of lumbar degeneration. J Biomech. 2016;49(4):586–93.
29. Kerttula LI, et al. Post-traumatic findings of the spine after earlier vertebral fracture in young patients: clinical and MRI study. Spine. 2000;25(9):1104–8.
30. Carragee E, et al. ISSLS Prize Winner: does discography cause accelerated progression of degeneration changes in the lumbar disc: a ten-year matched cohort study. Spine (Phila Pa 1976). 2009;34:2338–45. This study suggests that modern discography techniques using small needles and low pressures may result in accelerated disc degeneration, 2009.
31. Osti O, Vernon-Roberts B, Fraser R. 1990 Volvo Award in experimental studies. Anulus tears and intervertebral disc degeneration. An experimental study using an animal model. Spine. 1990;15(8):762–7.
32. Holm S, et al. Experimental disc degeneration due to endplate injury. Clin Spine Surg. 2004;17(1):64–71.
33. Pfeiffer M, et al. Degeneration model of the porcine lumbar motion segment: effects of various intradiscal procedures. Eur Spine J. 1994;3(1):8–16.
34. Adams MA. Biomechanics of back pain. Acupunct Med. 2004;22(4):178–88.
35. Dolan P, et al. Intervertebral disc decompression following endplate damage: implications for disc degeneration depend on spinal level and age. Spine. 2013;38(17):1473–81.
36. Przybyla A, et al. Outer annulus tears have less effect than endplate fracture on stress distributions inside intervertebral discs: relevance to disc degeneration. Clin Biomech. 2006;21(10):1013–9.
37. Ishihara H, et al. Effects of hydrostatic pressure on matrix synthesis in different regions of the intervertebral disk. J Appl Physiol. 1996;80(3):839–46.
38. Adams MA, et al. *The Biomechanics of Back Pain-E-Book*. Elsevier health sciences; 2012.
39. Walter B, et al. Complex loading affects intervertebral disc mechanics and biology. Osteoarthr Cartil. 2011;19(8):1011–8.
40. Stefanakis M, et al. Annulus fissures are mechanically and chemically conducive to the ingrowth of nerves and blood vessels. Spine. 2012;37(22):1883–91.
41. Jelec V, et al. Facet orientation and tropism: association with accelerated degeneration of stabilizing structures in lower lumbar spine. Acta Clin Croat. 2016;55(1):117–24.
42. Sengupta DK, Fan H. The basis of mechanical instability in degenerative disc disease: a cadaveric study of abnormal motion versus load distribution. Spine (Phila Pa 1976). 2014;39(13):1032–43.

43. Homminga J, et al. Posteriorly directed shear loads and disc degeneration affect the torsional stiffness of spinal motion segments: a biomechanical modeling study. Spine (Phila Pa 1976). 2013;38(21):E1313–9.
44. Melnyk AD, et al. The effect of disc degeneration on anterior shear translation in the lumbar spine. J Orthop Res. 2015;33(4):450–7.
45. Hutton WC, Cyron BM. Spondyloysis. The role of the posterior elements in resisting the intervertebral compressive force. Acta Orthop Scand. 1978;49(6):604–9.
46. Kim YE, Choi HW. Effect of disc degeneration on the muscle recruitment pattern in upright posture: a computational analysis. Comput Methods Biomech Biomed Eng. 2015;18(15):1622–31.
47. Hammouri QM, et al. The utility of dynamic flexion-extension radiographs in the initial evaluation of the degenerative lumbar spine. Spine (Phila Pa 1976). 2007;32(21):2361–4.
48. Modic MT, et al. Degenerative disk disease: assessment of changes in vertebral body marrow with MR imaging. Radiology. 1988;166(1 Pt 1):193–9.
49. Xia W, et al. The influence of spinal-pelvic parameters on the prevalence of endplate Modic changes in degenerative thoracolumbar/lumbar kyphosis patients. PLoS One. 2018;13(5):e0197470.
50. Lotz JC, Fields AJ, Liebenberg EC. The role of the vertebral end plate in low back pain. Glob Spine J. 2013;3(3):153–64.
51. Green TP, Allvey JC, Adams MA. Spondylolysis. Bending of the inferior articular processes of lumbar vertebrae during simulated spinal movements. Spine (Phila Pa 1976). 1994;19(23):2683–91.
52. Cyron B. The shearing stiffness of the lumbar intervertebral joint. Acta Orthop Belg. 1979;45:459–69.
53. Cyron BM, Hutton WC, Troup JD. Spondylolytic fractures. J Bone Joint Surg Br. 1976;58-b(4):462–6.
54. Skrzypiec DM, et al. Estimation of shear load sharing in moderately degenerated human lumbar spine. J Biomech. 2013;46(4):651–7.
55. During J, et al. Toward standards for posture. Postural characteristics of the lower back system in normal and pathologic conditions. Spine (Phila Pa 1976). 1985;10(1):83–7.
56. Amin DB, et al. Mechanisms of failure following simulated repetitive lifting: a clinically relevant biomechanical cadaveric study. Spine (Phila Pa 1976). 2020;45(6):357–67.
57. Chamoli U, Chen AS, Diwan AD. Interpedicular kinematics in an in vitro biomechanical assessment of a bilateral lumbar spondylolytic defect. Clin Biomech (Bristol, Avon). 2014;29(10):1108–15.
58. Grobler LJ, et al. L4–5 isthmic spondylolisthesis. A biomechanical analysis comparing stability in L4–5 and L5-S1 isthmic spondylolisthesis Spine (Phila Pa 1976). 1994;19(2):222–7.
59. El-Rich M, et al. A biomechanical study of L5-S1 low-grade isthmic spondylolisthesis using a personalized finite element model. Stud Health Technol Inform. 2006;123:431–4.
60. Melnyk AD, et al. An in vitro model of degenerative lumbar spondylolisthesis. Spine (Phila Pa 1976). 2013;38(14):E870–7.
61. Konz RJ, et al. The pathomechanism of spondylolytic spondylolisthesis in immature primate lumbar spines: in vitro: and finite element assessments. Spine. 2001;26(4):E38–49.
62. Patwardhan A, et al. An experimental model of adult-onset slip progression in isthmic spondylolistesis. Stud Health Technol Inform. 2002;91:322–4.
63. Sairyo K, et al. The pathomechanism of isthmic lumbar spondylolisthesis: a biomechanical study in immature calf spines. Spine. 1998;23(13):1442–6.
64. Crawford NR, et al. Biomechanics of grade I degenerative lumbar spondylolisthesis. Part 1: in vitro model. J Neurosurg. 2001;94(1 Suppl):45–50.
65. Suzuki K, et al. Posterior stabilization of degenerative lumbar spondylolisthesis with a Leeds-Keio artificial ligament: a biomechanical analysis in a porcine vertebral model. Spine. 1999;24(1):26–31.
66. Beadon K, et al. A repeatable ex vivo model of spondylolysis and spondylolisthesis. Spine. 2008;33(22):2387–93.
67. Melnyk AD, et al. Load transfer characteristics between posterior spinal implants and the lumbar spine under anterior shear loading: an in vitro investigation. Spine (Phila Pa 1976). 2012;37(18):E1126–33.
68. Foreman P, et al. L5 spondylolysis/spondylolisthesis: a comprehensive review with an anatomic focus. Childs Nerv Syst. 2013;29(2):209–16.
69. Leone A, et al. Lumbar spondylolysis: a review. Skeletal Radiol. 2011;40(6):683–700.
70. Hu SS, et al. Spondylolisthesis and spondylolysis. J Bone Joint Surg Am. 2008;90(3):656–71.
71. Taillard WF. Etiology of spondylolisthesis. Clin Orthop Relat Res. 1976;117:30–9.

4 Lumbar Segmental Instability

Venkata Paruchuri, Veronica Pajnic,
Muhammad Moazzam, Dean Matthysen,
Nicholas Green, and Deniz U. Erbulut

4.1 Introduction

Spinal stability refers to the spine's ability to endure physiological loads without inducing pain, deformity, or neurological impairments. It encompasses the precise alignment, arrangement, and interconnections of the vertebrae within a spinal motion segment during both static and dynamic phases. On the other hand, segmental instability denotes an abnormal displacement or lack of stability within a spinal motion segment. This condition typically arises from disruptions in the structural integrity and functional dynamics of the spine, including trauma, degenerative alterations, or underlying pathologies. The consequences of instability within a spinal motion segment manifest as a distorted distribution of loads, heightened stress on various structures, and irregular patterns of movement. As a result, patients may experience persistent pain, restricted range of motion, and functional limitations. Furthermore, instability can contribute to the development or progression of other pathological conditions, such as disc degeneration, spondylolisthesis, or spinal stenosis.

4.2 Biomechanics

The lumbar spine is a complex biomechanical structure responsible for providing both stability and mobility. It is composed of individual functional spinal units (FSUs) that consist of two adjacent vertebrae, the intervertebral disc, and connecting ligaments and muscles. Each FSU functions as an independent entity while contributing to the overall stability and movement of the lumbar spine.

4.2.1 Structure and Function of the Lumbar Spine

The spinal motion segment (SMS), also referred to as the functional spinal unit (FSU), serves as the fundamental building block of the lumbar spine's biomechanical system. It plays a vital role in facilitating load transmission, motion

V. Paruchuri · M. Moazzam
Ochsner Clinical School, University of Queensland, Brisbane, QLD, Australia
e-mail: v.paruchuri@uq.net.au; m.moazzam@uq.net.au

V. Pajnic · N. Green
Metro North Health, Herston Biofabrication Institute, Brisbane, QLD, Australia
e-mail: Veronica.Pajnic@health.qld.gov.au; nicholas.green@health.qld.gov.au

D. Matthysen
University of Queensland Mayne Medical School, Brisbane, QLD, Australia
e-mail: d.matthysen@uq.net.au

D. U. Erbulut (✉)
Herston Biofabrication Institute, Metro North Hospital and Health Service, Brisbane, QLD, Australia
e-mail: deniz.erbulut@health.qld.gov.au; erbulutdeniz@gmail.com

A. F. Özer et al. (eds.), *Dynamic Lumbar Spine Stabilization*,
https://doi.org/10.1007/978-3-032-12122-6_4

control, and stability within the spine. The FSU comprises two neighbouring vertebrae, an intervertebral disc, and the surrounding ligaments and muscles. It is under constant monitoring and regulation by a neural system to modulate its functions. The structural integrity of the FSU is upheld by several components, including intervertebral cartilaginous joints such as discs (consisting of the annulus fibrosus and nucleus pulposus), zygapophyseal synovial joints, anterior and posterior spinal ligaments, and, to a lesser extent, intertransverse, interspinous, and ligamentum flavum ligaments. Furthermore, the paraspinal muscles play a crucial role in supporting inertial loading [1, 2].

4.2.2 Functional Roles and Biomechanical Properties of Lumbar Spine Components

Vertebrae

The lumbar vertebrae, consisting of vertebral bodies, pedicles, laminae, and spinous processes, play an essential role in the biomechanics of the lumbar spine (Fig. 4.1). The shape and orientation of each of these structures contribute to load distribution, stability, and range of motion within each FSU [3].

Vertebral Body

The vertebral body is the weight-bearing portion of each vertebra and is composed of cancellous bone within a thin outer layer of cortical bone. Its primary role is to withstand compressive forces and distribute loads evenly along the spinal column. The vertebral body achieves this through a system of trabeculae (Fig. 4.2). The cancellous portion of the vertebral body is composed of vertical, horizontal, and two oblique systems of trabeculae. The vertical trabecular columns transmit compressive forces between the endplates and transmit load to the horizontal lamellae, dispersing the load radially [4].

Pedicles and Laminae

Pedicles project posteriorly from the vertebral body, forming the lateral boundaries of the vertebral arch (Fig. 4.1). The laminae are flat plates that connect the pedicles posteriorly, completing the vertebral arch, and together forming the vertebral canal [5]. In the lumbar spine, the laminae are integrated with the articular processes and serve to diffuse loads between the superior and inferior articular facets [6, 7]. These loads are distributed via the oblique trabecular systems to the endplates, as well as to the cortex by vertical trabeculae in the processes [6, 8].

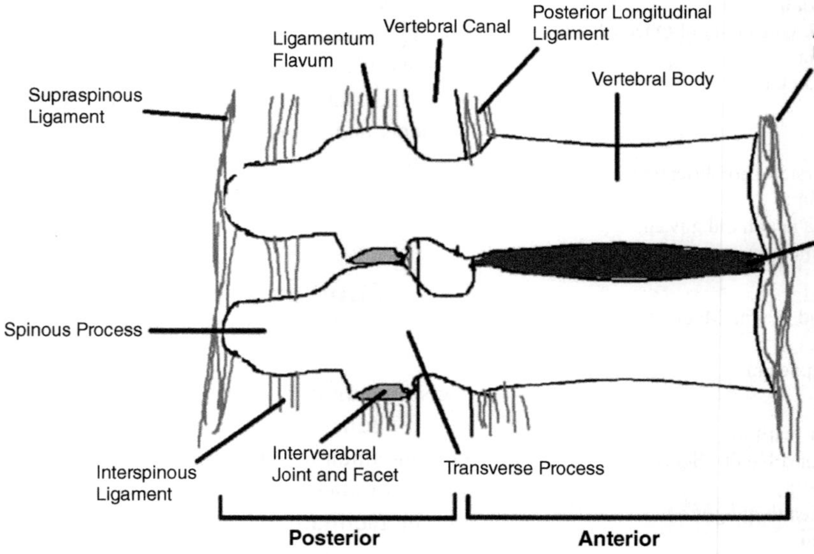

Fig. 4.1 Lateral view of a functional spinal unit

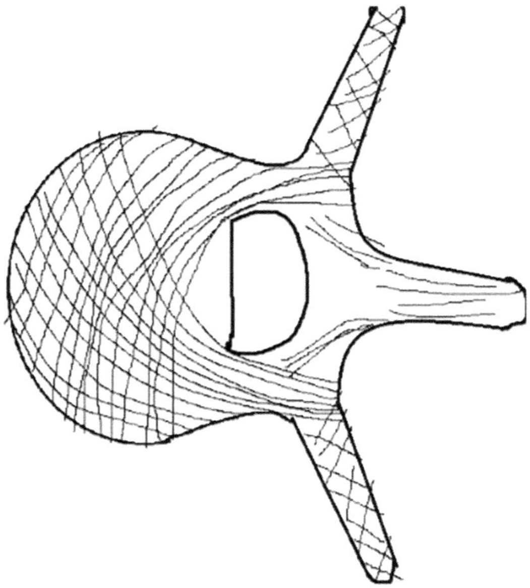

Fig. 4.2 Pattern of trabeculation in the vertebral body

Facet Joints

The facet joints, also known as zygapophyseal joints, are diarthrodial synovial joints located between the articular processes of adjacent vertebrae (Fig. 4.1). In the lumbar spine, each vertebra has two superior and two inferior facet joints, forming a paired joint complex. This joint complex forms the articular triad with the intervertebral disc [9]. Compressive loads are transmitted through this joint complex, with loads experienced by the facet joints varying based on the degree of extension [7]. Between 3% and 25% of axial compressive load may be carried by the facet joints, with increasing forces, disc height loss and increased extension [10, 11]. The axial compressive loads are borne by the articular joint surfaces, capsular ligaments, and contact between the tips of the articular process [7]. These joints influence the range of motion and stability in multiple planes, guiding flexion/extension, lateral bending, and axial rotation [7].

Spinous Processes and Transverse Processes

The spinous processes extend posteriorly from the conjunction of the laminae and serve as attachment sites for various ligaments and muscles involved in spinal stability (Fig. 4.1). The transverse processes project laterally from the vertebral arch and similarly provide attachment sites for ligaments and muscles.

Intervertebral Discs

The intervertebral discs exhibit complex behaviour under physiologic load conditions. These fibrocartilaginous structures are located between adjacent vertebral bodies and consist of three main components: the annulus fibrosus, the nucleus pulposus, and the cartilaginous endplates.

Annulus Fibrosus

The annulus fibrosus is the outer ring-shaped structure of the intervertebral disc (Fig. 4.3). It is composed of 15–25 concentric layers of fibrocartilaginous lamellae, consisting mainly of type 1 collagen fibres. These collagen fibres are arranged obliquely between 25° and 45° in the transverse plane and alternate in different directions between adjacent lamellae. This arrangement creates a tensile structure capable of withstanding circumferential stresses arising from the nucleus pulposus [12].

Nucleus Pulposus

The nucleus pulposus is the viscoelastic, gel-like core of the intervertebral disc and is composed of a hydrated matrix primarily consisting of water, proteoglycans, and type II collagen fibres (Fig. 4.3). It forms approximately 50% of the volume of the mature intervertebral disc. The proteoglycans within the nucleus pulposus ensure a high water content, creating a hydrostatic pressure that increases with compressive loads, and maintain disc height and flexibility. The type II collagen fibres provide a loose network for structural integrity [12]. Loss of proteoglycans and, therefore, water content is a component of early disc degeneration due to the reduced capacity to withstand and distribute compressive loads [13].

Cartilaginous Endplates

The endplates are thin cartilaginous layers located on the superior and inferior surfaces of the intervertebral disc. They provide a connection between the disc and the adjacent vertebral bod-

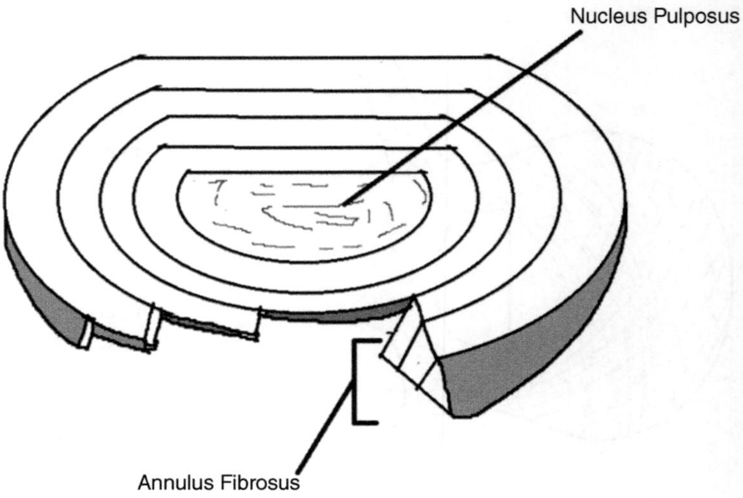

Fig. 4.3 Depiction of the nucleus pulposus and annulus fibrosus

ies, facilitating nutrient exchange and thereby supporting the structural integrity of the disc. Moreover, they play a role in load transfer, ensuring the effective distribution of mechanical forces throughout the intervertebral disc. The endplate comprises type II collagen and proteoglycans and contains approximately 60% water [12].

Ligamentous Structures

Ligaments in the lumbar spine provide passive stability and limit excessive motion within the FSU. These are divided into four groups:

1. Connect the posterior elements of the vertebrae: interspinous ligaments, supraspinous ligament, and ligamentum flavum [5]
2. Ligaments that interconnect the vertebrae: anterior longitudinal and posterior longitudinal ligaments [5]
3. The iliolumbar ligament
4. The false ligaments: the mamillo-accessory ligament, intertransverse ligaments, transforaminal ligaments and the annulus fibrosus [5]

Interspinous Ligament

The interspinous ligament is a thick, fibrous structure that connects adjacent spinous processes along the posterior aspect of the vertebral column (Fig. 4.4). It resists excessive flexion and limits separation of the spinous processes, contributing approximately 6% to spinal stability in all directions [13]. Histologically, it is composed of dense connective tissue with predominantly collagen fibres, providing mechanical strength and stability to the spine [14].

Supraspinous Ligament

The supraspinous ligament is a continuation of the interspinous ligament, extending from the tip of one spinous process to another (Fig. 4.4). It runs along the posterior midline of the vertebral column and limits flexion and anterior translation of the spine. The supraspinous ligament is thicker and stronger in the lumbar region compared to the thoracic and cervical regions, reflecting the greater demands for stability in the lower back. Despite this, it contributes only approximately 2% to stability in all directions [13].

Ligamentum Flavum

The ligamentum flavum is a paired ligament located between the laminae of adjacent vertebrae (Fig. 4.4). It consists of elastic fibres embedded in a matrix of collagen fibres. The ligamentum flavum plays a significant role in spinal stability by maintaining the upright posture of the spine and limiting excessive flexion, providing approximately 22% of stability in flexion [13]. The elastic fibres allow it to stretch during flexion and then recoil to its resting position [14].

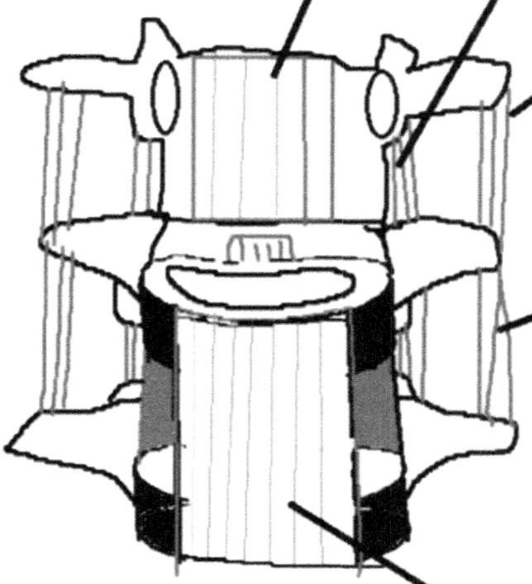

Fig. 4.4 Depiction of the ligaments of the spinal column

Anterior Longitudinal Ligament (ALL)

The anterior longitudinal ligament is a broad band of fibrous tissue that runs along the anterior aspect of the vertebral bodies (Fig. 4.4). It extends from the sacrum to the axis (C2) and provides stability against excessive anterior translation, limiting hyperextension of the spine (40%). It further contributes to stability in lateral bending (15%) [13]. The ALL is composed of dense collagen fibres, orientated longitudinally along the spine, allowing it to resist tensile forces [14].

Posterior Longitudinal Ligament (PLL)

The posterior longitudinal ligament is situated within the vertebral canal, running along the posterior aspect of the vertebral bodies. It limits excessive flexion and posterior translation of vertebrae, contributing 16% of stability in flexion [13]. Histologically, the PLL consists of fibrous tissue rich in collagen fibres, providing strength and stability to the posterior vertebral column.

Iliolumbar Ligament

The iliolumbar ligaments are present bilaterally, connecting the transverse processes of the fifth lumbar vertebra to the anteromedial surface of the ilium. The posterior band of the iliolumbar ligament limits flexion, while the anterior band constrains lateral bending [15].

Muscles

The muscles and tendons surrounding and imparting forces on the spinal column constitute the active stabilising subsystem. These structures may be considered as acting locally and globally. The local active stabilisers act on the FSU, while the global stabilisers act across multiple FSUs.

Psoas Major

The psoas major is the muscle that is responsible for the flexion of the hip. It originates in the anterolateral aspect of the lumbar spine and inserts into the lesser trochanter of the femur while descending through the brim of the pelvis. Its actions in facilitating the flexion and extension of the lumbar spine are minuscule—its fibres are arranged such that they flex the lower lumbar segments and extend the upper lumbar segments [16]. Instead, it has been determined to use the lumbar spine as a base to stabilise its actions on the hip joint. Despite its minimal influence on the movement of the lumbar spine, the psoas has been shown to exert significant compressive pressure on the lower lumbar discs, being capable of exerting compression loads equivalent to 100 kg of weight on the L5–S1 segment [16].

Multifidus Muscle

The multifidus muscle is a deep intrinsic muscle of the back that spans several vertebral levels. It is composed of multiple fascicles that originate from the sacrum, ilium, and lumbar vertebrae and insert into the spinous processes of the vertebrae above. The multifidus muscle is particularly important for segmental stability due to its segmental and contralateral activation patterns. It is composed of short fibres, with a high proportion of type I slow-twitch muscle fibres, providing capacity for fine adjustment of segmental movement [17]. The multifidus acts as a local stabiliser, providing segmental control and increasing spinal stiffness during dynamic movements [18]. It is primarily responsible for stability in the lumbar spine, resisting excessive flexion, extension, lateral bending, and rotation.

Erector Spinae Muscles

The erector spinae muscles, including the iliocostalis, longissimus, and spinalis muscles, are a group of large superficial muscles located on either side of the vertebral column. These muscles have a broad span and provide global stability. They play a significant role in generating trunk extension forces and resisting forward flexion [19].

Transversus Abdominis and Internal Oblique Muscles

The deep abdominal muscles, including the transversus abdominis and internal oblique muscles, contribute to the local stability of the lumbar spine. They form part of the anterior part of the lumbar core musculature and regulate intra-abdominal pressure. The activation of these muscles contributes to axial compression and intervertebral stiffness, preventing excessive lordosis and shear forces [20].

Other Relevant Muscles

Furthermore, the gluteus maximus, gluteus medius, quadratus lumborum and hip flexors play a role in lumbar stability during movements and in postural control. The gluteus maximus, for example, assists in hip extension and contributes to stabilising the lumbar spine during activities such as standing and walking. The gluteus medius plays a role in pelvic stability and contributes to the control of lateral bending and rotation. The hip flexors contribute to rotational movement control. The deep spinal extensors provide segmental stability, while the abdominal and hip muscles contribute to global stability and controlled movement [1, 2, 7].

The coordinated action of these structures is essential for controlled movement, load transmission, and protection of neural structures. Understanding the functional roles and biomechanical properties of the components of the lumbar spine is essential in defining the stability, mobility, and load-bearing characteristics of the lumbar spine.

Neural Input

The neural control unit is responsible for monitoring and regulating the activity of the passive and active stabilisers of the lumbar spine. Transducers in spinal ligaments observe position and load changes and convey this information to the control unit, which modifies the action of the corresponding muscles to prevent extreme motions and instability.

4.2.3 Load Transmission

Load transmission involves the transfer of forces throughout spinal structures. The spine's ability to support the body's weight and transmit external loads while maintaining stability and mobility relies on multiple mechanisms.

Compressive Forces

Compression forces are primarily borne by the vertebral bodies. The forces are transferred through the cartilaginous endplates and distributed across adjacent intervertebral discs.

Tensile Forces

Tensile forces are managed by the annulus fibrosus, the outer fibrous ring of the intervertebral disc. It withstands tension and prevents disc bulging or rupture during load transmission.

Shear Forces

Shear forces in the spine result from various movements, including bending and twisting. The combination of ligaments, facet joints, and intervertebral discs works synergistically to distribute these forces and prevent excessive stress on individual structures.

Effective load transmission within the spine is vital for preventing excessive stress on individual structures and maintaining spinal integrity. Altered load transmission can contribute to conditions such as disc degeneration, facet joint arthrosis, or vertebral fractures. Understanding the intricate mechanisms of load transmission helps clinicians diagnose and manage these conditions effectively, allowing for targeted interventions to restore proper load distribution and reduce the risk of further damage.

4.2.4 Stability

The spine achieves stability through the combined action of passive and active stabilisation mechanisms modulated by a neuromuscular control system, which work together to limit excessive motion and maintain the integrity of its structure. In this section, we will explore the concepts of stability in the spine, focusing on the passive and active mechanisms involved.

Passive Stabilisation

The passive stabilisation mechanism (osteoligamentous system) refers to the anatomical structures that provide inherent stability to the spine. The passive stabilising system of the spine comprises the vertebrae, discs, and ligaments of the FSU. This system is considered passive, as it does not create spinal motion; however, it provides feedback for the neuromuscular control system [1, 21]. The osteoligamentous system includes:

1. Ligaments: The spine is supported by a network of ligaments that connect the vertebrae and play a crucial role in limiting excessive motion. Ligaments, such as the anterior and posterior longitudinal ligaments, ligamentum flavum, and interspinous ligaments, provide passive resistance to forces acting on the spine.
2. Intervertebral discs: The intervertebral discs act as passive stabilisers by providing stability and distributing forces evenly throughout the spine. The fibrous annulus fibrosus and gel-like nucleus pulposus of the discs resist compressive, shear, and torsional forces.
3. Bony structures: The shape and alignment of the vertebrae themselves contribute to spinal stability. The interlocking nature of the vertebral bodies and the orientation of the facet joints provide inherent stability and limit excessive motion in the spine.

Active Stabilisation

Active stabilisation mechanisms involve the coordinated action of muscles and neural control to provide dynamic stability to the spine [1, 21]. These mechanisms include:

1. Deep muscles: Deep muscles, such as the multifidus and transversospinalis groups, are local stabilisers that span individual vertebral segments. They provide segmental stability and fine control of spinal movements, working to maintain proper alignment and limit excessive motion.
2. Superficial muscles: Superficial muscles, including the erector spinae and abdominal muscles, contribute to global spinal stability. They generate forces that stabilise the spine during dynamic activities and help control movement in multiple planes.
3. Neural control: The nervous system plays a vital role in maintaining spinal stability through neural control mechanisms. Proprioceptive feedback from specialised receptors within the muscles, tendons, and

ligaments provides information about the position and movement of the spine. This feedback regulates muscle activation and controls spinal posture and movement.

By combining passive and active stabilising mechanisms, the spine achieves an optimal balance between stability and mobility. The passive structures provide inherent stability, while the active muscles and neural control systems dynamically adapt to changing conditions and provide precise control over spinal movements.

Disruptions in the passive or active stabilisation mechanisms can lead to spinal instability, increased risk of injuries, and the development of spinal disorders. Therefore, maintaining the integrity and function of both the passive and active stabilisation mechanisms is crucial for preserving spinal health and overall well-being.

4.2.5 Neutral Zone and Stiffness

The neutral zone and stiffness are fundamental concepts in spinal biomechanics that play a crucial role in maintaining spinal stability and function. The neutral zone refers to the range of motion around the neutral or resting position where minimal resistance or force is required to initiate movement in the spine [21]. It represents a region of low resistance to movement, characterised by minimal tension or compression in the spinal structures.

It may be further characterised as a non-linear load-displacement curve, including a neutral zone (NZ) and an elastic zone (EZ). The NZ describes a range of intervertebral motion about the neutral posture with little passive resistance from surrounding structures. The EZ demonstrates increasing resistance to displacement subject to increasing tension in surrounding musculature, tendons, ligaments, and connective tissue. The EZ is a region of high stiffness, requiring more load per unit displacement. The neutral zone is influenced by various factors, including age, spinal health, and the presence of spinal disorders [22].

Stiffness, on the other hand, refers to the resistance of the spine to deformation or movement. It represents the ability of the spinal structures, including the intervertebral discs, ligaments, and muscles, to withstand external forces and maintain stability [23, 24]. Stiffness is crucial for load distribution and protection of the spinal structures.

The stiffness of the spine varies depending on several factors. The lumbar spine, for instance, tends to exhibit greater stiffness compared to the cervical and thoracic regions due to its role in supporting the weight of the upper body and facilitating weight-bearing activities [25]. Factors such as age-related degeneration, spinal pathology, and muscle tone can also influence spinal stiffness [24].

An optimal balance between the neutral zone and stiffness is essential for spinal stability and function. A large neutral zone indicates increased spinal instability, while excessive stiffness can restrict spinal motion and reduce adaptability [23]. Imbalances in the neutral zone and stiffness can lead to abnormal movement patterns, increased stress on spinal structures, and potential injury [24].

4.3 Segmental Instability

Instability in the FSU occurs with abnormal displacement (translation, rotation, or coupled) under physiologic loads, due to failure or dysfunction of the spine stabilising system. Biomechanically, segmental instability has been defined as the increase in intervertebral neutral zone range secondary to decreased capacity of the spinal stabilising systems in maintaining ROM within physiological limits [26]. Stabilising system dysfunction may arise due to injury, degeneration, or disease processes. The progression of instability may be described in three phases [27]:

1. Stage of dysfunction
2. Stage of instability
3. Stage of restabilisation

Despite maintaining stability, compensatory mechanisms may result in degeneration, injury and/or fatigue and therefore increase the risk of chronic dysfunction.

4.3.1 Passive/Osteoligamentous Dysfunction

Lumbar segmental instability may arise due to disruption or damage to the passive stabilising structures of the spine. This may arise due to degenerative disc disease, ligamentous laxity, facet joint degeneration, or trauma. Degenerative changes on the intervertebral discs and facet joints can lead to reduced disc height, facet joint osteoarthritis, and loss of joint congruity [28].

4.3.2 Active/Musculotendinous Dysfunction and Neuromuscular Control

Muscle dysfunction and impaired neuromuscular control play a crucial role in lumbar segmental instability. Research has shown that patients with segmental instability exhibit altered activation patterns and delayed or inadequate muscle recruitment, particularly in the deep stabilising muscles (transversus abdominis and multifidus) [29]. This muscle dysfunction leads to inadequate spinal stability and an increased reliance on the passive structures for support, further exacerbating the instability.

4.3.3 Factors Contributing to Instability

Several factors contribute to the development and progression of lumbar segmental instability. These include age-related degenerative changes, repetitive microtrauma, excessive or abnormal loading of the lumbar spine, poor posture, obesity, and genetic predisposition. Repetitive or excessive loading can lead to microinstability, causing progressive wear and tear of the passive structures [30]. Genetic factors may influence the structural integrity of the discs, ligaments, and facet joints, making individuals more susceptible to segmental instability [31].

4.3.4 Classifications of Segmental Instability

Various classification systems have been proposed to categorise lumbar segmental instability based on clinical presentation, radiographic findings, and functional impairment. These classification systems aid in diagnosing and guiding the management of lumbar segmental instability.

Radiographic Classification
The radiographic classification system focuses on dynamic assessment of the lumbar spine using imaging techniques, allowing for the evaluation of segmental instability based on objective measurements. To date, radiographic signs have been the mainstay of confirmatory testing of clinical features of segmental instability. Radiographic indicators of instability include parameters such as pathological features in neutral images or translation and angulation in flexion/extension images. Additionally, abnormal motion patterns, such as hypermobility or abnormal motion at adjacent levels, may also be considered in the evaluation. Radiographic classification provides valuable information regarding the structural integrity of the spine and the extent of segmental instability [32].

Clinical Classification
The clinical classification system focuses on the patient's subjective symptoms, functional limitations, and physical examination findings to categorise lumbar segmental instability It takes into account patient-reported pain, disability, and the impact on daily activities.

Clinical assessment should consider both subjective and objective measures to categorise patients with lumbar segmental instability. Pain intensity may be evaluated using visual analogue scales or numerical rating scales, such as the Oswestry Disability Index or the Roland-Morris Disability Questionnaire. One should also perform examinations for the presence of neurological deficits. In addition, functional tests such as the prone instability test and the aberrant movement pattern test may be employed to assess segmental instability during specific movements. These tests involve evaluating abnormal movement patterns, such as excessive segmental motion or pain reproduction, which are indicative of instability.

4.4 Imaging and Examination

4.4.1 Radiographs

Several structural changes indicative of spinal instability may be noted on neutral radiographs, including the presence of a vacuum phenomenon at the intervertebral disc, moderate disc degeneration with mild disc space narrowing, osteosclerosis and traction spurs caused by increased tensile stresses in the ligamentous attachment of the lumbar vertebrae [32–36]. A number of findings associated with various stages of stabilisation may be detected in neutral radiographs; these include marked disc space narrowing (Kirkaldy-Willis and Farfan) and claw osteophytes, which are thought to be due to the same aetiology as traction spurs [27, 37]. Discussion of intercrestal line position is a controversial finding that may warrant discussion, but the literature at this point is not definitive.

Lateral projection functional radiographs with patients in either flexion or extension are a key tool used for the detection of lumbar instability, although additional techniques such as axial traction and compression are often utilised. Questions have been raised as to the diagnostic value of these techniques [38–45]. Flexion-extension radiographs are the most widely used imaging diagnosis of lumbar intervertebral instability; however, several shortfalls are present, including difficulty in reproducibility, with slight misalignments resulting in a 10%–15% variation in the measured lumbar displacement and a lack of standardisation in the methods of obtaining the image and diagnosing lumbar instability [27, 45–47]. Patients are typically imaged in a standing position or a lateral decubitus position. Typically, intervertebral motion is found to be larger when imaging is conducted in a standing position; however, in cases of unstable spondylolisthesis, evidence suggests that the lateral decubitus position is preferred. This is thought to be due to splinting of the spine by paraspinal and/or abdominal muscles [43, 48, 49]. While the lateral flexion-extension imaging allows for investigation of vertebral translation and rotation in the sagittal plane, a number of other techniques exist for detecting instability in other planes; these include side bending for the detection of instability of axial rotation and lateral translation in the coronal plane [27, 46, 47].

4.4.2 Computed Tomography Imaging

Computed Tomography (CT) provides detailed imaging of abnormal spinal anatomy that may predispose a patient to spinal instability, such as abnormal facet joint orientation [27, 50]. CT is most often conducted in a neutral position; however, techniques such as the one described by Kirkaldy-Willis and Farfan, in which the patient is imaged while being strapped at the pelvis and rotating their torso, may be used to investigate abnormal joint motion. This increased motion may be detected at the facet joint as a vacuum phenomenon; however, the clinical relevance of this finding is uncertain [27, 51]. Due to the relatively high exposure to ionising radiation, CT imaging is rarely used for large patient series, hence limiting its use in functional imaging.

4.4.3 Magnetic Resonance Imaging

The use of magnetic resonance imaging (MRI) in cases of lumbar spine instability is best suited for the investigation of degenerative changes in the spine. The degenerative changes which MRI is best suited to investigate include degeneration of the vertebral end plate, traction spurs, annular tears, degenerative disc disease, facet joint osteoarthritis and stenosis of the spinal canal [52–54].

While these findings are associated with spinal instability, they are not diagnostic in themselves and are an indication for further imaging, such as flexion-extension radiography. It should be noted that due to the nature of MRI, patients are typically imaged in a supine position, hence removing the normal compressive loading applied to the lumbar spine. While some efforts have been made to conduct erect images, these are not standard practice.

4.4.4 Physical Examination

A wide range of physical examinations may be employed for the detection of lumbar spine instability; these tests generally provide a higher level of specificity than sensitivity, with specificities found ranging from 48% in the case of the posterior draw test up to 100% for the sit-to-stand test [55, 56]. Sensitivities ranging from as low as 5% in the case of passive physiological intervertebral movements up to 84% for the passive lumbar extension test have been observed [57, 58]. A systematic review of 11 different physical examinations by Alqarni et al. [5] found the passive lumbar extension test to have the highest positive likelihood ratio (8.8) and lowest negative predictive value (0.2), with a corresponding sensitivity and specificity of 89% and 90%, respectively.

4.5 Spinal Instability and Lumbar Pathology

The previously discussed factors of lumbar spinal instability can be applied to better understand various pathologies found in clinical medicine. While Panjabi, in his instability hypothesis, believed an excess of degrees in the neutral zone represented injury and suggested that a decrease in NZ degrees represented degeneration, the reality is not as simple [26]. Later research demonstrated that degenerated spines not only showed variation in the degree of the NZ but actually had additional axes of motion, suggesting a component of erraticity in pathology. This section will explore enlightening pathologies linked to changes in the neutral zone to better assess the potential limitations in Panjabi's hypothesis and expand on how perspectives on instability can be further applied.

4.5.1 Displacement Pathology

The simplest pathological states of the lumbar spine to explore are those related to displacement. Changes in either the passive or active stabilisation system will lead to abnormalities in how the spinal units move [1]. Scoliosis, or an irregular lateral curvature of the spine, highlights this process well. In a more specific application of the NZ definition, there is a respective NZ for axial rotation of the spine and another for lateral bending, both of which were reasonably hypothesised to play a role in the development of scoliosis. Research was done that supported that hypothesis, with the NZ for axial rotation being significantly increased in scoliosis patients [59]. In neutral posture, this meant that the increase in axial twist and lateral bending led to the changes in the overall curvature. This is because the normal stress distribution is altered to fit the scoliotic state [59]. To fit the changes in stresses and curvature during scoliosis, the muscles of the lumbar trunk change in bulk and posture. Similarly, the muscles on both sides of a scoliotic spine have to adapt to the positional changes of the spine, and it is shown that there are bilateral differences in muscle fibre diameter [59]. From our prior discussion of how diverse and significant balancing forces are to maintaining a healthy spine, it stands to reason that adaptation in pathologies makes necessary changes in the various stabilisation systems. In the scoliotic state, that involved both muscular and fatty changes.

Spondylolisthesis is a related displacement pathology that is defined as the slippage of a vertebral body from its normal position (Fig. 4.5). Changes in the stability system can lead to an increased range of motion and, therefore, a neutral zone. Studies show that there is an inverse relationship between the stiffness of the disc and the amount of neutral zone [60]. Biomechanics of slippage can be calculated

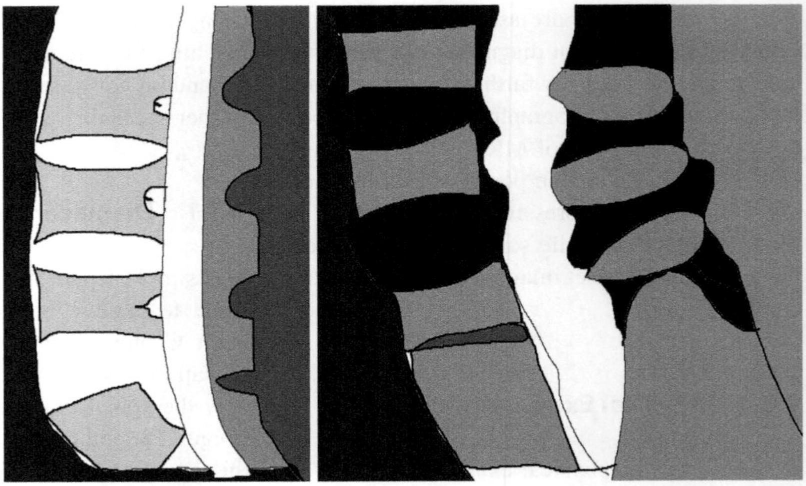

Fig. 4.5 Depiction of L4 spondylolisthesis and corresponding deformation changes

from the cyclic displacement produced by flexion-extension of the segment [60]. Load deformation data can be used to calculate stiffness, absorption energy, and neutral zone values (the range a spinal segment moves with minimal resistance [60, 61]. The suggested maximum bending of the lumbar spine from simulation was 27°, which was from a shear force of 1.9 kN [62]. However, a lumbar spine graded W9 in slip grade has a maximum bending of 34° from a shear force of 5.5 kN [62]. Effectively, a lumbar spine with spondylolisthesis exhibited greater bending and overall mobility [62].

4.5.2 Compression Pathology

Another major type of spinal pathology to consider is compression-related injuries. Compression fractures of the lumbar spine occur during axial loads that overcome stability structures and lead to trauma. The origin of how these axial loads occur is what differentiates pure compression fractures, flexion-compression fractures, and extension-compression fractures [26]. Interestingly, the NZ for flexion-compression fractures was found to be increased compared to the other types. Compression-related fractures were found to show. Notably, when comparing the NZ changes between compression fractures and burst fractures, where the bone breaks into multiple pieces upon loading, burst fractures had significantly greater NZ increases in lateral bending and flexion. This suggests that the degree of trauma is related to increases in NZ, which supports Panjabi's original hypothesis [63].

4.5.3 Degeneration Pathology

Degenerative pathologies shine a light on potential unexpected variations in the NZ theory. Assessing degenerative disc disease showed that an increase in NZ was not what defined the pathology. Rather, the axis of rotations for the spinal segments was changed altogether [64, 65]. Specifically, the instantaneous axis of rotation was moved depending on how the degenerative disease progressed and where the degeneration was in the FSU [64, 65].

Some examples of degeneration include intervertebral disc degeneration and facet joint degeneration. Intervertebral disc degeneration involves articular tropism, or the asymmetrical orientation of the lumbar zygapophysial joints may play a role [61]. Asymmetrical zygapophysial joints have unequal resistance to posteroanterior shear stresses applied [61]. Unequal load sharing leads to intervertebral joint rotation and ultimately damage in the annulus fibrosus.

Facet joint degeneration involves compressive forces acting on the spine but does not cause loading of facet joints to a significant degree. Zygapophyseal joints lose intervertebral disc height through persistent axial load transmission, particularly when the back is extended. Curvature of the articular surfaces can predispose the facet joints to damage in varied spinal positions [7]. The facet joint has a capsule surrounding it, which is composed of densely packed collagen fibres in a parallel arrangement and elastic fibres that are irregularly arranged [7]. The significance of the capsule lies in its ability to allow for significantly greater applied external force compared to a lumbar spine without an intact capsule [7].

4.6 Conclusion

Lumbar segmental instability can occur due to the breakdown of active or passive stabilising forces. Changes in the structural components of the lumbar spinal segments themselves can lead to dysfunction in the osteoligamentous system. Dysfunction in the neurological or musculotendinous components relevant to the spine is another pathway toward instability. If any of the stabilising forces fail, then that is represented by changes in the neutral zone according to Panjabi [1, 21–26]. Pathologies can be separated into displacement, compression, and degenerative categories. Each lumbar spinal disease has a unique pathogenesis related to failure of normal biomechanical equilibrium stemming from breakdown of the stabilising forces discussed earlier. Imaging, including CT, radiographs, and MRI, and physical examination, such as musculoskeletal testing, can help physicians detect lumbar instability and diagnose pathology.

References

1. Panjabi MM. The stabilizing system of the spine. Part I. Function, dysfunction, adaptation, and enhancement. J Spinal Disord. 1992;5(4):383–9; discussion 397. https://doi.org/10.1097/00002517-199212000-00001.
2. O'Sullivan PB. Lumbar segmental 'instability': clinical presentation and specific stabilizing exercise management. Man Ther. 2000;5(1):2–12. https://doi.org/10.1054/math.1999.0213.
3. Poluyi T. Control system development for six degree of freedom spine simulator. PhD thesis. 2014.
4. Izzo R, Guarnieri G, Guglielmi G, Muto M. Biomechanics of the spine. Part I: spinal stability. Eur J Radiol. 2013;82(1):118–26. https://doi.org/10.1016/j.ejrad.2012.07.024.
5. Bogduk N, Bogduk N. Clinical and radiological anatomy of the lumbar spine. 5th ed. Edinburgh/New York: Churchill Livingstone; 2012. p. 260.
6. Pal GP, Routal RV. Transmission of weight through the lower thoracic and lumbar regions of the vertebral column in man. J Anat. 1987;152:93–105.
7. Inoue N, Orias AAE, Segami K. Biomechanics of the lumbar facet joint. Spine Surg Relat Res. 2020;4(1):1–7. https://doi.org/10.22603/ssrr.2019-0017.
8. Drews S, Matsuura M, Putz R. The trabecular architecture of the superior articular process of the lumbar spine (L2-S1). Surg Radiol Anat. 2008;30(3):209–13. https://doi.org/10.1007/s00276-008-0317-6.
9. Gellhorn AC, Katz JN, Suri P. Osteoarthritis of the spine: the facet joints. Nat Rev Rheumatol. 2013;9(4):216–24. https://doi.org/10.1038/nrrheum.2012.199.
10. Dunlop RB, Adams MA, Hutton WC. Disc space narrowing and the lumbar facet joints. J Bone Joint Surg Br. 1984;66(5):706–10. https://doi.org/10.1302/0301-620X.66B5.6501365.
11. Yang KH, King AI. Mechanism of facet load transmission as a hypothesis for low-back pain. Spine (Phila Pa 1976). 1984;9(6):557–65. https://doi.org/10.1097/00007632-198409000-00005.
12. Newell N, Little JP, Christou A, Adams MA, Adam CJ, Masouros SD. Biomechanics of the human intervertebral disc: a review of testing techniques and results. J Mech Behav Biomed Mater. 2017;69:420–34. https://doi.org/10.1016/j.jmbbm.2017.01.037.
13. Widmer J, Cornaz F, Scheibler G, Spirig JM, Snedeker JG, Farshad M. Biomechanical contribution of spinal structures to stability of the lumbar spine-novel biomechanical insights. Spine J. 2020;20(10):1705–16. https://doi.org/10.1016/j.spinee.2020.05.541.
14. Scapinelli R, Stecco C, Pozzuoli A, Porzionato A, Macchi V, De Caro R. The lumbar Interspinous ligaments in humans: anatomical study and review of the literature. Cells Tissues Organs. 2006;183(1):1–11. https://doi.org/10.1159/000094901.
15. Yamamoto I, Panjabi MM, Oxland TR, Crisco JJ. The role of the iliolumbar ligament in the lumbosacral junction. Spine (Phila Pa 1976). 1990;15(11):1138–41. https://doi.org/10.1097/00007632-199011010-00010.
16. Bogduk N, Pearcy M, Hadfield G. Anatomy and biomechanics of psoas major. Clin Biomech (Bristol, Avon). 1992;7(2):109–19. https://doi.org/10.1016/0268-0033(92)90024-X.
17. Agten A, Stevens S, Verbrugghe J, Eijnde BO, Timmermans A, Vandenabeele F. The lumbar mul-

tifidus is characterised by larger type I muscle Fibres compared to the erector spinae. Anat Cell Biol. 2020;53(2):143–50. https://doi.org/10.5115/acb.20.009.
18. Ding JZ, Kong C, Li XY, Sun XY, Lu SB, Zhao GG. Different degeneration patterns of paraspinal muscles in degenerative lumbar diseases: a MRI analysis of 154 patients. Eur Spine J. 2022;31(3):764–73. https://doi.org/10.1007/s00586-021-07053-2.
19. Aspden RM. Review of the functional anatomy of the spinal ligaments and the lumbar erector spinae muscles. Clin Anat. 1992;5(5):372–87.
20. Arjmand N, Shirazi-Adl A. Role of intra-abdominal pressure in the unloading and stabilization of the human spine during static lifting tasks. Eur Spine J. 2006;15(8):1265–75. https://doi.org/10.1007/s00586-005-0012-9.
21. Panjabi MM, White AA. Basic biomechanics of the spine. Neurosurgery. 1980;7(1):76–93. https://doi.org/10.1227/00006123-198007000-00014.
22. Panjabi MM. A hypothesis of chronic back pain: ligament subfailure injuries lead to muscle control dysfunction. Eur Spine J. 2006;15(5):668–76. https://doi.org/10.1007/s00586-005-0925-3.
23. Adams MA. Biomechanics of back pain. Acupunct Med. 2004;22(4):178–88. https://doi.org/10.1136/aim.22.4.178.
24. Gardner-Morse MG, Stokes IA. Physiological axial compressive preloads increase motion segment stiffness, linearity and hysteresis in all six degrees of freedom for small displacements about the neutral posture. J Orthop Res. 2003;21(3):547–52. https://doi.org/10.1016/S0736-0266(02)00199-7.
25. Cholewicki J, Silfies SP, Shah RA, Greene HS, Reeves NP, Alvi K, Goldberg B. Delayed trunk muscle reflex responses increase the risk of low Back injuries. Spine (Phila Pa 1976). 2005;30(23):2614–20. https://doi.org/10.1097/01.brs.0000188273.27463.bc.
26. Panjabi MM. The stabilizing system of the spine. Part II. Neutral zone and instability hypothesis. J Spinal Disord. 1992;5(4):390–6; discussion 397. https://doi.org/10.1097/00002517-199212000-00002.
27. Kirkaldy-Willis WH, Farfan HF. Instability of the lumbar spine. Clin Orthop Relat Res. 1982;165:110–23.
28. Nachemson AL. Disc pressure measurements. Spine (Phila Pa 1976). 1981;6(1):93–7. https://doi.org/10.1097/00007632-198101000-00020.
29. Hodges P, Richardson C, Jull G. Evaluation of the relationship between laboratory and clinical tests of transversus abdominis function. Physiother Res Int. 1996;1(1):30–40. https://doi.org/10.1002/pri.45.
30. Wilke HJ, Wolf S, Claes LE, Arand M, Wiesend A. Stability increase of the lumbar spine with different muscle groups. a biomechanical in vitro study. Spine (Phila Pa 1976). 1995;20(2):192–8. https://doi.org/10.1097/00007632-199501150-00011.
31. Battie MC, Videman T, Levalahti E, Gill K, Kaprio J. Genetic and environmental effects on disc degeneration by phenotype and spinal level: a multivariate twin study. Spine (Phila Pa 1976). 2008;33(25):2801–8. https://doi.org/10.1097/BRS.0b013e31818043b7.
32. Knutsson F. The instability associated with disk degeneration in the lumbar spine. Acta Radiol. 1944;25(5–6):593–609. https://doi.org/10.3109/00016924409136488.
33. Frymoyer JW, Selby DK. Segmental instability. Rationale for treatment. Spine (Phila Pa 1976). 1985;10(3):280–6. https://doi.org/10.1097/00007632-198504000-00017.
34. Macnab I. The traction spur. An indicator of segmental instability. J Bone Joint Surg Am. 1971;53(4):663–70.
35. Nachemson A. Lumbar spine instability. A critical update and symposium summary. Spine (Phila Pa 1976). 1985;10(3):290–1.
36. Pitkanen MT, Manninen HI, Lindgren KA, Sihvonen TA, Airaksinen O, Soimakallio S. Segmental lumbar spine instability at flexion-extension radiography can be predicted by conventional radiography. Clin Radiol. 2002;57(7):632–9. https://doi.org/10.1053/crad.2001.0899.
37. Axelsson P, Karlsson BS. Intervertebral mobility in the progressive degenerative process. A radiostereometric analysis. Eur Spine J. 2004;13(6):567–72. https://doi.org/10.1007/s00586-004-0713-5.
38. Boden SD, Wiesel SW. Lumbosacral segmental motion in normal individuals. Have we been measuring instability properly? Spine (Phila Pa 1976). 1990;15(6):571–6. https://doi.org/10.1097/00007632-199006000-00026.
39. Hayes MA, Howard TC, Gruel CR, Kopta JA. Roentgenographic evaluation of lumbar spine flexion-extension in asymptomatic individuals. Spine (Phila Pa 1976). 1989;14(3):327–31. https://doi.org/10.1097/00007632-198903000-00014.
40. Dvorak J, Panjabi MM, Chang DG, Theiler R, Grob D. Functional radiographic diagnosis of the lumbar spine. Flexion-extension and lateral bending. Spine (Phila Pa 1976). 1991;16(5):562–71. https://doi.org/10.1097/00007632-199105000-00014.
41. Tallroth K, Alaranta H, Soukka A. Lumbar mobility in asymptomatic individuals. J Spinal Disord. 1992;5(4):481–4. https://doi.org/10.1097/00002517-199212000-00014.
42. McGregor AH, McCarthy ID, Hughes SP. Motion characteristics of the lumbar spine in the normal population. Spine (Phila Pa 1976). 1995;20(22):2421–8. https://doi.org/10.1097/00007632-199511001-00009.
43. Friberg O. Lumbar instability: a dynamic approach by traction-compression radiography. Spine (Phila Pa 1976). 1987;12(2):119–29. https://doi.org/10.1097/00007632-198703000-00007.
44. Kalebo P, Kadziolka R, Sward L. Compression-traction radiography of lumbar segmental instability. Spine (Phila Pa 1976). 1990;15(5):351–5. https://doi.org/10.1097/00007632-199005000-00002.
45. Pitkanen M, Manninen HI, Lindgrer KA, Turunen M, Airaksinen O. Limited usefulness of traction-compression films in the radio-

graphic diagnosis of lumbar spinal instability. Comparison with flexion-extension films. Spine (Phila Pa 1976). 1997;22(2):193–7. https://doi.org/10.1097/00007632-199701150-00012.
46. Dupuis PR, Yong-Hing K, Cassidy JD, Kirkaldy-Willis WH. Radiologic diagnosis of degenerative lumbar spinal instability. Spine (Phila Pa 1976). 1985;10(3):262–76. https://doi.org/10.1097/00007632-198504000-00015.
47. Pitkanen M, Manninen H. Sidebending versus flexion-extension radiographs in lumbar spinal instability. Clin Radiol. 1994;49(2):109–14. https://doi.org/10.1016/s0009-9260(05)83451-8.
48. Lowe RW, Hayes TD, Kaye J, Bagg RJ, Luekens CA. Standing roentgenograms in spondylolisthesis. Clin Orthop Relat Res. 1976;117:80–4.
49. Pennal GF, Conn GS, McDonald G, Dale G, Garside H. Motion studies of the lumbar spine: a preliminary report. J Bone Joint Surg Br. 1972;54(3):442–52.
50. Trammell TR, Schroeder RD, Reed DB. Rotatory olisthesis in idiopathic scoliosis. Spine (Phila Pa 1976). 1988;13(12):1378–82. https://doi.org/10.1097/00007632-198812000-00009.
51. Nizard RS, Wybier M, Laredo JD. Radiologic assessment of lumbar intervertebral instability and degenerative spondylolisthesis. Radiol Clin North Am. 2001;39(1):55–71, v–vi. https://doi.org/10.1016/s0033-8389(05)70263-3.
52. Modic MT, Masaryk TJ, Ross JS, Carter JR. Imaging of degenerative disk disease. Radiology. 1988;168(1):177–86. https://doi.org/10.1148/radiology.168.1.3289089.
53. Bram J, Zanetti M, Min K, Hodler J. MR abnormalities of the intervertebral disks and adjacent bone marrow as predictors of segmental instability of the lumbar spine. Acta Radiol. 1998;39(1):18–23. https://doi.org/10.1080/02841859809172143.
54. Murata M, Morio Y, Kuranobu K. Lumbar disc degeneration and segmental instability: a comparison of magnetic resonance images and plain radiographs of patients with low Back pain. Arch Orthop Trauma Surg. 1994;113(6):297–301. https://doi.org/10.1007/BF00426175.
55. Fritz JM, Piva SR, Childs JD. Accuracy of the clinical examination to predict radiographic instability of the lumbar spine. Eur Spine J. 2005;14(8):743–50. https://doi.org/10.1007/s00586-004-0803-4.
56. Maigne JY, Lapeyre E, Morvan G, Chatellier G. Pain immediately upon sitting down and relieved by standing up is often associated with radiologic lumbar instability or marked anterior loss of disc space. Spine (Phila Pa 1976). 2003;28(12):1327–34. https://doi.org/10.1097/01.BRS.0000065569.76853.E9.
57. Abbott JH, McCane B, Herbison P, Moginie G, Chapple C, Hogarty T. Lumbar segmental instability: a criterion-related validity study of manual therapy assessment. BMC Musculoskelet Disord. 2005;6:56. https://doi.org/10.1186/1471-2474-6-56.
58. Kasai Y, Morishita K, Kawakita E, Kondo T, Uchida A. A new evaluation method for lumbar spinal instability: passive lumbar extension test. Phys Ther. 2006;86(12):1661–7. https://doi.org/10.2522/ptj.20050281.
59. Voinier SD, Agnew MJ, Carmouche JJ. Passive stiffness characteristics and neutral zone quality of the scoliotic lumbar torso in the principle anatomical planes of motion. Clin Biomech (Bristol, Avon). 2020;80:105162. https://doi.org/10.1016/j.clinbiomech.2020.105162.
60. Hasegewa K, Kitahara K, Hara T, Takano K, Shimoda H. Biomechanical evaluation of segmental instability in degenerative lumbar spondylolisthesis. Eur Spine J. 2009;18(4):465–70. https://doi.org/10.1007/s00586-008-0842-3.
61. Smit TH, van Tunen MS, van der Veen AJ, Kingma I, van Dieen JH. Quantifying intervertebral disc mechanics: a new definition of the neutral zone. BMC Musculoskelet Disord. 2011;12:38. https://doi.org/10.1186/1471-2474-12-38.
62. Joszko K, Gzik M, Wolański W, Gzik-Zroska B, Kawlewska E. Biomechanical evaluation of human lumbar spine in spondylolisthesis. J Appl Biomed. 2018;16(1):51–8.
63. Ching RP, Tencer AF, Anderson PA, Daly CH. Comparison of residual stability in thoracolumbar spine fractures using neutral zone measurements. J Orthop Res. 1995;13(4):533–41. https://doi.org/10.1002/jor.1100130408.
64. Beazell JR, Mullins M, Grindstaff TL. Lumbar instability: an evolving and challenging concept. J Man Manip Ther. 2010;18(1):9–14. https://doi.org/10.1179/106698110X12595770849443.
65. Gertzbein SD, Seligman J, Holtby R, Chan KH, Kapasouri A, Tile M, Cruickshank B. Centrode patterns and segmental instability in degenerative disc disease. Spine (Phila Pa 1976). 1985;10(3):257–61. https://doi.org/10.1097/00007632-198504000-00014.

Adult Deformity Classifications and Dynamic Stabilization

5

Ali Fahir Özer and Turgut Akgül

5.1 Introduction

Instrumentation and fusion surgery is the only indisputable method for the treatment of all kinds of deformity surgery. However, spinal deformity is quite common in individuals over the age of 65 years. Patients in this age group typically have a high rate of multiple comorbid conditions (reported prevalence: 32%–68%) [1]. Indeed, adult deformity surgery can lead to potentially fatal complications. The reported complication rates in adult deformity surgery range from 13% to 41%. Advanced age, smoking, and osteoporosis are risk factors for perioperative complications [2–7].

Revision surgery in patients with complications may cause more serious problems. Therefore, patients who are not willing to undergo surgery at an early stage are liable to develop fixed deformities over time, seriously affecting surgical success.

5.2 Overview of Classifications of Spinal Curves

In the medical sciences, classification systems are used to standardize the staging, treatment, and outcomes of pathological conditions. This helps create a universal common terminology. As with other pathologies, an increased understanding of spine deformities has enabled their classification, fostering a common approach to understanding the pathology and its treatment.

King reported the classification system for adolescent idiopathic scoliosis (AIS) in 1983 [8]. This system was based on Moe's experience in the surgical treatment of AIS patients with Harrington rod instrumentation. The curves were divided into five types, and guidelines and recommendations were provided as to what levels should be instrumented according to the type of curve in order to enable maximal preservation of the motion. For the first time, King et al. developed some very important definitions, some of which are still widely used: (1) stable vertebra: vertebra most closely bisected by the central sacral vertical line (CSVL); (2) structural and compensatory curves: defined according to their flexibility in side bending films [8]. The five types of curves identified by King and Moe are presented in Fig. 5.1.

A. F. Özer (✉)
Department of Neurosurgery, Koc University School of Medicine, Istanbul, Turkey

T. Akgül
Faculty of Medicine Department of Orthopaedics and Traumatology, Koç University Hospital Spine Center, Istanbul, Turkey
e-mail: takgul@kuh.ku.edu.tr

A. F. Özer et al. (eds.), *Dynamic Lumbar Spine Stabilization*,
https://doi.org/10.1007/978-3-032-12122-6_5

Fig. 5.1 King Moe classification. (Adapted from King et al. [8])

Location	Type	Description
Thoracic	I	Principal lumbar, secondary thoracic curve
	II	Principal thoracic, secondary lumbar curve
	III	Thoracic curve only (apex≥T10)
	IV	Long thoracic curve (extends to L4)
	V	Double thoracic curve
Double major		Equally structural thoracic&lumbar curves
Lumbar		Apex in lumbar spine
Thoracolumbar		Apex at thoracolumbar junction

- Type 1: An "S" shape deformity where both curves are structural and cross the CSVL, with the lumbar curve greater than the thoracic curve.
- Type 2: An "S" shape deformity where both curves are structural and cross the CSVL, with the thoracic curve greater than or equal to the lumbar curve.
- Type 3: Major thoracic curve where only the thoracic curve is structural and crosses the CSVL.
- Type 4: A long "C"-shaped thoracic curve with the fifth lumbar vertebra centered on the sacrum and the fourth lumbar vertebra inclined toward the thoracic curve.
- Type 5: Double thoracic curve.

With the increasing preference for segmental instrumentation systems over Harrington rods, this classification system failed to provide accurate and reliable results at appropriate levels for fusion [9–11]. Moreover, this classification system was shown to have low inter- and intra-observer reliability [12, 13].

This prompted the development of a new classification system by Lenke in 2001 [14]. In the Lenke classification, the spinal curve is defined according to the curve type and proposes a lumbar modifier definition; in addition, this was the first classification system for scoliosis to include global sagittal balance. Several new definitions have been made with this classification: (1) main curve: the largest curve and always structural; (2) small curve: a smaller curve, either structural or nonstructural; and (3) nonstructural curve: a curve that bends <25° in side-tilting radiographs.

According to these definitions, there are six different types of curves (Fig. 5.2):

- Type 1: The main thoracic (MT) is the only structural curve, while the others (proximal thoracic and lumbar or thoracolumbar) are not structural.
- Type 2: Double thoracic, where MT is the main curve, proximal thoracic (PT) is the minor but structural curve, and thoracolumbar (TL) or lumbar (L) curves are minor and nonstructural.
- Type 3: Double main curve model where MT is the main curve and the lumbar is the minor but structural curve, while PT is nonstructural.
- Type 4: Triple master curve pattern wherein MT is the main curve, but all three curves are structural.
- Type 5: The TL or L curve is the main and only structural curve, while PT and/or MT curves are small and nonstructural.
- Type 6: The TL or L curve is the major curve that is at least 5° greater than the minor but structural curve MT.

Curve type

Type	Proximal thoracic	Main thoracic	Throacolumbar/lumbar	Description
1	Nonstructural	Structural (major)	Nonstructural	Main thoracic (MT)
2	Structural	Structural (major)	Nonstructural	Double thoracic (MT)
3	Nonstructural	Structural (major)	Structural	Double major (DM)
4	Structural	Structural (major)	Structural (major)	Triple major (TM)§
5	Nonstructural	Nonstructural	Structural (major)	Thoracolumbar/lumbar (TL/L)
6	Nonstructural	Structural	Structural (major)	Thoracolumbar/lumbar-main thoracic (TL/L-MT)

Structural criteria
(Minor curves)

Proximal thoracic – Side bending cobb ≥25°
– T2-T5 kyphosis ≥+20°

Main thoracic – Side bending cobb ≥25°
– T10-L2 kyphosis ≥+20°

Thoracolumbar/lumbar – Side bending cobb ≥25°
– T10-L2 kyphosis ≥+20°

Location of apex
(SRS definition)

Curve	Apex
Thoracic	T2-T11/12 disk
Thoracolumbar	T12-L1
Thoracolumbar/lumbar	L1/2 disk-L4

Modifiers

Lumbar spine modifier	CSVL to lumbar apex
A	CSVL between pedicles
B	CSVL touches apical body(ies)
C	CSVL completely medial

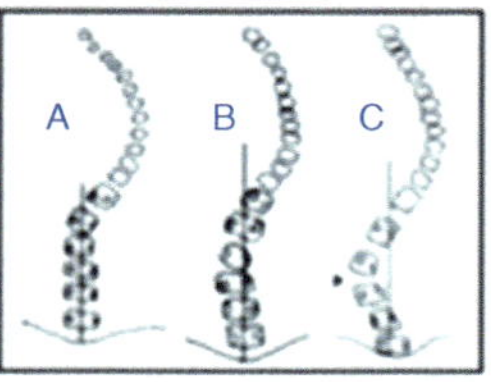

Thoracic sagittal profile T5-T12	
– (hypo)	<10°
N (normal)	10°–40°
+ (hyper)	>10°

Curve type (1–6) + lumbar spine modifier (A, B, C) + thoracic sagittal modifier (–, N, +)
Classification (eg, 1B+): ________

Fig. 5.2 Lenke classification [14]

A lumbar spine modifier is added to this sub-baseline curve type. This modifier is defined by the position of the CVSL on the apical vertebra of the lumbar curve. Lenke identified three lumbar modifiers:

- Modifier A: CSVL is located between the pedicles of the lumbar apical vertebra.
- Modifier B: CSVL is located between the medial border of the lumbar concave pedicle and the lateral edge of the apical vertebral body.
- Modifier C: The CSVL passes medially to the fully concave apical vertebral body.

As mentioned, a thoracic sagittal profile modifier is also included in the Lenke classification. Thoracic kyphosis is measured between T5 and T12 and is defined as follows:

- + (plus): when thoracic kyphosis is 40°
- N (normal): when thoracic kyphosis is between 10° and 40°
- – (minus): when thoracic kyphosis is <10°

The Lenke classification showed higher inter- and intra-rater reliability than the King classification. It is also a more reliable method to assist surgeons in choosing the best treatment method for each curve pattern. Types 1 and 5 Lenke curves can be treated anteriorly or posteriorly. Lenke Types 2, 3, 4, and 6 should be treated completely via the posterior approach. In patients with lumbar modifier A or B, a selective thoracic fusion is recommended to avoid fusion of the lumbar vertebrae as much as possible.

Although the Lenke classification is more comprehensive and reliable than the King classification, it is still far from perfect. Surgeons still deviate by 15% from the given algorithm for selecting fusion levels [15]. In addition, the classification fails to address the rotational component of the deformity. The classification was mainly developed for AIS, and predominantly thoracic curvatures were prioritized, whereas in adult degenerative scoliosis (ADS), the curvature is predominantly in the lumbar region and extends to the thorax. This draws the center of gravity to the lumbar region, unlike Lenke. This underlines the need to develop new classifications for ADS.

ADS is characterized by an abnormal spinal curvature >10°, which is usually observed in children and adolescents after skeletal maturity [16]. ADS is common in individuals aged >40 years. The progressive population aging has led to an increase in the incidence of ADS, making it an important public health problem. In patients older than 40 years, the incidence of ADS increases with age (6%–68%) [17]. Previous studies have focused on the etiology, patient statistics, clinical features, imaging findings, and treatment modalities for ADS. Recent research has suggested that sagittal imbalance, coronal changes, and rotational deformity in ADS have a major impact on the health-related quality of life (HRQoL) of patients [18–21].

Many studies have been conducted to develop classification systems. The common goal of these studies was to standardize the pathology and treatment. Aebi developed a classification for the etiology of adult deformity in 2005 but did not contribute to treatment recommendations [22].

Schwab et al. (2005) proposed a radiographic classification system based on the degree of lordosis (L1-S1) and frontal plane obliqueness of L3 on standing radiographs. A total of 98 adult patients with scoliosis with at least 2 years of follow-up were included in this study. Curve patterns were classified as thoracic/thoracolumbar/lumbar/thoracic and lumbar; the mean Cobb angle (± standard deviation) was 30° ± 19° [23]. This classification is only a radiological classification and does not involve clinical evaluation. We will discuss the importance of this later.

In 2006, the Scoliosis Research Society (SRS) published a largely descriptive classification system that includes seven curve types and three modifiers describing regional sagittal and lumbar degenerative curvature [24]. This classification system is essentially descriptive and does not take into account the clinical parameters, making it less valuable in practice. Later in 2012, Schwab and SRS published a hybrid classification system (SRS-Schwab classification) [25]. Similar to the initial classification of Schwab et al., this classification of the radiographic deformity was found to be associated with patient-reported satisfaction with outcomes. However, the new classification included several radiographic pelvic parameters such as pelvic incidence, lumbar lordosis, pelvic tilt, and sagittal vertical axis, which are closely related to the clinical manifestations [26]. The rationale behind the SRS-Schwab classification is that pelvic alignment is associated with spinal sagittal alignment, and postoperative pelvic parameters are closely related to both pain and spine-related disability [27] (Fig. 5.3).

The sagittal modifiers incorporated in this classification add to its clinical relevance since patient satisfaction is closely related to the correction of these parameters.

The first sagittal modifier uses these two radiographic parameters to calculate the difference between pelvic incidence and lumbar lordosis. This measurement is important for obtaining appropriate postoperative lumbar alignment and for surgical planning in patients with low lumbar lordosis relative to pelvic incidence [25]. Lumbar lordosis is the sagittal Cobb angle between the upper endplate of S1 and the upper endplate of L1. Pelvic incidence is the angle between the per-

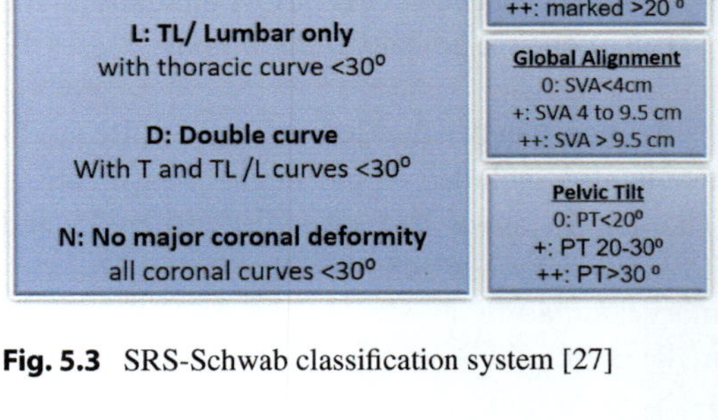

Fig. 5.3 SRS-Schwab classification system [27]

pendicular line passing through the midpoint of the upper sacral endplate and the line joining the axis of the femoral head to this midpoint. The pelvic incidence is classified as "–". If the discrepancy is <10°, the lumbar lordosis modifier is "0"; if it is between 10° and 20°, the modifier is "+"; and if it is >20°, the modifier is classified as "++".

The pelvic tilt is another important sagittal modifier because a high pelvic tilt reflects a compensatory mechanism to reduce marked global sagittal alignment [27]. Patients with greater pelvic tilt often need larger corrections (osteotomies) to reduce the risk of postoperative failure [25]. Pelvic tilt assesses the degree of retroversion by measuring the angle between the line from the midpoint on the sacral endplate to the bixofemoral axis and the vertical axis through the bixofemoral axis. Patients are classified as pelvic tilt modifier "0" if pelvic tilt is <20°, modifier "+" if between 20° and 30°, and modifier "++" if pelvic tilt is >30°.

The final sagittal modifier is the modifier of the global alignment based on the sagittal vertical axis. An increase in the sagittal vertical axis is associated with increased pain and disability [25]. SVA is defined as the distance between the posterosuperior corner of the sacrum and the sagittal C7 line. Patients are classified as SVA "0" if the measurement is <40 mm, modifier "+" if between 40 and 95 mm, and modifier "++" if >95 mm.

Compared to previous systems, the SRS-Schwab system focuses more on spinopelvic parameters because they are associated with better HRQoL scores after surgery [27, 28]. Schwab et al. (2010) conducted a study evaluating the relationship between spinal alignment parameters and modifiers and surgical planning [29]. Their data informed the recommendations for the extent of surgical correction required to achieve the best HRQoL scores.

Another study showed that the classification system can predict patient disability and preferences for surgical versus nonsurgical treatment [25, 30]. Patients with thoracolumbar and primary sagittal deformities have worse health status and greater disability than other curve types. A recent study found that patients operated on with a higher sagittal modifier had a worse prognosis [25, 26]. Studies investigating the achievement of sagittal alignment in the surgical treatment of adult spinal deformity are potentially the most important contribution to the SRS-Schwab classification, given its strong correlation with postoperative disability and pain. These studies highlight the utility of the SRS-Schwab system for treatment decisions and prognostic assessment.

Apart from these, two more important classifications should be mentioned. The first of these is the Silva–Lenke classification [31]. This classification system classifies ADS into six levels based on the patient's clinical symptoms and radiological findings. In the clinical evaluation, this system accepts neurogenic claudication or radiculopathy as a group and includes low back pain as a separate group; the remaining five parameters are evaluated radiologically. In two of the radiological evaluations, anterolisthesis and olisthesis are considered as the basis for determining degeneration, and the remaining three evaluation criteria are radiological parameters, i.e., lumbar kyphosis, coronal Cobb angle, and global imbalance. The system specifies the findings that are required at each level, and the number of findings increases with each level. In this classification, a separate section is not allocated to lumbar curvatures as in the SRS-Schwab system, but an attempt has been made to overcome this shortcoming with spinal parameters. Although it is not as detailed a classification as SRS-Schwab, it has more practical implications.

While simple decompression is recommended at Levels II and III, short fusion with decompression is recommended at Level IV. The need for fusion and long stabilization for Levels V and VI is particularly emphasized (Fig. 5.4).

The most striking point in this classification is that there is a global imbalance at Level 5, and it is emphasized that the deformity is also flexible. However, the recommended treatment is again long instrumentation and fusion. It is thought-provoking that the same treatment should be applied to two different pathologies, flexible or rigid. It turns out that there is a gap in between.

Symptom	Nonop Management	Level I	Level II	Level III	Level IV	Level V	Level VI
neurogenic claudication/ radiculopathy	minimal	+	+	+	+	+	+
back pain	minimal	minimal	+/-	+	+	+	+
ant osteophytes	+	+	-	-	-	-	-
olisthesis	-	-	-	+	+	+	+
coronal Cobb (<30º)	-	-	-	+	+	+	+
lumbar kyphosis	-	-	-	-	+	+	+
global imbalance	-	-	-	-	-	+(flexible)	+ (stiff/fused)

Fig. 5.4 Silva–Lenke classification. (Adapted from Silva and Lenke [31])

The last classification we will focus on is the Berjano–Lamartina classification. This classification is based on radiological evaluation, while clinical evaluations, such as those in Silva–Lenke classifications, are inconspicuous. This classification was developed mainly to facilitate surgical planning.

There are four main categories in the classification: Type I (limited apical segment disease); Type II (limited apical segment disease); Type III (enlarged segment disease—apical and non-apical); and Type IV (unstable spine): IVa, sagittally unstable; IVb, sagittal and coronally unstable [32].

For treatment, the detection of the pathological area of the Type I and II curves and the fusion of this area are sufficient. Type III requires the fusion of the entire extension of the coronal curve. Type IV usually requires aggressive corrective procedures, often including posterior tricolumnar osteotomies. Type IV is divided into two groups. In Type IVa, there is a severe sagittal imbalance but no coronal imbalance. In Type IVb, there is a severe sagittal and coronal imbalance (Fig. 5.5). This classification was later developed with additional articles, and more detailed surgical recommendations were made, especially in the mobile segment [33].

Type I: localized nonapical DSD (balanced)	Symptomatic DSD is present at nonapical segments of the main coronal curve	The deformity does not affect the surgical plan. Selective fusion can be performed, at the same levels that would be done in simple degenerative disease. Decompression without fusion in selected patients can be an alternative. In some cases, fusion should be extended to the sacrum
Type II: localized apical DSD (balanced)	Symptomatic DSD is present at the apical segments of the main coronal curve	Selective fusion is possible, but it should extend at both sides of the apex of the curve. An exception is single-level DSD with the degenerated disc being at the apex of the coronal curve. Correction of the curve with short fusion permits restoring the alignment of adjacent flexible discs
Type III: extensive (apical and nonapical) DSD (balanced)	Symptomatic DSD is present all over the main curve or beyond (frequently into the lumbosacral junction)	Fusion should include all the main curve and extend if needed to the lumbosacral junction
Type IV: imbalanced spine	Loss of lordosis is >25° and the sagittal deformity does not correct in extension films	Powerful correction methods (tricolumnar osteotomies or aggressive release) are needed
Type IVa: sagitally imbalanced	Severe sagittal imbalance with no or slight coronal imbalance	
Type IVb: coronally and Sagitally imbalanced	Severe imbalance both in the coronal and sagittal planes	

Fig. 5.5 Berjano–Lamartina classification. (Adapted from Berjano and Lamartina [32])

5.3 Overview and Criticism of Classifications

Kuntz et al. (2008) conducted a detailed study involving volunteer subjects of all ages. Standing upright, neutral upright spinal alignment was assessed using all spinopelvic parameters from occiput to pelvis, which we can consider as a classification [34]. This classification revealed age-related spinal deterioration. The study determined the location, shape, size, and flexibility of the deformity curve and the global sagittal array. Based on the findings of the literature review, the authors concluded that despite a wide variation in regional curves from the occiput to the pelvis in asymptomatic volunteers, the horizontal gaze emphasizes that the global sagittal alignment of the spine on the pelvis and femoral heads is maintained in a narrow range in order to maintain balance. This is a very important finding, which shows that it is not easy to maintain spinal sagittal balance with age-related deterioration in the spine.

Duval-Beaupere et al. reported three main pelvic sagittal parameters, pelvic incidence (PI), pelvic tilt (PT), and sacral tilt (SS), as important parameters [35, 36]. It is accepted that these parameters constantly change to maintain the PI constant in order to provide sagittal balance and maintain the horizontal gaze with the advancement of age. PI is somewhat of a relatively constant morphological parameter with slight changes throughout adulthood. However, recent studies have reported that PI changes with age, especially in women [37]. In this study, PI was found to be higher in women aged over 40 years who had given birth. As PI increases, lumbar lordosis increases proportionally to maintain sagittal vertical balance because PT and SS are posture-dependent parameters that vary with pelvic rotation on the hip axis. The relation between these three pelvic parameters is represented by the equation PI = PT + SS. The basic facts accepted in this determination are shocking.

In a study conducted in Japan, normative values for both sagittal alignment and HRQoL scores were found to vary according to age [37, 38]. A study described the normal reference range for global sagittal balance parameters in healthy individuals in different age groups [37]. This study included 626 asymptomatic volunteers of both sexes who were divided into 10-year age groups from the third to eighth decade of life, with at least 50 subjects in each age group.

Advancing age was found to lead to an increase in PT and SVA and a decrease in LL and thoracic kyphosis. From the seventh decade to the eighth decade, a remarkable change was observed in the spinopelvic sagittal alignment. This natural history of sagittal spinopelvic alignment should be included in the surgical planning of adult scoliotic deformity (ASD) patients.

As more and more ASD patients are treated surgically, the data obtained is of great importance. This has led to the development of the concept of age-adjusted fitness goals for ASD patients [39]. The SRS-Schwab classification provides a framework for surgeons to define spinopelvic malalignment and realignment targets using a global sagittal array and spinopelvic parameters. Unfortunately, despite achievement of the ideal goals for the radiological parameters described in the SRS-Schwab classification, the rate of complications such as proximal junction failure (PJF) and revision surgery for it is higher in these patients. In a significant number of patients, more intraoperative correction is required due to the severe deformity [40]. In another important study, patients who developed PJF had significantly greater corrections in SVA and more postoperative LL [41].

It was assumed that overcorrection of ASD would be required to counteract the effects of continued degeneration in the elderly; however, over time, several studies have identified advanced age and surgical overcorrection of SVA as independent risk factors for proximal junction kyphosis (PJK) and revision surgery [42–45].

However, none of the current classification systems take into account the patient's age, and the treatment guidelines do not specify age-specific alignment targets.

Studies have shown that the implementation of identical sequencing goals for all patients without consideration of elderly age and clinical comorbidities, and attempting to create a radiographically perfect spine, is doomed to fail in the long run. Realistic radiographic reconstruction of sagittal balance for physicians concerned with achieving age-specific global sagittal balance will be critical in establishing future ASD classification systems.

Patients with ASD have been treated conservatively for several years because of the high risk of major surgery, given their advanced age, lack of powerful instrumentation tools, and poor bone quality for a major corrective spinal surgery [46, 47].

Advances in anesthesia for spine surgery and advances in surgical techniques and technology supported by diagnostic imaging have helped advance the surgical treatment of ASD patients. Although treatment protocols for ASD patients have evolved over the past two decades, ongoing efforts to develop a widely accepted adult deformity classification system are evidence of the inherent difficulty of treating patients with ASD due to clinical variability [48].

It should not be forgotten that the classical approach for the treatment of ASD is associated with very high complication rates ranging from 25% to 80% [49, 50]. A prospective multicenter evaluation of 291 patients who underwent ASD surgery (minimum follow-up of 2 years reported a high rate of complications) [51]. A total of 469 complications were documented (207 minor; 262 major), and 203 patients (69.8%) were affected. The most common categories of complications were implant-related, radiological, and neurological, while intraoperative complications were associated with three-column osteotomies. The most common implant-related and radiological complications were rod breakage and PJK, respectively. Other frequent complications were cardiopulmonary, infection, gastrointestinal, vascular, musculoskeletal, and renal complications. Several other studies have reported similar data related to complications.

Despite the developments in surgical techniques in the last two decades, especially efforts to treat scoliosis with minimally invasive surgical methods, technological advances in instrumentation design and placement, and advances in medical treatment for hemorrhage control, there has not been a significant decrease in complication rates [51–54]. This prompts us to look for other approaches besides fusion and rigid stabilization and shows that the future of spine surgery can be improved by improving the treatment for mobile deformity, for which there is a lack of robust classification systems.

Above, we have explained in detail that efforts to restore the ideal parameters in elderly patients with a broken spine using fusion and rigid stabilization do not yield the expected results in terms of PJK or HRQoL, even if the radiological outcomes are good. The spine that the patient has at a young age and the one at later ages are two different spines in terms of their attributes. The spine that we try to achieve with surgery is a completely different third spine, and it is very different from the slowly deteriorating spine that the individual lives with. "Is it right to create this third spine or to bring the existing one closer to the maximum level that it can recover as it is?" The answer to the question is important, and in our opinion, the correct thing is to use the existing backbone without changing it.

While adhering to the classifications, the personal characteristics of each patient should not be ignored. Body mass index, nicotine use, and the severity of osteoporosis are important factors that do not stand out in the classifications. More importantly, most of these patients present to the outpatient clinic with symptoms of root irritation due to neurogenic claudication or foraminal stenosis. Investigations reveal ASD in most cases. Again, a large proportion of the patients state that they are able to maintain an upright posture when they start walking but lean forward after a while. Whether or not the global sagittal balance is impaired, this is the period when the patient has a golden opportunity. The patient can achieve global sagittal balance using the muscle compartment. It has the ability to insert the SVA into the sacrum. The biggest mistake made during this period was to follow this patient as if it were normal, to apply pain procedures, and to send him to FTR. However, a simple dynamic stabilization surgery at this stage, which can immensely benefit these patients, is often ignored. In almost all classifications, it is mentioned that the deformity is mobile, but its only importance in treatment is to perform symmetric or asymmetric osteotomy for the fixed deformity, and then fusion and rigid stabilization meet at the common denominator. We think there is a shortcoming here: why should we fix the mobile deformity of the mobile patient? The common answer provided in the classifications is fix and fix. In our opinion, the answer should be "fix the mobile deformity, but leave it as mobile as possible," and it should be a much simpler, less risky, and age-appropriate surgical option, and this is exactly where the shortcoming is.

Patient expectations are very important. The greatest wish of a patient who cannot see the opposite is to be able to see the opposite. Having a straight spine is a secondary problem for the patient. It is debatable how rational it is to bring an elderly person to the values of a normal young person. Except for a very advanced deformity, most patients do not come to the doctor for straightening the spine. Most of the time, these patients present with mild neurological findings and low back pain. In fact, simple decompression surgeries save the moment, but in most cases, they do not save the future. In order to correct these deformities in a patient who can correct his own deformity, the choice between "doing fusions between vertebrae, descending to the iliac bones, and restoring the ideal parameters" or "intervening in the problematic areas by decompression, correcting the deformity while ensuring maximal mobility, without forcing the parameters" is a pertinent issue. Whether to stabilize it or not is the biggest dilemma facing spine surgery. As already stated, we recommend the latter option.

5.4 Pedicular Dynamic Stabilization and ASD Classifications

It is pertinent to mention here that there are no serious shortcomings in the current classifications, but that only the point of view should change. They are classifications that have lasted for years and have developed over time with accumulating evidence. In the foreseeable future, classifications that provide three-dimensional information and other more detailed parameters without overwhelming the surgeon are likely to be made. For now, modifying the classification systems with respect to the treatment recommendations is of much relevance.

First of all, examinations are important to us. The main problem here is that the age-related spinal deterioration prevents the spine from keeping the trunk upright, and any treatment that keeps the spine upright helps to carry the trunk. Lateral bending films should be obtained to assess whether the deformity is mobile or not. Another important issue is to assess the extent of improvement in deformity by comparing lying down and standing X-rays. This determines whether this deformity is mobile and the extent to which it is amenable to surgical correction. Depending on the patient's medical condition during the surgery, we can only correct the deformity with Ponte osteotomies if necessary; however, we do not consider this necessary. These limits are the limits that the patient can comfortably tolerate. Another important examination is to determine the extent to which the patient can lean forward. If the patient is able to cooperate well, side X-rays should be taken to assess how he is standing straight and how much he bends while walking. In patients who cannot cooperate, first, it is necessary to take a straight side view, as much as possible, and then, after 15–30 min of walking, one more lateral X-ray should be obtained to assess the extent of loss of global sagittal balance. This can help determine the extent of improvement in sagittal balance that can be achieved with the use of a dynamic stabilization system.

Sagittal modifiers are important in SRS-Schwab ASD classification in groups with thoracic curves, lumbar curves, and only scoliotic curves without sagittal balance disorder. Fusion surgery rigid stabilization is not required for patients with PI-LL of 10°–20°, patients with SVA of 4–9.5 cm, and patients with PT of 20°–30°. Their deformities are mobile, so the first groups in the modifiers are ideal candidates for dynamic stabilization, and those in the second group should be supported by Ponte osteotomies at most or corrected and left as much as possible, depending on the patient's condition. In the Silva–Lenke classification, the same approach should be applied for Levels I–IV. Dynamic systems up to Types I–III should be considered in the Berjano–Lamartina approach, which is a similar classification [55–57] (Fig. 5.6).

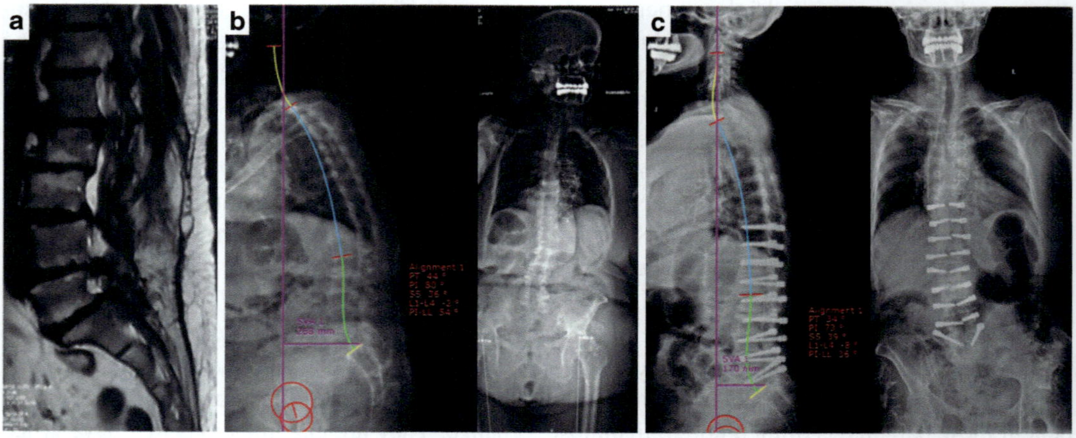

Fig. 5.6 A 63-year-old woman. Three years back, she underwent an operation for lumbar disc herniation. In the last 2 years, she experienced increasing back pain and difficulty walking. Investigations revealed impaired sagittal balance. (**a**) MRI showed multilevel degenerative changes, resulting in a multilevel lumbar narrow canal. (**b**) Curve type according to SRS-Schwab classification: N, modifiers; PI-LL within 54° (++), global alignment SVA 26.8 cm (++), and PT 44° (++). Silva–Lenke, Level III, Berjano–Lamartina Type III. (**c**) A radiograph obtained on postoperative day 8 shows no problem (Dynesys system)

5.5 Long-Segment Surgical Methods in Pedicular Dynamic System

Dynamic System: We use two systems for long-segment surgery: Orthrus and dynamic screw and double PEEK rod. We have used the Dynesys system for a long time and noticed that its tethers loosened over time. It can be used in deformities without balance issues, but the forward bending moments on the tethers in the deformity cause increased loads, and excessively loaded rods (tethers) to maintain balance easily loosen and lose their function. Therefore, when we revised these cases, we used double rods (tethers) using perforated screw blockers and spacers to avoid disrupting the healthy osteosynthesis of the screws into the bone and avoiding the need for new screws. We have not yet observed any problems in the two patients we revised this way, despite the two-year follow-up. The biggest problem with the use of the dynamic system is loosening of the screws, as patients are older and have poor bone quality. Although the screw does not bear the entire load, as in rigid systems, even if it does share the load, there is a risk of loosening if the bone quality is poor. Therefore, we use these screws in a two-stage surgery. This topic is discussed in detail in another chapter of the book. We first place the screws, wait 4-6 months depending on the patient's T-score, and after the osteosynthesis is completed, the rods are tightened in the second stage. The Orthrus system is a modular system that uses a short rod for the double-headed screws. Rod fracture is not an issue with this system, but screw loosening can occur. Because it is a modular system, revision is very easy. The system can be used in two stages. The use of this system has been described in previous sections (Fig. 5.7).

Screw loosening can be a problem, especially in patients undergoing long-segment stabilization if the T score is above -1.5. This problem becomes more serious with age and increasing levels [58, 59]. Dynamic stabilization should be applied to patients with slowly developing instability in the deformity. Acceptable results can be achieved with dynamic stabilization applied to single-level pathologies [60] (Fig. 5.8).

However, screw loosening also occurs, especially as the level increases [61] The system we routinely use for deformity is the dynamic screw and double PEEK rod system, and so far, our two-year results have been uneventful. In a finit element thesis study, which has not yet been published as an article, it was observed that the double-rod system did not significantly compromise

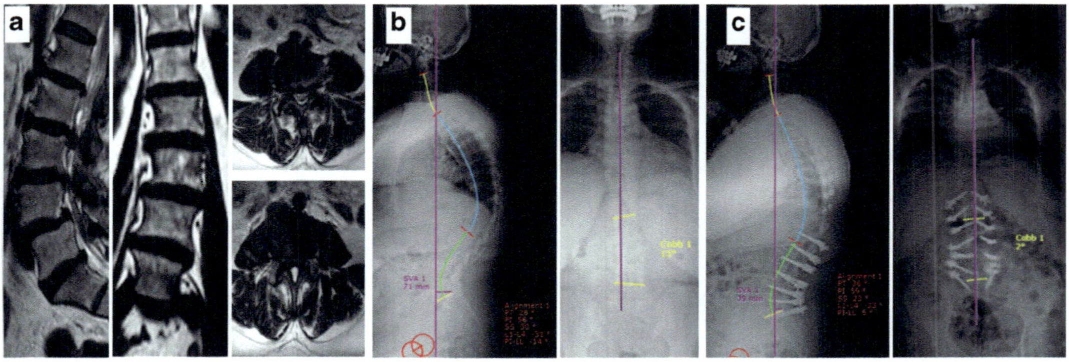

Fig. 5.7 A 69-year-old woman presented with the inability to stand due to pain and severe pain while walking and especially when standing. Neurological examination was normal. (**a**) MRI shows advanced degenerative disk disease in all disks between L1 and S1; the L4 spine has shifted forward over L5. Coronal sections show a right-facing 15° scoliosis. (**b**) This case was classified as SRS-Schwab, coronal curve type N, modifiers: PI-LL 14 (+), global alignment SVA 7.1 cm (+), and PT 26 (+). Silva–Lenke Level III, Berjano–Lamartina Type II. (**c**) The patient underwent two-stage surgery and was stabilized with the T12 and S1 Orthrus system. The patient is in the second year postoperatively and has no complaints

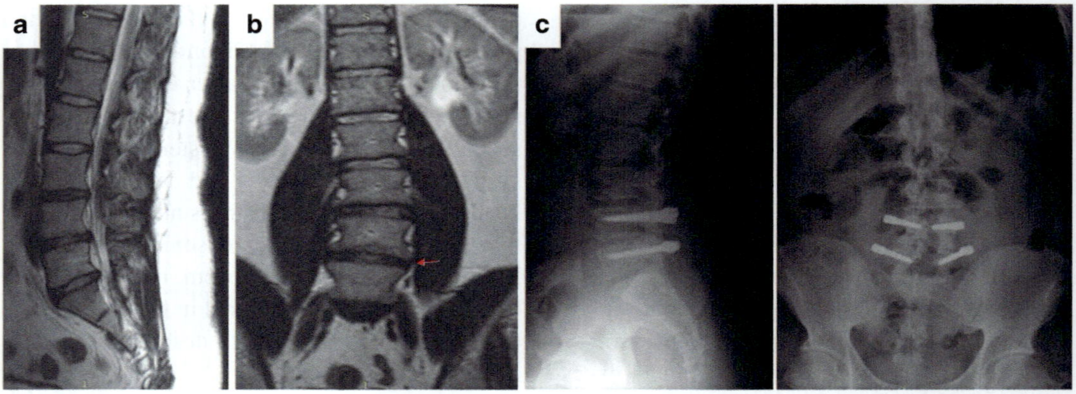

Fig. 5.8 A 30-year-old man was operated on for low back pain. (**a**) Preoperative sagittal MRI shows no pathology; (**b**) MR coronal section shows a decrease in disk height and minimal olisthesis in L4–5 (red arrow). This case was classified as follows: SRS-Schwab, coronal curve type N, modifiers; PI-LL within 10°, global alignment SVA < 4 cm, and PT < 20° Silva–Lenke Level III, Berjano-Lamartine Type II. (**c**) Only this distance is dynamically stabilized. The patient is in the postoperative fifth year

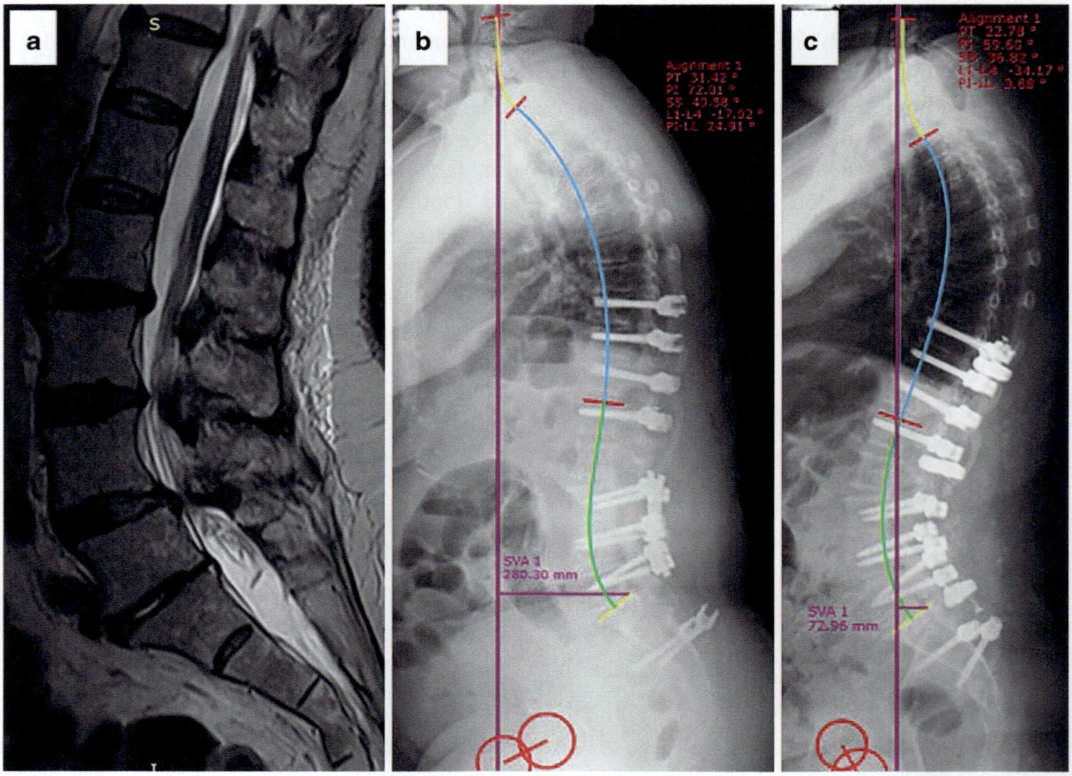

Fig. 5.9 A 72 year old, woman, she had low back pain, numbness in both feet when he started walking, and after a while, her trunk leaned forward. (**a**) MRI showed flattening of lumbar lordosis, transitional vertebra at L5, and degenerative spondylolisthesis and spinal stenosis at L4-5. (**b**) Sagittal radiography of the entire spine taken in the patient's first stage surgery showed significant sagittal imbalance. (**c**) Sagittal balance was observed to have improved in the second stage surgery performed with double PEEK rods and dynamic screws. The clinical outcome was also successful postoperatively 2 years

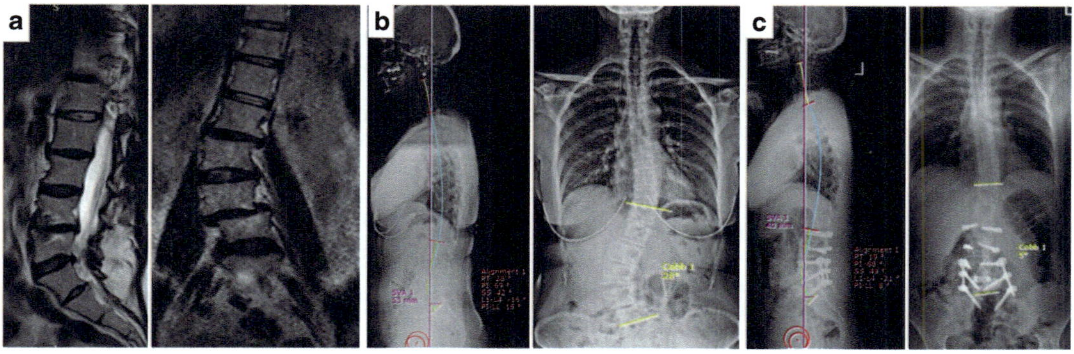

Fig. 5.10 A 48-year-old woman presenting with low back and right hip-right leg pain that increased with activity and affected her daily life. (**a**) On MRI, the lowest vertebra is the transitional vertebra, and there are widespread degenerative changes, the most common being the disc above it. In the lumbar spine, there is widespread degenerative base, olisthesis is observed at multiple levels, and degenerative scoliosis is clearly seen in coronal MRI sections of the lumbar spine. (**b**) Curve type according to SRS-Schwab classification: N, modifiers; PI-LL within 18° (+), global alignment SVA 5.3 cm (+), and PT 28° (+). Silva–Lenke Level III, Berjano-Lamartine Type II. ph obtained (**c**) on postoperative day 8 shows no problem (Dynesys system)

spinal flexibility compared to the single-rod system. The double-peek rod system is flexible enough to accommodate deformities and is easy to use. After the main rod is placed in the system, the accessory rod is connected to the main rod at three points. (Fig. 5.9). In this way, it can be seen that SV is effectively corrected and other pelvic parameters come to acceptable levels.

In elderly patients, a decrease in bone density, an increase in BMI, and atrophy with fatty degeneration in muscles increase the load on the instrument, and just like the development of pseudoarthrosis, osteosynthesis is not sufficient, and loosening of screws easily develops in these patients. This problem can be addressed by performing the surgery in two stages if the patient does not have an obvious neurological deficit and the pain is tolerable [62] (Fig. 5.10).

Especially in patients with coronal imbalance, if the trunk is bent forward and corrected during surgery, an additional load will be exerted on the rod. A single rod in the form of a rope may not be enough to meet this. Therefore, in these patients, a two-rod system is used via two-hole screws.

5.6 Conclusion

Use of dynamic systems in ADS surgery can greatly reduce the mortality and morbidity rates in appropriately selected patients. It is important to perform surgery at an early stage before the deformity has progressed, and these patients should be closely followed up. The period when the deformity is mobile is the golden period, and the patient's time should not be wasted with physiotherapy, algology, or osteopathic methods at this stage. It is a simpler surgery compared to fusion and rigid stabilization. The surgery can be performed in two stages, and in appropriate cases, both stages can be performed under spinal anesthesia. This can greatly reduce the probability of complications such as screw loosening, breakage, PJK, and pseudoarthrosis, which are the biggest problems in fusion and rigid stabilization. Naturally, it is necessary to wait for the experiences and results of other surgeons in this regard. We are hopeful for the future with our own data.

References

1. Kebaish KM, Neubauer PR, Voros GD, Khoshnevisan MA, Skolasky RL. Scoliosis in adults aged forty years and older: prevalence and relationship to age, race, and gender. Spine (Phila Pa 1976). 2011;36(9):731–6.
2. Glassman SD, Hamill CL, Bridwell KH, Schwab FJ, Dimar JR, Lowe TG. The impact of perioperative complications on clinical outcome in adult deformity surgery. Spine. 2007;32(24):2764–70.
3. Núñez-Pereira S, Vila-Casademunt A, Domingo-Sàbat M, et al. Impact of early unanticipated revision surgery on health-related quality of life after adult spinal deformity surgery. Spine J. 2018;18(6):926–34.
4. Veeravagu A, Li A, Swinney C, Tian L, Moraff A, Azad TD, Cheng I, Alamin T, Hu SS, Anderson RL, Shuer L, Desai A, Park J, Olshen RA, Ratliff JK. Predicting complication risk in spine surgery: a prospective analysis of a novel risk assessment tool. J Neurosurg Spine. 2017;27(1):81–91.
5. Yoshida G, Hasegawa T, Yamato Y, Kobayashi S, Oe S, Banno T, Mihara Y, Arima H, Ushirozako H, Yasuda T, Togawa D, Matsuyama Y. Predicting perioperative complications in adult spinal deformity surgery using a simple sliding scale. Spine (Phila Pa 1976). 2018;43(8):562–70.
6. Elsamadicy AA, Adogwa O, Ongele M, Sergesketter AR, Tarnasky A, Lubkin DET, Drysdale N, Cheng J, Bagley CA, Karikari IO. Preoperative hemoglobin level is associated with increased health care use after elective spinal fusion (≥3 levels) in elderly male patients with spine deformity. World Neurosurg. 2018;112:e348–54.
7. Dinizo M, Dolgalev I, Passias PG, Errico TJ, Raman T. Complications after adult spinal deformity surgeries: all are not created equal. Int J Spine Surg. 2021;15(1):137–43.
8. King HA, Moe JH, Bradford DS, Winter RB. The selection of fusion levels in thoracic idiopathic scoliosis. J Bone Joint Surg Am. 1983;65(9):1302–13.
9. Richards BS. Lumbar curve response in type II idiopathic scoliosis after posterior instrumentation of the thoracic curve. Spine (Phila Pa 1976). 1992;17(8 Suppl):282–6.
10. Roye DP Jr, Farcy JP, Rickert JB, Godfried D. Results of spinal instrumentation of adolescent idiopathic scoliosis by King type. Spine (Phila Pa 1976). 1992;17(8 Suppl):S270–3.
11. Knapp DR Jr, Price CT, Jones ET, Coonrad RW, Flynn JC. Choosing fusion levels in progressive thoracic idiopathic scoliosis. Spine (Phila Pa 1976). 1992;17(10):1159–65.
12. Cummings RJ, Loveless EA, Campbell J, Samelson S, Mazur JM. Interobserver reliability and intraobserver reproducibility of the system of King et al. for the classification of adolescent idiopathic scoliosis. J Bone Joint Surg Am. 1998;80(8):1107–11.
13. Behensky H, Giesinger K, Ogon M, Krismer M, Hannes B, Karlmeinrad G, Michael O, Martin K. Multisurgeon assessment of coronal pattern classification systems for adolescent idiopathic scoliosis: reliability and error analysis. Spine (Phila Pa 1976). 2002;27(7):762–7.
14. Lenke LG, Betz RR, Haher TR, Lapp MA, Merola AA, Harms J, Shufflebarger HL. Multisurgeon assessment of surgical decision-making in adolescent idiopathic scoliosis: curve classification, operative approach, and fusion levels. Spine (Phila Pa 1976). 2001;26(21):2347–53.
15. Newton PO, Faro FD, Lenke LG, Betz RR, Clements DH, Lowe TG, Haher TR, Merola AA, D'Andrea LP, Marks M, Wenger DR. Factors involved in the decision to perform a selective versus nonselective fusion of Lenke 1B and 1C (King-Moe II) curves in adolescent idiopathic scoliosis. Spine (Phila Pa 1976). 2003;28(20):S217–23.
16. Du JP, Fan Y, Liu JJ, Zhang JN, Chang Liu S, Hao D. Application of gelatin sponge impregnated with a mixture of 3 drugs to intraoperative nerve root block combined with robot-assisted minimally invasive transforaminal lumbar interbody fusion surgery in the treatment of adult degenerative scoliosis: a clinical observation including 96 patients. World Neurosurg. 2017;108:791–7.
17. Uddin OM, Haque R, Sugrue PA, Ahmed YM, El Ahmadieh TY, Press JM, Koski T, Fessler RG. Cost minimization in treatment of adult degenerative scoliosis. J Neurosurg Spine. 2015;23(6):798–806.
18. Sun XY, Zhang XN, Hai Y. Optimum pelvic incidence minus lumbar lordosis value after operation for patients with adult degenerative scoliosis. Spine J. 2017;17:983–9.
19. Yagi M, Kaneko S, Yato Y, Asazuma T. Standing balance and compensatory mechanisms in patients with adult spinal deformity. Spine (Phila Pa 1976). 2017;42(10):E584–91.
20. Chen RQ, Hosogane N, Watanabe K, Funao H, Okada E, Fujita N, Hikata T, Iwanami A, Tsuji T, Ishii K, Abe T, Toyama Y, Nakamura M, Matsumoto M. Reliability analysis of Spino-pelvic parameters in adult spinal deformity: a comparison of whole spine and pelvic radiographs. Spine (Phila Pa 1976). 2016;41(4):320–7.
21. Hayden AM, Hayes AM, Brechbuhler JL, Israel H, Place HM. The effect of pelvic motion on spinopelvic parameters. Spine J. 2018;18(1):173–8.
22. Aebi M. The adult scoliosis. Eur Spine J. 2005;14(10):925–48.
23. Schwab F, El-Fegoun AB, Gamez L, Goodman H, Farcy JP. A lumbar classification of scoliosis in the adult patient: preliminary approach. Spine (Phila Pa 1976). 2005;30(14):1670–3.
24. Lowe T, Berven SH, Schwab FJ, Bridwell KH. The SRS classification for adult spinal deformity: building on the King/Moe and Lenke classification systems. Spine. 2006;31:S119–25.
25. Schwab F, Ungar B, Blondel B, Buchowski J, Coe J, Deinlein D, DeWald C, Mehdian H, Shaffrey C, Tribus C, Lafage V. Scoliosis Research Society-Schwab adult spinal deformity classification: a validation study. Spine. 2012;37:1077–82.

26. Mundis GM, Turner JD, Deverin V, Uribe JS, Nunley P, Mummaneni P, Anand N, Park P, Okonkwo DO, Wang MY, Bess S, Kanter AS, Fessler R, Nguyen S, Akbarnia BA, International Spine Study Group. A critical analysis of sagittal plane deformity correction with minimally invasive adult spinal deformity surgery: a 2-year follow-up study. Spine Deform. 2017;5:265–71.
27. Lafage V, Schwab F, Patel A, Hawkinson N, Farcy JP. Pelvic tilt and truncal inclination: two key radiographic parameters in the setting of adults with spinal deformity. Spine (Phila Pa 1976). 2009;34(17):E599–606.
28. Ames CP, Smith JS, Scheer JK, Bess S, Bederman SS, Deviren V, Lafage V, Schwab F, Shaffrey CI. Impact of spinopelvic alignment on decision making in deformity surgery in adults: a review. J Neurosurg Spine. 2012;16:547–64.
29. Schwab F, Patel A, Ungar B, Farcy J-P, Lafage V. Adult spinal deformity-postoperative standing imbalance: how much can you tolerate? An overview of key parameters in assessing alignment and planning corrective surgery. Spine. 2010;35:2224–31.
30. Schwab FJ, Lafage V, Shaffrey CI, Smith JS, Moal B, Klineberg EO, Ames CP, Hostin R, Fu K-MG, Kebaish KM, Burton DC, Akbarnia BA, Gupta MC, Deviren V, Mundis GM, Boachie-Adjei O, Hart RA, Bess RS. The Schwab-SRS adult spinal deformity classification: assessment and clinical correlations based on a prospective operative and nonoperative cohort. Spine J. 2012;12:S18.
31. Silva FE, Lenke LG. Adult degenerative scoliosis: evaluation and management. Neurosurg Focus. 2010;28(3):E1.
32. Berjano P, Lamartina C. Classification of degenerative segment disease in adults with deformity of the lumbar or thoracolumbar spine. Eur Spine J. 2014;23(9):1815–24.
33. Obeid I, Berjano P, Lamartina C, Chopin D, Boissière L, Bourghli A. Classification of coronal imbalance in adult scoliosis and spine deformity: a treatment-oriented guideline. Eur Spine J. 2019;28(1):94–113.
34. Kuntz C 4th, Shaffrey CI, Ondra SL, Durrani AA, Mummaneni PV, Levin LS, Pettigrew DB. Spinal deformity: a new classification derived from neutral upright spinal alignment measurements in asymptomatic juvenile, adolescent, adult, and geriatric individuals. Neurosurgery. 2008;63(3 Suppl):25–39.
35. Duval-Beaupère G, Schmidt C, Cosson P. A Barycentremetric study of the sagittal shape of spine and pelvis: the conditions required for an economic standing position. Ann Biomed Eng. 1992;20(4):451–62.
36. Legaye J, Duval-Beaupère G, Hecquet J, Marty C. Pelvic incidence: a fundamental pelvic parameter for three-dimensional regulation of spinal sagittal curves. Eur Spine J. 1998;7(2):99–103.
37. Yukawa Y, Kato F, Suda K, Yamagata M, Ueta T, Yoshida M. Normative data for parameters of sagittal spinal alignment in healthy subjects: an analysis of gender specific differences and changes with aging in 626 asymptomatic individuals. Eur Spine J. 2018;27(2):426–32.
38. Lafage R, Schwab F, Challier V, Henry JK, Gum J, Smith J, Hostin R, Shaffrey C, Kim HJ, Ames C, Scheer J, Klineberg E, Bess S, Burton D, Lafage V, International Spine Study Group. Defining spino-pelvic alignment thresholds: should operative goals in adult spinal deformity surgery account for age? Spine (Phila Pa 1976). 2016;41(1):62–8.
39. Lafage R, Schwab F, Glassman S, Bess S, Harris B, Sheer J, Hart R, Line B, Henry J, Burton D, Kim H, Klineberg E, Ames C, Lafage V, International Spine Study Group. Age-adjusted alignment goals have the potential to reduce PJK. Spine (Phila Pa 1976). 2017;42(17):1275–82.
40. Yagi M, Akilah KB, Boachie-Adjei O. Incidence, risk factors and classification of proximal junctional kyphosis: surgical outcomes review of adult idiopathic scoliosis. Spine (Phila Pa 1976). 2011;36(1):E60–8.
41. Kim HJ, Bridwell KH, Lenke LG, Park MS, Song KS, Piyaskulkaew C, Chuntarapas T. Patients with proximal junctional kyphosis requiring revision surgery have higher postoperative lumbar lordosis and larger sagittal balance corrections. Spine (Phila Pa 1976). 2014;39(9):E576–80.
42. Kim YJ, Bridwell KH, Lenke LG, Glattes CR, Rhim S, Cheh G. Proximal junctional kyphosis in adult spinal deformity after segmental posterior spinal instrumentation and fusion: minimum five-year follow-up. Spine (Phila Pa 1976). 2008;33(20):2179–84.
43. Lau D, Clark AJ, Scheer JK, Daubs MD, Coe JD, Paonessa KJ, LaGrone MO, Kasten MD, Amaral RA, Trobisch PD, Lee JH, Fabris-Monterumici D, Anand N, Cree AK, Hart RA, Hey LA, Ames CP, SRS Adult Spinal Deformity Committee. Proximal junctional kyphosis and failure after spinal deformity surgery: a systematic review of the literature as a background to classification development. Spine (Phila Pa 1976). 2014;39(25):2093–102.
44. Kim HJ, Bridwell KH, Lenke LG, Park MS, Ahmad A, Song KS, Piyaskulkaew C, Hershman S, Fogelson J, Mesfin A. Proximal junctional kyphosis results in inferior SRS pain subscores in adult deformity patients. Spine (Phila Pa 1976). 2013;38(11):896–901.
45. Kim HJ, Lenke LG, Shaffrey CI, Van Alstyne EM, Skelly AC. Proximal junctional kyphosis as a distinct form of adjacent segment pathology after spinal deformity surgery: a systematic review. Spine (Phila Pa 1976). 2012;37(22 Suppl):S144–64.
46. Ascani E, Bartolozzi P, Logroscino CA, Marchetti PG, Ponte A, Savini R, Travaglini F, Binazzi R, Di Silvestre M. Natural history of untreated idiopathic scoliosis after skeletal maturity. Spine (Phila Pa 1976). 1986;11(8):784–9.
47. Briard JL, Jegou D, Cauchoix J. Adult lumbar scoliosis. Spine (Phila Pa 1976). 1979;4(6):526–32.

48. Bridwell KH, Berven S, Edwards C 2nd, Glassman S, Hamill C, Schwab F. The problems and limitations of applying evidence-based medicine to primary surgical treatment of adult spinal deformity. Spine (Phila Pa 1976). 2007;32(19 Suppl):S135–9.
49. Acosta FL Jr, McClendon J Jr, O'Shaughnessy BA, Koller H, Neal CJ, Meier O, Ames CP, Koski TR, Ondra SL. Morbidity and mortality after spinal deformity surgery in patients 75 years and older: complications and predictive factors. J Neurosurg Spine. 2011;15(6):667–74.
50. Yadla S, Maltenfort MG, Ratliff JK, Harrop JS. Adult scoliosis surgery outcomes: a systematic review. Neurosurg Focus. 2010;28(3):E3.
51. Smith JS, Klineberg E, Lafage V, Shaffrey CI, Schwab F, Lafage R, Hostin R, Mundis GM Jr, Errico TJ, Kim HJ, Protopsaltis TS, Hamilton DK, Scheer JK, Soroceanu A, Kelly MP, Line B, Gupta M, Deviren V, Hart R, Burton DC, Bess S, Ames CP, International Spine Study Group. Prospective multicenter assessment of perioperative and minimum 2-year postoperative complication rates associated with adult spinal deformity surgery. J Neurosurg Spine. 2016;25(1):1–14.
52. Weiss HR, Goodall D. Rate of complications in scoliosis surgery—a systematic review of the Pub Med literature. Scoliosis. 2008;3:9.
53. Christiansen PA, LaBagnara M, Sure DR, Shaffrey CI, Smith JS. Complications of surgical intervention in adult lumbar scoliosis. Curr Rev Musculoskelet Med. 2016;9(3):281–9.
54. Sciubba DM, Yurter A, Smith JS, Kelly MP, Scheer JK, Goodwin CR, Lafage V, Hart RA, Bess S, Kebaish K, Schwab F, Shaffrey CI, Ames CP, International Spine Study Group (ISSG). A comprehensive review of complication rates after surgery for adult deformity: a reference for informed consent. Spine Deform. 2015;3(6):575–94.
55. Ozer AF, Akyoldaş G. Dynamic instrumentation for spinal deformities-chapter 35. In: Zileli M, Yaman O, Aebi M, editors. Correction techniques for spinal deformity. Noida: Thieme; 2024.
56. Korkmaz M, Ozer AF. Dynamic stabilization and deformity surgery. In: Sharif S, Peev N, Steinmetz M, editors. Spinal deformity surgery: tips from the masters. Thieme Medical and Scientific Publishers Private; 2022. ISBN: 978-93-90553-33-4/eISBN: 978-93-90553-41-9.
57. Silvestre M, Lolli F, Bakaloudis G, Parisini P. Dynamic stabilization for degenerative lumbar scoliosis in elderly patients. Spine (Phila Pa 1976). 2010;35(2):227–34. https://doi.org/10.1097/BRS.0b013e3181bd3be6.
58. Kuo CH, Chang PY, Tu TH, Fay LY, Chang HK, Wu JC, Huang WC, Cheng H. The effect of lumbar lordosis on screw loosening in Dynesys dynamic stabilization: four-year follow-up with computed tomography. Biomed Res Int. 2015;2015:152435.
59. Ko CC, Tsai HW, Huang WC, Wu JC, Chen YC, Shih YH. Screw loosening in the Dynesys stabilization system: radiographic evidence and effect on outcomes. Neurosurg Focus. 2010;28(6):E10.
60. Ozer AF, Oktenoglu T, Egemen E, Sasani M, Yilmaz A, Erbulut DU, Yaman O, Suzer T. Lumbar single-level dynamic stabilization with semi-rigid and full dynamic systems: a retrospective clinical and radiological analysis of 71 patients. Clin Orthop Surg. 2017;9(3):310–6.
61. Ciplak NM, Suzer T, Senturk S, Yaman O, Sasani M, Oktenoglu T, Yilmaz A, Erbulut DU, Özer AF. Complications of 2-level dynamic stabilization: a correlative clinical and radiological analysis at two-year follow-up on 103 patients. Turk Neurosurg. 2018;28(5):756–62.
62. Ozer AF, Başak AT, Özbek MA, Hekimoğlu M, Aydın AL, Ateş Ö, Günerbüyük C, Akgül T, Sasani M, Öktenoğlu T. Lumbar dynamic stabilization with 2-stage surgery: early results. Int J Spine Surg. 2022;16(4):638–45.

Spinal Fusion Surgery Advantages and Disadvantages

6

Mehmet Yiğit Akgün, Melihcan Savaşçı, and Özkan Ateş

6.1 Introduction

The indications for spinal fusion have expanded over time since the surgery was originally developed for the treatment of instability due to spine pathologies, traumatic injuries, or deformities. Since the earliest description of spinal fusion with iliac crest graft performed by Dr. Russell A. Hibbs in 1911 and tibial graft by Dr. Fred H. Albee for tuberculosis, it has become famous and popular day by day. Over time, with the development and progress of surgical techniques, the indications have gradually increased [1–3]. When the distribution of surgical pathologies is examined, lumbar degenerative disc disease and cervical disc replacement are among the most common causes of fusion [4].

These techniques required prolonged bed rest after surgery and the use of braces and casts for immobilization, and their use was complex, with a rate of pseudoarthrosis of at least 20%. Surgical implants for the spine were developed later in the century to improve the rate of fusion and hasten the recovery of patients after surgery. Today, the population of patients in whom surgeons use arthrodesis has changed greatly. Several studies and systematic reviews have been published. The literature showed that spinal fusion procedures have a positive effect on patient outcomes.

The use of surgical implants with current surgical technology aims to improve deformity, manage pain, and improve arthrodesis by immobilization of the spine. In addition, it provides the formation of new bone trabeculae by increasing osteoblastic activity through fusion. One of the studies related to fusion in the literature is the Spine Patient Outcomes Research Trial (SPORT). The aim of this publication is to investigate the efficacy of operative and nonoperative managements in the treatment of spinal stenosis and degenerative spondylolisthesis and to present the

M. Y. Akgün (✉) · Ö. Ateş
Department of Neurosurgery, Koc University Hospital, Istanbul, Turkey

Koc University Hospital, Spine Center, Istanbul, Turkey
e-mail: makgun@kuh.ku.edu.tr; oates@kuh.ku.edu.tr

M. Savaşçı
Bakırköy Prof. Dr. Mazhar Osman Training and Research Hospital for Neurology, Neurosurgery and Psychiatry, Istanbul, Turkey

A. F. Özer et al. (eds.), *Dynamic Lumbar Spine Stabilization*,
https://doi.org/10.1007/978-3-032-12122-6_6

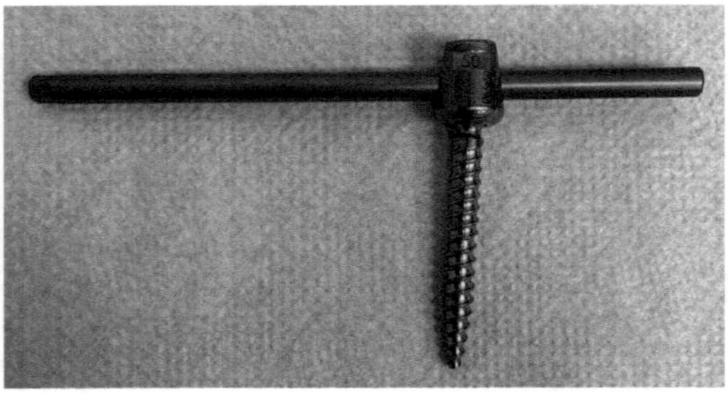

Fig. 6.1 Screw and rod system

clinical results. The benefit of spinal operations performed for fusion purposes in the postoperative 2, 4, and 8 years has been reported [5]. In addition, it has been shown that decompression with instrumentation gives better results than decompression alone in tumor patients with cord compression caused by spinal metastases [6].

When the trend in spinal fusion surgery around the world is examined, what draws attention is the increase in the number of fusion procedures. Kim et al. It evaluated the use of spine surgery in Japan, Korea, and the United States and found that the incidence of spine surgery was highest in the United States. Likewise, it has been reported that fusion surgery has increased approximately two times in Canada, the United Kingdom, Australia, and Norway [7, 8]. The increase in spinal fusion procedures could not be associated with higher surgical rates among specialties [1, 4]. When considering cervical, thoracic, and lumbar spine fusion procedures, it was observed that fusion procedures increased in all regions of the spine. According to Rajaee et al., primary lumbar fusion emerges as the spine region with the highest increase rate compared to cervical and thoracic fusion procedures, with a 2.7-fold increase (170.9%) in this time period [1] (Fig. 6.1).

After the detailed description of the biomechanical and pathophysiological features of the human spine, advanced diagnostic imaging techniques have contributed to the increasing rates of spinal fusion use. The contribution of many factors, such as the increase in the availability of spinal fixation devices, the expansion of surgical indications, the development of new surgical approaches, and various instrumentation techniques, together with minimally invasive surgery (MIS), cannot be ignored. In addition, significant technological advances, increasing numbers of well-trained spine specialists, an increase in population life expectancy, and the overall improved safety profile of spinal fusion procedures over time may be additional reasons for a continued upward trend in spinal fusion [1, 4]. The overall increased safety of spinal fusion procedures with lower complication rates may also explain the decrease in reoperation rates [8]. Of course, the risk of complications from existing procedures should not be overlooked. Management of potential complications such as neurological injuries, dural tears, implant-related problems, pseudarthrosis, infections, and wound problems is equally important. It is important to be aware of the evaluation and management of patients, especially in multilevel spinal fusions that carry a higher risk of complications [9, 10]. Despite the increasing number of spine fusion procedures, it is extremely important to make individual decisions for each patient, taking into account the patient's condition and risk of complications (Fig. 6.2).

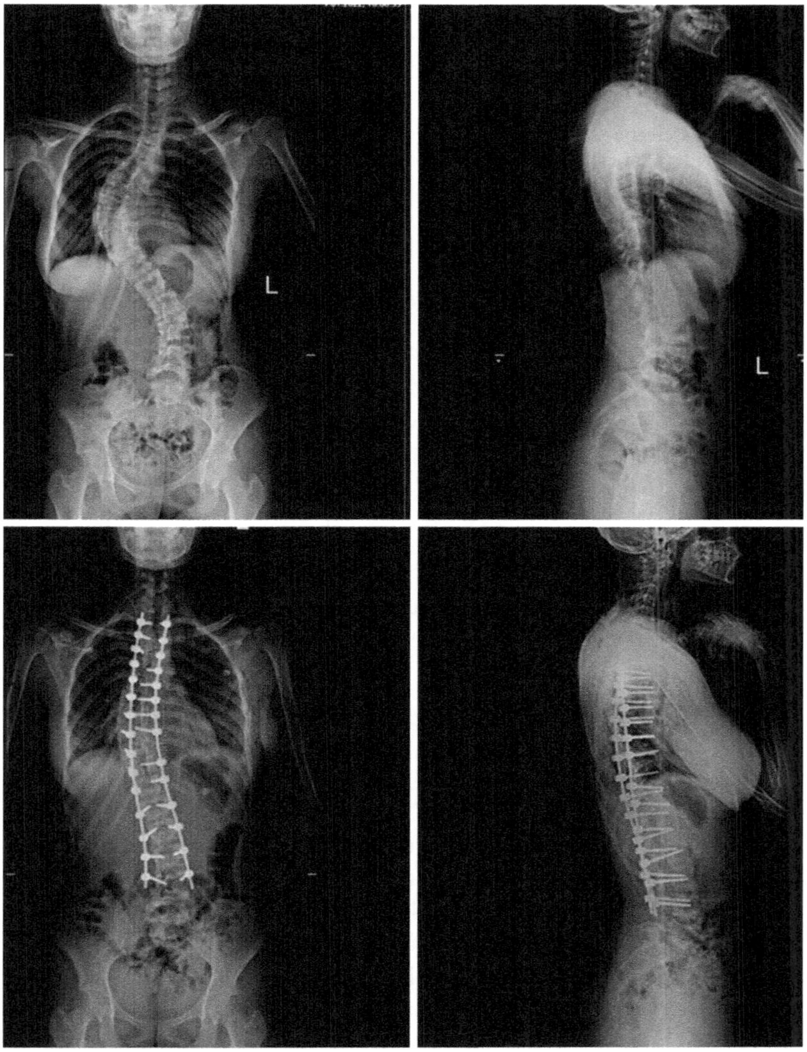

Fig. 6.2 A case of left-facing scoliosis in the thoracic vertebrae with a Cobb angle of approximately 68°

6.2 Advantages

One of the effective treatment methods for stabilizing painful segment movement and providing sagittal balance with lordosis is surgical fusion [11]. Regardless of the approach (anterior/lateral/posterior), depending on the surgeon's preference and the patient's condition, there are a wide variety of fusion methods, from interbody fusion with cage to internal fixation. In light of biomechanical principles, new technologies, and developments in materials, pedicle fixation spinal stabilization systems have evolved over the years. Pedicle screw design (single axis vs polyaxial), screw-rod system attachment (side loading vs top loading), and the biomaterials that are used are some of the differences of each system [12].

The FDA's approval of intervertebral fusion cages in 1996 was one of the important developments for fusion surgery. Thus, significant progress has been made in fusion rates. In addition, the use of conventional autografts, as well as titanium and polyetheretherketone (PEEK) cages, improved osseointegration and postoperative results [13]. Today, with the increase in lumbar spinal fusion procedures, the method has become

Table 6.1 Interbody fusion techniques and their general uses

Technique	Indications	Advantages	Disadvantages
PLIF	Degenerative Segmental instability Deformity and stenosis Recurrent disc hernia Pseudoarthrosis	Good height restoration Common technique Posterior visualization and decompression possibility Option for 360-degree stabilization	Paraspinal muscle damage Neural/dural injury Difficult restoration of spinal alignment
TLIF	Degenerative Segmental instability Deformity and stenosis Recurrent disc hernia Pseudoarthrosis	Increase in biomechanical stability secondary to muscle and ligament preservation Option for 360-degree stabilization Reduced rates of nerve root damage and dural injury	Limited overall view Difficult restoration of spinal alignment
LLIF	Lumbar laterolisthesis Degenerative and deformity (combined with posterolateral fusion)	Minimal muscle-splitting, faster mobilization Correction of lordosis higher cage size, height restoration	Injury of lumbar plexus and iliac vessels Need for neuromonitoring Not suitable for L5/S1 fusion Not suitable for adverse vascular anatomy
ALIF	Osteochondrosis Oblique access for disc disease Ant. approach for L4-5-S1 disc herniation	Efficient anterior discectomy Sparing neural structures Correction of lordosis higher cage size, height restoration	Retrograde ejaculation Not suitable for adverse vascular anatomy Visceral injuries Need for additional posterolateral fusion

more familiar. It is widely adopted as the surgical treatment of various spinal disorders such as congenital or degenerative deformities, degenerative disc disease, spondylolisthesis, spinal stenosis, trauma, infection, and tumor [11, 14]. Currently, there are different approaches to lumbar interbody fusion, including ALIF, PLIF, lateral or extreme lateral lumbar interbody fusion (LLIF), and TLIF (Table 6.1). In the literature, there is still no clear evidence of clinical superiority of one approach over the other. Indications for each approach vary depending on surgeon preference, spinal fusion levels, and the patient's condition [11, 15]. With the evolution of MIS techniques, these fusion approaches have also become usable in MIS surgery and are a possible reason for the increasing number of spinal fusion procedures [11, 16].

A number of new bone graft substitutes have been introduced to improve spine fusion rates as alternate methods to autograft harvesting [17]. Bone graft substitutes such as bone marrow aspirate (BMA), mesenchymal stem cells (MSCs), allograft (i.e., cortico-cancellous allograft), and demineralized bone matrix (DBM) are often used in combination with synthetic grafts, ceramics, or growth factors such as recombinant human bone morphogenetic proteins (rhBMPs) [18]. Despite the progress of developments, the use of autografts continues to be the first choice of surgeons in general. Tissue engineering products, such as bone growth factors, have the potential to lower the rate of pseudarthrosis [18]. Also, recombinant human parathyroid hormone (rhPTH) has been studied clinically for improving spinal fusion [19]. Although there are some contradictions in the studies, it has been reported that BMP-2 provides an increase in posterolateral fusion rates and additionally reduces clinical morbidity [20]. In the study, it was reported that local autograft application in combination with BMA had the highest fusion rates for most bone graft materials in posterolateral lumbar fusion applications [21]. However, the higher costs and restricted approval for the use of new bone grafts can prohibit their utilization despite improved clinical outcomes.

After decompression surgery, more space is created around the spinal cord and nerve roots,

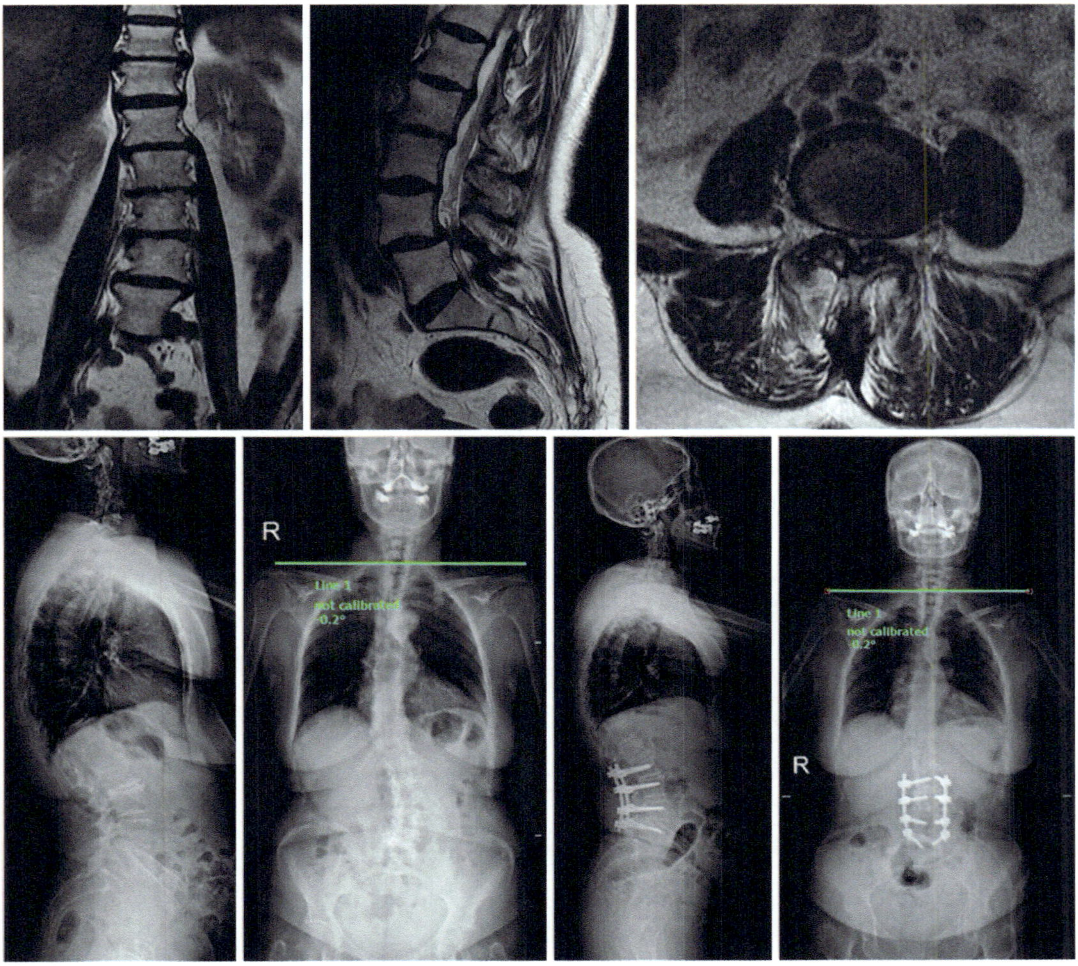

Fig. 6.3 The sagittal and coronal balance of the patient with neurogenic claudication and spinal stenosis showed significant improvement after decompression and stabilization

resulting in significant relief from nerve pain. However, instability can be observed at the affected levels after decompression. Discs and facet joints cannot maintain proper stability after procedures such as total facetectomy, which are applied to relieve the nerve roots sufficiently. When this happens, the spine begins to move in abnormal ways. As a result, satisfactory results cannot occur in patients after the operation. If we look at the advantages of preventing this abnormal movement with fusion techniques, by fusing the level, there is less concern that the patient will need surgery again at that level. Discs and/or facets are often one of the potential causes of low back pain. Thanks to the fusion, the same level of movement can be stopped, and serious relief can be achieved in the symptoms of the patients. Another advantage is that it minimizes the risk of deformity that may develop after decompression (Fig. 6.3). Some patients develop post-laminectomy kyphosis, which is an abnormal alignment of the spine. This can often lead to additional surgery. Similarly, with fusion, the patient's existing deformity can be corrected, helping to restore the normal alignment of the spine. This can reduce wear and tear (and the need for future surgery) at adjacent levels.

6.3 Disadvantages

On the other hand, there are some potential disadvantages that can be seen with this surgery. In order to reveal the necessary anatomical landmarks in fusion surgeries (lateral facet joints and transverse processes), more muscle dissection is required. In addition, after more bone resection, longer recovery time and back/low back pain can be seen. Depending on the prolongation of the duration of the surgery, an increase in bleeding may be observed. Additional problems such as dural tear, nerve injury, and increased infection rates may be encountered. Bone grafts or bone substitutes are also placed in the spine to help your bones gradually fuse together, but inflammation can result and potentially lead to more scarring (arachnoiditis) and subsequent pain. Most fusions involve inserting rods and screws aimed at stabilizing the spine until the bone fusion has solidified. However, it should be noted that this equipment itself can cause nerve damage and the development or worsening of neurological deficits. In addition, the segment that develops fusion may cause additional stresses above or below its level in some cases, and adjacent segment disease may develop in the patient (Fig. 6.4). Pseudoarthrosis and adjacent segment disease are among the most controversial topics of the current procedure. It is thought that the segment with the missile creates additional stresses on the mobile segment in its conduit, potentially leading

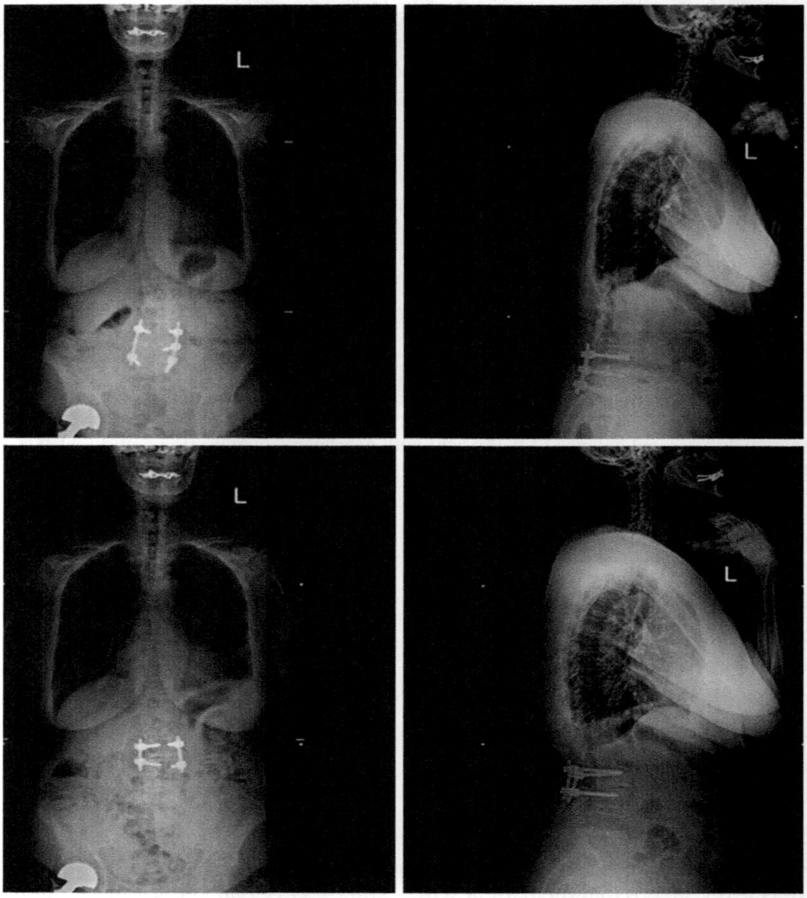

Fig. 6.4 The patient who was operated on five times for LDH has neurogenic claudication. The patient has significant stenosis in the adjacent segment and in the segment with listeria. After removing the old system and decompression + stabilization at the upper levels, there is a significant improvement in the patient's posture

to degeneration of the mobile segment. However, many theorize that because degenerative spine disease is a chronic condition that typically encompasses many levels, neighboring levels can wear out regardless.

Mobility is one of the most discussed topics. It is rare for patients to experience movement restriction after one or two levels of fusion. Often, patients with back pain with their stenosis have increased mobility when the painful segments are immobilized. It is known that even the cases with multilevel fusion can perform their activities without detecting a significant decrease in their quality of life. Among the reasons for this, we can cite that most of the bending on the trunk occurs at the hips. For this reason, it should be noted that the main affected movement in multi-level fusions is rotation. However, as we mentioned, patients can perform sports such as golf after single- or two-level fusion surgeries.

6.4 Conclusion

The current goals and situations of spinal fusion surgery remain similar to those of the fifth century: to correct deformity and degeneration of the spine in order to improve quality of life. With the advancement of technology and the abundance of studies on this subject, there has been a great increase in the number of patients undergoing surgical correction of their spinal deformities. As surgical treatment has become less invasive, patients have reported greater comfort with spinal fusion options.

However, the lack of guidelines and evidence for the treatment of different surgical indications has led to wide variability in surgical management. High-quality, prospective studies are needed to better evaluate clinical outcomes and revision surgery rates. A worldwide comparison between increases in short and long segment fusion rates will provide additional procedural evidence that may be informative about the potential impact on surgical outcomes.

Considering the rapid developments in the history of medicine and some practices in the past, it is observed that the approach to some diseases has changed drastically. Perhaps in centuries to come, physicians will remember little of a time when screws and rods were standard care in spinal deformity management.

References

1. Rajaee SS, Bae HW, Kanim LEA, Delamarter RB. Spinal fusion in the United States: analysis of trends from 1998 to 2008. Spine (Phila Pa 1976). 2012;37:67–76.
2. Deyo RA, Nachemson A, Mirza SK. Spinal-fusion surgery the case for restraint. N Engl J Med. 2004;350:722–6.
3. Camillo FX. Arthrodesis of the spine. In: Campbell WC, Canale ST, Beaty JH, editors. Campbell's operative orthopaedics. 11th ed. Philadelphia: Mosby/Elsevier; 2008.
4. Sheikh SR, Thompson NR, Benzel E, et al. Can we justify it? Trends in the utilization of spinal fusions and associated reimbursement. Neurosurgery. 2020;86:E193–202.
5. Ilyas H, Udo-Inyang I Jr, Savage J. Lumbar spinal stenosis and degenerative spondylolisthesis: a review of the SPORT literature. Clin Spine Surg. 2019;32:272–8.
6. Laufer I, Sciubba DM, Madera M, et al. Surgical management of metastatic spinal tumors. Cancer Control. 2012;19:122–8.
7. Kim P, Kurokawa R, Itoki K. Technical advancements and utilization of spine surgery—international disparities in trend-dynamics between Japan, Korea, and the USA. Neurol Med Chir (Tokyo). 2010;50:853–8.
8. Grotle M, Småstuen MC, Fjeld O, et al. Lumbar spine surgery across 15 years: trends, complications and reoperations in a longitudinal observational study from Norway. BMJ Open. 2019;9:e028743.
9. Al-Mohrej OA, Aldakhil SS, Al-Rabiah MA, et al. Surgical treatment of adolescent idiopathic scoliosis: complications. Ann Med Surg (Lond). 2020;52:19–23.
10. Yavin D, Casha S, Wiebe S, et al. Lumbar fusion for degenerative disease: a systematic review and meta-analysis. Neurosurgery. 2017;80:701–15.
11. Mobbs RJ, Phan K, Malham G, et al. Lumbar interbody fusion: techniques, indications and comparison of interbody fusion options including PLIF, TLIF, MI-TLIF, OLIF/ATP, LLIF and ALIF. J Spine Surg. 2015;1:2–18.
12. Warburton A, Girdler SJ, Mikhail CM, et al. Biomaterials in spinal implants: a review. Neurospine. 2020;17:101–10.
13. MacBarb RF, Lindsey DP, Bahney CS, et al. Fortifying the bone-implant interface part 1: an in vitro evaluation of 3D-printed and TPS porous surfaces. Int J Spine Surg. 2017;11:15.

14. Provaggi E, Capelli C, Leong JJH, et al. A UK-based pilot study of current surgical practice and implant preferences in lumbar fusion surgery. Medicine (Baltimore). 2018;97:e11169.
15. Lee N, Kim KN, Yi S, et al. Comparison of outcomes of anterior, posterior, and transforaminal lumbar Interbody fusion surgery at a single lumbar level with degenerative spinal disease. World Neurosurg. 2017;101:216–26.
16. Mobbs RJ, Sivabalan P, Li J. Minimally invasive surgery compared to open spinal fusion for the treatment of degenerative lumbar spine pathologies. J Clin Neurosci. 2012;19:829–35.
17. Stark JR, Hsieh J, Waller D. Bone graft substitutes in single-or double-level anterior cervical discectomy and fusion: a systematic review. Spine (Phila Pa 1976). 2019;44:E618–28.
18. Reisener MJ, Pumberger M, Shue J, Girardi FP, Hughes AP. Trends in lumbar spinal fusion-a literature review. J Spine Surg. 2020;6(4):752–61.
19. Cottrill E, Ahmed AK, Lessing N, et al. Investigational growth factors utilized in animal models of spinal fusion: systematic review. World J Orthop. 2019;10:176–91.
20. Mariscal G, Nuñez JH, Barrios C, et al. A meta-analysis of bone morphogenetic protein-2 versus iliac crest bone graft for the posterolateral fusion of the lumbar spine. J Bone Miner Metab. 2020;38:54–62.
21. Morris MT, Tarpada SP, Cho W. Bone graft materials for posterolateral fusion made simple: a systematic review. Eur Spine J. 2018;27:1856–67.

7 Total Disc Replacement and Posterior Dynamic Stabilization in the Treatment of Degenerative Disc Disease

Tunç Öktenoğlu

7.1 Introduction

Low back pain is one of the most common problems that observed in adult population. The prevalence rate is as high as 84% [1] and almost half of the cases are due to degenerative disc disease (DDD) [2]. The DDD is one of the leading causes of pain and disability in adults. The direct and indirect socioeconomic impact on annual health costs is estimated over 50 billion USD in USA [3].

The DDD may cause some other spinal problems to develop over time, such as disc herniation, subsidence, narrowing of neural foramens, lumbar canal stenosis, facet arthropathy, lumbar spondylolisthesis, and lumbar deformity.

7.1.1 Natural History of Disc Degeneration

The aging process causes alterations in the cellular matrix of the disc nucleus. The normal ratio of glycoproteins, chondroitin sulfate, and keratin sulfate starts to invert. The chondroitin sulfate molecules are much more hydrophilic structures compared to keratin sulfate molecules. The diminishing of chondroitin sulfate and increase in keratin sulfate in the annulus nucleus result in a decrease of fluid content in disc material (Fig. 7.1).

This biochemical alteration leads to some structural changes in intervertebral disc material, such as a decrease in height [4–6].

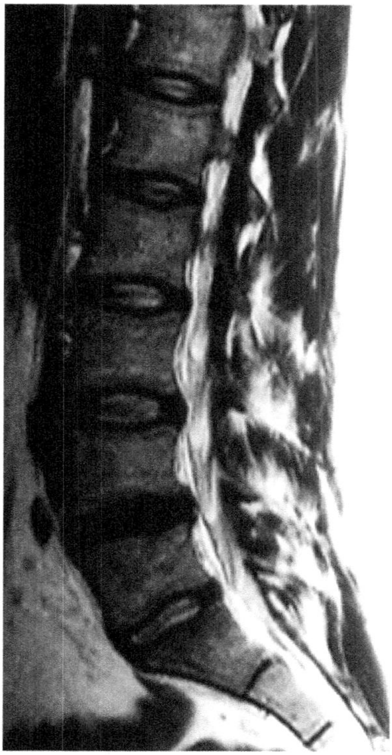

Fig. 7.1 T2-weighted sagittal lumbar MR shows L4–5 degenerative disk (black disk)

T. Öktenoğlu (✉)
Neurosurgery, Koc University School of Medicine, Istanbul, Turkey

A. F. Özer et al. (eds.), *Dynamic Lumbar Spine Stabilization*,
https://doi.org/10.1007/978-3-032-12122-6_7

In the 1970s, Kirkaldy-Willis [7] described the degenerative cascade of an intervertebral disc tissue. He divided the degenerative cascade into three stages.

1. *Dysfunctional stage*: Small circumferential tears in the outer layer of the disc grow inward. The mobility of the motion segment may be limited following an injury.
2. *Relative instability stage*: The inner material of the disc begins to protrude outward through the tears, leading to decreased disc height.
3. *Restabilization stage*: Osteophytes form at the margins of the disc, and the changes in the disc become fixed. The vertebral motion segment restabilizes.

The clinical complaints that are low back pain and/or leg pain are generally observed in the first two stages. The development of a disc herniation usually occurs in the instability stage.

The progress of disc height loss in the unstable stage might result in two different patterns. In the first pattern, the vertebral body develops subluxation over an adjacent vertebra, resulting in either spondylolisthesis or retrolisthesis. The direction of translation is probably determined by the segmental and global anatomical and biomechanical features of the spine. The orientation of the facet joints at each level, the mobility capacity of the degenerated disc, and the level of the degenerated disc along the lordotic posture of the lumbar spine [8, 9] and sagittal balance of the spine are critical in the type of deformity. The lower segments usually show spondylolisthesis, whereas the upper segments have a predisposition to retrolisthesis. The second pattern observed in the restabilization stage is vertical subsidence of disc space without translational deformity. As the disc space becomes severely narrow, the two adjacent end plates of the vertebral bodies come closer to each other. This type of vertical subluxation might cause loss of lordosis and stretch annular structures [7, 10]. Preservation of lordosis might cause neural foramen stenosis.

The clinical complaints may also be in the restabilization stage. Facet arthrosis, osteophyte formation, and thickening of ligamentous structures (particularly ligamentum flavum) develop to stabilize the unstable segment. On the other hand, these alterations might cause central canal and/or neural foramen stenosis and may compress neural elements. Additionally, loss of motion segment due to severe degeneration and loss of disc height might cause hypermobility at adjacent segments, which can be considered as accelerating the degenerative cascade at adjacent segments.

7.1.2 Pain Mechanism

The pain mechanism in DDD with disc herniation and/or translational deformity or with stenosis (central canal and/or neural foramen) is clear. On the other hand, the pain originating in pure DDD is open to debate.

Currently, there are two different theories accepted as pain mechanisms in DDD.

The first theory was described by Panjabi in 1992 [11]. Panjabi defined spinal instability as increased motion at the "neutral zone." The range of motion of a spinal unit can be divided into two zones: neutral and elastic (Fig. 7.2).

The neutral zone is where the initial motion starts against minimal internal resistance, whereas the motion at the elastic zone is produced against maximal internal resistance. The increased motion at the neutral zone might be due to injury, degenerative disc disease, and/or muscle weakness (Fig. 7.3).

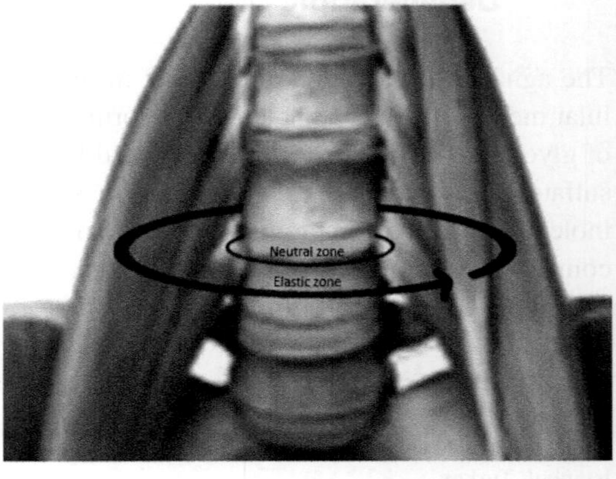

Fig. 7.2 The neutral and elastic zones are depicted in a functional segmental unit of a spine

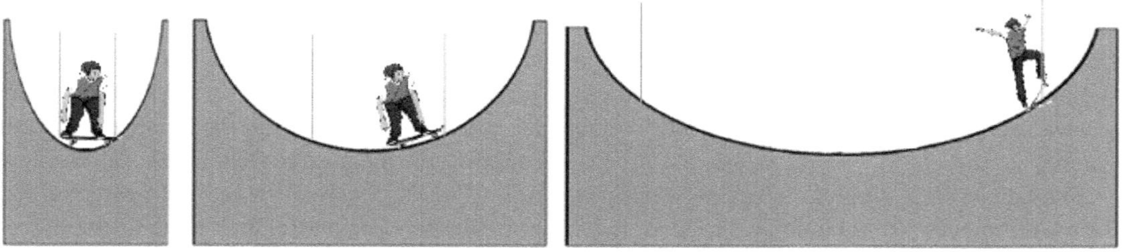

Fig. 7.3 A narrow skateboarding site allows limited movement, while the expansion of the site will allow the skateboard to move more. The skateboard site can be considered a neutral zone. (Courtesy of Dr. Tunç Öktenoğlu)

Abnormal, excessive segmental motion may cause pain with overstretching of soft tissues and/or entrapment of nerve roots.

The second theory was described by Mulholland and Sengupta in 2002 [12]. The intervertebral disc is normally rich in fluid and thus distributes the load evenly to the end plates. However, with the degeneration process, proteoglycan content is reduced, and thus, fluid content of the disc is also reduced. In such circumstances, the intervertebral disk material may not distribute the loads evenly. Therefore, the normal physiological loads may produce stress concentrations higher and more uneven loading compared to a healthy disc. This uneven distribution of loads may cause fragmentation at the endplates and annulus, which causes pain. This is described as "stone in the shoe."

7.1.3 Treatment

The treatment of a patient with DDD without a neurologic deficit starts with conservative methods. Physiotherapy exercise methods increase the strength of muscles and support the spine more effectively. The weight loss of a patient also helps by decreasing the load applied to the spine. In recent years, the pain procedures, either epidural or nerve root block injections, have become popular due to these injections offering acute pain relief. However, a significant number of patients do not respond to these conservative and/or interventional procedures. In this group of patients, surgical treatment is needed. Additionally, some patients show neurologic deficits or develop neurologic deficits during conservative treatment that require a decompression procedure.

Currently, there are three different surgical methods available in the treatment of DDD.

This chapter focuses on dynamic stabilization techniques.

7.1.4 Fusion Surgery

In the early years of the twentieth century, surgical fusion of a spinal motion segment was described and performed in the treatment of spinal infection [13–16]. After the 1950s, the indication of fusion was broadened, and the fusion procedure was applied in the surgical treatment of spinal deformities, fractures, and tumors [17–22].

The main goal of this method was to preserve or reestablish the spinal stability and to correct the deformity in situ. The development of spinal instrumentation in the 1970s and 1980s enabled surgeons to effectively restore spinal curvature and increase disc and neural foramen height [23–25]. The advances in spinal instrumentation increased the popularity and success of this technique.

The improvement of implants offered immediate stability so that the patient could be mobilized in the postoperative period and discharged soon after the operation. The postoperative complications due to long hospitalization are decreased. The fusion procedure has become a standard procedure for DDD, degenerative spondylolisthesis, degenerative scoliosis, post-discectomy syndrome, or segmental instability adjacent to previous fusion [26–30].

Fritzell et al. [31] demonstrated that the patients who received a fusion procedure for DDD showed better outcomes compared to a similar group of patients who were treated conservatively. This study won the 2001 Volvo Award.

The advances in surgical techniques, such as the development of minimally invasive techniques, have decreased the complications due to muscle injury, long operation time, blood loss, and infection. Moreover, the fusion techniques are also improved. Historically, posterior fusion methods evolved to posterolateral fusion procedures. Anterior lumbar fusions (anterior lumbar interbody fusion (ALIF)), anterior fusion through a posterior approach (posterolateral interbody fusion (PLIF)), and transforaminal interbody fusion (TLIF) have become popular. All these techniques offered higher fusion rates, better restoration of disc height, and maintained proper sagittal balance [32–34].

Despite all the advances in surgical implants and improvements in surgical methods, there is still a persistent disassociation between a radiographically successful fusion and successful pain relief. Today, it is easily achieved with 95% radiographic fusion rates; however, the clinical pain relief success is in the 60%–80% range [35]. Long-term studies documented that as many as 29% of patients who were treated with a fusion procedure in the past will have a return of pain [36]. This pain is usually due to adjacent segment disease [37–39].

These side effects of fusion surgery and a relatively significant number of patients with fair or moderate outcomes despite the development of solid fusion motivated the authors to explore different surgical techniques to eliminate the risks related to the fusion procedure and to achieve better outcomes.

7.2 Disc Prosthesis

There are several different descriptions used in literature for this technique: lumbar disc prosthesis, lumbar arthroplasty, lumbar disc arthroplasty, lumbar artificial disc, and total lumbar disc replacement (TDR). All indicate the motion preservation technique.

The main factors that allow TDR to be used in surgical treatment for DDD are (1) relief of pain by preserving motion at the applied segment (opposite to the fusion technique), (2) elimination of risks observed in the per-operative and postoperative periods related to the fusion procedure, and (3) less stress increase at adjacent segments compared to fusion (less adjacent segment disease risk).

7.2.1 TDR History

The concept and clinical application of disc replacement techniques started in the 1950s [40, 41]. In those days, the diagnosis of disc herniation was mainly based on myelography. A plain X-ray was the only diagnostic tool in the evaluation of low back pain. The physicians who operated on the patients for lumbar disc herniation noticed the continuation of backache in a significant number of patients following the operation, who showed progressive disc space collapse following surgery in follow-up serial radiographic studies.

The relation between the continuation of low back pain with progressive disc space collapse following a discectomy procedure caused surgeons to focus on the prevention of disc collapse following a discectomy procedure. Cleveland [40] and Hamby and Glaser [41] inserted an acrylic substance into the disc space following discectomy to prevent disc collapse. The clinical advantage of this method could not be documented. In 1974, Froming [42] described a nucleus replacement device that was a fluid-filled elastic chamber between two metal cup endplates. There is no data regarding the biomechanical properties of this device. Edeland [43] and Fassio and Ginestie [44] designed a nucleus replacement device that was silicon fluid or silicone rubber contained in a plastic tube. Urbaniak et al. [45] and Stubstad et al. [46] designed a disc-shaped device. The center of the device consisted of a silicon material with an outer covering made of Dacron (Invista, Wichita, KS). The preliminary animal model test results were promising.

The modern designs for lumbar disc prosthesis started in the 1960s with Fernström [47]. He implanted a stainless-steel ball into the disc spaces. Fernström applied his device to 191 lumbar and 13 cervical regions of 125 patients. The early outcomes were similar to the fusion procedure. However, in the late postoperative period, there were significant complications related to device extrusions and subsidence.

In France, at Charité hospital, Dr. Karin Buettner-Janz, an orthopedic surgeon as well as a former Olympic gymnast, and Kurt Schellnack, an engineer, published their first experiences with the Charité artificial disc prosthesis for the lumbar spine in the early 1980s [48]. This technique started the modern lumbar arthroplasty period. They have modified the device several times, and finally, the first clinical experience of the final version, that is, SB Charité III (DePuy Spine Inc., Raynham, Massachusetts, USA), was documented in 1994 [49]. Later on, several different lumbar arthroplasty devices were developed. ProDisc-L (Centinel Spine, West Chester, Pennsylvania, USA), activeL (Aesculap Implant Systems, Center Valley, Pennsylvania, USA), Acroflex (Acromed Corporation, Cleveland, Ohio, USA), Maverick (Medtronic, Dublin, Ireland), Kineflex (Spinal Motion, Mountain View, California, USA), FlexiCore (Stryker, Kalamazoo, Michigan, USA), and M6-L (Orthofix, Lewisville, Texas, USA) lumbar discs have either completed or are ongoing their clinical trials; some of them have been discontinued or withdrawn without FDA approval. On the other hand, all of them are available outside of the USA. In recent years, new designs have been developed to eliminate the risks related to the anterior approach insertion of artificial disk prosthesis. The XL TDR (NuVasive, San Diego, California, USA) is designed to place the artificial disc through a lateral approach, and the Triumph (Globus Medical, Audubon, Pennsylvania, USA) is designed to place it through a posterior approach. These implants are still in the investigational period in the USA but are available outside the United States.

7.2.2 Classification of Disc Prosthesis

The artificial disc prosthesis can be classified depending on either its material properties or biomechanical properties (Fig. 7.4).

7.2.2.1 Material Properties

Some artificial disk prostheses are made of metal-on-metal, such as Maverick, Kineflex, and FlexiCore. On the other hand, some artificial disk prostheses contain a polyethylene core (a core made of ultra-high molecular weight polyethylene: UHMWPE) between metal articulating surfaces, such as Charité, ProDisk-L, and activeL.

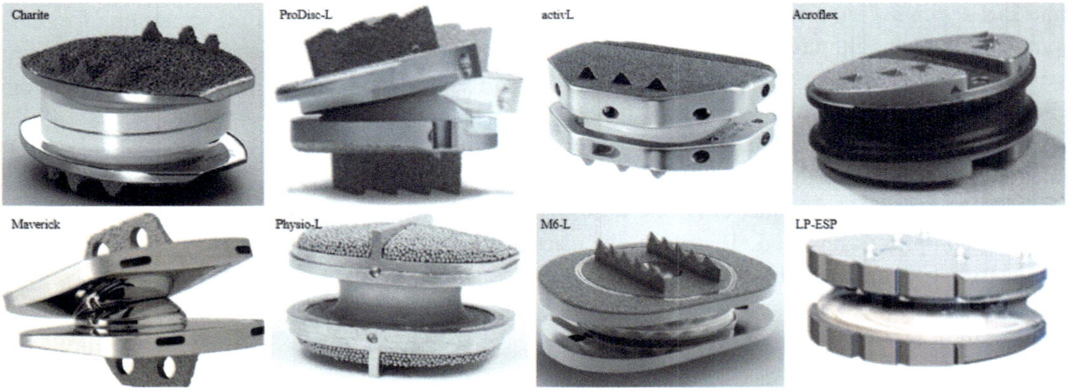

Fig. 7.4 Numerous different types of disc prosthesis have been developed

7.2.2.2 Biomechanical Properties

The normal three-joint (an intervertebral disk and a pair of facet joints) of a functional spinal unit has six degrees of freedom. The motion segment shows flexion and extension movements in the sagittal plane, right and left lateral bendings in the coronal plane, and in the axial plane, right and left rotational movements. An ideal artificial disk prosthesis should absorb the load applied onto the motion segment and allow all six movements without any restrictions. An artificial disk device that allows hypermobility beyond the physiologic limits in a given mode without any mechanical limitation for that mode of motion is considered "unconstrained." A device that allows normal motion but shows restrictions to the movements that are beyond physiologic limits is defined as "semiconstrained." Any implant that limits the normal physiologic movements is defined as "constrained" [50, 51]. On the other hand, depending on the device design, an artificial disc may show different biomechanical properties for different movements. For example, a Charité disc is "unconstrained" in axial plane movements; that is, there is no mechanical limitation for axial rotational movements. On the other hand, due to device limits, the movements beyond physiologic limits in flexion-extension and lateral bending movements are then considered as "semiconstrained" [50].

One should keep in mind that a motion segment of the spine is totally different from the hip and knee joints. The functional spinal unit (motion segment) of a spine consists of three joints. Moreover, although the facet joints are synovial joints, the intervertebral disc is a synchondrosis. The biomechanical properties are also different. In hip or knee joint replacement technique, the whole joint is replaced; however, in disc replacement technique, only one-third of the joint complex is replaced. Therefore, the use of the terms "constrained," "semiconstrained," and "unconstrained" to describe the spinal segment motion is different from their usage in hip or knee replacement literature.

Finally, there is one additional movement that the lumbar disc has: axial compression. A healthy lumbar disc shows 0.5–1.5 mm axial compression. None of the intervertebral disc prostheses has this feature. Therefore, in regard to the axial compression mode, all devices can be considered as "constrained" [52].

Table 7.1 Structure and biomechanical properties of artificial lumbar disc implants

Device	Biomechanics	Structure
Charité	Unconstrained	Metal on polymer
ProDisc-L	Semiconstrained	Metal on polymer
activL	Semiconstrained	Metal on polymer
Flexicore	Constrained	Metal-on-metal
Kineflex-L	Semiconstrained	Metal-on-metal
Acroflex	Constrained	Elastic core
Maverick	Semiconstrained	Metal-on-metal
Triumph	Semiconstrained	Metal-on-metal
XL TDR	One piece	Laterally placed
M6-L	One piece	Elastomeric

The normal anatomy of a functional spinal unit with surrounding soft tissues (ligaments and muscles) offers a "semiconstrained" pattern of mobility. The system allows physiologic movements and restrains the excessive motion.

The material and biomechanical properties of disc prostheses are depicted in Table 7.1.

7.2.3 Biomechanics of Disc Prosthesis

Biomechanical studies comparing the device with "unconstrained" (e.g., Charité) vs. "constrained" (e.g., ProDisc-L) showed no significant advantage over each other. As expected, "unconstrained" devices have a higher range of motion (ROM) in axial and lateral bending movements and conversely show less ROM in flexion-extension [53].

On a theoretical basis, the "constrained" devices might cause an increase in facet loads during extension, whereas the "unconstrained" prosthesis that is free to translate in extension might cause better load sharing between facet joint loading and capsuloligamentous tension [54]. Moreover, it is postulated that the "constrained" devices might increase facet loads due to impingement in flexion-extension, whereas the ability to show translational movements offered by "unconstrained" devices might unload the facet joints. On the other hand, the "constrained" prosthesis absorbs the loads applied onto the spine better than the "unconstrained" prosthesis; therefore, it might offer better facet joint preservation. The "unconstrained" devices do not show any restriction to shear forces; restriction forces against translational movements are only offered by posterior elements. Therefore, in the long term, the facet joints and ligamentous structures are prone to develop degenerative changes [55].

There is a strong correlation between intervertebral disc height and ROM following disc replacement. Moreover, an increase in ROM correlates with clinical outcome parameters (Oswestry Disability Index (ODI) and Visual Analog Scale (VAS)). Tournier et al. [56] compared the ROM of Charité, ProDisc-L, and Maverick prostheses and found no significant difference at the index level and also documented maintenance *of* sagittal balance.

Adjacent segment disease (ASDis) following a fusion procedure is a common problem. The disc prosthesis offers the advantages of preservation of motion, maintaining disc height, restoring lumbar lordosis, preserving paravertebral muscles, and thus decreasing the forces applied onto adjacent segments. Long-term studies with ProDisc-L [57] and with Charité [58] showed the advantages of disc prostheses in regard to ASDis and adjacent segment degeneration (ASDeg). A systematic review study compared over 1732 fusion patients with 758 arthroplasty patients. There was significantly less ASDeg observed in the arthroplasty group; additionally, the development of ASDis is strongly correlated with the fusion procedure. This study is graded as an IC recommendation for using arthroplasty instead of fusion to decrease the risk of ASDis [59]. A more recent meta-analysis of 13 studies showed the difference in ASDeg is more significant after a 5-year follow-up period [60]. The retrospective radiologic analysis of the patients from the activeL investigational device exemption (IDE) trial documented that the ASDeg at 5-year follow-up was 9.7% and reoperation for ASDis is 2.3% [61]. There was an inverse correlation with the occurrence of ASDeg and motion preservation. 10.6% of patients with preservation of 0–1° of motion showed adjacent segment alteration; on the other hand, there were no adjacent segment alterations in patients with 6 degrees or more of motion [61].

Similar results are achieved with the use of TDR at two levels. Radcliff et al. published a prospective randomized study and compared the reoperation rates between two-level TDR and fusion surgery. They reported that the reoperation rate in patients with fusion surgery was higher in the 5-year follow-up [62]. Dmitriev et al. conducted an in vitro biomechanical study using human cadavers. They reported that the specimens with L3–4 and L4–5 TDR showed better ROM compared to the fusion group and similar intradiscal pressure and ROM at adjacent segments with intact specimens [63].

The beneficial effect of the TDR technique on the adjacent segment disc has been documented. However, facet load changes following TDR application are not clear. The main causes of unsatisfactory outcome following application of Charité disc prosthesis were related to subsidence, device migration, and degeneration of facet joints either at the operated level or adjacent segments [64]. Siepe et al. reported a prospective clinical trial using the ProDisc device. They found that at 53 months postoperative, the facet degeneration rate at the operated level was higher than at the other levels. The rate of facet degeneration was significantly higher at the L5-S1 segment compared to other segments. They also noted that the development of facet degeneration decreased the ODI scores and ROM [65]. A biomechanical study using ball-socket-type TDR in cadavers showed the importance of device placement. The TDR implanted anteriorly increased the facet loads 2.5 times more compared to intact segment facet joints, and conversely, the posteriorly placed device resulted in a decrease in facet loads [66]. It is documented that anterior- and posterior-placed TDRs influenced the muscle forces more than laterally placed devices [67]. In a 2-year follow-up study using the Maverick disc prosthesis, a satisfactory outcome was achieved in patients with moderate facet degeneration; moreover, the shift of the center of rotation posteriorly decreased the facet loads [68].

7.2.4 Clinical Outcome with TDR

The Charité Artificial Disc is the first modern artificial disc that has FDA approval and is widely used all around the world. The FDA-controlled investigational device exemption (IDE) study documented that at 2-year follow-up, the overall success was 63% for TDR and 53% for fusion [69]. There was no complication related to the device, and the reoperation rates for the TDR group were 5.4% and 9.1% for the fusion group. Hospital stay was also significantly shorter in TDR compared to the fusion group [70, 71]. The IDE study was extended to a 5-year follow-up, and the clinical outcome (ODI and VAS) parameters were similar to the 2-year outcome [72, 73]. On the other hand, there were some criticisms of this promotion of results. Major criticism was that the high failure rate in the fusion group is due to the disused surgical technique that was used in the fusion procedure. The clinical success criteria were determined by only a 25% improvement in ODI score, no device failure, no neurological deterioration, and no major complication. Only 57% of the TDR group achieved these criteria, whereas 46% of the fusion group met these criteria. Finally, it was observed that in both groups a significant number of patients were still using narcotics at the 2-year follow-up [74, 75].

Lemaire (100 patients, 54 single-level, 45 patients 2 level, and one patient 3 level) [76] and David (106 patients with one level) [58] documented their results with a 10-year follow-up. Lemaire reported 90% and David reported 82.1% excellent or good clinical outcomes. Both studies showed that TDR is a strong option for the surgical treatment of DDD.

ProDisc-L is designed by Marnay. He reported 78% good-excellent outcomes at 8–10-year follow-up in 58 patients [51]. There were no device-related complications or subsidence. Moreover, there was no significant difference in outcome between one-level and two-level applications. However, the IDE trial results at 5-year follow-up showed that there was no clinical advantage between TDR and fusion. The TDR group showed a significant advantage only in regard to adjacent segment degeneration (9% in the TDR vs 28% in the fusion group). ROM decreased by 0.5°, and the reoperation rates were similar for the operated level (8% for TDR and 12% for fusion) and for adjacent segments (1.9% for TDR and 4% for fusion) [77]. Surgical time and blood loss were significantly less in the TDR group [77, 78].

ActivL is a recent FDA-approved device. It is considered a third-generation device. The UHMWP core allows 2 mm translation in the anterior and posterior direction; thus, it is considered a "semiconstrained" prosthesis. The IDE trial of the implant was based on comparing it with the other FDA-approved TDR devices (Charité and ProDisc-L). In a randomized study, a total of 218 patients received activL, and 106 patients received the other TDR devices. The patients operated on with activL showed better ODI scores. 5-year follow-up results demonstrated the safety and efficacy with satisfactory outcomes compared to other TDR devices [79]. A recent meta-analysis compared the numerous TDR devices with each other and also with fusion and conservative treatment. This study showed that the actvL offered better outcomes compared to other TDR devices, fusion, and conservative treatment in regard to pain control, disability, and quality of life [80]. Maverick is a metal-on-metal type disc prosthesis (Figs. 7.4 and 7.5).

The first study, published in 2005, had 2-year follow-up results of 64 patients [81]. The study documented favorable clinical outcomes. The IDE trial compared the Maverick device with ALIF. Satisfactory outcome at 2-year follow-up for Maverick was 73.5% and 55.3% for the fusion group [82].

Sasani et al. documented their clinical results in 2009 with the Maverick device [83]. The authors observed satisfactory outcomes in 16 patients with DDD; 4 also had lumbar disk herniation. The mean follow-up was 2.4 months.

There are some other studies for other TDR devices that documented favorable outcomes [84, 85].

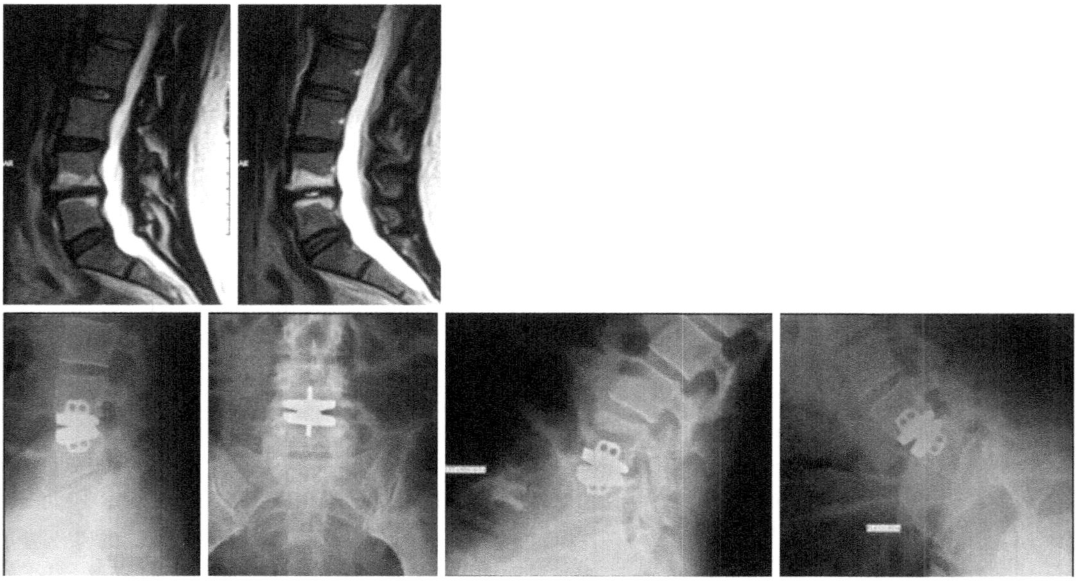

Fig. 7.5 Maverick TDR device applied to the L4–5 segment with degenerative disc disease

7.2.5 Complications

The complications of a new technology and technique might be observed at the early postoperative term or at the late postoperative term. The complications observed with the application of TDR can be categorized into three subgroups: (a) due to technique, (b) due to device, or (c) due to approach.

There are numerous reports documenting the complications related to the technique. Putzier et al. [86] reported 23% fusion at the index level in a 17-year follow-up. Development of vertebral fracture, pedicle fracture, and deformity has been documented [81, 87–89]. Facet joint disease was observed in 20% of patients at 4.4-year follow-up [65]. Heterotopic ossification is also a common problem. Tortolani et al. [90] reported 4.3% at 2-year follow-up, and Park et al. [91] observed 50% heterotopic ossification at 8-year follow-up. The development of the adjacent segment problem is another problem observed with this technique. Harrop et al. [59] reported 9.7% ASDeg following TDR application, whereas Zigler et al. [61] published only 1% ASDis. Osteolysis and acquired spondylolysis were also documented as case reports [92, 93].

There are numerous reports documenting the complications directly related to the device. Device dislocation was observed with ProDisc-L and Charité [64, 94, 95]. The application of TDR made of metal-on-metal might cause metallosis (Maverick) [96–98]. Subsidence is a significant complication. There was a 53%–59% revision operation due to subsidence with the use of Charité and ProDisc [64, 99].

The technique is applied through the anterior approach. The presence of an experienced general and/or vascular surgeon in the surgical team helps to decrease complication rates. The complications observed with TDR in regard to approach-related issues are similar to complications documented with the ALIF technique. The neurologic complications observed with the anterior approach were reported as 9% in a meta-analysis study [100]. The most common neurologic problem is retrograde ejaculation due to injury to the hypogastric plexus, reported in 0.42–6% of cases [101]. The incidence of major vein injuries is 1.4%–3% [99]. The risk of vascular injury increases with prolonged retraction, previous abdominal surgery, and multilevel surgery [102]. In recent years, new TDR designs have been developed to insert the device through a lateral or posterior approach to eliminate the risks related to the anterior approach.

In our clinic, we have designed a new minimally invasive anterior approach method to minimize the risks related to the anterior approach [103].

The overall complications after TDR application can reach 18% [55, 104–106].

7.3 Posterior Dynamic Stabilization

Posterior dynamic stabilization (PDS) technique is an alternative surgical method to fusion procedure and TDR in the treatment of low back problems. PDS devices are classified into three types: (1) posterior interspinous spacers, (2) total facet replacement devices, and (3) posterior pedicle screw-based systems. This chapter focuses on pedicle screw-based systems. The PDS abbreviation is used for pedicle screw-based posterior dynamic stabilization methods. The PDS technique is totally different from the fusion and TDR techniques. Basically, the fusion procedure eliminates the movement (abnormal and normal) at the index level and offers stability. Depending on the surgical method, some fusion procedures remove intervertebral disc material to achieve better fusion (ALIF, PLIF, TLIF). The TDR technique removes the pain-originating disc material and inserts an artificial disc prosthesis to work as an intervertebral disc. The technique is designed to preserve motion at the index level. Most TDR devices are inserted through the anterior approach. However, the PDS (pedicle screw-based) is different from the other two methods. The PDS does not eliminate the motion at the index level as does the fusion method but controls the abnormal motion. The PDS supports the spine and works with the intervertebral disc, instead of removing it as does TDR. Therefore, it is expected to serve lifelong. This is the most challenging part for PDS. On the other hand, the application through the posterior approach is more familiar to spine surgeons.

7.3.1 PDS History and Classification

There are numerous different pedicular screw-based PDS techniques available. These systems can be categorized into two subgroups: (a) rigid screw with dynamic rod and (b) dynamic screw with rigid rod.

7.3.1.1 Rigid Screw-Dynamic Rod

These systems allow motion through a dynamic rod. Mostly applied systems are Graf Ligament, Dynesys, Accuflex, Bioflex, Transition, and any rod made of *polyetheretherketone* (PEEK) (Fig. 7.6).

Graf Ligament (SEM Co., Mountrouge, France). In 1992, Graf [107] described the application of a soft elastic rod named the Graf Ligament in the treatment of low back pain. The system consists of rigid pedicle screws and soft rods that are made of polyester-threaded bands (Fig. 7.6).

Dynamic Neutralization System (*Dynesys*) (Dynesys-Zimmer, Minneapolis, MN, USA). The Dynasis system was developed by Dubois in 1994 [108]. The system is a modification of the Graf Ligament system. In this system, spacers between screws are used to eliminate the risk of subsidence that is observed with the Graf Ligament system. The Dynesys system consists of titanium alloy pedicle screws with spacers that are made of polycarbonate urethane, surrounded by tensioned polyethylene terephthalate cords [109] (Fig. 7.6).

Accuflex Rod System (*Globus Medical Inc., Audubon, PA*, USA). The system consists of a metallic rod with helical cuts that allow some flexibility, particularly in flexion-extension mode (Fig. 7.6).

CD-Horizon Legacy PEEK Rod (Medtronic Sofamor Danek, Memphis, TN, USA). The system used a dynamic rod made of polyetheretherketone. The stiffness of the PEEK rod is less than the metallic rod, which allows some motion (Fig. 7.6).

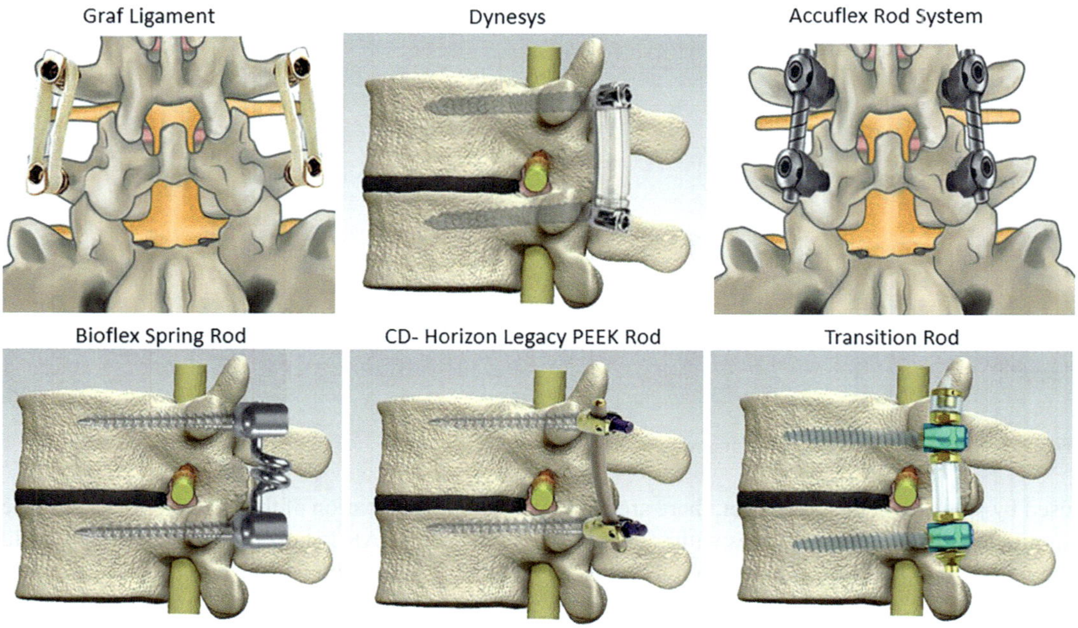

Fig. 7.6 Posterior pedicle screw-based dynamic stabilization systems with dynamic rod. (Illustrated by Prof. Ali Fahir Özer)

Bioflex Spring Rod (Biospine Corp., Seoul, Korea). The system uses a Nitinol rod that is an alloy of titanium and nickel. The rod has elasticity. Moreover, it is also called "memory metal" because it is a metal that has the ability to return to its original shape after deformation. The system acts as a tension band at the posterior column (Fig. 7.6).

Fulcrum Assisted Soft Stabilization System (*FASS*) (Neoligaments, Leads, UK). The technique was developed by Sengupta and Mullholland [110]. The system consists of a fulcrum between the screws and anterior to the elastic rod.

7.3.1.2 Dynamic Screw-Rigid Rod

The flexibility with this configuration is obtained by a hinged screw. Cosmic is the first system in this field. Later, Saphina's system was designed (Fig. 7.7).

Cosmic System (GmBH & Co, KG, Ulm, Germany). The technique was designed by von Strempel, and the author published clinical experience in 2006 [111]. The characteristic of this technique is the use of a pedicle screw with a hinge at the head of the screw. Therefore, the system allows some movements in the sagittal plane. The composition enables the load sharing between the Cosmic and the vertebral column (Fig. 7.7).

Saphinas System (Tıpsan A.Ş., İzmir, Turkey). The system is a modification of the Cosmic system. Similar to the Cosmic system, the Saphinas system also consists of a hinge screw. However, Saphina's system allows 1° of rotational movement in addition to flexion-extension movements (Fig. 7.7).

Posterior pedicle screw-based dynamic stabilization technique has increasing popularity. Therefore, there are new designs developed and

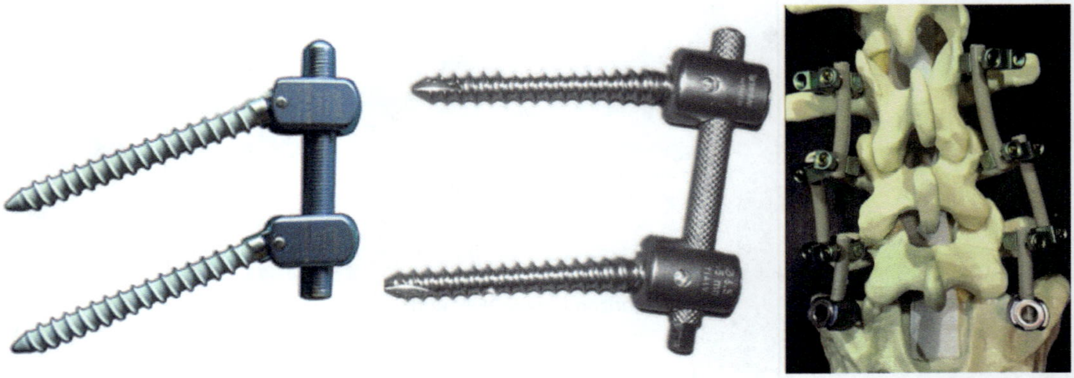

Fig. 7.7 PDS systems with a dynamic screw

used by spine surgeons. However, there are also a significant number of techniques withdrawn from the market due to unacceptable complications.

7.4 Biomechanics of PDS Systems

Pedicle screw-based PDS systems have been biomechanically well studied. On the other hand, one should keep in mind that all systems have different material properties, particularly in the use of dynamic rods. Therefore, all rods have different stiffness and thus different elasticity properties. These different material properties naturally stabilize the segment differently. It is documented that PDS with high stiffness shows similar stabilization as rigid systems [109, 112–115]. Recent studies documented that the PDS with lower stiffness may stabilize the segment effectively [114, 116]. Dynamic spinal implants with minimal stiffness of 45 N/mm axially and 30 N/mm bending are enough to reduce ROM by 30% of the intact ROM, and this is considered optimal motion restriction [114]. Panjabi documented that the optimal axial stiffness value for the longitudinal rods is approximately 50 N/mm for effective dynamic stabilization [117].

The application of PDS systems alters the position of the instantaneous axis of rotation (IAR). The posteriorly applied systems cause a posterior shift of IAR [112, 118, 119]. In an ideal system, the location of the IAR should be as close to the intact IAR localization as possible to avoid pathological loading of the spine.

Perez-Orribo et al. [118] performed a biomechanical study. They have compared the biomechanical behavior of rigid instrumentation and PDS in a cadaver model. They concluded that PDS shifted the IAR less than rigid stabilization. The study documented that PDS restored the destabilized segmental motion close to intact ROM.

Sengupta et al. [120] analyzed the load sharing between the anterior and posterior columns and also load distribution alterations at the intervertebral space following rigid stabilization and PDS with PEEK and Transition (Globus Medical, Audubon, PA, USA) rods. They observed that the rigid screw-PEEK rod combination showed similar biomechanical properties as a rigid fixation system in regard to load sharing between anterior and posterior columns. The anterior column loading was 55% for the rigid system and 59% for the PEEK rod; however, the PDS system with the Transition rod, which is a more dynamic rod compared to the PEEK rod, offered 75% anterior column loading. This result showed that the PDS system offered the closest load sharing between anterior and posterior columns to the intact spine, with an 80%–20% load distribution between anterior and posterior columns as described by Panjabi (Table 7.2) [120].

The evaluation of ROM following stabilization demonstrated that the rigid system causes a significantly greater decrease in ROM compared to the two PDS systems. There was no significant difference between the PEEK rod and the Transition system in regard to ROM following stabilization. The most interesting result was observed in the intervertebral load distribution analysis. The PDS with a Transition rod offered more uniform load distribution at the intervertebral space compared to other fixation methods. This biomechanical study demonstrated that although the PEEK rods are considered as dynamic (or semi-rigid), they only offer preservation of some motion compared to a rigid rod; however, when load sharing between anterior and posterior columns and load distribution at the intervertebral space are concerns, then they show similar biomechanical properties as a rigid rod. The Transition PDS offered similar kinematics as the PEEK rod in regard to motion preservation; however, the load sharing between anterior-posterior columns and load distribution at the intervertebral space were similar to an intact spine.

Table 7.2 Load distribution between anterior and posterior columns

Normal	Anterior %: 80	Posterior %: 20 (White, Panjabi)
Rigid	Anterior %: 55	Posterior %: 45
PEEK	Anterior %: 59	Posterior %: 41
PDS	Anterior %: 75	Posterior %: 25

Öktenoğlu et al. [121] compared the biomechanical effects of three different stabilization methods on a destabilized human cadaver. The authors compared the rigid system (rigid screw-rigid rod) with the semi-rigid system (rigid screw-dynamic rod; Talin Rod, Tıpsan, İzmir, Turkey) and with the full dynamic system (dynamic screw (hinge screw, Saphinas)-dynamic rod). As expected, the rigid system offered the most effective stabilization to the destabilized segment. The two PDS systems also effectively stabilized the destabilized segment while preserving some motion. However, the full dynamic method (dynamic screw-dynamic rod) combination stabilized the spine most closely to intact ROM limits (Fig. 7.8).

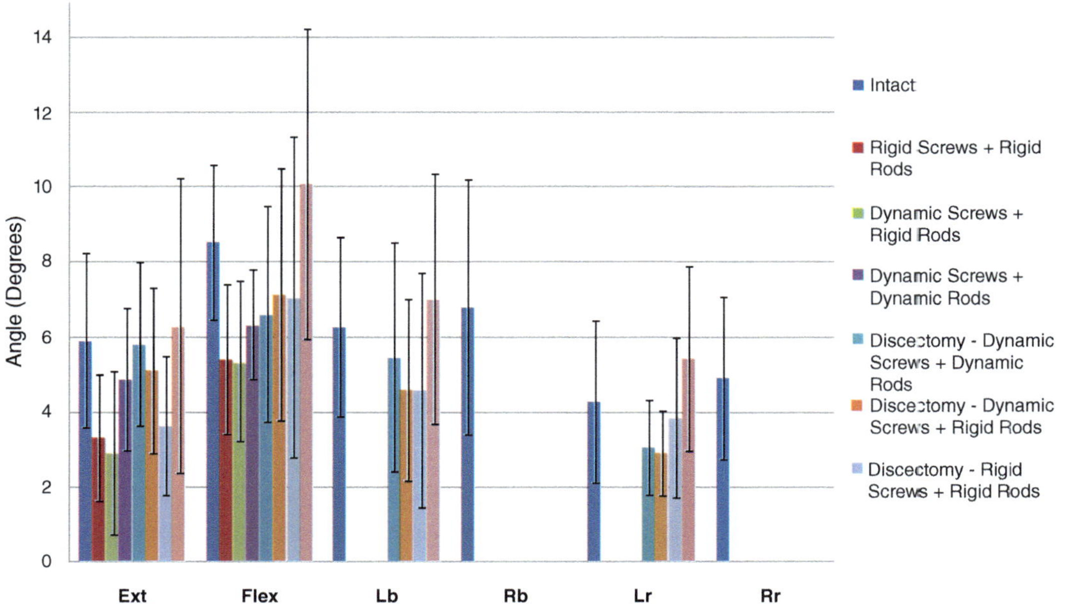

Fig. 7.8 The comparison of three different stabilization methods with regard to the preservation of motion. The dynamic screw-dynamic rod combination offered effective stabilization with preservation of ROM most close to the intact segment

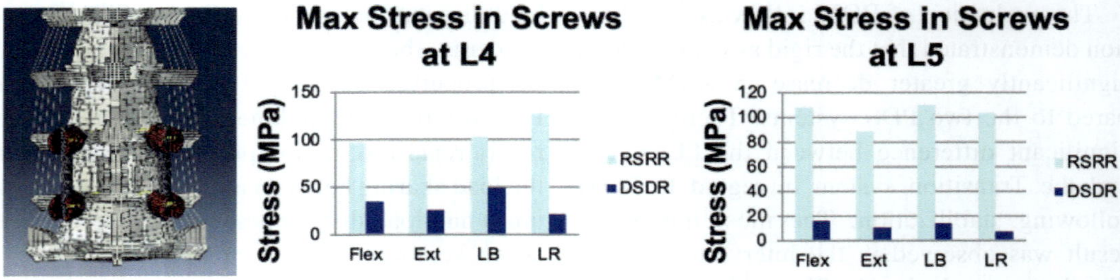

Fig. 7.9 The finite element study showed that the stress on the dynamic screw is less than on the rigid screw

The same study was also conducted as a finite element study [122]. Similar results were achieved. Moreover, the stress on the dynamic screw was less than on the rigid screw (Fig. 7.9).

As per the author's knowledge, these studies are the only biomechanical studies that evaluate the biomechanical effects of a dynamic screw-dynamic rod combination on a destabilized spinal segment.

There are numerous biomechanical studies with different types of PDS documents that show the PDS systems effectively stabilize the spine [118, 120, 123–129].

7.4.1 Clinical Outcome with PDS

The first system with pedicle screw-based PDS applied for low back pain is called the Graf Ligament. The implants employed screws to attach an artificial "ligament" to the spine. The biomechanical study [130] documented that the system only limits flexion-extension, but without limiting translational movements. Results from early studies were very promising, with one paper showing Graf Ligament stabilization resulting in a higher satisfaction rate (93%) when compared to the traditional fusion method (78%) [131]. However, on a longer follow-up, clinical outcomes showed mixed outcomes at different intervals [131–133]. The use of the Graf Ligament was found to be associated with high revision rates [131, 134]. Kanayama et al. [135] applied Graf Ligament to 64 patients with degenerative spondylolisthesis. Clinical and radiological evaluations showed that although in 80% of patients, lordosis was maintained, the system was unable to correct sagittal plane deformity.

Sánchez et al [136] reported the 2-year follow-up results of 20 patients. In this study the Accuflex rod system was used as PDS. They observed satisfactory clinical outcome and they noticed no progression of disc degeneration in 83% of patients. Moreover, three patients (16%) showed disc rehydration with one grade higher on the Pfirmann classification by MRI study at follow-up. On the other hand, they observed relatively high revision rate (22.22%).

Luo et al. [137] documented the results of 23 patients with degenerative disk disease who were treated with the Dynesys system. They observed a satisfactory clinical outcome at a mean follow-up of 39 months. Moreover, in the operated segment, 47.4% of the flexion/extension range of motion was retained.

Akyoldaş et al. [138] published their experiences with the use of the Dynesys system for multilevel degenerative low back problems. The clinical outcomes in regard to VAS and ODI were satisfactory. They found the screw-loosening rate as 6% and the breakage rate as 3.6%. They also observed ASDeg in 4.8% of patients. No reoperations were required due to ASDis. In this study, the infection rate was 5.9%. The reoperation rate was 8.4%. Three patients underwent reoperation due to screw breakage, and four patients due to operation site infection. In this study, the overall complication rate was 20.4%. These results were comparable to the fusion procedure.

Öktenoğlu et al. [139] reported the clinical outcomes of 20 patients with single-level DDD. A dynamic screw-rigid rod construct (Cosmic) PDS system was applied. We found satisfactory clinical outcomes at post-op 24 months, and there was no construct-related complication. Similar satisfactory outcomes were reported [138, 140].

von Strempel developed the dynamic screw-rigid rod construct (Cosmic). He documented his experiences in 139 patients with a follow-up of 2 years. He found that ODI improved from 49.0% preoperatively to 22.5% and VAS from 7.3 preoperatively to 2.5 after 2 years. There was no alteration of the lordosis. Eleven revision surgeries (7.9%) were performed. They observed 2 broken screws (0.3%) and 17 screws (2.5%) with a radiolucent halo [141].

7.4.2 Complications with PDS

There are numerous types of pedicle screw-based PDS techniques available, and each has different biomechanical properties. Therefore, the complications related to hardware, such as screw loosening and screw breakage, and complications related to biomechanical properties, such as ASDeg and/or ASDis, may differ. Dynesys' system was evaluated more than the other PDS systems because the technique is one of the pioneer methods applied in surgical treatment for DDD.

Pham et al. [142] reviewed the literature to document the complications observed following application of Dynesys. They found 21 studies with a total of 1166 patients (mean age of 55.5 years, range 39–71) and a mean follow-up period of 33.7 months (range 12.0–81.6). In this review, the infection rate was found to be 4.3% over a mean follow-up period of 34.8 months. This is similar to the literature on infection rates for lumbar fusion (range 1%–5%) [143–147]. This review study showed that 11.7% of patients developed pedicle screw loosening and 1.6% of patients were found to have a pedicle screw breakage (mean follow-up period of 30 months). The screw fracture rate of 1.6% is on the lower border of reported screw breakages for lumbar fusion, which are reported from 1.3% to 21% but are mostly within the 4%–6% range [148–153]. This might be the flexibility offered by Dynesys that minimizes the incidence of screw fracture [113, 154]. On the other hand, this flexibility might be the cause of screw loosening, which was found in a significant number of patients. One of the goals of the Dynesys system is to avoid ASDeg/is by using dynamic stabilization to reduce stress on adjacent segments [155, 156]. In this review of Dynesys' dynamic stabilization, the rate of ASD was 7% of patients over a mean follow-up period of 33.5 months. The rate of ASDeg/is following the fusion procedure is highly variable. Park et al. published a systematic review on ASDeg of the lumbar spine following a fusion procedure and found the incidence of radiographically diagnosed ASDeg to be 8%–100%, whereas in studies focusing on ASDis, the incidence ranged from 5.2% to 18.5% [157]. In another review study, Radcliff et al. found ASDeg rates after lumbar fusion between 1.9% and 30.3% at 5 years, with the largest study reporting 13% at 5 years and 22% at 10 years, with a mean annual incidence of 2.5% [158]. Lawrence et al. reported a review manuscript that focused on survival analyses. They documented that clinically relevant ASDeg occurred at a mean annual incidence of 0.6%–3.9% after lumbar fusion [159].

The revision surgery following Dynesys' method was observed in 117 patients (a total of 1032 patients, 11.3%). 40.6% of patients who developed ASDeg had a reoperation for this complication. Other reasons for revision surgery were infection, hardware revision, or hardware removal; usually, a fusion procedure was applied in revision. This is fairly consistent with reoperation rates with lumbar fusion reported in the literature. Radcliff et al. performed a subgroup analysis of the Spine Patient Outcomes Research Trial (SPORT) and found a 13% reoperation rate within 4 years for patients who had undergone surgery for lumbar spinal stenosis [160]. Lad et al. reviewed 16,556 patients with spondylolisthesis through a database search and found overall reoperation rates ranging from 10.6% to 18.4%, depending on whether patients underwent decompression alone versus instrumented and uninstrumented arthrodesis [161]. Many other studies on lumbar fusion have reported similar reoperation rates [37, 162–168].

Özer et al. [140] documented their clinical findings with three different types of pedicle screw-based PDS in the surgical treatment of DDD: (1) Dynesys method, (2) dynamic screw with dynamic rod (PEEK rod), and (3) dynamic screw with dynamic rod (CD-HORIZON BalanC™, Medtronic, Inc., USA). In post-op 30 months, they observed one screw loosening in the Dynesys group (at post-op 1 year, in 23 patients, 4%), one screw loosening in the PEEK rod group (at post-op 2 years in 31 patients, 3%), and one screw breakage in the Dynesys group (at post-op 30 months, in 23 patients, 4%). Although there was not any complication related to the BalanC rod in that study, later, due to a significant rod breakage complication rate, the rod was withdrawn from the market.

Ciplak et al. documented the complication rates of 2-level PDS at postoperative 2 years [169]. A total of 103 patients were included in the study. The authors applied dynamic screws (hinged) with a rigid rod. Although the clinical outcomes were satisfactory, 8.7% of patients developed screw breakage, 3.9% of patients developed screw loosening, and 0.9% of patients developed screw fracture and loosening together. Development of ASDeg was also studied, and 11.7% (12/103) of patients developed ASDeg. Depending on clinical complaints, a total of 14 patients (13.5%) needed revision surgery. Revision surgery was mostly (8/14 patients) performed for ASDis. The complication rates were significantly higher compared to single-level PDS application. The authors concluded that this high rate of complication was probably due to the use of a rigid rod. The longer use of a rigid rod diminishes the dynamism of the construct. Therefore, the use of a dynamic rod instead of a rigid rod with dynamic screws might offer lower complication rates.

PDS is expected to work lifelong. Therefore, they should keep dynamic properties and be strong enough to bear loads lifelong. The dynamic screws are made of metal (titanium); however, the structure and design of dynamic rods differ. Some rods even showed satisfactory capacity in biomechanical tests; after use in clinics, they failed and were withdrawn from the market (Fig. 7.10). *Research on new rod designs is still ongoing.*

7.4.3 Comparison of TDR with PDS

Both methods (TDR and PDS) offer satisfactory outcomes in the surgical treatment of DDD. However, there are some factors that bring an advantage to pedicle screw-based PDS. It is generally accepted that the presence of spondylosis, spondylolisthesis, facet arthropathy (or previous facet removal), or central or lateral recess stenosis is considered a contraindication for TDR application. On the other hand, the PDS system can be applied even with the presence of these pathologies. If there is a need, the first decompression procedure (microdiscectomy, lumbar central canal, and/or foraminal microdecompression) is performed, then the PDS system can be applied.

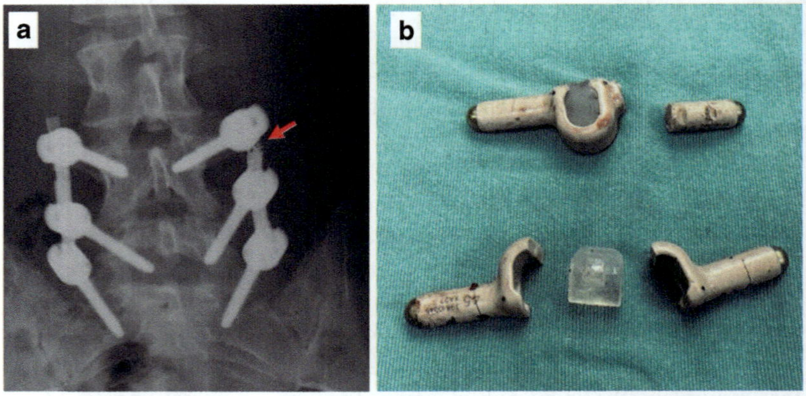

Fig. 7.10 The failure of dynamic rods: (**a**) Talin rod and, (**b**) BalanC rod

The application route of the PDS system is also less traumatic than TDR. If there is no need for decompression, then the pedicular screws can be inserted through muscles [170], without performing paravertebral muscle dissection (Fig. 7.11). Thus, the complications related to muscle dissection are eliminated.

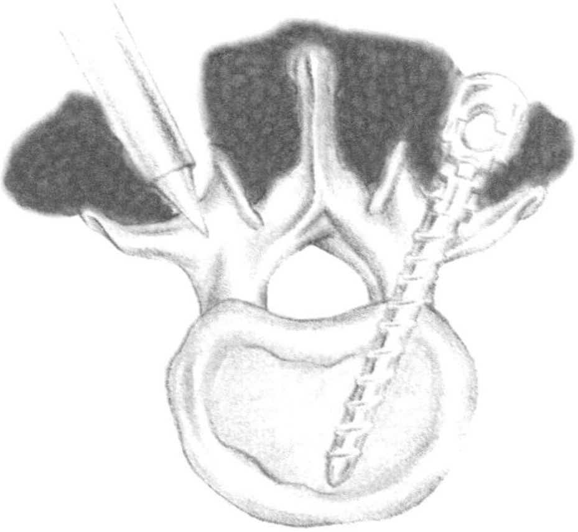

Fig. 7.11 The insertion of pedicular screws as per the Wiltse method. (Illustrated by Prof. Ozer)

As mentioned above, the PDS does not replace the intervertebral disc structure but supports the spine and restores the disrupted load distribution [121, 122]. Rehydration of a degenerated intervertebral disc following PDS application has been found in a limited number of literature [171, 172]. Yilmaz et al. [173] analyzed the MRI changes at postoperative 12 months following PDS (hinge screw with rigid rod) for DDD. They found that 34% of patients (20/59 patients) showed improvements in regard to disc degeneration, and 13.5% of patients (8/59 patients) showed progression in disc degeneration (Figs. 7.12 and 7.13).

The authors concluded that the offer of physiological movement and balanced load distribution by PDS may decelerate the degeneration and appear to facilitate the regeneration process. Moreover, in this study, the authors used a rigid rod; however, the use of a dynamic rod with a dynamic screw (hinged) may offer better load distribution and better kinematics [121, 122]. Therefore, it is reasonable to achieve better results with more dynamic constructs.

The TDR system can be applied to one or two levels; however, the PDS system can be applied to multi-segment pathologies. Moreover, the PDS system is not only for DDD but can be applied to numerous degenerative spine prob-

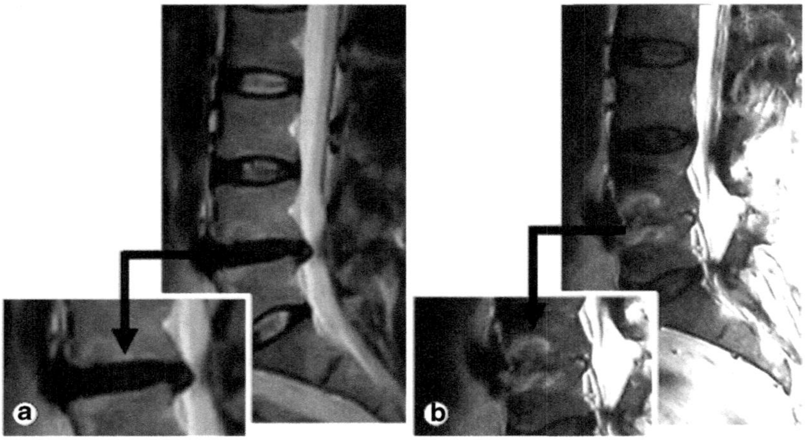

Fig. 7.12 Representative case of fusion development in a female patient with back pain caused by an extensive posterior annulus rupture. (**a**) Preoperative T2-weighted (T2W) magnetic resonance imaging (MRI). Decreased signal intensity in the disc space at the L4–L5 level (Pfirrmann grade 3). (**b**) Postoperative T2W MRI. Fusion at the same level is visible after 12 months postoperatively (Pfirrmann grade 5)

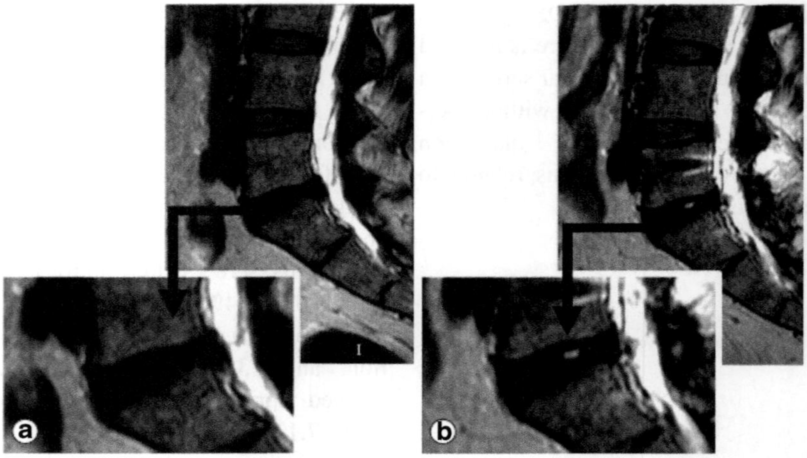

Fig. 7.13 Representative case of no change in a male patient with severe, chronic episodes of back pain and recent leg pain caused by a foraminal disc herniation. (**a**) Preoperative T2-weighted (T2W) magnetic resonance imaging (MRI). Decreased signal intensity in the disc space at the L5–S1 level (Pfirrmann grade 4). (**b**) Postoperative T2W MRI. No change in signal intensity at the same level after 12 months postoperatively (Pfirrmann grade 4)

lems. Today, there is an increasing number of studies documenting the use of the PDS system for spondylolisthesis, lumbar canal stenosis, recurrent disc herniation, unstable osteoporotic compression fracture, degenerative deformity, and facet replacement [129, 138–140, 174–178].

The PDS system appears to have a slightly lower complication rate profile compared with published literature on lumbar fusion and is associated with a slightly lower incidence of ASDed/is. One should keep in mind that the application of PDS is not as aggressive a procedure as the fusion procedure. PDS has favorable outcomes with shorter hospital stays compared to spinal fusion [108, 147, 172, 179–184]. This stabilization method also provides enough stability to prevent progression of low-grade spondylolistheses [108, 154, 156, 185]. The preservation of mobility in the lumbar spine plays a significant role in patient quality of life, and dynamic stabilization helps to maintain this mobility [31, 108, 181, 182, 186]. Without the need for fusion, there are no risks of bone graft donor-site complications such as pain, hematoma, or fracture. No allograft materials are required, also preventing the already low risk of disease transmission associated with these products [156, 183, 187, 188]. Therefore, to achieve similar clinical success with a lower complication rate with a relatively easy procedure compared to fusion is also an advantage.

References

1. Punnett L, Prüss-Utün A, Nelson DI, et al. Estimating the global burden of low back pain attributable to combined occupational exposures. Am J Ind Med. 2005;48(6):459–69.
2. Fardon DF, Williams AL, Dohring EJ, Murtagh FR, Gabriel Rothman SL, Sze GK. Lumbar disc nomenclature: version 2.0. Spine J. 2014;14(11):2525–45.
3. Frymoyer JW. The economics of spinal disorders. In: Frymoyer JW, editor. The adult spine: principles and practice. 2nd ed. Philadelphia: Lippincott-Raven; 1997. p. 143–50.
4. Crean JK, Roberts S, Jaffray DC, Eisenstein SM, Duance VC. Matrix metalloproteinases in the human intervertebral disc: role in disc degeneration and scoliosis. Spine. 1997;22:2877–84.
5. Duance VC, Crean JK, Sims TJ, et al. Changes in collagen crosslinking in degenerative disc disease and scoliosis. Spine. 1998;23:2345–51.
6. Hukins DW. A simple model for the function of proteoglycans and collagen in the response to compression of the intervertebral disc. Proc R Soc Lond B Biol Sci. 1992;249:281–5.
7. Kirkaldy-Willis WH. The pathology and pathogenesis of low back pain, and the three phases of the spectrum of degenerative disease. In: Kirkaldy-

Willis WH, editor. Managing low back pain. 2nd ed. New York: Churchill-Livingstone; 1988. p. 49–75, 117–131.
8. Boden SD, Riew KD, Yamaguchi K, et al. Orientation of the lumbar facet joints: association with degenerative disc disease. J Bone Joint Surg. 1996;78A:403–11.
9. Dai LY. Orientation and tropism of lumbar facet joints in degenerative spondylolisthesis. Int Orthop. 2001;25:40–2.
10. Andersson GB. What are the age-related changes in the spine? Baillieres Clin Rheumatol. 1998;12:161–73.
11. Panjabi MM. The stabilizing system of the spine. Part II. Neutral zone and instability hypothesis. J Spinal Disord. 1992;5:390–7.
12. Mulholland RC, Sengupta DK. Rationale, principles and experimental evaluation of the concept of soft stabilization. Eur Spine J. 2002;11(Suppl 2):S198–205.
13. Crock HV. Anterior lumbar interbody fusion. Clin Orthop. 1982;165:157–63.
14. Harmon PH. Anterior extraperitoneal disc excision and interbody fusion. Clin Orthop. 1960;18:169–98.
15. Hodgson AR, Wong AK. A description of a technique and evaluation of results in anterior fusion for deranged intervertebral disc and spondylolisthesis. Clin Orthop. 1968;56:133–61.
16. Stauffer RN, Coventry MB. Anterior interbody lumbar spine fusion. J Bone Joint Surg Am. 1972;54-A:756–68.
17. Bohlman HH, Eismont FJ. Surgical techniques of anterior decompression and fusion for spinal cord injuries. Clin Orthop. 1981;154:57–67.
18. Gertzbein SD, Court-Brown CM, Jacobs RR, et al. Decompression and circumferential stabilization of unstable spinal fractures. Spine. 1988;13:892–5.
19. Gertzbein SD. Fractures of the thoracic and lumbar spine. Baltimore: Williams & Wilkins; 1992.
20. Kostuik JP. Decision making in adult scoliosis. Spine. 1979;4:520–5.
21. Kostuik JP, Weinstein JN. Differential diagnosis and surgical treatment of metastatic spine tumors. In: Frymoyer JW, editor. The adult spine. New York: Raven Press; 1991. p. 861–88.
22. Weinstein JN. Differential diagnosis and surgical treatment of primary benign and malignant spine tumors. In: Frymoyer JW, editor. The adult spine. New York: Raven Press; 1991. p. 829–86.
23. Dick W. The 'fixateur interne' as a versatile implant for spine surgery. Spine. 1987;12:882–900.
24. Magerl FP. Stabilization of the lower thoracic and lumbar spine with external skeletal fixation. Clin Orthop. 1984;189:125–41.
25. Roy-Camille R, Saillant G, Berteaux D, Marie-Anne S, Mamoudy P. Vertebral osteosynthesis using metal plates. Chirurgie. 1979;105:597–603. (in French).
26. Grobler LJ, Wiltse LL. Classification, non-operative, and operative treatment of spondylolisthesis. In: Frymoyer JW, editor. The adult spine. New York: Raven Press; 1991. p. 1655–704.
27. Kostuik JP, Frymoyer JW. Failures after spinal fusion: causes and surgical treatment. In: Frymoyer JW, editor. The adult spine. New York: Raven Press; 1991. p. 2027–68.
28. Kozak JA, Heilman AE, O'Brien JP. Anterior lumbar fusion options: technique and graft materials. Clin Orthop. 1994;300:45–51.
29. Leong JCY, Hoper G, Fang D, Chun SY. Disc excision and anterior spinal fusion for lumbar disc protrusion in the adolescent. Spine. 1982;7:623–6.
30. Mayer HM, Korge A. Non-fusion technology in degenerative lumbar spinal disorders: facts, questions, challenges. Eur Spine J. 2002;11(Suppl 2):85–91.
31. Fritzell P, Hagg O, Wessberg P, Nordwall A. Chronic low back pain and fusion: a comparison of three surgical techniques: a prospective multicenter randomized study from the Swedish lumbar spine study group. Spine. 2002;27:1131–41.
32. Humphreys SC, Hodges SD, Patwardhan AG, et al. Comparison of posterior and transforaminal approaches to lumbar interbody fusion. Spine. 2001;26:567–71.
33. Miyamoto M, Genbum Y, Ito H. Diagnosis and treatment of lumbar spinal canal stenosis. J Nippon Med Sch. 2002;69:583–7.
34. Mukhtar AM, Farghaly MM, Ahmed SH. Surgical treatment of thoracic and lumbar tuberculosis by anterior interbody fusion and posterior instrumentation. Med Princ Pract. 2003;12:92–6.
35. West JL III, Bradford DS, Ogilvie JW. Results of spinal arthrodesis with pedicle screw-plate fixation. J Bone Joint Surg. 1991;73A:1179–84.
36. Finnegan WJ, Fenlin JM, Marvel JP, Nardini RJ, Rothman RH. Results of surgical intervention in the symptomatic multiply-operated back patient. Analysis of sixty-seven cases followed for three to seven years. J Bone Joint Surg Am. 1979;61(7):1077–82.
37. Ghiselli G, Wang JC, Bhatia NN, Hsu WK, Dawson EG. Adjacent segment degeneration in the lumbar spine. J Bone Joint Surg. 2004;86A:1497–503.
38. Hilibrand AS, Carlson GD, Palumbo MA, Jones PK, Bohlman HH. Radiculopathy and myelopathy at segments adjacent to the site of a previous anterior cervical arthrodesis. J Bone Joint Surg. 1999;81A:519–28.
39. Javedan SP, Dickman CA. Cause of adjacent-segment disease after spinal fusion. Lancet. 1999;354:530–1.
40. Cleveland DA. The use of methylacrylic for spinal stabilization after disc operations. Marquette Med Rev. 1955;20:62–4.
41. Hamby WB, Glaser HT. Replacement of spinal intervertebral discs with locally polymerizing methyl methylacrylic. J Neurosurg. 1959;16:311–3.
42. Froming N. Artificial intervertebral disc. United States Patent File. 1974.

43. Edeland HG. Some additional suggestions for an intervertebral disc prosthesis. J Biomech Eng. 1985;7:7–62.
44. Fassio B, Ginestie JF. Discal prosthesis made of silicone: experimental study and first clinical cases. Nouv Presse Med. 1978;7:207. [French].
45. Urbaniak JR, Bright DS, Hopkins JE. Replacement of intervertebral discs in chimpanzees by silicon-Dacron implants: a preliminary report. J Biomed Mater Res. 1973;7:165–86.
46. Stubstad JA, Urbaniak JR, Kahn P. Prosthesis for spinal repair. United States Patent File. 1975.
47. Fernström U. Arthroplasty with intercorporal endoprothesis in herniated disc and in painful disc. Acta Chir Scand Suppl. 1966;357:154–9.
48. Büttner-Janz K, Schellnack K, Zippel H. Biomechanics of the SB Charité lumbar intervertebral disc endoprosthesis. Int Orthop. 1989;13(3):173–6.
49. Griffith SL, Shelokov AP, Büttner-Janz K, LeMaire JP, Zeegers WS. A multicenter retrospective study of the clinical results of the LINK SB Charité intervertebral prosthesis. The initial European experience. Spine. 1994;19(16):1842–9.
50. Bono CM, Lee CK. Critical analysis of trends in fusion for degenerative disc disease over the past 20 years: influence of technique on fusion rate and clinical outcome. Spine. 2004;29:455–63.
51. Marnay T. Lumbar disc replacement: 7–11 year clinical experience. New York, Spine Solutions, Inc., 2000.
52. Errico TJ. Lumbar disc arthroplasty. Clin Orthop Relat Res. 2005;435:106–17.
53. Wilke H-J, Schmidt R, Richter M, Schmoelz W, Reichel H, Cakir B. The role of prosthesis design on segmental biomechanics. Eur Spine J. 2012;21(S5):577–84.
54. Cunningham BW, McAfee PC, Geisler FH, et al. Distribution of in vivo and in vitro range of motion following 1-level arthroplasty with the CHARITE artificial disc compared with fusion. J Neurosurg Spine. 2008;8(1):7–12.
55. Huang RC, Girardi FP, Cammisa FP, Wright TM. The implications of constraint in lumbar total disc replacement. J Spinal Disord Tech. 2003;16(4):412–7.
56. Tournier C, Aunoble S, Le Huec JC, et al. Total disc arthroplasty: consequences for sagittal balance and lumbar spine movement. Eur Spine J. 2007;16(3):411–21.
57. Huang RC, Tropiano P, Marnay T, Girardi FP, Lim MR, Cammisa FP. Range of motion and adjacent level degeneration after lumbar total disc replacement. Spine J. 2006;6(3):242–7.
58. David T. Long-term results of one-level lumbar arthroplasty: minimum 10-year follow-up of the CHARITE artificial disc in 106 patients. Spine. 2007;32(6):661–6.
59. Harrop JS, Youssef JA, Maltenfort M, et al. Lumbar adjacent segment degeneration and disease after arthrodesis and total disc arthroplasty. Spine. 2008;33(15):1701–7.
60. Ren C, Song Y, Liu L, Xue Y. Adjacent segment degeneration and disease after lumbar fusion compared with motion-preserving procedures: a meta-analysis. Eur J Orthop Surg Traumatol. 2014;24(S1):245–53.
61. Zigler JE, Blumenthal SL, Guyer RD, Ohnmeiss DD, Patel L. Progression of adjacent-level degeneration after lumbar total disc replacement: results of a posthoc analysis of patients with available radiographs from a prospective study with 5-year follow-up. Spine. 2018;43(20):1395–400.
62. Radcliff K, Spivak J, Darden B, Janssen M, Bernard T, Zigler J. Five-year reoperation rates of 2-level lumbar total disk replacement versus fusion: results of a prospective, randomized clinical trial. Clin Spine Surg. 2018;31(1):37–42.
63. Dmitriev AE, Gill NW, Kuklo TR, Rosner MK. Effect of multilevel lumbar disc arthroplasty on the operative- and adjacent-level kinematics and intradiscal pressures: an in vitro human cadaveric assessment. Spine J. 2008;8(6):918–25.
64. van Ooij A, Oner FC, Verbout AJ. Complications of artificial disc replacement. J Spinal Disord Tech. 2003;16(4):369–83.
65. Siepe CJ, Zelenkov P, Sauri-Barraza J-C, et al. The fate of facet joint and adjacent level disc degeneration following total lumbar disc replacement: a prospective clinical, X-ray, and magnetic resonance imaging investigation. Spine. 2010;35(22):1991–2003.
66. Dooris AP, Goel VK, Grosland NM, Gilbertson LG, Wilder DG. Load-sharing between anterior and posterior elements in a lumbar motion segment implanted with an artificial disc. Spine. 2001;26(6):E122–9.
67. Han K-S, Kim K, Park WM, Lim DS, Kim YH. Effect of centers of rotation on spinal loads and muscle forces in total disk replacement of lumbar spine. Proc Inst Mech Eng H J Eng Med. 2013;227(5):543–50.
68. Le Huec J-C, Basso Y, Aunoble S, Friesem T, Bruno MB. Influence of facet and posterior muscle degeneration on clinical results of lumbar total disc replacement: two-year follow-up. J Spinal Disord Tech. 2005;18(3):219–23.
69. Hochschuler SH, Ohmeiss, Guyer RD, Blumenthal SL. Artificial disc: preliminary results of a prospective study in the United States. In: Gunzburg R, Mayer HM, Szpalski M, Aebi M, editors. Arthroplasty of the spine. Berlin: Springer-Verlag; 2004. p. 44–8.
70. Blumenthal S, McAfee PC, Guyer RD, et al. A prospective, randomized, multicenter Food and Drug Administration investigational device exemptions study of lumbar total disc replacement with the CHARITE artificial disc versus lumbar fusion: part I: evaluation of clinical outcomes. Spine. 2005;30(14):1565–75. discussion E387–391.

71. McAfee PC, Cunningham B, Holsapple G, et al. A prospective, randomized, multicenter Food and Drug Administration investigational device exemption study of lumbar total disc replacement with the CHARITE artificial disc versus lumbar fusion: part II: evaluation of radiographic outcomes and correlation of surgical technique accuracy with clinical outcomes. Spine. 2005;30(14):1576–83. discussion E388–390.
72. Guyer RD, McAfee PC, Banco RJ, et al. Prospective, randomized, multicenter food and drug administration investigational device exemption study of lumbar total disc replacement with the CHARITE artificial disc versus lumbar fusion: five-year follow-up. Spine J. 2009;9(5):374–86.
73. Geisler FH, McAfee PC, Banco RJ, et al. Prospective, randomized, multicenter FDA IDE study of CHARITÉ artificial disc versus lumbar fusion: effect at 5-year follow-up of prior surgery and prior discectomy on clinical outcomes following lumbar arthroplasty. SAS J. 2009;3(1):17–25.
74. van den Eerenbeemt KD, Ostelo RW, van Royen BJ, Peul WC, van Tulder MW. Total disc replacement surgery for symptomatic degenerative lumbar disc disease: a systematic review of the literature. Eur Spine J. 2010;19(8):1262–80.
75. Mirza SK. Point of view: commentary on the research reports that led to Food and Drug Administration approval of an artificial disc. Spine. 2005;30(14):1561–4.
76. Lemaire J-P. Clinical and radiological outcomes with the Charité artificial disc: a 10-year minimum follow-up. J Spinal Disord Tech. 2005;18(4):353–9.
77. Zigler J, Delamarter R, Spivak JM, et al. Results of the prospective, randomized, multicenter Food and Drug Administration investigational device exemption study of the ProDisc-L total disc replacement versus circumferential fusion for the treatment of 1-level degenerative disc disease. Spine. 2007;32(11):1155–62. discussion 1163
78. Zigler JE, Delamarter RB. Five-year results of the prospective, randomized, multicenter, Food and Drug Administration investigational device exemption study of the ProDisc-L total disc replacement versus circumferential arthrodesis for the treatment of single-level degenerative disc disease. J Neurosurg Spine. 2012;17(6):493–501.
79. Yue JJ, Garcia R, Blumenthal S. Five-year results of a randomized controlled trial for lumbar artificial discs in single-level degenerative disc disease. Spine (Phila Pa 1976). 2017;17(10):S70.
80. Zigler J, Ferko N, Cameron C, Patel L. Comparison of therapies in lumbar degenerative disc disease: a network meta-analysis of randomized controlled trials. J Comp Eff Res. 2018;7(3):233–46.
81. Le Huec JC, Mathews H, Basso Y, et al. Clinical results of maverick lumbar total disc replacement: two-year prospective follow-up. Orthop Clin North Am. 2005;36(3):315–22.
82. Gornet MF, Burkus JK, Dryer RF, Peloza JH. Lumbar disc arthroplasty with maverick disc versus stand-alone interbody fusion: a prospective, randomized, controlled, multicenter investigational device exemption trial. Spine. 2011;36(25):E1600–11.
83. Sasani M, Oktenoğlu T, Tuncay K, Canbulat N, Carilli S, Ozer FA. Total disc replacement in the treatment of lumbar discogenic pain with disc herniation: a prospective clinical study. Turk Neurosurg. 2009;19(2):127–34.
84. Guyer RD, Pettine K, Roh JS, et al. Five-year follow-up of a prospective, randomized trial comparing two lumbar total disc replacements. Spine. 2016;41(1):3–8.
85. Sasso RC, Foulk DM, Hahn M. Prospective, randomized trial of metal-on-metal artificial lumbar disc replacement: initial results for treatment of discogenic pain. Spine. 2008;33(2):123–31.
86. Putzier M, Funk JF, Schneider SV, et al. Charité total disc replacement–clinical and radiographical results after an average follow-up of 17 years. Eur Spine J. 2006;15(2):183–95.
87. Shim CS, Lee S, Maeng DH, Lee S-H. Vertical split fracture of the vertebral body following total disc replacement using ProDisc: report of two cases. J Spinal Disord Tech. 2005;18(5):465–9.
88. Sott AH, Harrison DJ. Increasing age does not affect good outcome after lumbar disc replacement. Int Orthop. 2000;24(1):50–3.
89. Chung SK, Kim YE, Wang K-C. Biomechanical effect of constraint in lumbar total disc replacement: a study with finite element analysis. Spine. 2009;34(12):1281–6.
90. Tortolani PJ, Cunningham BW, Eng M, McAfee PC, Holsapple GA, Adams KA. Prevalence of heterotopic ossification following total disc replacement. A prospective, randomized study of two hundred and seventy-six patients. J Bone Joint Surg Am. 2007;89(1):82–8.
91. Park S-J, Kang K-J, Shin S-K, Chung S-S, Lee C-S. Heterotopic ossification following lumbar total disc replacement. Int Orthop. 2011;35(8):1197–201.
92. McAfee PC, Cunningham BW, Devine J, Williams E, Yu-Yahiro J. Classification of heterotopic ossification (HO) in artificial disk replacement. J Spinal Disord Tech. 2003;16(4):384–9.
93. Schulte TL, Lerner T, Hackenberg L, Liljenqvist U, Bullmann V. Acquired spondylolysis after implantation of a lumbar ProDisc II prosthesis: case report and review of the literature. Spine. 2007;32(22):E645–8.
94. Siepe CJ, Mayer HM, Heinz-Leisenheimer M, Korge A. Total lumbar disc replacement: different results for different levels. Spine. 2007;32(7):782–90.
95. Aunoble S, Donkersloot P, Le Huec JC. Dislocations with intervertebral disc prosthesis: two case reports. Eur Spine J. 2004;13(5):464–7.
96. François J, Coessens R, Lauweryns P. Early removal of a Maverick disc prosthesis: surgical findings

and morphological changes. Acta Orthop Belg. 2007;73(1):122–7.

97. Zeh A, Planert M, Siegert G, Lattke P, Held A, Hein W. Release of cobalt and chromium ions into the serum following implantation of the metal-on-metal maverick-type artificial lumbar disc (Medtronic Sofamor Danek). Spine. 2007;32(3):348–52.
98. Gornet MF, Burkus JK, Harper ML, Chan FW, Skipor AK, Jacobs JJ. Prospective study on serum metal levels in patients with metal-on-metal lumbar disc arthroplasty. Eur Spine J. 2013;22(4):741–6.
99. Brau SA, Delamarter RB, Kropf MA, et al. Access strategies for revision in anterior lumbar surgery. Spine. 2008;33(15):1662–7.
100. Härtl R, Joeris A, McGuire RA. Comparison of the safety outcomes between two surgical approaches for anterior lumbar fusion surgery: anterior lumbar interbody fusion (ALIF) and extreme lateral interbody fusion (ELIF). Eur Spine J. 2016;25(5):1484–521.
101. Sasso RC, Kenneth Burkus J, LeHuec J-C. Retrograde ejaculation after anterior lumbar interbody fusion: transperitoneal versus retroperitoneal exposure. Spine. 2003;28(10):1023–6.
102. Tropiano P, Huang RC, Girardi FP, Cammisa FP, Marnay T. Lumbar total disc replacement. Surgical technique. J Bone Joint Surg Am. 2006;88(Suppl 1 Pt 1):50–64.
103. Carilli S, Sasani M, Ozer AF. Pitfalls of the anterior approach to lumbar vertebrae. WSJ. 2007;2(3):139–43.
104. Bertagnoli R, Yue JJ, Shah RV, et al. The treatment of disabling single-level lumbar discogenic low back pain with total disc arthroplasty utilizing the ProDisc prosthesis: a prospective study with 2-year minimum follow-up. Spine. 2005;30(19):2230–6.
105. Bertagnoli R, Yue JJ, Fenk-Mayer A, Eerulkar J, Emerson JW. Treatment of symptomatic adjacent-segment degeneration after lumbar fusion with total disc arthroplasty by using the prodisc prosthesis: a prospective study with 2-year minimum follow up. J Neurosurg Spine. 2006;4(2):91–7.
106. Adams C, McKinley K, Freeman BJC. Does total disc replacement reduce stress in the adjacent level disc when compared to fusion? A biomechanical study on the human cadaver lumbar spine. Eur Spine J. 2005;14(1):S12.
107. Graf H. Evaluation of the therapeutic effect of the Graf stabilisation system. Second meeting, European Spine Society, Rome, Italy. 1991.
108. Stoll TM, Dubois G, Schwarzenbach O. The dynamic neutralization system for the spine: a multi-center study of a novel non-fusion system. Eur Spine J. 2002;11(Suppl 2):S170–8.
109. Rohlmann A, Burra NK, Zander T, Bergmann G. Comparison of the effects of bilateral posterior dynamic and rigid fixation devices on the loads in the lumbar spine: a finite element analysis. Eur Spine J. 2007;16(8):1223–31.
110. Sengupta DK, Mulholland RC. Fulcrum assisted soft stabilization system: a new concept in the surgical treatment of degenerative low back pain. Spine (Phila Pa 1976). 2005;30(9):1019–29.
111. von Strempel A, Moosman D, Stoss C, Martin A. Stabilization of the degenerated lumbar spine in the non fusion technique with cosmic posterior dynamic system. World Spine J. 2006;1(1):40–7.
112. Niosi CA, Zhu QA, Wilson DC, Keynan O, Wilson DR, Oxland TR. Biomechanical characterization of the three-dimensional kinematic behaviour of the Dynesys dynamic stabilization system: an in vitro study. Eur Spine J. 2006;15(6):913–22.
113. Schmoelz W, Huber JF, Nydegger T, Claes L, Wilke HJ. Dynamic stabilization of the lumbar spine and its effects on adjacent segments: an in vitro experiment. J Spinal Disord Tech. 2003;16(4):418–23.
114. Schmidt H, Heuer F, Wilke HJ. Which axial and bending stiffnesses of posterior implants are required to design a flexible lumbar stabilization system? J Biomech. 2009;42(1):48–54.
115. Schulte TL, Hurschler C, Haversath M, Liljenqvist U, Bullmann V, Filler TJ, Osada N, Fallenberg EM, Hackenberg L. The effect of dynamic, semi-rigid implants on the range of motion of lumbar motion segments after decompression. Eur Spine J. 2008;17(8):1057–65.
116. Wilke HJ, Heuer F, Schmidt H. Prospective design delineation and subsequent in vitro evaluation of a new posterior dynamic stabilization system. Spine (Phila Pa 1976). 2009;34(3):255–61.
117. White A, Panjabi M. Physical properties and functional biomechanics of the spine in clinical biomechanics of the spine, chapter 1, Lippincott Williams & Wilkins, Philadelphia, 1990.
118. Perez-Orribo L, Zucherman JF, Hsu KY, Reyes PM, Rodriguez-Martinez NG, Crawford NR. Biomechanics of a posterior lumbar motion stabilizing device: in vitro comparison to intact and fused conditions. Spine (Phila Pa 1976). 2016;41(2):E55–63.
119. Bozkuş H, Senoğlu M, Baek S, Sawa AG, Ozer AF, Sonntag VK, Crawford NR. Dynamic lumbar pedicle screw-rod stabilization: in vitro biomechanical comparison with standard rigid pedicle screw-rod stabilization. J Neurosurg Spine. 2010;12(2):183–9.
120. Sengupta DK, Bucklen B, McAfee PC, Nichols J, Angara R, Khalil S. The comprehensive biomechanics and load-sharing of semirigid PEEK and semirigid posterior dynamic stabilization systems. Adv Orthop. 2013;2013:745610.
121. Oktenoglu T, Erbulut DU, Kiapour A, Ozer AF, Lazoglu I, Kaner T, Sasani M, Goel VK. Pedicle screw-based posterior dynamic stabilisation of the lumbar spine: in vitro cadaver investigation and a finite element study. Comput Methods Biomech Biomed Eng. 2015;18(11):1252–61.
122. Erbulut DU, Kiapour A, Oktenoglu T, Ozer AF, Goel VK. A computational biomechanical investigation of posterior dynamic instrumentation: combination of dynamic rod and hinged (dynamic) screw. J Biomech Eng. 2014;136(5):051007.

123. Cook DJ, Yeager MS, Thampi SS, Whiting DM, Cheng BC. Stability and load sharing characteristics of a posterior dynamic stabilization device. Int J Spine Surg. 2015;9:9.
124. Sengupta D, Bucklen B, Ingalhalikar A, Muzumdar A, Khalil S. Does semi-rigid instrumentation using both flexion and extension dampening spacers truly provide an intermediate level of stabilization? Adv Orthop. 2013;2013:738252.
125. Yu AK, Siegfried CM, Chew B, et al. Biomechanics of posterior dynamic fusion systems in the lumbar spine: implications for stabilization with improved arthrodesis. J Spinal Disord Tech. 2016;29:E325–30.
126. Lin HM, Pan YN, Liu CL, Huang LY, Huang CH, Chen CS. Biomechanical comparison of the K-ROD and Dynesys dynamic spinal fixator systems—a finite element analysis. Biomed Mater Eng. 2013;23(6):495–50.
127. Shih SL, Liu CL, Huang LY, Huang CH, Chen CS. Effects of cord pretension and stiffness of the Dynesys system spacer on the biomechanics of spinal decompression—a finite element study. BMC Musculoskelet Disord. 2013;14:191.
128. Schmoelz W, Onder U, Martin A, von Strempel A. Non-fusion instrumentation of the lumbar spine with a hinged pedicle screw rod system: an in vitro experiment. Eur Spine J. 2009;18(10):1478–85.
129. Chien CY, Tan CH, Lu TH, Lin SC, Chuang WH, Chiang MC, Luh YP, Chen YJ. Pretension effects of the Dynesys cord on the tissue responses and screw-spacer behaviors of the lumbosacral construct with hybrid fixation. Spine (Phila Pa 1976). 2013;38(13):E775–82.
130. Strauss PJ, Novotny JE, Wilder DG, Grobler LJ, Pope MH. Multidirectional stability of the Graf system. Spine (Phila Pa 1976). 1994;19(8):965–72.
131. Madan S, Boeree NR. Outcome of the Graf ligamentoplasty procedure compared with anterior lumbar interbody fusion with the Hartshill horseshoe cage. Eur Spine J. 2003;12(4):361–8.
132. Hashimoto T, Oha F, Shigenobu K, Kanayama M, Harada M, Ohkoshi Y, Tada H, Yamamoto K, Yamane S. Mid-term clinical results of Graf stabilization for lumbar degenerative pathologies. A minimum 2-year follow-up. Spine J. 2001;1(4):283–9.
133. Grevitt MP, Gardner AD, Spilsbury J, Shackleford IM, Baskerville R, Pursell LM, Hassaan A, Mulholland RC. The Graf stabilisation system: early results in 50 patients. Eur Spine J. 1995;4(3):169–75. discussion 135.
134. Askar Z, Wardlaw D, Muthukumar T, Smith F, Kader D, Gibson S. Correlation between intervertebral disc morphology and the results in patients undergoing Graf ligament stabilisation. Eur Spine J. 2004;13:714–8.
135. Kanayama M, Hashimoto T, Shigenobu K. Rationale, biomechanics, and surgical indications for Graf ligamentoplasty. Orthop Clin N Am. 2005;36(3):373–7.
136. Reyes-Sánchez A, Zárate-Kalfópulos B, Ramírez-Mora I, Rosales-Olivarez LM, Alpizar-Aguirre A, Sánchez-Bringas G. Posterior dynamic stabilization of the lumbar spine with the Accuflex rod system as a stand-alone device: experience in 20 patients with 2-year follow-up. Eur Spine J. 2010;19(12):2164–70.
137. Luo L, Zhang C, Zhou Q, Zhao C, Wang L, Liang L, Tu B, Ouyang B, Gan Y. Effectiveness of Transpedicular dynamic stabilization in treating Discogenic low Back pain. World Neurosurg. 2018;111:e192–8.
138. Akyoldas G, Cevik OM, Suzer T, Sasani M, Oktenoglu T, Ozer AF. Dynamic stabilization of the lumbar spine using the Dynesys® system. Turk Neurosurg. 2020;30(2):190–3.
139. Oktenoglu T, Ozer AF, Sasani M, Kaner T, Canbulat N, Ercelen O, Sarioglu AC. Posterior dynamic stabilization in the treatment of lumbar degenerative disc disease: 2-year follow-up. Minim Invasive Neurosurg. 2010;53(3):112–6.
140. Ozer AF, Oktenoglu T, Egemen E, Sasani M, Yilmaz A, Erbulut DU, Yaman O, Suzer T. Lumbar single-level dynamic stabilization with semi-rigid and full dynamic systems: a retrospective clinical and radiological analysis of 71 patients. Clin Orthop Surg. 2017;9(3):310–6.
141. von Strempel A. Dynamische dorsale Stabilisierung mit dem Cosmic-System. Orthop Traumatol. 2010;22:561–72.
142. Pham MH, Mehta VA, Patel NN, Jakoi AM, Hsieh PC, Liu JC, Wang JC, Acosta FL. Complications associated with the Dynesys dynamic stabilization system: a comprehensive review of the literature. Neurosurg Focus. 2016;40(1):E2.
143. Chaichana KL, Bydon M, Santiago-Dieppa DR, Hwang L, McLoughlin G, Sciubba DM, Wolinsky JP, Bydon A, Gokaslan ZL, Witham T. Risk of infection following posterior instrumented lumbar fusion for degenerative spine disease in 817 consecutive cases. J Neurosurg Spine. 2014;20(1):45–52.
144. Fang A, Hu SS, Endres N, Bradford DS. Risk factors for infection after spinal surgery. Spine (Phila Pa 1976). 2005;30(12):1460–5.
145. Olsen MA, Mayfield J, Lauryssen C, Polish LB, Jones M, Vest J, Fraser VJ. Risk factors for surgical site infection in spinal surgery. J Neurosurg. 2003;98(2 Suppl):149–55.
146. Olsen MA, Nepple JJ, Riew KD, Lenke LG, Bridwell KH, Mayfield J, Fraser VJ. Risk factors for surgical site infection following orthopaedic spinal operations. J Bone Joint Surg Am. 2008;90(1):62–9.
147. Putzier M, Schneider SV, Funk J, Perka C. Die Anwendung eines dynamischen Pedikelschraubensystems (DYNESYS) bei lumbalen Segmentdegenerationen—in Vergleich klinischer und radiologischer Ergebnisse bei unterschiedlichen Indikationen [application of a dynamic pedicle screw system (DYNESYS) for lumbar segmental degenerations—comparison of clinical and radiological results for different indications]. Z Orthop Ihre Grenzgeb. 2004;142(2):166–73. (Ger)

148. Dickman CA, Fessler RG, MacMillan M, Haid RW. Transpedicular screw-rod fixation of the lumbar spine: operative technique and outcome in 104 cases. J Neurosurg. 1992;77(6):860–70.
149. Esses SI, Sachs BL, Dreyzin V. Complications associated with the technique of pedicle screw fixation. A selected survey of ABS members. Spine (Phila Pa 1976). 1993;18(15):2231–8. discussion 2238–9.
150. Matsuzaki H, Tokuhashi Y, Matsumoto F, Hoshino M, Kiuchi T, Toriyama S. Problems and solutions of pedicle screw plate fixation of lumbar spine. Spine (Phila Pa 1976). 1990;15(11):1159–65.
151. Suda K, Ito M, Abumi K, Haba H, Taneichi H, Kaneda K. Radiological risk factors of pseudoarthrosis and/or instrument breakage after PLF with the pedicle screw system in isthmic spondylolisthesis. J Spinal Disord Tech. 2006;19(8):541–6.
152. Yahiro MA. Comprehensive literature review. Pedicle screw fixation devices. Spine (Phila Pa 1976). 1994;19(20 Suppl):2274–8.
153. Yuan HA, Garfin SR, Dickman CA, Mardjetko SM. A historical cohort study of pedicle screw fixation in thoracic, lumbar, and sacral spinal fusions. Spine (Phila Pa 1976). 1994;19(20 Suppl):2279–96.
154. Ko CC, Tsai HW, Huang WC, Wu JC, Chen YC, Shih YH, Chen HC, Wu CL, Cheng H. Screw loosening in the Dynesys stabilization system: radiographic evidence and effect on outcomes. Neurosurg Focus. 2010;28(6):E10.
155. Freudiger S, Dubois G, Lorrain M. Dynamic neutralisation of the lumbar spine confirmed on a new lumbar spine simulator in vitro. Arch Orthop Trauma Surg. 1999;119(3–4):127–32.
156. Schaeren S, Broger I, Jeanneret B. Minimum four-year follow-up of spinal stenosis with degenerative spondylolisthesis treated with decompression and dynamic stabilization. Spine (Phila Pa 1976). 2008;33(18):E636–42.
157. Park P, Garton HJ, Gala VC, Hoff JT, McGillicuddy JE. Adjacent segment disease after lumbar or lumbosacral fusion: review of the literature. Spine (Phila Pa 1976). 2004;29(17):1938–44.
158. Radcliff KE, Kepler CK, Jakoi A, Sidhu GS, Rihn J, Vaccaro AR, Albert TJ, Hilibrand AS. Adjacent segment disease in the lumbar spine following different treatment interventions. Spine J. 2013;13(10):1339–49.
159. Lawrence BD, Wang J, Arnold PM, Hermsmeyer J, Norvell DC, Brodke DS. Predicting the risk of adjacent segment pathology after lumbar fusion: a systematic review. Spine (Phila Pa 1976). 2012;37(22 Suppl):S123–32.
160. Radcliff K, Curry P, Hilibrand A, Kepler C, Lurie J, Zhao W, Albert TJ, Weinstein J. Risk for adjacent segment and same segment reoperation after surgery for lumbar stenosis: a subgroup analysis of the spine patient outcomes research trial (SPORT). Spine (Phila Pa 1976). 2013;38(7):531–9.
161. Lad SP, Babu R, Baker AA, Ugiliweneza B, Kong M, Bagley CA, Gottfried ON, Isaacs RE, Patil CG, Boakye M. Complications, reoperation rates, and health-care cost following surgical treatment of lumbar spondylolisthesis. J Bone Joint Surg Am. 2013;95(21):e162.
162. Ciol MA, Deyo RA, Kreuter W, Bigos SJ. Characteristics in Medicare beneficiaries associated with reoperation after lumbar spine surgery. Spine (Phila Pa 1976). 1994;19(12):1329–34.
163. Hu RW, Jaglal S, Axcell T, Anderson G. A population-based study of reoperations after back surgery. Spine (Phila Pa 1976). 1997;22(19):2265–70.
164. Jansson KA, Németh G, Granath F, Blomqvist P. Spinal stenosis re-operation rate in Sweden is 11% at 10 years—a national analysis of 9,664 operations. Eur Spine J. 2005;14(7):659–63.
165. Malter AD, McNeney B, Loeser JD, Deyo RA. 5-year reoperation rates after different types of lumbar spine surgery. Spine (Phila Pa 1976). 1998;23(7):814–20.
166. Martin BI, Mirza SK, Comstock BA, Gray DT, Kreuter W, Deyo RA. Reoperation rates following lumbar spine surgery and the influence of spinal fusion procedures. Spine (Phila Pa 1976). 2007;32(3):382–7.
167. Taylor VM, Deyo RA, Ciol M, Kreuter W. Surgical treatment of patients with back problems covered by workers compensation versus those with other sources of payment. Spine (Phila Pa 1976). 1996;21(19):2255–9.
168. Taylor VM, Deyo RA, Goldberg H, Ciol M, Kreuter W, Spunt B. Low back pain hospitalization in Washington state: recent trends and geographic variations. J Spinal Disord. 1995;8(1):1–7.
169. Ciplak NM, Suzer T, Senturk S, Yaman O, Sasani M, Oktenoglu T, Yilmaz A, Erbulut DU, Özer AF. Complications of 2-level dynamic stabilization: a correlative clinical and radiological analysis at two-year follow-up on 103 patients. Turk Neurosurg. 2018;28(5):756–62.
170. Wiltse LL, Bateman JG, Hutchinson RH, et al. The paraspinal sacrospinalis-splitting approach to the lumbar spine[J]. J Bone Joint Surg Am. 1968;50(5):919–26.
171. Cho BY, Murovic J, Park KW, Park J. Lumbar disc rehydration postimplantation of a posterior dynamic stabilization system. J Neurosurg Spine. 2010;13:576–80.
172. Bordes-Monmeneu M, Bordes-Garcia V, Rodrigo-Baeza F, Saez D. Sistema de neutralización dinámica en la coluna lumbar. SISTEMA DYNESYS. Experiencia en 94 casos [System of dynamic neutralization in the lumbar spine: experience on 94 cases]. Neurocirugia (Astur). 2005;16(6):499–506. (Spanish)
173. Yilmaz A, Senturk S, Sasani M, Oktenoglu T, Yaman O, Yildirim H, Suzer T, Ozer AF. Disc rehydration after dynamic stabilization: a report of 59 cases. Asian Spine J. 2017;11(3):348–55.
174. Ozer AF, Goel VK, Alanay A, Sasani M, Oktenoglu T, Erbulut D. Posterior transpedicular dynamic sys-

tems in the treatment of chronic lumbar instability. Adv Orthop. 2013;2013:432520.

175. Oktenoglu T, Hekimoglu M, Aydin AL, Sasani M, Cerezci O, Ozer AF. Kyphoplasty with posterior dynamic stabilization in the surgical treatment of unstable thoracolumbar osteoporotic vertebral compression fractures. Turk Neurosurg. 2021;31(6):924–30.
176. Di Silvestre M, Lolli F, Bakaloudis G, Parisini P. Dynamic stabilization for degenerative lumbar scoliosis in elderly patients. Spine (Phila Pa 1976). 2010;35(2):227–34.
177. Di Silvestre M, Lolli F, et al. Adult's degenerative scoliosis: midterm results of dynamic stabilization without fusion in elderly patients-is it effective? Adv Orthop. 2013;2013:1.
178. Lee SE, Jahng TA, Kim HJ. Decompression and nonfusion dynamic stabilization for spinal stenosis with degenerative lumbar scoliosis: clinical article. J Neurosurg Spine. 2014;21(4):585–94.
179. Cienciala J, Chaloupka R, Repko M, Krbec M. Osetrení degenerativního onemocnení bederní pátere metodou dynamické neutralizace systémem Dynesys [Dynamic neutralization using the Dynesys system for treatment of degenerative disc disease of the lumbar spine]. Acta Chir Orthop Traumatol Cechoslov. 2010;77(3):203–8. (Czech)
180. Hu Y, Gu YJ, Xu RM, Zhou LJ, Ma WH. Short-term clinical observation of the Dynesys neutralization system for the treatment of degenerative disease of the lumbar vertebrae. Orthop Surg. 2011;3(3):167–75.
181. Sapkas G, Mavrogenis AF, Starantzis KA, Soultanis K, Kokkalis ZT, Papagelopoulos PJ. Outcome of a dynamic neutralization system for the spine. Orthopedics. 2012;35(10):e1497–502.
182. Schwarzenbach O, Berlemann U. Dynamische dorsale Stabilisierung mithilfe des Pedikelschrauben-systems DYNESYS® [dynamic posterior stabilization with the pedicle screw system DYNESYS®]. Oper Orthop Traumatol. 2010;22(5–6):545–57. (Ger)
183. Welch WC, Cheng BC, Awad TE, Davis R, Maxwell JH, Delamarter R, Wingate JK, Sherman J, Macenski MM. Clinical outcomes of the Dynesys dynamic neutralization system: 1-year preliminary results. Neurosurg Focus. 2007;22(1):E8.
184. Yang M, Li C, Chen Z, Bai Y, Li M. Short term outcome of posterior dynamic stabilization system in degenerative lumbar diseases. Indian J Orthop. 2014;48(6):574–81.
185. Schnake KJ, Schaeren S, Jeanneret B. Dynamic stabilization in addition to decompression for lumbar spinal stenosis with degenerative spondylolisthesis. Spine (Phila Pa 1976). 2006;31(4):442–9.
186. Putzier M, Schneider SV, Funk JF, Tohtz SW, Perka C. The surgical treatment of the lumbar disc prolapse: nucleotomy with additional transpedicular dynamic stabilization versus nucleotomy alone. Spine (Phila Pa 1976). 2005;30(5):E109–14.
187. Payer M, Smoll NR, Oezkan N, Tessitore E. Dynamic transpedicular stabilisation and decompression in single-level degenerative anterolisthesis and stenosis. Acta Neurochir. 2014;156(2):221–7.
188. Yu SW, Yang SC, Ma CH, Wu CH, Yen CY, Tu YK. Comparison of Dynesys posterior stabilization and posterior lumbar interbody fusion for spinal stenosis L4L5. Acta Orthop Belg. 2012;78(2):230–9.

8 Anesthesia in Lumbar Dynamic Stabilization Surgeries

Mete Manici

Pain in lumbar disc herniations is described as lower back pain radiating to the leg. Mixter and Barr performed the first successful discectomy operation in 1934 [1, 2]. Strempel developed the first dynamic screw in 1999. The increasingly complex surgical procedures have necessitated advancements in anesthesia techniques and drug development. However, in spinal surgeries, anesthesia management should be carefully evaluated as a process that encompasses the intraoperative and postoperative periods, taking into consideration all neurological, cardiovascular, and respiratory system issues accompanying the surgery. Additionally, an anesthetist may face challenges such as significant blood loss, prolonged surgery, position-related complications, and difficulties in pain control, depending on the magnitude of the surgery.

A comprehensive preoperative assessment, informing the patient, and obtaining their consent enable the anticipation of all issues that may arise during surgery. Enhanced Recovery After Surgery (ERAS) is a concept that involves a contemporary, evidence-based perioperative care approach, encompassing multimodal strategies aimed at reducing hospital stay and complications. These protocols, which promote faster recovery, increased patient satisfaction, shorter hospital stays, and reduced healthcare expenditures, are commonly employed in spinal surgery today [3].

Considering all these factors, a comprehensive preoperative assessment in thoracic spine surgeries is crucial. Safe perioperative management extending throughout the operation and even into the post-discharge period is highly important for the secure completion of the procedure. This necessitates a harmonious and collaborative effort between the surgical and anesthesia teams, ensuring the safety of the entire process, lasting from the operation period to the patient's discharge.

8.1 Preoperative Assessment

Patients should undergo a detailed anesthesia examination in advance of surgery. First of all, it is crucial to establish a connection with the patient, answer their questions, provide information about the surgery, and obtain their consent. Completion of consultations, organization of blood and blood products, and intensive care are of utmost importance for reducing intraoperative and postoperative complications.

Assessing mouth opening and neck movements during the preoperative period will prepare us for potential difficulties in managing the airway. Patients with borderline lung functions may require postoperative ventilator support. Consultation should be sought for potential cardiovascular complications.

M. Manici (✉)
Koc University School of Medicine, Istanbul, Turkey
e-mail: mmanici@kuh.ku.edu.tr

A. F. Özer et al. (eds.), *Dynamic Lumbar Spine Stabilization*,
https://doi.org/10.1007/978-3-032-12122-6_8

Considering the high risk of bleeding during surgery in these patients, an adequate reserve of blood and blood products should be prepared. It should be noted that the use of nonsteroidal analgesics for pain management can lead to bleeding disorders. Perioperative assessment and prophylaxis should also be conducted for deep vein thrombosis that may occur due to prolonged bed rest.

At this stage, a decision should be made on whether premedication will be administered and which agents will be used. It is known that administering 600 mg of gabapentin before surgery reduces postoperative pain scores and provides mild sedation [4]. For preoperative anxiety, oral administration of 0.5 mg alprazolam or 5 mg diazepam the night before the operation (0.05–0.2 mg/kg) is highly effective. The amnestic and sedative effects of midazolam can be utilized by administering it intravenously just before the surgery.

All preexisting medical conditions of patients should be documented at this stage. All procedures to be applied to the patient must be explained in detail, information must be provided, and consents must be obtained.

8.2 Monitoring

All patients, as in other surgeries, should be monitored according to the standards accepted by the American Society of Anesthesiology (ASA), including a minimum pulse oximeter, EKG, arterial blood pressure, capnography, and body temperature. Patients with comorbidities or predicted bleeding during surgery may require more invasive monitoring. Arterial cannulation, an invasive monitoring method, can be used to assess blood pressure without being dependent on position, and blood gas sampling can be performed to evaluate the current hemodynamic status. Application of a large central venous line is a necessary intervention for rapid transfusion and for providing inotropic support through infusion. Monitoring body temperature is essential because a decrease can affect intraoperative blood loss and neurophysiological monitoring.

Especially in spine surgeries, neurological monitoring is necessary to reduce spinal surgical injury. The simplest methods for evaluating spinal cord functions and nerve root damage include somatosensory-evoked potentials (SSEP), motor-evoked potentials (MEP), arousal testing, and electromyography (EMG). Anesthetic agents can suppress SSEP signals. In the absence of neurological monitoring techniques, the incidence of postoperative motor deficits or paraplegia after correcting scoliosis ranges from 3.7% to 6.9%, while it can be reduced to 0.5% with intraoperative monitoring. Surgical injury or hemodynamic changes can lead to neuronal damage. SSEP and MEP monitoring are stated to be useful tools in monitoring spinal cord perfusion and physiological status.

8.3 Premedication and Induction

An appropriate dose of alprazolam or diazepam can be used as premedication one night before the surgery. Similarly, midazolam can be used for this purpose immediately before the operation. Gabapentin and pregabalin, started before the operation and continued afterward, are supportive for pain control. For the induction and maintenance of anesthesia, if there is no significant difficulty with the airway, an intravenous hypnotic (propofol (2.5 mg/kg), thiopental (3–5 mg/kg), or etomidate (0.1–0.4 mg/kg)) and a non-depolarizing neuromuscular blocker (rocuronium (0.6–1.2 mg/kg), vecuronium (0.08–0.1 mg/kg)) are administered to start. After intubation, anesthesia maintenance can continue in the form of inhaled or total intravenous anesthesia (TIVA). Preoperative prophylactic antibiotics are given at an appropriate time. Considering the postoperative bleeding risk in patients, routine use of low-molecular-weight heparin or low-dose warfarin is recommended. However, compression stockings and intermittent pneumatic compression devices (SCD) are routinely recommended for use.

Nausea and vomiting are significant anesthesia-related side effects that can impact patient comfort and the patient's metabolic state. For induction, dexamethasone or a 5-HT3 receptor antagonist at the end of the surgery is recommended in high-risk groups. Additionally, droperidol or metoclopramide may be suggested to prevent nausea and vomiting.

Hypothermia is a condition characterized by a decrease in body temperature associated with the stress response that disrupts patient stability and increases the risk of wound infection, blood loss, and metabolic disturbances during the perioperative period. To mitigate this condition, devices blowing heated air, heated intravenous fluids, and heated humidified gases should be used, and the patient's body temperature should be monitored throughout the entire perioperative period.

After spinal surgery, the infection rate has been shown to range from 0.4% to 12% in the literature. Risk factors for infection may include the patient's age, smoking, diabetes, a history of surgical infections, high body mass index, and chronic alcohol use. As antibiotic prophylaxis, a single dose of a first-generation cephalosporin is recommended [5].

8.4 Regional Anesthesia in Lumbar Dynamic Stabilization

Although studies have not conclusively demonstrated the superiority of general anesthesia over regional anesthesia techniques in vertebral surgery, there is evidence in research showing several advantages of regional anesthesia, including perioperative hemodynamic stability, reduced mortality, decreased intraoperative blood loss, decreased hospital stay, and decreased cognitive function impairment. Especially in the geriatric group, neuroaxial blocks have become increasingly preferred [6]. When deciding which anesthesia method to use, an appropriate anesthesia plan should be made, taking into account the patient, the planned surgery, and all other risks. Recently, the lumbar erector spinae plane block, included in the popular plane blocks, has been suggested for selected patients undergoing vertebral surgeries and can also be used in postoperative analgesia; however, further studies are recommended in this regard [7]. Regional anesthesia directly affects the spinal cord, causing a delay in somatosensory-evoked potentials. Therefore, it is contraindicated in monitored patients [8]. When deciding which anesthesia method to use in lumbar dynamic surgical operations, an appropriate anesthesia plan should be made, considering the patient and all other risks associated with the surgery.

8.5 Position

In lumbar dynamic stabilization surgeries, the patient's position is crucial for anesthesia. The patient is in a prone position. Intraoperative access to the airway is limited, and the head is fixed. While prioritizing corneal pressure and optic nerve damage, careful control should be maintained for all possible body pressure sores. It is vital for the patient to maintain a neutral position. Especially, preventing venous and lymphatic return from the prone position can lead to edema in the neck, face, and airway. Ensuring the eyes are carefully closed will prevent corneal damage. Properly placed pillows in the chest and abdomen area will ease abdominal and chest movements and facilitate mechanical ventilation.

8.6 Transfusion and Fluid Management

During dynamic stabilization surgery, fluid management has two main objectives: maintaining normovolemia and preventing a decrease in serum osmolality. Maintaining normovolemia aims to keep hemodynamics stable. Preventing a decrease in serum osmolality helps prevent the development of tissue edema [9].

In cases where a significant amount of blood loss is expected, central venous catheters should be placed if necessary. Cannulas should be securely fixed to prevent dislodgement in the prone position. The decision to invasively monitor arterial pressure should be made based on the planned operation, expected blood loss, patient comorbidities, and postoperative care. Surgeries related to spinal deformities are generally associated with large amounts of blood loss. To reduce blood loss, appropriate management of blood conservation strategies should be applied. Controlled hypotension has been used in the past to minimize blood loss. A decrease in systemic blood pressure reduces spinal perfusion pressure. Hypotension can lead to spinal ischemia even without spinal cord manipulation, resulting in neurological deficits and even blindness. Therefore, the potential risks of hypotension should be considered. Avoiding hypotension is crucial, and normotension should be carefully maintained with necessary fluid and blood replacements. Perioperative phlebotomy, hemodilution, and the administration of antifibrinolytics should be considered to reduce blood loss. It has been shown that a loading dose of 10–15 mg/kg of tranexamic acid, followed by an infusion of 1 mg/kg/h until skin closure, reduces intraoperative bleeding by 30% [10].

In recent years, the perioperative management of fluid therapy has gained significant importance with the use of Enhanced Recovery After Surgery (ERAS) protocols. The ERAS spine protocol is known to play a crucial role in achieving faster recovery, increasing patient satisfaction, reducing hospital stay, and lowering healthcare expenses.

8.7 Pain Control

In lumbar dynamic stabilization surgeries, pain control is of critical importance, and a multimodal pain management approach is the most suitable method for postoperative analgesia. Pain can hinder effective breathing in patients, increasing the risk of atelectasis. The use of high doses of narcotics to alleviate pain can lead to respiratory depression. Patient-controlled analgesia (PCA) devices prepared with intravenous opioids can be used to ensure that patients experience at least 48 hours of a pain-free period after surgery. In addition to intravenous opioid drugs, the use of nonsteroidal analgesics is known to reduce opioid consumption. Oral or intravenous acetaminophen has also been shown to reduce opioid consumption after surgery. Finally, studies have shown that starting gabapentin preoperatively and continuing it postoperatively reduces patients' pain scores and opioid consumption. However, the potential side effects, such as dizziness and sedation, should be considered. Local anesthetic infiltration is another method that can be used. Blocks such as the erector spinae plane block performed preoperatively can reduce postoperative pain. It is known that dexmedetomidine leads to less fentanyl consumption and a lower incidence of delirium, according to studies.

References

1. Barker FG. The Massachusetts General Hospital. Early history and neurosurgery to 1939. J Neurosurg. 1998;79:948–59.
2. Mixter WJ, Barr JS. Rupture of the intervertebral disc with involvement of the spinal canal. N Engl J Med. 1934;211:210–5.
3. Dagal A, Bellabarba C, Bransford R, et al. Enhanced perioperative care for major spine surgery. Spine (Phila Pa 1976). 2019;44:959–66.
4. Pandey CK, Navkar DV, Giri PJ, et al. Evaluation of the optimal preemptive dose of gabapentin for postoperative pain relief after lumbar diskectomy: a randomized, double-blind, placebo controlled study. J Neurosurg Anesthesiol. 2005;17(2):65–8.
5. Parchi PD, Evangelisti G, Andreani L, Girardi F, Darren L, Sama A, Lisanti M. Postoperative spine infections. Orthop Rev (Pavia). 2015;7(3):5900.
6. Lee JK, Park JH, Hyun SJ, Hodel D, Hausmann ON. Regional anesthesia for lumbar spine surgery: can it be a standard in the future? Neurospine. 2021;18(4):733–40.
7. Örükoğlu HU, İçli D, Aksu C, Cesur S, Kuş A, Gürkan Y. Erector spinae block for postoperative pain management in lumbar disc hernia repair. J Anesth. 2021;35(3):420–5.
8. Klasen J, Thiel A, Detsch O, et al. The effect of epidural and intravenous lidocaine on somatosensory evoked potentials after stimulation of the posterior tibialis nerve. Anesth Analg. 1995;81(2):332–7.
9. Bajwa SJS, Kulshresth A. Challenging aspects and implications for anaesthesia. J Spine Neurosurg. 2013;2(3):2–8.
10. Tejskal P, Trnka Š, Hrabálek L, Wanek T, Jablonský J, Novák V. Effects of Tranexamic acid on perioperative blood loss and wound hematoma development in lumbar spine surgery: a prospective randomized study. Acta Chir Orthop Traumatol Cechoslov. 2023;90(3):176–80.

Further Reading

Strempel AV, Moosmann D, Stoss C, Martin A. Stabilisation of the degenerated lumbar spine in the nonfusion technique with cosmic posterior dynamic-system. WSJ. 2006;1(1):40–7.

Nuwer MR, Dawson EG, Carlson LG, et al. Somatosensory evoked potential monitoring reduces neurological defcits after scoliosis surgery: results of a large multicenter study. Electroenceph Clin Neurophysiol. 1995;96:6–11.

Aydogan MS, Korkmaz MF, Ozgül U, Erdogan MA, Yucel A, Karaman A, et al. Pain, fentanyl consumption and delirium in adolescents after scoliosis surgery: dexmedetomidine vs midazolam. Paediatr Anaesth. 2013;23:446–52.

9 Posterior Dynamic Systems as Facet Replacement System

Hakan Bozkus

9.1 The Role of Lumbar Facet Joints

The zygapophyseal, or facet, joints are symmetrically positioned bilaterally posterolateral to the mid-sagittal plane within each functional spine unit (FSU), contributing significantly to the mechanical behavior of the spine. These facet joints are typically classified as diarthrodial synovial joints, characterized by low friction between the cartilaginous surfaces. This unique structure enables rotational and translational movements between adjacent vertebrae, limited by the extent of motion permitted by the capsular ligament. Within the FSU, the space between the upper vertebra's inferior facet surface and the lower vertebra's superior facet surface is referred to as the articular pillar. In a healthy spine, the articular pillars on both sides experience compression loads, while the capsular ligament functions to resist tensile forces.

Typically, the inclination angle between the lumbar facet joint surfaces ranges from 82° to 86° in the sagittal plane and 85° to 120° in the axial plane. Morphologically, the superior facet surface exhibits convexity, whereas the inferior facet surface is concave. Furthermore, the facet joint surfaces become increasingly vertically oriented from L1 to S1 [1]. This specific morphological characteristic grants the lumbar facet joints greater resistance against axial rotation and lateral bending motions while facilitating a wider range of flexion and extension movements.

Under normal conditions, the FSU maintains stability according to the three-column theory. The posterior column comprises the facet joints, facet capsules, laminae, pedicles, spinous processes, and interspinous ligaments [2].

Roughly 16–25% of the axial compressive loads experienced by the spine are borne by the posterior column, specifically through the facet force. Furthermore, the load transmitted through the facet joints tends to increase with the progression of intervertebral disc degeneration [3, 4]. Similarly, considering the physiological presence of lordosis in the lumbar region, studies have indicated that approximately 25% of the compressive loads directed toward the lumbar region are transferred to the posterior column when accounting for the gravity line [5].

When examining the force and pressure transmitted across the facet articular surfaces, varying outcomes arise due to different loading conditions and measurement techniques employed, primarily because the shape of the facet articular surfaces is nonuniform.

Notably, the following data have been documented: when applying a compressive load of 1000 N and a shear load ranging between 200 and 400 N using pressure-sensitive paper, pres-

H. Bozkus (✉)
American Outpatient Medical Center,
Istanbul, Turkey
e-mail: mhakanb@amerikanhastanesi.org

A. F. Özer et al. (eds.), *Dynamic Lumbar Spine Stabilization*,
https://doi.org/10.1007/978-3-032-12122-6_9

sure readings of 3.7 MPa at 4° of flexion and 6.1 MPa at 6° of extension were recorded [6]. Furthermore, employing a flat electroresistive pressure sensor array at a moment loading of 7.5 Nm (with ±600 N preload), facet forces of 4 N in flexion, 14 N in extension, 16 N in lateral bending, and 56 N in axial rotation were measured [7]. However, when utilizing the strain-gauge technique in the L1-2 FSU with a moment loading of 7.5 Nm in all directions and a 400 N compressive follower load, the facet loading results showed variability, with standard deviations being notably high. Nonetheless, the facet loading results aligned reasonably well with existing literature, particularly in sagittal plane movements [8].

The resection of the facet capsule enhances facet mobility. However, it is important to note that this resection does not lead to a significant alteration in measurements during extension, as there is no load exerted on the facet capsule. Nonetheless, when considering flexion, axial rotation, and lateral bending movements, the resection of the facet capsule becomes particularly significant [9].

The mechanical loading of facet joints triggers a cascade of mechanical, physiological, and chemical events within the facet joint tissues. These physiological responses are mediated through the mechanotransduction mechanism, operating at the cellular and molecular levels within the macroscopic tissues. However, if there is an imbalance or disruption in the mechanotransduction mechanism within the tissue, it can lead to dysfunction and degeneration of the facet joints [9].

When assessing the location of the instantaneous axis of rotation (IAR) during physiological movements within the lumbar FSU, distinct patterns emerge. In the sagittal plane, during flexion movement, the IAR is positioned on the anterior side of the intervertebral disc tissue, while during extension movement, it is situated on the posterior side, in close proximity to the facet joints. In the axial plane, the IAR is typically found within the central region of the intervertebral disc tissue during axial rotation. In the coronal plane, the IAR is positioned on the left side of the intervertebral disc tissue when the lateral bending movement is toward the right, and conversely, on the right side of the intervertebral disc tissue when the lateral bending movement is toward the left.

Therefore, the IAR is not a fixed point but is dynamically shifted during movement. Especially in cases of degeneration, trauma, or facetectomy that result in destabilization of the spine, the location of the IAR may change, and some stabilization techniques may need to be applied to restore the IAR to its original position when instability occurs.

Approximately, the range of flexion-extension motion in the lumbar region expands from 12° at the L1-2 level to 18° at L5-S1. Each segment allows for a rotational movement of approximately 3° in axial rotation and a lateral bending movement of around 7° [10].

Biomechanically, alterations in certain movement modes can occur when unilateral or bilateral facetectomy is performed to varying degrees.

Specifically, statistically significant increases in flexion movement are observed following unilateral partial facetectomy (involving more than 50% resection of the facet joint) and bilateral total facetectomy. On the other hand, axial rotation motion does not experience a significant increase following unilateral or bilateral partial facetectomy. However, axial rotation toward the opposite side is increased after unilateral total facetectomy. In cases of unilateral total facetectomy, the axial rotation movement toward the facetectomized side does not show an increase due to the preservation of facet joint integrity on the other side. In instances of bilateral total facetectomy, there is a significant increase in axial rotation movement in both directions, while extension and lateral bending movement do not display significant changes [11].

Hence, unilateral partial facetectomy (less than 50%) generally does not induce destabilization in the FSU, given that the supra/interspinous ligaments remain undamaged. Nonetheless, if there is preexisting segmental instability in the vicinity of the partial facetectomy, it may contribute to destabilization. It is important to consider that unilateral total facetectomy holds the potential for destabilizing the FSU [11].

Moreover, distinct biomechanical changes arise following laminectomy and resection of the supra/interspinous ligaments in multiple FSUs, depending on whether the lumbar facet joint is preserved or entirely removed. Complete removal of the lumbar facet joint has been found to significantly augment motion in all directions beyond the normal range. Following both surgical techniques, axial rotation demonstrates the highest susceptibility to instability, while lateral bending is the least affected. Additionally, both surgical techniques result in a forward shift of the IAR, with the shift being more prominent in cases of total facet joint removal. Consequently, the increased motion associated with the complete removal of the facet joint has the potential to heighten the predisposition of that segment to instability [12]. Comparable biomechanical changes have been corroborated through finite element model (FEM) studies [13, 14].

9.2 Lumbar Posterior Dynamic Systems

Posterior lumbar stabilization and fusion surgery is commonly employed for treating degenerative diseases, tumors, infections, and trauma affecting the lumbar region. While technological advancements have improved bone fusion rates, potential complications such as pseudarthrosis and, more commonly, adjacent segment disease (ASD) continue to be acknowledged. Pseudarthrosis is characterized by the absence of a solid bone fusion one year after surgery and can occur in approximately 15% or more cases following primary lumbar fusion surgery [15, 16]. ASD manifests as abnormal symptomatic changes, including disc herniation, lumbar instability, stenosis, or facet joint arthropathy, in segments neighboring the level of the successfully fused segment [17]. While ASD does not always present with clinical symptoms, it frequently manifests as back pain and/or radiculopathy [18]. Typically, ASD occurs in the segment above the fused level, known as the rostral segment. However, it can also manifest in the segment below, particularly following L4-5 fusion [19]. Additionally, it has been reported that in cases where there is preoperative degeneration in the adjacent segments to the one intended for fusion, additional surgical intervention may be necessary [20].

Posterior dynamic systems have been developed with the goal of stabilizing the FSU while preserving its physiological range of motion, thereby optimizing the IAR. Furthermore, these systems aim to distribute the load within the FSU, thereby mitigating stress accumulation on the instrumentation. By working on these principles, they also aim to minimize the risk of complications such as pseudarthrosis and ASD.

This chapter focuses specifically on pedicle screw-based systems, which are commonly utilized in posterior dynamic systems as an alternative to facet joints. It is important to note that interspinous devices and disc prostheses applied with a posterior approach are excluded from the scope of this discussion.

9.2.1 Graf Ligament

The Graf ligament (SEM Co, Mountrouge, France) is a system that employs an inelastic polyester ligament (dacriline) to connect rigid pedicle screws, aiming to address abnormal rotational instability within the FSU. These systems exert compression on the facet joints and restrict FSU motion to extension while allowing limited flexion. However, the use of this ligament may lead to significant narrowing of the lateral canal, orientation of the ligamentum flavum toward the spinal canal, and an increased lordotic curvature of the FSU (Fig. 9.1).

Moreover, in terms of load distribution within the FSU, the Graf ligament bears the load transmitted through the disc to the posterior annulus and facet joints, potentially contributing to disc degeneration [21, 22].

Application of the Graf ligament following in vitro laminectomy results in a notable limitation of flexion, extension, and lateral bending movements. Conversely, axial rotation movement demonstrates a significant increase of 107–132% compared to the normal range [23].

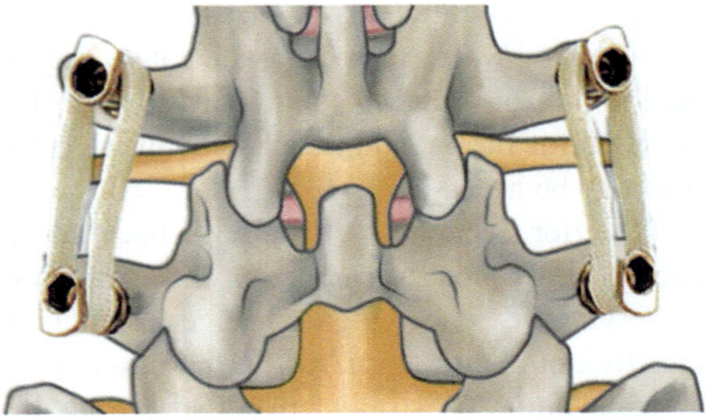

Fig. 9.1 The Graf ligament (SEM Co, Mountrouge, France) is a system that employs an inelastic polyester ligament (dacriline) to connect rigid pedicle screws, aiming to address abnormal rotational instability within the FSU. (Courtesy of Prof. Ali Fahir Özer)

In a published clinical series spanning a 10-year period and utilizing the Graf ligament, approximately 33% of patients experienced facet arthrodesis, while 7% developed ASD. It is important to note that this technique is not recommended for use in cases of degenerative scoliosis and laterolisthesis [24]. It is worth mentioning that no recent literature has been published regarding this technique since 2009 [25].

9.2.2 Dynamic Neutralization System (Dynesys)

Dynesys (Zimmer Spine, IN, US) is comprised of titanium pedicle screws (Protasul 100), polycarbonate-urethane (Sulene-PCU) tubing, and polyester (Sulene-PET) bands housed within these tubes. This system aims to provide mobility to the load within the FSU while ensuring stabilization. The tubes within the system restrict compression during extension, while the bands resist tension during flexion (Fig. 9.2).

Consequently, when the extensor muscles are engaged, the Dynesys system promotes segmental lordosis within the FSU and reduces the load transmitted through the disc, thus functioning predominantly as a load-bearing mechanism. Clinically, the Dynesys system has undergone extensive examination in the literature, with studies focusing on short- and medium-term results.

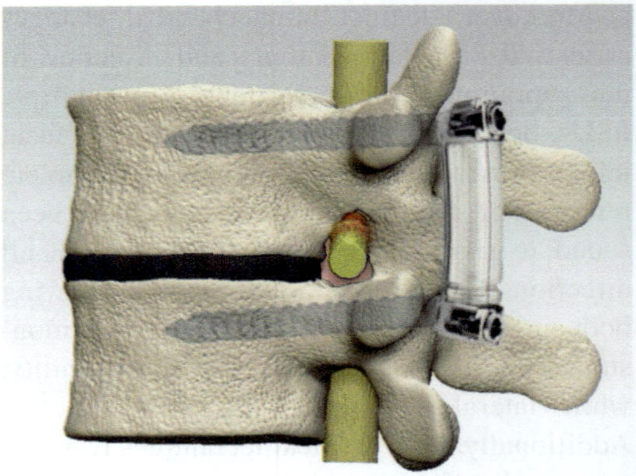

Fig. 9.2 Dynesys (Zimmer Spine, IN, US) is comprised of titanium pedicle screws (Protasul 100), polycarbonate-urethane (Sulene-PCU) tubing, and polyester (Sulene-PET) bands housed within these tubes. (Courtesy of Prof. Ali Fahir Özer)

These systems have been developed for use without fusion. In a comparison between patient groups who underwent lumbar microdiscectomy with and without the Dynesys system, it was reported that the group with the Dynesys system exhibited a halt in disc degeneration, attributed to the reduced load on the facet joints [26, 27]. Likewise, reports have indicated that the use of Dynesys systems can contribute to a reduction in the occurrence of ASD. Additionally, patients undergoing treatment with Dynesys systems may experience improved clinical recovery, as the absence of fusion requirements minimizes unnecessary tissue destruction [28, 29].

When the Dynesys system is applied in vitro after resection of the posterior ligaments, ligamentum flavum, facet capsules, and posterolateral nucleotomy, it results in a decrease in flexion and lateral bending movements compared to normal, while maintaining extension movement at a normal level. However, axial rotation movement increases beyond normal parameters. In comparison to rigid instrumentation, the Dynesys system exhibits a similar decrease in flexion movement but shows a greater increase in extension, lateral bending, and axial rotation movements compared to the normal range. There was no significant difference observed in the range of motion (ROM) and neutral zone at the adjacent segments between stabilization with both types of instrumentation [30].

When comparing the Dynesys system and rigid instrumentation in terms of their effect on intradiscal pressure, both stabilizations showed no significant difference in intradiscal pressure in neutral and flexion positions. However, a decrease in intradiscal pressure was observed with both types of instrumentation in the extension position. The increase in intradiscal pressure during flexion and the decrease during extension can be theoretically explained by the posterior displacement of the axis of rotation. There was no significant difference in intradiscal pressure at the adjacent segments between both types of stabilization [31].

In cases where the Dynesys system was applied at multiple distances, a significant increase in axial rotation was observed at the stabilized distance. When the Dynesys system was applied at two distances and anterior column support was added to the lower distance, the hybrid dynamic stabilization allowed for greater motion at the adjacent segments [32].

On the other hand, in an FEM study, it was observed that when the Dynesys system was applied with total facetectomy, flexion movement increased by 40% compared to normal, and axial rotation movement increased by 200% compared to normal. This significant increase in movement imposed higher stress on the implant, increasing the risk of implant failure [33]. Furthermore, approximately 19% of patients with the Dynesys system required revision surgery, indicating the importance of careful patient selection when considering the use of these systems [34, 35].

9.2.3 IsoBar TTL and AccuFlex Dynamic Rod Systems

In the IsoBar TTL (Scient'X, Beaurains, France) and AccuFlex (Globus Medical, PA, US) rod systems, the titanium rods between the pedicle screws offer flexibility and facilitate load sharing with the anterior column. In the case of IsoBar, the disc-shaped compressed titanium located in the middle of the rod functions as a shock absorber. In an FEM study involving the IsoBar TTL system, it was observed that when a rigid and dynamic IsoBar TTL rod was applied to the L4-5 segment after L5-S1 fusion, the maximum stress in the adjacent segment (L3-4) decreased by 5.5% during flexion with dynamic stabilization (Fig. 9.3).

However, it increased by 17% at the L4-5 level. Furthermore, the decrease in rod stiffness and the increase in axial rotation motion indicate that the IAR is maintained in its physiological position at the stabilized segment [36].

In the AccuFlex system, the presence of helical incisions in the middle of the rod allows for its semi-rigid behavior (Fig. 9.4).

However, it is important to consider that over time, tissue may enter these spiral incisions, potentially hindering the rod's functioning. Both systems have been approved by the FDA as fusion facilitators. In terms of single-level lumbar fusion patients who received the AccuFlex system, their outcomes were comparable to those who received rigid rods. On the other hand, when used independently in patients who underwent

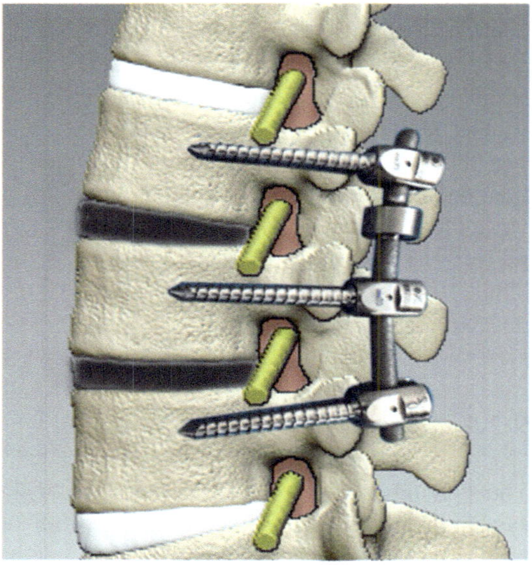

Fig. 9.3 In the IsoBar TTL (Scient'X, Beaurains, France), the titanium rods between the pedicle screws offer flexibility and facilitate load sharing with the anterior column, and the disc-shaped compressed titanium located in the middle of the rod functions as a shock absorber. (Courtesy of Prof. Ali Fahir Özer)

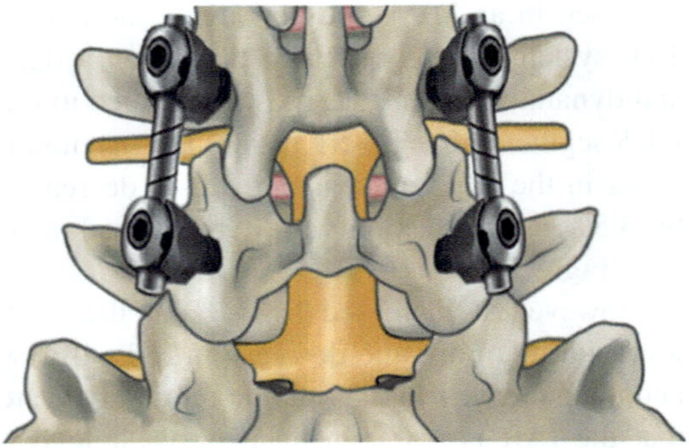

Fig. 9.4 In the AccuFlex system, the presence of helical incisions in the middle of the rod allows for its semi-rigid behavior. (Courtesy of Prof. Ali Fahir Özer)

lumbar decompression without fusion, clinical improvement was reported in 83% of patients, although hardware fatigue was detected in approximately 22% of cases during the 2-year follow-up period [37, 38].

9.2.4 Stabilimax NZ Rod System

The Stabilimax NZ (Applied Spine Technologies Inc., CT, US) rod system was designed with dual concentric springs and incorporated a ball-and-socket joint on each end, enabling dynamization at the rod and rod screw junction. Biomechanical studies, including both cadaveric and FEM analyses, have demonstrated its ability to restore neutral zone motion in both normal and destabilized spines [39]. However, despite undergoing FDA review, the company decided to terminate the clinical application of this product, leading to its discontinuation.

9.2.5 PercuDyn System

The PercuDyn (Interventional Spine, CA, US) system comprises a pedicle anchor with a polycarbonate-urethane stabilizer, which acts as a mechanical stop between the inferior and superior facets to enhance the stiffness of the facet column (Fig. 9.5).

Bilateral fixation with this system provides stabilization during extension and lateral bending movements, while reducing the load on the facet joints and intradiscal pressure through the use of the tampon. In patients with lumbar discogenic pain associated with facet pain and spinal stenosis, significant clinical improvement of around 70% was observed in the early period. However, it is important to note that approximately 10% of patients required revision surgery, and in the long term, 46% of patients reported clinically unsuccessful outcomes [40, 41].

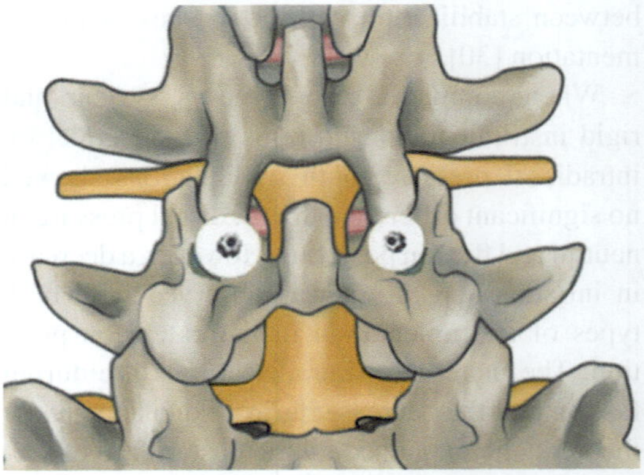

Fig. 9.5 The PercuDyn (Interventional Spine, CA, US) system comprises a pedicle anchor with a polycarbonate-urethane stabilizer, which acts as a mechanical stop between the inferior and superior facets to enhance the stiffness of the facet column. (Courtesy of Prof. Ali Fahir Özer)

9.2.6 PEEK Rod Systems

The CD-Horizon Legacy PEEK rod (Medtronic Sofamor Danek, TN, US) has received FDA approval for use in spinal surgery as a supplement to single-level interbody fusion. Unlike titanium rods, PEEK rods are designed to facilitate load sharing between spinal segments. PEEK (polyetheretherketone) is a fully biocompatible and inert semi-crystalline thermoplastic polymer with minimal toxicity. It possesses a modulus of elasticity that falls between that of cortical and cancellous bone, significantly lower than that of titanium [42].

The modulus of elasticity for titanium rods (Ti, Ti6Al4V alloy), which are commonly used in spine surgery, is 114 GPa, whereas the modulus of elasticity for PEEK is 3.2 GPa. When evaluating the pedicle screw-rod system made of these two materials under a 400 N axial compression load, the Ti rod carries 266.8 N of load, while the PEEK rod carries 109.8 N of load. In terms of the load transmitted through the facets, the Ti rod allows 71% of the load to pass through the facets, whereas the PEEK rod allows 33% of the load to pass through the facets. These results indicate that rigid rod systems experience higher stress due to carrying a greater load, while dynamic or semi-rigid rod systems can potentially experience less stress by distributing the load [43, 44].

In an FEM study that simulated L4-5 cage fusion using a Ti rod and a PEEK rod, it was observed that PEEK rod stabilization increased the risk of cage subsidence and cage damage while promoting fusion. Additionally, the use of a PEEK rod was associated with a higher risk of rod breakage but a lower risk of screw breakage [45].

An in vivo animal study involving PEEK rod application demonstrated increased bone fusion around the screw; however, it did not enhance screw-bone integration. Therefore, based on these findings, the potential risk of screw loosening should be taken into consideration in clinical practice [46].

In a recent systematic review and meta-analysis, it was found that patients in clinical series who received PEEK rods had statistically significantly better outcomes in terms of ODI, JOA, and VAS scores, as well as bone fusion rates, compared to those who received Ti rods [47]. Additionally, in patients with single-level lumbar degenerative disc disease who underwent Dynesys with a PEEK rod and dynamic pedicle screw combination without fusion, similar successful clinical and radiological results were observed [48].

9.2.7 Dynamic Pedicle Screws

This type of pedicle screw is designed to allow a certain degree of flexion and extension movements in the sagittal plane. Biomechanical studies conducted with these screws have demonstrated their effectiveness. For instance, in a T12-L5 calf spine model, L2-4 stabilization was performed using both types of screws after creating a highly unstable segment with L3-4 discectomy, facetectomy, and laminectomy. The results showed that both screws stabilized flexion and extension by 65% and lateral bending by 90% compared to normal in the L3-4 segment. However, they only provided close-to-normal stabilization in axial rotation movement [49]. In another study using a T10-L4 human cadaver model, T12-L2 stabilization was performed using 0°, ±5°, and ±10° movable screw types in an unstable model created by performing L1 anterior wedge-style resection. The findings indicated that rigid pedicle screws provide more stabilization than dynamic pedicle screws in flexion and extension. On the other hand, dynamic pedicle screws offer near-normal stabilization in all ranges of motion and allow movement in the FSU [50].

When investigating the changes in intra-disc pressure using dynamic and rigid pedicle screws, an L1-5 pig cadaver model was utilized. Stabilization was performed at the L2-4 two-distance level, and pressure values were examined in both the stabilized disc distance and adjacent disc levels under flexion-compression cyclic loading (24,000 cycles/5 Hz). The dynamic pedicle screw used in this study allowed ±15° movement in the sagittal plane. In the stabilized L2-3 cranial segment, the intra-disc pressure increased 9.1 times more than normal with the use of a rigid system, while this increase was 6.8 times with the dynamic system. At the L3-4 distance (caudal level), the increase in intradiscal pressure was 2.7 times higher than normal with the rigid system and 1.7 times higher than normal with the dynamic system. In this experimental model, the intra-disc pressure at the adjacent segments L1-2 and L4-5 without stabilization was found to be significantly higher when the rigid system was used compared to the dynamic system. These findings suggest that dynamic pedicle screw systems result in less increase in disc pressure at adjacent disc levels, potentially reducing the risk of disc degeneration [51].

Cosmic (Ulrich Medical, Ulm, Germany) and Safinaz (Medikon Medikal, Ankara, Turkey) screw systems are examples of dynamic pedicle screw systems that are currently used in clinical practice (Fig. 9.6).

The clinical application of dynamic pedicle screws has shown favorable outcomes in conditions such as degenerative disc disease, spinal stenosis, recurrent disc herniation, and painful segmental instability [52–57]. However, it is important to note that in patients undergoing surgery with both dynamic screws at two distances, complications such as ASD, screw breakages, and screw loosening have been reported. These complications may be attributed to the rigid behavior of these screw systems [58].

In the FEM study comparing Dynesys and Cosmic systems, the rigid system was applied to the L4-5 level in the L1-S1 model, while both systems were separately applied in the transition region at L3-4. It was observed that the Cosmic screw and rigid rod provided better protection and restricted movement of the intervertebral disc and facet joints in the transitional segment, whereas Dynesis allowed movement in this segment. Both systems were shown to cause distortion in the adjacent segments (L1-2, L2-3, L5-S1). Moreover, the study demonstrated a higher risk of screw pullout and fatigue failure due to the high stress distribution in Cosmic screws. Based on these findings, it is recommended to use Cosmic screws in severe degenerative conditions within the transitional segment, while the Dynesys system is more suitable for application in healthy discs or cases of mild degeneration [59].

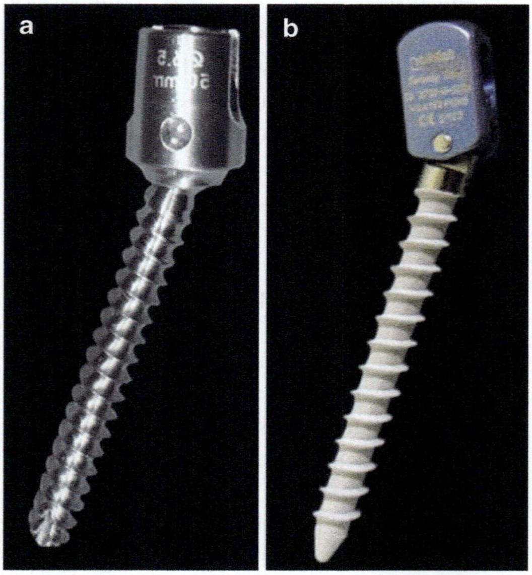

Fig. 9.6 This type of pedicle screw is designed to allow a certain degree of flexion and extension movements in the sagittal plane. (**a**) Safinaz Screw (without hydroxyapatite) (**b**) Cosmic Screw (coated by hydroxyapatite)

In the first biomechanical study using Safinaz, another dynamic screw, the effects of dynamic and rigid pedicle screw stabilization and load sharing were examined in an L3-S1 human cadaver model after L4-5 discectomy. Strain-gauge technology was utilized to measure the strain in the system. The dynamic pedicle screw used in the experiment allowed ±10° movement in the sagittal plane and ±1° movement in the axial plane. In this experimental model, bilateral L4-5 discectomy was performed, involving the removal of the ligamentum flavum, posterior longitudinal ligament, and a maximum amount of disc tissue, while preserving the anterior longitudinal ligament, facet joints and capsules, laminae, and interspinous ligament. The study demonstrated that dynamic screws provided a 30% greater reduction in the range of motion in the FSU compared to normal, while still allowing an average of 160% more motion in flexion, extension, lateral bending, and axial rotation than rigid pedicle screws. On the other hand, it was found that the axial loading and bending moment borne by the rod in the rigid pedicle screw-rod system were significantly higher than in the dynamic pedicle screw-rod system. During flexion, the dynamic pedicle screw-rod system experiences approximately 40% less axial compressive load compared to the rigid system. However, during extension, both systems bear an equal load. Both systems demonstrate a posterior shift of the IAR of approximately 1 cm compared to the normal spine. Notably, the dynamic pedicle screw-rod system redistributes the load passing through the FSU, whereas the rigid pedicle screw-rod system concentrates the load on the system itself [60].

Initially, dynamic pedicle screws were used in conjunction with rigid rods. However, in clinical practice, they are now often combined with certain dynamic rods, such as the PEEK rod.

Unilateral dynamic pedicle screws, combined with either rigid or dynamic rods, have emerged as a viable treatment option for unilateral total facetectomy procedures. This approach offers clinically adequate stability and proves to be a cost-effective alternative, with the potential to protect against ASD [61]. However, further comprehensive biomechanical studies are necessary to enhance our understanding of this subject.

9.2.8 Posterior Lumbar Facet Replacement and Arthroplasty Systems

In patients with facet tropism, facet hypertrophy, facet arthropathy, and spinal stenosis, surgical treatment often involves partial or full laminectomy and facetectomy to alleviate back and leg pain. While decompression and/or fusion procedures lead to clinical improvement, rigid stabilization and solid fusion may result in decreased spinal motion and ASD.

To address these concerns, it is crucial for these systems to establish strong connections with both the cranial and caudal spinal distances. Since fusion is not employed, these systems must be designed to seamlessly integrate and replicate the natural motion of facet joints at the treated segment.

9.2.9 Anatomic Facet Replacement System

The Anatomic Facet Replacement System (AFRS, Facet Solutions Inc., UT, US) was specifically designed to be anatomically compatible with facet morphology.

This system utilizes conventional titanium pedicle screw fixation to secure the superior and inferior facet implants, which are connected via cross-linking members to provide stability. The implant is made from a cobalt-chromium-molybdenum alloy. Furthermore, the surface of the implant that interacts with the bone is coated with titanium plasma and hydroxyapatite to promote increased bone growth.

In the in vitro cadaveric and FEA study of the AFRS, a bilateral total facetectomy was performed at the L4-5 level in the L3-S1 model to simulate destabilization. It was shown that AFRS can restore the range of motion and intradiscal pressure under physiologic loads to approximate the intact spine. The screw-to-bone interface stress with AFRS was found to be minimal, indicating the potential for lasting hardware stability [62].

In an Investigational Device Exemption (IDE) study conducted under the supervision of the FDA, AFRS was applied to 390 patients, and the clinical outcomes were reported as a viable alternative to posterolateral fusion and instrumentation. The first 2- and 4-year results of 213 randomly selected patients indicated promising clinical results for the AFRS treatment option [63].

In the literature, there have been reported cases of tissue reaction and neurological deterioration occurring approximately 2 years after the implantation of AFRS due to cobalt allergy [64]. These cases have raised concerns regarding the possibility of metal-on-metal facet replacement devices, including AFRS, releasing fine debris that may trigger an immune reaction and ultimately result in implant failure.

9.2.10 Total Facet Arthroplasty System

The Total Facet Arthroplasty System (TFAS; Archus Orthopedics Inc., WA, US) consists of cephalad "L"-shaped stems secured to a caudal bearing system that allows for motion. The bearing system resembles a sphere sliding along a curved plate. The construct is anchored via pegs passing into the vertebral body along the same course as traditional pedicle screws and is secured using polymethyl methacrylate bone cement. It is

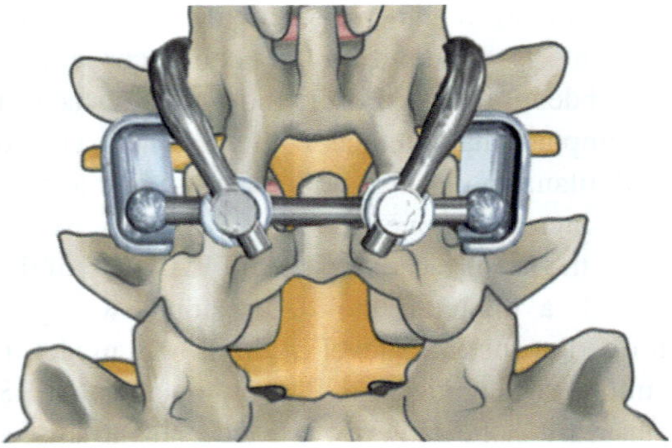

Fig. 9.7 The bearing system resembles a sphere sliding along a curved plate. The construct is anchored via pegs passing into the vertebral body along the same course as traditional pedicle screws and is secured using polymethyl methacrylate bone cement. (Courtesy of Prof. Ali Fahir Özer)

composed of implant-grade metal and is offered in a range of sizes to accommodate the specific anatomy of each patient (Fig. 9.7).

Several biomechanical studies conducted on human cadaveric models have indicated that TFAS allows for normal spinal motion and maintains normal disc pressure following wide decompressive laminectomy and bilateral facetectomy [65–68].

In a clinical prospective study with a follow-up period of approximately 4 years, clinical improvement was observed in a limited number of patients. However, it is important to note that degeneration occurred in both the treated segment and adjacent segments [69].

Furthermore, a case report documented TFAS fracture occurring at 9 and 27 months postoperatively, leading to the need for salvage operation through an anterior approach [70].

Overall, while TFAS has shown promise in terms of providing normal spinal motion and disc pressure, its potential for segmental and ASD, as well as the risk of implant fracture, should be carefully considered and closely monitored in clinical practice.

Unfortunately, due to financial difficulties, the phase 3 randomized controlled IDE clinical trial (NCT00418197) for TFAS could not be completed, and the initial results of the trial have not been published.

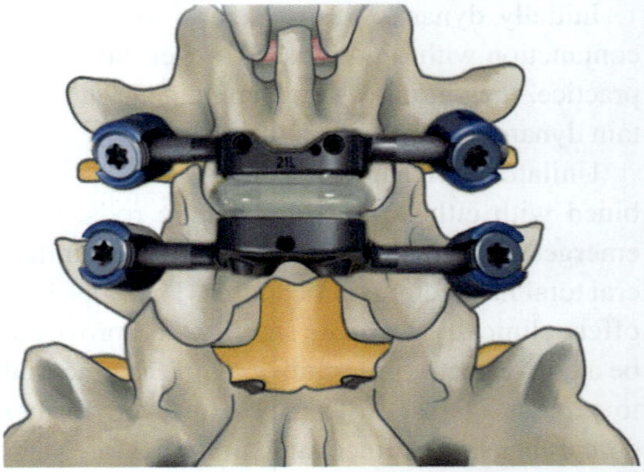

Fig. 9.8 Total posterior arthroplasty system (TOPS, Premia Spine, PA, US) is a unitary device consisting of titanium plates connected by a polycarbonate-urethane (PCU) articulating core. The plates have protrusion arms that are secured to cephalad and caudal vertebrae with pedicle screws. (Courtesy of Prof. Ali Fahir Özer)

9.2.11 Total Posterior Arthroplasty System

Total posterior arthroplasty system (TOPS, Premia Spine, PA, US) is a unitary device consisting of titanium plates connected by a polycarbonate-urethane (PCU) articulating core. The plates have protrusion arms that are secured to cephalad and caudal vertebrae with pedicle screws, which are coated with hydroxyapatite to promote bony ingrowth. The PCU core provides a limited range of motion to the construct but also absorbs shock, decreasing load transfer to adjacent spinal levels and to the implant-bone interface, lowering the risk of construct failure. Moreover, it covers articulating surfaces, preventing the release of possible debris from wear (Fig. 9.8).

In a human cadaveric study involving the TOPS system, it was observed that when applied following laminectomy and bilateral facetectomy, it preserved the normal ROM in the treated segment and did not significantly impact the motion of adjacent segments. This preservation of ROM was attributed to the system's ability to distribute the load in conjunction with the natural intervertebral disc [71].

A comparison of the biomechanical behavior between the TOPS system and the Dynesys system revealed notable differences. When the Dynesys system was utilized, the ROM in flexion, extension, and lateral bending movements was restricted. However, with the application of the TOPS system, the ROM in these movements was preserved, closely resembling the normal range. Additionally, an evaluation of the moment exerted on the screws demonstrated that the Dynesys system experienced 56% higher forces in flexion-extension and 86% higher forces in lateral bending compared to the TOPS system [72].

In a multicenter prospective pilot study, 29 patients diagnosed with spinal stenosis and/or spondylolisthesis at the L4-5 level demonstrated clinical improvement after one year of undergoing the TOPS procedure. Furthermore, no instances of radiologic hardware malfunction were detected [73].

In a nonrandomized prospective clinical study, the outcomes of 10 patients who received the TOPS procedure were evaluated after 11 years. All patients experienced clinical improvement, demonstrating the efficacy of the intervention. However, it should be noted that one patient exhibited asymptomatic spinal canal stenosis in the adjacent segment. Additionally, except for one patient, no device malfunctions were reported. The patient who experienced hardware failure at an early stage underwent a subsequent posterolateral fusion procedure to address the issue [74].

A phase 3 clinical trial (NCT00405691) evaluating the effectiveness of TOPS versus pedicle screw in patients with moderate or severe spinal stenosis between L3-5 and undergoing posterolateral spinal fusion has been conducted. However, the results of this trial have not yet been reported [75].

9.3 Conclusion

In order to address the limitations of spinal fusion, such as reduced motion and the risk of ASD, several dynamic implants based on posterior pedicle screws have been developed over the past two decades. These implants offer potential for motion preservation. Additionally, some of these systems can be combined with rigid stabilization, creating hybrid systems. Ongoing biomechanical studies and clinical trials are evaluating the effectiveness of these systems compared to each other and traditional posterior spinal fusion surgery. When considering the application of these systems, factors such as appropriate patient selection, cost-effectiveness, and ease of surgical application should be taken into account.

References

1. Panjabi MM, Oxland T, Takata K, Goel V, Duranceau J, Krag M. Articular facets of the human spine. Qzuantitative three-dimensional anatomy. Spine. 1993;18(10):1298–310.
2. Denis F. Spinal instability as defined by the three-column spine concept in acute spinal trauma. Clin Orthop Relat Res. 1984;189:65–76.
3. Yang KH, King AI. Mechanism of facet load transmission as a hypothesis for low back pain. Spine. 1984;9(6):557–65.
4. Adams MA, Hutton WC. The effect of posture on the role of the apophyseal joints in resisting intervertebral compressive force. J Bone Joint Surg. 1980;62 [Br]:358–62.
5. Pal GP, Routal RV. Transmission of weight through the lower thoracic and lumbar regions of the vertebral column in man. J Anat. 1987;152:93–105.
6. Dunlop RB, Adams MA, Wc H. Disc space narrowing and the lumbar facet joints. J Bone Jt Surg Br. 1984;66(5):706–10.
7. Niosi CA, Wilson DC, Zhu QA, Keynan O, Wilson DR, Oxland TR. The effect of dynamic posterior stabilization on facet joint contact forces: an in-vitro investigation. Spine. 2008;33(1):19–26.
8. Sawa AG, Crawford NR. The use of surface strain data and a neural networks solution method to determine lumbar facet joint loads during in vitro spine testing. J Biomech. 2008;41(12):2647–53.
9. Jaumard NV, Welch WC. Spinal facet joint biomechanics and mechanotransduction in normal, injury and degenerative conditions. J Biomech Eng. 2011;133:1–31.
10. Panjabi MM, Oxland TR, Yamamoto I, Crisco JJ. Mechanical behavior of the human lumbar and lumbosacral spine as shown by three-dimensional load-dissplacement curves. J Bone Joint Surg Am. 1994;76A:413–24.
11. Abumi K, Panjabi MM, Kramer KM, Duranceau J, Oxland T, Crisco JJ. Biomechanical evaluation of lumbar spinal stability after graded facetectomies. Spine. 1990;15:1142–7.

12. Detwiler PW, Spetzler CB, Taylor SB, Crawford NR, Porter RW, Sonntag VKH. Biomechanical comparison of facet-sparing laminectomy and Christmas tree laminectomy. J Neurosurg Spine. 2003;99(2 Suppl):214–20.
13. Lee KK, Teo EC. Effects of laminectomy and facetectomy on the stability of the lumbar motion segment. Med Eng Phys. 2004;26:183–92.
14. Zander T, Rohlmann A, Klöckner C, Bergmann G. Influence of graded facetectomy and laminectomy on spinal biomechanics. Eur Spine J. 2003;12:427–34.
15. Larsen JM, Capen DA. Pseudarthrosis of the lumbar spine. J Am Acad Orthop Surg. 1997;5:153–62.
16. Turner JA, Ersek M, Herron L, Haselkorn J, Kent D, Ciol MA, Deyo R. Patient outcomes after lumbar spinal fusions. JAMA. 1992;268:907–11.
17. Park P, Garton HJ, Gala VC, Hoff JT, McGillicuddy JE. Adjacent segment disease after lumbar or lumbosacral fusion: review of the literature. Spine. 2004;29:1938–44.
18. Etebar S, Cahill DW. Risk factors for adjacent-segment failure following lumbar fixation with rigid instrumentation for degenerative instability. J Neurosurg. 1999;90(2 Suppl):163–9.
19. Mashaly H, Paschel EE, Khattar NK, Goldschmidt E, Gerszten PC. Posterior lumbar dynamic stabilization instead of arthrodesis for symptomatic adjacent-segment degenerative stenosis: description of a novel technique. Neurosurg Focus. 2016;40(1):E5.
20. Putzier M, Hoff E, Tohtz S, Gross C, Perka C, Strube P. Dynamic stabilization adjacent to single-level fusion: part II. No clinical benefit for asymptomatic, initially degenerated adjacent segments after 6 years follow-up. Eur Spine J. 2010;19:2181–9.
21. Grevitt MP, Gardner AD, Spilsbury J, Shackleford IM, Baskerville R, Pursell LM, Hassaan A, Mulholland RC. The Graf stabilisation system: early results in 50 patients. Eur Spine J. 1995;4:169–75.
22. Mulholland RC, Sengupta DK. Rationale, principles and experimental evaluation of the concept of soft stabilization. Eur Spine J. 2002;2(11 Suppl):S198–205.
23. Strauss PJ, Novotny JE, Wilder DG, Pope MH. Multidirectional stability of Graf system. Spine. 1994;19(8):965–72.
24. Kanayama M, Hashimoto T, Shigenobu K, Togawa D, Oha F. A minimum 10-year follow-up of posterior dynamic stabilization using Graf artificial ligament. Spine. 2007;32(18):1992–6.
25. Nagano A, Miyamoto K, Nishimoto H, Hosoe H, Suzuki N, Shimizu K. Transforaminal lumbar interbody fusion for failed Graf ligamentoplasty: a report of two cases. J Orthop Surg. 2009;17(2):220–2.
26. Putzier M, Schneider SV, Funk JF, Tohtz SW, Perka C. The surgical treatment of the lumbar disc prolapse: nucleotomy with additional transpedicular dynamic stabilization versus nucleotomy alone. Spine. 2005;30(5):E109–14.
27. Stoll TM, Dubois G, Schwarzenbach O. The dynamic neutralization system for the spine: a multi-center study of a novel non-fusion system. Eur Spine J. 2002;2(11 Suppl):S170–8.
28. Nohara H, Kanaya F. Biomechanical study of adjacent intervertebral motion after lumbar spinal fusion and flexible stabilization using polyethylene-terephthalate bands. J Spinal Disord Tech. 2004;17:215–9.
29. Welch WC, Cheng BC, Awad TE, Davis R, Maxwell JH, Delamarter RD, Wingate JK, Sherman J, Macenski MM. Clinical outcomes of the Dynesys dynamic neutralization system: 1-year preliminary results. Neurosurg Focus. 2007;22(1):E8.
30. Schmoelz W, Huber JF, Nydegger T, Claes L, Wilke HJ. Dynamic stabilization of the lumbar spine and its effects on adjacent segments: an in vitro experiment. J Spinal Disord Tech. 2003;16:418–23.
31. Schmoelz W, Huber JF, Nydegger T, Claes L, Wilke HJ. Influence of a dynamic stabilization system on load bearing of bridged disc: an in vitro study of intradiscal pressure. Eur Spine J. 2006;15:1276–85.
32. Cheng BC, Gordon J, Cheng J, Welch WC. Immediate biomechanical effects of lumbar posterior dynamic stabilization above a circumferential fusion. Spine. 2007;32:2551–7.
33. Kiapour A, Ambati D, Hoy RW, Goel VK. Effect of graded facetectomy on biomechanics of Dynesys dynamic stabilization system. Spine. 2012;37(10):E581–9.
34. Grob D, Benini A, Junge A, Mannion AF. Clinical experience with the Dynesys semirigid fixation system for the lumbar spine: surgical and patient-oriented outcome in 50 cases after an average of 2 years. Spine. 2005;30(3):324–31.
35. Anand N, Baron EM. Role of Dynesys as pedicle-based nonfusion stabilization for degenerative disc disorders. Adv Orthop. 2012;2012:2183855.
36. Castellvi AE, Huang H, Vestgaarden T, Saigal S, Clabeaux DH, Pienkowski d. Stress reduction in adjacent level discs via dynamic instrumentation: a finite element analysis. Int J Spine Surg. 2007;1(2):74–81.
37. Mandigo CE, Sampath P, Kaiser MG. Posterior dynamic stabilization of the lumbar spine: pedicle-based stabilization with the AccuFlex rod system. Neursurg Focus. 2007;22(1):E9.
38. Reyes-Sanchez A, Zarate-Kalfopulos B, Ramirez-Mora I, Rosales—Olivarez LM, Alpizar-Aguirre A, Sanches-Bringas G. Posterior dynamic stabilization of the lumbar spine with Accuflex rod system as a stand-alone device: experience in 20 patients with 2-year follow-up. Eur Spine J. 2010;19(12):2164–70.
39. Panjabi MM, Timm JP. Development of Stabilimax NZ from biomechanical principles. SAS J. 2007;1:2–7.
40. Canero G, Carbone S. The results of a consecutive series of dynamic posterior stabilizations using the PercuDyn device. Eur Spine J Suppl. 2015;7:865–71.
41. Kareem H, Ulbricht C. A prospective long-term follow-up study of posteior dynamic stabilizing system to treat back pain associated with degenerative disc disease. Global Spine J. 2020;10(1):30–8.

42. Mayrogenis AF, Vottis C, Triantafyllopoulos G, Papagelopoulos PJ, Pneumaticos SG. PEEK rod systems for the spine. Eur J Orthop Surg Traumatol. 2014;24(Suppl 1):S111–6.
43. Highsmith JM, Tumialan LM, Rodts GE. Flexible rods and the case for dynamic stabilization. Neurosurg Focus. 2007;22(1):E11.
44. Ahn YH, Chen WM, Lee KY, Park KW, Lee SJ. Comparison of the load-sharing characteristics between pedicle-based dynamic and rigid rod devices. Biomed Mater. 2008;3(4):44101.
45. Fan W, Guo LX, Zhang M. Biomechanical analysis of lumbar interbody fusion supplemented with various posterior stabilization systems. Eur Spine J. 2021;30(8):2342–50.
46. Wu J, Shi L, Liu D, Wu Z, Gao P, Liu W, Li X, Guo Z. Evaluating screw stability after pedicle screw fixation with PEEK rods. Global Spine J. 2023;13(2):393–9.
47. Li W, Zhao H, Li C, Liu T, Guan J, Yang Y, Yu X. Polyetheretherketone (PEEK) rods versus titanium rods for posterior lumbar fusion surgery: a systematic review and meta-analysis. J Orthop Surg Res. 2023;18:348.
48. Ozer AF, Oktenoglu T, Egemen E, Sasani M, Yilmaz A, Erbulut DU, Yaman O, Suzer T. Lumbar single-level dynamic stabilization with semi-rigid and full dynamic systems: A retrospective clinical and radiological analysis of 71 patients. Clin Orthop Surg. 2017;9(3):310–6.
49. Scifert JL, Sairyo K, Goel VK, Grobler LJ, Grosland NM, Spratt KF, Chesmel KD. Stability analysis of an enhanced load sharing posterior fixation device and its equivalent conventional device in a calf spine model. Spine. 1999;24(21):2206–13.
50. Xu HZ, Wang XY, Chi YL, Zhu QA, Lin Y, Huang QS, Dai LY. Biomechanical evaluation of a dynamic pedicle screw fixation device. Clin Biomech. 2006;21(4):330–6.
51. Dath R, Sirkett DM, Gheduzzi S, Miles AW. Intradiscal pressure changes with dynamic pedicle screw systems. J Spinal Disord Tech. 2008;21(4):241–6.
52. Kaner T, Dalbayrak S, Oktenoglu T, Sasani M, Aydin AL, Ozer AF. Orthopedics. 2010;33(5):309.
53. Ozer AF, Crawford NR, Sasani M, Oktenoglu T, Bozkus H, Kaner T, Aydin S. Dynamic lumbar pedicle screw-rod stabilization: two- year follow-up and comparison with fusion. Open Orthop J. 2010;4:137–41.
54. Kaner T, Sasani M, Aydin AL, Ozer AF. Clinical outcomes of degenerative lumbar spinal stenosis treated with lumbar decompression and the cosmic "semi-rigid" posterior system. SAS J. 2010;4(4):99–106.
55. Kaner T, Sasani M, Oktenoglu T, Aydin AL, Ozer AF. Minimum two-year follow-up of cases with recurrent disc herniation treated with microdiscectomy and posterior dynamic transpedicular stabilization. Open Orthop J. 2010;4:120–5.
56. von Strampel A, Moosman D, Stoss C, Martin A. Stabilization of degenerated lumbar spine in the nonfusion technique with cosmic posterior dynamic system. World Spine J. 2006;1(1):40–7.
57. Stoffel M, Behr M, Reinke A, Stüer C, Ringel F, Meyer B. Pedicle screw-based dynamic stabilization. Of the thoracolumbar spine with the Cosmic-system: a prospective observation. Acta Neurochir. 2010;152(5):835–43.
58. Ciplak NM, Suzer T, Senturk S, Yaman O, Sasani M, Oktenoglu T, Yilmaz A, Erbulut DU, Ozer AF. Complications of 2-level dynamic stabilization: a correlative clinical and radiological analysis at two-year follow-up on 103 patients. Turk Neurosurg. 2018;28(5):756–62.
59. Chien CY, Kuo YJ, Lin SC, Chuang WH, Luh YP. Kinematic and mechanical comparisons of lumbar hybrid fixation using Dynesys and Cosmic systems. Spine. 2014;39(15):E878–84.
60. Bozkus H, Senoglu M, Baek S, Sawa AGU, Ozer AF, Sonntag VKH, Crawford NR. Dynamic lumbar pedicle screw-rod stabilization: in vitro biomechanical comparison with standard rigid pedicle screw-rod stabilization. J Neurosurg Spine. 2010;12(2):183–9.
61. Bozkus H, Sasani M, Oktenoglu T, Aydin AL, Ozer AF. Unilateral dynamic stabilization for unilateral lumbar spinal pathologies; a new surgical concept. Turk Neurosurg. 2012;22(6):718–23.
62. Goel VK, Mehta A, Jangra J, Faizan A, Kiapour A, Hoy RW, Fauth AR. Anatomic facet replacement system (AFRS) restoration of lumbar segment mechanics to intact: a finite element study and in vitro cadaver inverstigation. SAS J. 2007;1(1):46–54.
63. Myer J, Youssef JA, Rahn KA, Lorio MP, McKee DJ. ACADIA facet replacement system IDE study: preliminary outcomes at two-and four-years postoperative. Spine J. 2014;14(11):S160–1.
64. Goodwin ML, Spiker WR, Brodke DS, Lawrence BD. Failure of facet replacement system with metal-on-metal bearing surface and subsequent discovery of cobalt allergy: report of 2 cases. J Neurosurg Spine. 2018;29(1):81–4.
65. Philips FM, Tzermiadianos MN, Voronov LI, Havey RM, Carandang G, Renner SM, Rosler DM, Ochoa JA, Patwaardhan AG. Effect of the total facet arthroplasty system after complete laminectomy-facetectomy on the biomechanics of implanted and adjacent segments. Spine J. 2009;9(1):96–102.
66. Zhu Q, Larson CR, Sjovold SG, Rosler DM, Keynan O, Wilson DR, Cripton PA, Oxland TR. Biomechanical evaluation of the total facet arthroplasty system!: 3-dimensional kinematics. Spine. 2007;32(1):55–62.
67. Voronov LI, Havey RM, Rosler DM, Sjovold SG, Funk M, Carandang G, Zindrick D, Rosler DM, Patwaardhan AG. L5–S1 segmental kinematics after facet arthroplasty. Int J Spine Surg. 2009;3(2):50–8.
68. Sjovold SG, Zhu Q, Bowden A, Larson CR, Bakker PM, Villaraga ML, Ochoa JA, Rosler DM, Cripton PA. Biomechanical evaluation of the total facet arthroplasty system-(TFAS): loading as compared to a rigid posterior instrumentation system. Eur Spine J. 2012;21(8):1660–73.

69. Vermesan D, Prejbeanu R, Daliborca CV, Haragus H, Magureanu M, Marelli M, Promenzio L, Caprio M, Cagiano R, Tatullo M. A new device used in the restoration of kinematics after total facet arthroplasty. Med Devices (Auckl). 2014;7:157.
70. Palmer DK, Inceoglu S, Cheng WK. Stem fracture after total facet replacement in the lumbar spine: a report of two cases and review of the literature. Spine J. 2011;11(7):e15–9.
71. Wilke HJ, Schmidt H, Werner K, Werner S, Drumm J. Biomechanical evaluation of a new total posterior-element replacement system. Spine. 2006;31(24):2790–6.
72. Meyers K, Tauber M, Sudin Y, Fleischer S, Arnin U, Girardi F, Wright T. Use of instrumented pedicle screws to evaluate load sharing in posterior dynamic stabilization systems. Spine J. 2008;8(6):926–32.
73. McAfee P, Khoo LT, Pimenta L. Treatment of lumbar spinal stenosis with a total posterior arthroplasty prosthesis: implant description, surgical technique, and a prospective report on 29 patients. Neurosurg Focus. 2007;22(1):1–11.
74. Smorgick Y, Mirovsky Y, Floman Y, Rand N, Millgram M, Anekstein Y. Long-term results for total facet joint replacement in the management of lumbar degenerative spondylolisthesis. J Neurosurg Spine. 2019;4:1–6.
75. Gu BJ, Blue R, Yoon J, Welch WC. Posterior lumbar facet replacement and arthroplasty. Neurosurg Clin N Am. 2021;32:521–6.

10 Biomechanics of Posterior Dynamic Pedicular Stabilization Systems

Ali Fahir Özer, Deniz U. Erbulut, and Vijay K. Goel

10.1 Introduction

Lower back pain stands as a prevalent global health concern, affecting individuals across diverse demographics. Among its primary instigators lies the degeneration of intervertebral discs, often triggering a cascade of spinal disorders such as disc herniation, spondylolisthesis, spondylosis, and spinal stenosis. The manifestation of back pain commonly occurs when the posterior disc protrudes, exerting pressure on and impinging on nerve roots—a condition known as a herniated disc. Additionally, spinal stenosis, characterized by a narrowing of the spinal canal, can lead to nerve root impingement, exacerbating discomfort.

Vijay K. Goel died before publication of this work was completed.

A. F. Özer (✉)
Department of Neurosurgery,
Koc University School of Medicine,
Istanbul, Turkey

D. U. Erbulut
Herston Biofabrication Institute,
Metro North Hospital and Health Service,
Brisbane, QLD, Australia
e-mail: deniz.erbulut@health.qld.gov.au

V. K. Goel
Department of Bioengineering &
Orthopaedic Surgery,
University of Toledo,
Toledo, OH, USA
e-mail: goelshashi1@gmail.com

Treatment options for lower back pain vary depending on the severity of the case and encompass conservative measures or surgical techniques. Conservative treatments, including exercise regimens, medications, physiotherapy, and rehabilitation programs, are typically employed as initial interventions. Surgical treatment becomes a consideration for patients whose back pain significantly impedes daily activities and fails to respond to conservative therapies. Surgical methods may involve decompression with spinal fusion or nonfusion devices.

Spinal fusion, aided by rigid instrumentation, has emerged as a cornerstone in treating various spinal disorders since its introduction by Albee and Hibbs in 1911. The objective of fusion surgery is to achieve therapeutic goals while minimizing disruption to the normal structure and function of the spinal column [1, 2]. However, the use of rigid instrumentation has been associated with a notable amount of morbidity and complications, including adjacent disc degeneration. This phenomenon arises due to the immobility induced by fusion surgery, resulting in increased mechanical stress on adjacent segments and necessitating further interventions. Consequently, there has been a growing impetus to explore alternative procedures with novel concepts to address these concerns [3].

In recent times, posterior dynamic stabilization devices have emerged as a reliable alternative to fusion surgery and have garnered

A. F. Özer et al. (eds.), *Dynamic Lumbar Spine Stabilization*,
https://doi.org/10.1007/978-3-032-12122-6_10

increasing acceptance. These devices offer comparable benefits to fusion, including the preservation and safeguarding of intervertebral discs, earlier intervention, and minimally invasive techniques. The essence of dynamic stabilization lies in its focus on maintaining motion at the treated segment, thereby mitigating the risk of accelerated degeneration at adjacent levels—an issue of paramount concern in fusion surgeries, given the protective effects of ongoing segmental motion.

While dynamic stabilization has attracted considerable attention from researchers, the design of new spinal implant systems necessitates a cautious approach [4, 5]. Unlike fusion implants, which aim to provide stabilization until fusion occurs, dynamic stabilization systems must fulfill this role throughout the patient's lifetime [6]. Consequently, various posterior dynamic stabilization systems have been reported in the literature, primarily categorized as pedicle screw-based systems and posterior interspinous spacers. This paper provides a biomechanical evaluation of posterior spinal implants, offering insights into the biomechanical properties of several such devices.

10.2 Biomechanical Assessment of Dynamic Spinal Implants

The implantation of dynamic spinal implants inevitably alters segmental biomechanics, underscoring the importance of evaluating their effects on both treated and untreated spinal segments prior to clinical trials. This necessitates a comprehensive biomechanical evaluation of posterior dynamic stabilization systems, achievable through in vivo, in vitro, and finite element analysis (FEA) studies.

In vitro studies, utilizing spine specimens from humans or other species, play a pivotal role in biomechanical evaluation and should adhere to standardized protocols during specimen preparation and testing [7]. It is recommended to incorporate multi-spinal segments to encompass one free functional spinal unit (FSU) on each side of the implanted segment. Desired loads are then applied to the free end of the specimen, with motion data recorded accordingly. Two loading protocols—displacement control and flexibility control loading—are commonly employed, encompassing force loadings such as shear, pure moment, and complex loads.

Finite Element Analysis (FEA) plays a pivotal role in the biomechanical assessment of implants, offering insights into the structural analysis of both the implant and the bone, as well as their interactions. By simulating various loading scenarios, FE analysis provides a comprehensive understanding of load shearing, stresses, and strain within the construct of interest. This facilitates the prospective delineation of necessary parameters for the development of spinal implants, parameters that are not ascertainable through in vitro experimental studies alone. However, it is imperative to validate the finite element model through in vitro experimental studies to ensure its accuracy and reliability. Figure 10.1 illustrates the integration of in vitro

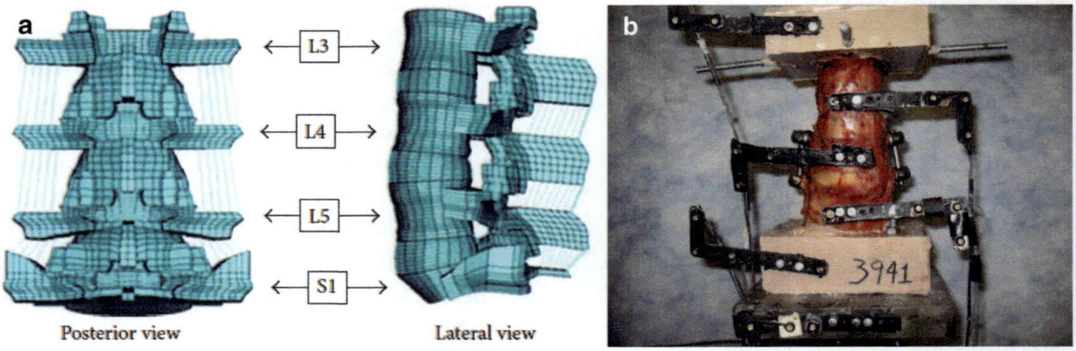

Fig. 10.1 (**a**) The finite element model of the lumbar spine. (Courtesy of Dr. Deniz Erbulut) and (**b**) the lumbar spine specimen equipped with a posterior dynamic stabilization system

cadaver studies and lumbar FE models, highlighting the complementary nature of these methodologies in advancing our understanding of spinal implant biomechanics.

10.3 Posterior Dynamic Stabilization Systems

10.3.1 Pedicle Screw-Based Stabilization Systems

The Dynesys, also known as the Dynamic Neutralization System for the Spine, represents a dynamic stabilization device offering an alternative approach to addressing degenerative lumbar disc issues (see Fig. 10.2a). First introduced in 1994 by Dubois et al. [8], the Dynesys functions as a pedicle screw-based system. Its primary objective is to serve as a flexible posterior spinal fixation system, aimed at either preserving intersegmental motions or reducing them to levels comparable to those observed in the intact spine, thereby mitigating adverse effects on adjacent segments. The Dynesys, a bilateral device, comprises titanium alloy pedicle screws and polycarbonate urethane (PCU) spacers surrounding tensioned polyethylene terephthalate (PET) cords [9].

Schmoelz et al. [10] conducted an in vitro study to assess the biomechanical impact of Dynesys on stabilization magnitudes at the treated segment. All six spines underwent testing across four stages: intact, with a defect in the middle segment, fixation with Dynesys, and fixation with an internal fixator. Cadavers were subjected to pure moments in three motion planes—flexion-extension, lateral bending, and axial rotation. Results demonstrated Dynesys' ability to stabilize the spine in the bridged segment, offering greater flexibility compared to the internal fixator. In a subsequent study under the same loading conditions, Schmoelz et al. [11] explored Dynesys' influence on the bridged intervertebral disc. Minimal alterations in disc load bearing were observed during axial rotation, while both devices provided adequate support to the anterior column, albeit slightly below the intact level, during flexion. Moreover, Dynesys showed no significant differences in intradiscal pressure compared to the internal fixator. Beastall

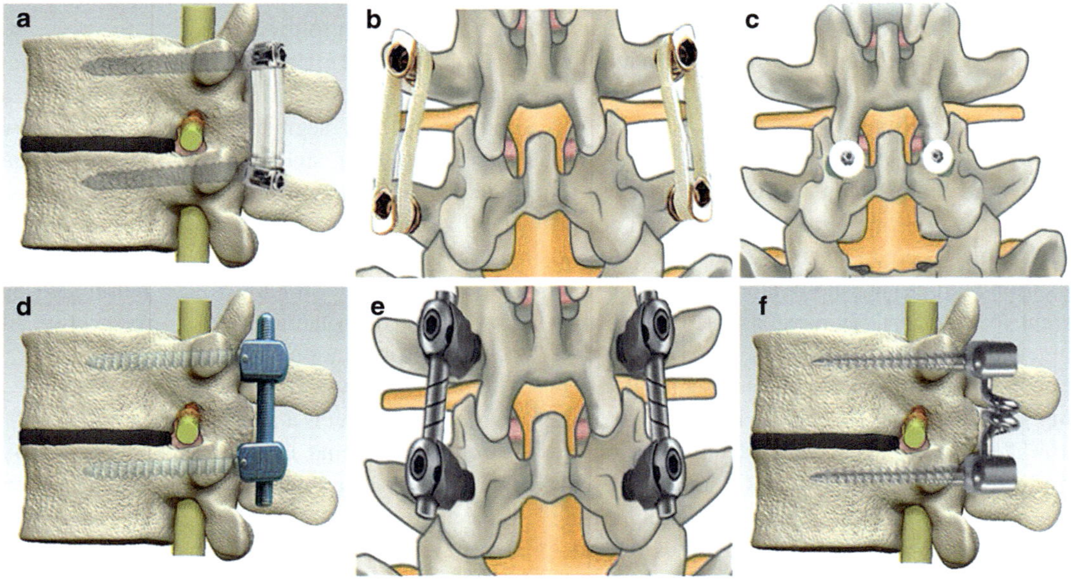

Fig. 10.2 Posterior dynamic stabilization systems illustrated include (**a**) Dynesys, (**b**) Graf system, (**c**) PercuDyn, (**d**) Cosmic, (**e**) AccuFlex, and (**f**) BioFlex. (Courtesy of Prof. Ali Fahir Özer)

et al. [12] investigated Dynesys' biomechanical effects on the lumbar spine, revealing a notable reduction in motion at the bridged segment post-implantation, without affecting the range of motion at the adjacent segment.

Biomechanical studies have revealed that certain posterior dynamic stabilization techniques exhibit comparable effects on flexion, extension, and lateral bending when compared to rigid instrumentation, owing to dynamic implants with high stiffness [4, 9, 10, 13, 14]. Recent research suggests that dynamic implants with lower stiffness may suffice to stabilize the spinal segment [13, 15]. Implants with minimal stiffness of 45 N/mm axially and 30 N/mm bending have been shown to reduce spinal flexibility by 30% of the intact range of motion, considered optimal for motion reduction [13]. Additionally, an optimal axial stiffness value of approximately 50 N/mm for longitudinal rods is recommended for effective pedicle screw-based dynamic implants [9]. For instance, studies have indicated that Dynesys (Dynesys-Zimmer, Minneapolis, MN, USA) exhibits higher stiffness than initially anticipated [10, 14]. However, posterior dynamic fixators with high stiffness may limit mobility in the treated segment, negating potential benefits. Conversely, dynamic rods with very low axial stiffness (<200 N/mm) have been shown to influence segmental kinematics and allow for increased mobility [9].

Schmoelz et al. [10] conducted an in vitro study on Dynesys' biomechanical impact, testing six spines across four stages: intact, with a middle segment defect, fixation with Dynesys, and fixation with an internal fixator. Cadavers underwent loading in flexion-extension, lateral bending, and axial rotation. Results indicated Dynesys effectively stabilized the bridged segment, offering greater flexibility than the internal fixator. In a related study [11], Dynesys' influence on the bridged intervertebral disc was examined, revealing minor alterations in disc load bearing during axial rotation. While both devices provided adequate support in flexion, Dynesys maintained intradiscal pressure levels comparable to the internal fixator. Additionally, Beastall et al. [12] explored Dynesys' impact on the lumbar spine, noting reduced motion at the bridged segment without affecting adjacent segment motion.

Biomechanical studies suggest that some posterior dynamic stabilization techniques mimic the effects of rigid instrumentation on spinal movement [4, 9, 10, 13, 14]. Recent research indicates that implants with lower stiffness may suffice for spinal stabilization [13, 15], with minimal stiffness of 45 N/mm axially and 30 N/mm bending reducing spinal flexibility by 30% [13]. Optimal axial stiffness for effective pedicle screw-based implants is around 50 N/mm [9]. Dynesys exhibits higher stiffness than anticipated [10, 14], while posterior dynamic fixators with high stiffness limit mobility, contrasting with dynamic rods with very low axial stiffness (<200 N/mm) that enhance segmental mobility [9].

Cosmic, from Ulrich GmbH & Co. KG, Ulm, Germany, is a posterior dynamic stabilization system using pedicle screws for nonrigid lumbar spine stability. The hinged head of the pedicle screws facilitates load sharing between the Cosmic and the anterior vertebral column [16]. In a study involving 103 patients, Cosmic demonstrated significant pain relief, improved stability, and mobility. However, a 10% reoperation rate was noted during follow-up.

Wilke et al. [15] proposed that a dynamic system offering 70% less range of motion than a non-degenerated segment could prevent screw loosening. Other studies support the idea that reducing the load in pedicle screw-based dynamic stabilization systems helps minimize the risk of screw loosening [17]. Additionally, studies indicate that screw loosening can be minimized by using hinged dynamic screws, irrespective of posterior stabilization systems [18, 19].

The PercuDyn (Interventional Spine Inc., Irvine, CA, USA) is a posterior dynamic stabilization implant that limits extension, primarily functioning as a bilateral facet augmentation system, as shown in Fig. 10.2d. It consists of two titanium screws anchoring to the pedicles and a polycarbonate urethane cushion bumper against the inferior auricular process, providing flexibility. Masala et al. [20] studied its effectiveness for lumbar stenosis treatment in 24 patients, with 83% showing improvement at the 1-year follow-up and no device-related complications reported.

The Accuflex (Globus Medical, Inc.) is another posterior dynamic stabilization system using helical cuts on the rod for flexibility, categorized as a pedicle screw-based system with 6.5 mm titanium alloy screws, as depicted in Fig. 10.2e. This design allows motion primarily in flexion-extension mode, with insertion feasible by most spine surgeons. Reyes-Sánchez et al. [21] reported clinical outcomes in lumbar spinal stenosis patients, with 83% experiencing benefits, though 22.22% required hardware removal due to fatigue failure.

BioFlex, similar to Dynesys, utilizes titanium pedicle screws connected by Nitinol rods with coiling, shown in Fig. 10.2f. Nitinol, a shape memory alloy, offers superelasticity and rigidity, acting as a tension band in the posterior spinal column. This system resists excessive deformation during extension, preserving physiological motion range [22].

10.4 Conclusions

While fusion remains the prevailing standard for treating lower back pain, clinical reports have highlighted numerous complications. These issues primarily stem from adjacent segment degeneration induced by the high stiffness of the stabilized segment. Consequently, nonfusion stabilization systems have gained traction as a means to preserve segment mobility and alleviate adjacent segment phenomena. Ongoing research underscores the necessity for long-term clinical assessments of dynamic stabilization systems.

Conversely, the stiffness of dynamic implants poses a significant concern as it may fail to provide the appropriate range of motion. Hence, optimizing the stiffness of dynamic implants is crucial to achieving the desired spinal range of motion effectively. This optimization process is pivotal for ensuring the efficacy and long-term success of dynamic stabilization systems in managing lower back pain.

References

1. White AA III, Panjabi MM. Clinical biomechanics of the spine. Lippincott-Raven; 1990.
2. Zhang QH, Teo EC. Finite element application in implant research for treatment of lumbar degenerative disc disease. Med Eng Phys. 2008;30(10):1246–56.
3. Schwarzenbach O, Berlemann U, Stoll TM, Dubois G. Posterior dynamic stabilization systems: DYNESYS. Orthop Clin N Am. 2005;36(3):363–72.
4. Niosi CA, Zhu QA, Wilson DC, Keynan O, Wilson DR, Oxland TR. Biomechanical characterization of the threedimensional kinematic behaviour of the Dynesys dynamic stabilization system: an in vitro study. Eur Spine J. 2006;15(6):913–22.
5. Sangiorgio SN, Sheikh H, Borkowski SL, Khoo L, Warren CR, Ebramzadeh E. Comparison of three posterior dynamic stabilization devices. Spine. 2011;36(19):E1251–8.
6. Molinari RW. Dynamic stabilization of the lumbar spine. Curr Opin Orthop. 2007;18(3):215–20.
7. Goel VK, Panjabi MM, Patwardhan AG, Dooris AP, Serhan H. Test protocols for evaluation of spinal implants. J Bone Joint Surg A. 2006;88(2):103–9.
8. Dubois G, De Germay B, Schaerer NS, Fennema P. Dynamic neutralization: a new concept for restabilization of the spine. In: Szpalski M, Gunzburg R, Pope MH, editors. Lumbar segmental instability. Philadelphia: Lippincott Williams &Wilkins; 1999. p. 233–40.
9. Rohlmann A, Burra NK, Zander T, Bergmann G. Comparison of the effects of bilateral posterior dynamic and rigid fixation devices on the loads in the lumbar spine: a finite element analysis. Eur Spine J. 2007;16(8):1223–31.
10. Schmoelz W, Huber JF, Nydegger T, Dipl-Ing, Claes L, Wilke HJ. Dynamic stabilization of the lumbar spine and its effects on adjacent segments: an in vitro experiment. J Spinal Disord Tech. 2003;16(4):418–23.
11. Schmoelz W, Huber JF, Nydegger T, Claes L, Wilke HJ. Influence of a dynamic stabilisation systemon load bearing of a bridged disc: an in vitro study of intradiscal pressure. Eur Spine J. 2006;15(8):1276–85.
12. Beastall J, Karadimas E, Siddiqui M, et al. The dynesys lumbar spinal stabilization system: a preliminary report on positional magnetic resonance imaging findings. Spine. 2007;32(6):685–90.
13. Schmidt H, Heuer F, Wilke HJ. Which axial and bending stiffnesses of posterior implants are required to design a flexible lumbar stabilization system? J Biomech. 2009;42(1):48–54.
14. Schulte TL, Hurschler C, Haversath M, et al. The effect of dynamic, semi-rigid implants on the range of motion of lumbar motion segments after decompression. Eur Spine J. 2008;17(8):1057–65.
15. Wilke HJ, Heuer F, Schmidt H. Prospective design delineation and subsequent in vitro evaluation of a new posterior dynamic stabilization system. Spine. 2009;34(3):255–61.

16. Stoffel M, Behr M, Reinke A, StÅNuer C, Ringel F, Meyer B. Pedicle screw-based dynamic stabilization of the thoracolumbar spine with the cosmic-system: a prospective observation. Acta Neurochir. 2010;152(5):835–43.
17. Meyers K, Tauber M, Sudin Y, et al. Use of instrumented pedicle screws to evaluate load sharing in posterior dynamic stabilization systems. Spine J. 2008;8(6):926–32.
18. Ozer A, Crawford N, Sasani M, et al. Dynamic lumbar pedicle screw-rod stabilization: two-year follow-up and comparison with fusion. Open Orthop J. 2010;4:137–41.
19. von Strempel A. Dynamic stabilisation: cosmic system. Interact Surg. 2008;3(4):229–36.
20. Masala S, Tarantino U, Nano G, et al. Lumbar spinal stenosis minimally invasive treatment with bilateral transpedicular 6 advances in orthopedics facet augmentation system. Cardiovasc Intervent Radiol. 2012;36(3):738–47.
21. Reyes-SÅLanchez A, ZÅLarate-KalfÅLopulos B, RamÅLırez-Mora I, Rosales-Olivarez LM, Alpizar-Aguirre A, SÅLanchez-Bringas G. Posterior dynamic stabilization of the lumbar spine with the Accuflex rod system as a stand-alone device: experience in 20 patients with 2-year follow-up. Eur Spine J. 2010;19(12):2164–70.
22. Cho BY, Murovic J, Park KW, Park J. Lumbar disc rehydration postimplantation of a posterior dynamic stabilization system: case report. J Neurosurg. 2010;13(5):576–80.

Stabilization with Polyaxial Dynamic Screw and Hinged Screw

11

Mehdi Sasani and Ali Fahir Özer

The lumbar spine degenerative disease affects adults in their fifth decade and the elderly. Lumbar degenerative disc disease has currently become a chronic health problem because of the aging population in the whole world. Low back pain is a crucial finding of lumbar degenerative disc disease in the aging spine. In general, low back pain may occur from the vertebral endplate disruption, disc annulus rupture, vertebral periosteum tension, or facet joint erosion. Pain is the leading symptom, such as low back pain and unilateral or bilateral leg radiating pain [1]. Load transmission across the columns of the lumbar spine is 20–25% in the anterior column, 20–25% in the posterior column, and 40–50% in the middle column for young men. In degenerative disk disease, this distribution is shifted such that 50% of load transmission occurs in the anterior column [2].

In the vast majority of individuals, conservative treatment is appropriate to treat the symptoms successfully. As a conventional surgical treatment, fusion was the first choice for chronic low back pain for many years. Fusion surgery is performed worldwide, and the long-term results of this procedure are slowly beginning to be published. With recent technological developments, the fusion rates have increased to 95%, although the same degree of patient satisfaction has not been observed. It is also true, however, that while striving to increase the quality of life for patients with chronic instability, when the mortality and morbidity rates are considered, fusion surgery performed with an instrument is undoubtedly risky. On the other hand, the clinical outcome of fusion has been shown to be worse than the radiological outcome [3]. Many patients have failed to improve after successful spinal fusion [4]. Additionally, fusion may accelerate degeneration of adjacent segments, making alternative treatments attractive [5].

Dynamic stabilization devices are a recent technological development over the last two decades. Their theoretical success is based on immobilization of the injured segment to protect it from further injury and the sharing of load across the bridged segment. The goals of dynamic stabilization devices are to:

1. Control the neutral posture of the segment.
2. Control sagittal plane bending of the treated level.
3. Unload the intervertebral disk at the treated level.
4. Modify the distribution of loads within the segment, in particular within the intervertebral disk [6].

In 1992, Henry Graf [7] was the first to use dynamic stabilization systems to treat the chronic

M. Sasani
Koc University School of Medicine, Istanbul, Turkey

A. F. Özer (✉)
Department of Neurosurgery, Koc University School of Medicine, Istanbul, Turkey

A. F. Özer et al. (eds.), *Dynamic Lumbar Spine Stabilization*,
https://doi.org/10.1007/978-3-032-12122-6_11

instability of rotational forces as a cause of lower back pain. The Graf theorized that the origin of chronic low back pain is abnormal rotational motion. Therefore, he stated that if rotation were prevented, there would be no pain. The device that gave his name to the Graf artificial ligament for stabilizing the spine with transpedicular screws instead of a rod. That was aimed at locking the lumbar facets with limited flexion movement. Moreover, it was intended to redistribute the transmission pathway for load across the painful disc by providing posterior tensioning.

After Graft, Dynesys defined the system to support the posterior tension band; moreover, many lumbar spinal dynamic systems have been described so far.

The Dynesys dynamic stabilization system is a posterior lumbar pedicular dynamic stabilization system that has been shown to achieve some of the goals of dynamic stabilization, namely, control of neutral posture, controlled (but not eliminated) motion, and unloading of the posterior portion of the disc [8]. Whether appropriate levels of reduction in motion and appropriately redistributed loading across the spine are achieved with the device is questionable, however, especially in light of poor results in the hands of some investigators [9].

Recently, the fulcrum-assisted soft stabilization system was improved, which was based on the same technique as the previous ones [2].

The second-generation dynamic stabilization system was developed, which unloads the disk by sharing 25% of the load off the disk at full flexion and extension [8]. Strempel designed and developed the first dynamic hinged screw system in 1999. This system (Cosmic) was developed as a stable and nonrigid implant with calcium phosphate-coated and hinged screws to maintain limited flexion and extension capability during stabilization [10]. The hinged screw of the Cosmic system prevents rotation, translational instability, and screw loosening as compared to the previous systems.

The Saphinaz screw utilized in this system was designed by Ozer [1]. The difference between a hinged screw and a polyaxial dynamic screw is that the hinged screw allows only flexion and extension movements but absolutely restricts rotation. The Saphinaz screw, on the other hand, has a polyaxial feature and allows the head to move in all directions when locked with the rod. Based on the fact that the posterior rod is rigid, and as the number of treated segments increases, the rigidity of the system will surpass the dynamic quantity, critics assert that this system is not fully dynamic but is semi-rigid. This judgment is correct; however, if pain eradication is the target, then this surgical intervention, which is much simpler, will biomechanically provide an almost stabilizing outcome in comparison to fusion. On the other hand, if the rod is chosen more dynamically, the system gradually becomes more dynamic depending on the flexibility of the rod. In this way, we used these screws with the Balance C rod, and in some patients, the rod was broken, but our early clinical results were very good [11]. This showed us that the system will work when there is a suitable rod. It turned out that the thinking was correct, but we had a problem with the appropriate material for the rod. Unfortunately, there is no ideal dynamic rod to use with these screws on the market right now.

Comparison of the components of these dynamic devices shows that the mechanism of dynamism differs among systems. The rods were chosen as the dynamic part in the Graf ligament, and Dynesys was the first generation of dynamic stabilization systems. Moreover, the hinged heads of the screws were chosen as the second generation of the dynamic stabilization system, while the fulcrum-assisted soft stabilization system used the neck of the screw as a fulcrum for movement. The hinged screw system was followed by the polyaxial dynamic screw system, in which the screw head was connected to the body with the ball socket mechanism. In the Cosmic and in the system studied here, the hinged head of the screw was chosen as the dynamic part to enable flexion and extension. In the Saphinaz (polyaxial screw dynamic rod), the screw head has the freedom to move in all directions, and there is no restriction. This will cause less load transfer from the screw body to the vertebral body due to the free screw head and will reduce the possibility of screw loosening in the vertebral body.

With the micro-dynamic pedicle screw developed by Liu et al. in recent years, it has the advantage of providing a better range of motion in flexion-extension than the traditional pedicle screw without sacrificing spinal stabilization.

It also has the potential to normalize the load transfer behavior of the fused segment and reduce the stress values of pedicle screws [12].

11.1 Biomechanics Behavior of Disc

A. Biomechanics of degenerative disc: Biochemical changes in disc degeneration begin with the basis of disc deterioration due to disc dehydration during hopeless efforts to repair the nuclear pulpous rather than initial structural changes in the proteoglycans. Biomechanical impairment evolves later. Later, local mechanical loading affects the distribution and type of collagen and the other macromolecules [13]. At the start of degeneration, the mechanical and elastic properties of the intervertebral disc are able to withstand any physiological load. The annulus is faced with loads coming from the nucleus, and attempts are made to meet the compressive loads that reach the annulus from the radial direction and the loads going through the annulus' lamellar structure. During the normal aging process, the time-dependent disc deformability and expansion increase by approximately two-fold. The increase in load causes extensive overflow from the disc as well as a decrease in disc height. The deterioration of the facet joints also begins simultaneously with disc degeneration. Subchondral sclerosis, osteophyte formation, and subarticular cartilage loss occur. Each functional unit becomes loose, and the chances of hyperactivity increase. Two vertebrae, one on top of the other, can move unevenly, causing the top vertebra to be either slightly in front of or behind the lower one. This change in the center of motion is called "segmental instability." Clinically, segmental instability, or "degenerative instability," can cause painful situations that must be studied and treated.
B. Biomechanics of lumbar pedicular dynamic stabilization: Load transmissions across the columns of the lumbar spine are 20–25% in the anterior column, 20–25% in the posterior column, and 40–50% in the middle column for young men. In degenerative disc disease, this distribution is shifted such that 50% of load transmission occurs in the anterior column [14]. The biomechanical study of the lumbar pedicular dynamic stabilization systems described here showed that load transmission across the posterior column was reduced relative to a rigid system. (Fig. 11.1). Although it is not possible to conclude what percent of the load is borne by each column from the biomechanical findings, the poste-

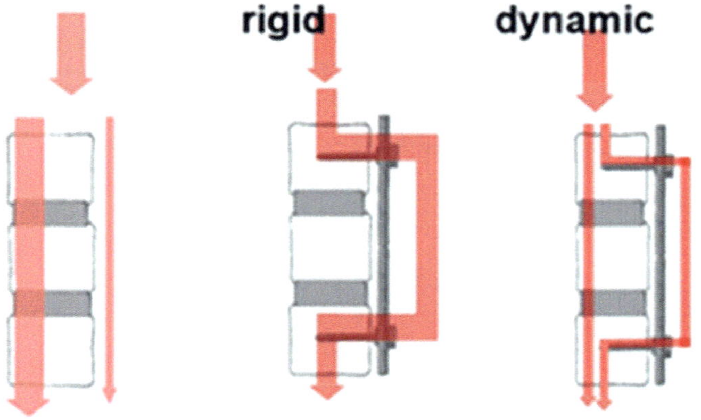

Fig. 11.1 The system in dynamic stabilization is based on sharing the load instead of bearing it. Dynamic stabilization, or semi-rigid stabilization, controls the abnormal motion while allowing motion in the spinal segment

rior shift in the axis of rotation that was observed shows that redistribution of loading toward the posterior column does occur. It is possible that less anterior load transmission provides a better chance for regeneration of degenerated discs [15]. In fact, follow-up in our institution of some cases after dynamic screw fixation with the Cosmic system has shown evidence of rehydration of previously degenerated discs [13].

11.2 Cosmic Screw

The Cosmic system consists of hinged pedicle screws with an outer diameter of 6 and 7 mm, respectively, and an inner diameter of 4 and 5 mm, respectively, and a rod with an outer diameter of 6.25 mm (Fig. 11.2). The base of the screw head and the rod are threaded to increase the rotational stability of the connection between the rod and screw. The threaded part of the screw is coated with Bonit. With greater instability, a transverse stabilizer can be mounted in addition. The screw thread is self-tapping and has a rounded tip. There are open and closed screws. The rod is connected tightly to the pedicle screw by a grub screw. The system was tested in the laboratory beforehand and was also tested clinically [10, 16]. The other designed form of the Cosmic screw system is the miacosmic cannula screw. Miacosmic is especially used in obese patients or when performed with the percutaneous Wiltse paramedian approach.

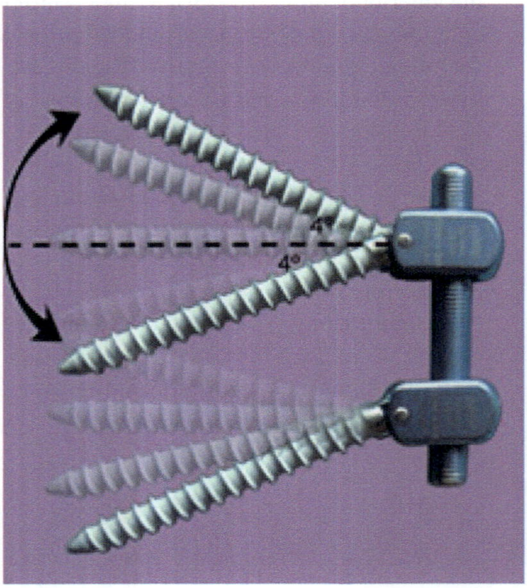

Fig. 11.2 Cosmic hinged screw

11.3 Saphinaz Screw

The Saphinaz screw has a polyaxial feature and allows the head to move in all directions when locked with the rod (Fig. 11.3).

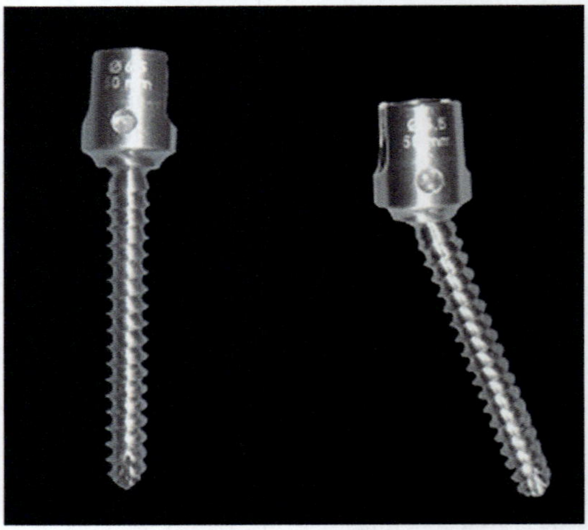

Fig. 11.3 Saphinaz hinged screw

11.4 Indication of Posterior Transpedicular Dynamic Stabilization

The posterior dynamic stabilization technique, either Cosmic or Saphinaz, applies to patients with:

- Laminectomy(ies) performed for unstable spinal stenosis.
- Degenerative spondylolisthesis.
- Recurrent disc herniation.
- Adjacent segment disease following fusion.
- In degenerative disc disease.

These patients present to the hospital with pain radiating to the lower back or legs and have difficulty maintaining their daily lives. The aim of the treatment is to eliminate the nerve compression that causes pain with microsurgical methods, that is, to perform nerve decompression. The second stage is also fixation with a posterior transpedicular dynamic screw if there is segmental instability before surgery or to prevent instability that may occur early or late after surgery due to bone removal, such as postoperative laminectomy or facetectomy. In noncompressive degenerative disc disease that does not compress on the neural elements, the patient only has back pain due to the degenerated disc. In other words, the patient has disc dehydration due to disc degeneration. In this case, only the posterior dynamic fixation carries the vertical load. Approximately more than one year later, follow-up lumbar MRI examinations show that the disc is hyperintense again in T2W-weighted MRI examinations, which indicates rehydration. (Fig. 11.4).

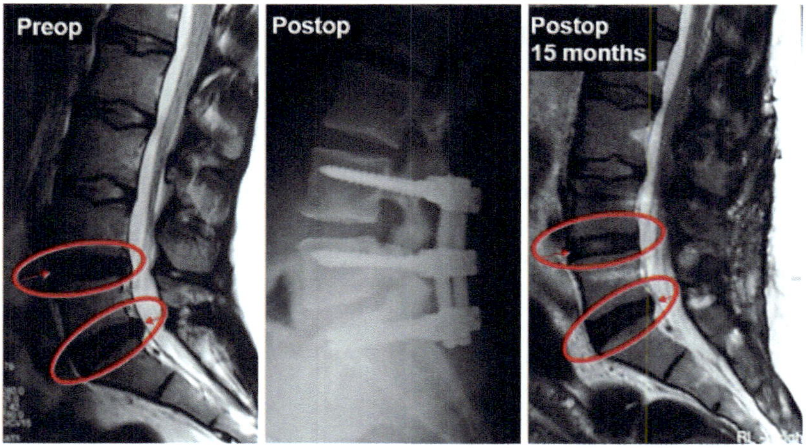

Fig. 11.4 Follow-up lumbar MRI examinations (T2W-weighted) showed that the disc was hyperintense again 15 months postoperatively

11.5 Surgical Procedure

Surgery is performed under general anesthesia in the knee-chest position to maintain lordosis of the lumbar vertebrae. The surgical approach was along the median line, opening the lumbar aponeurosis and rasping the paravertebral muscles through the facet joints. Facet joints and ligaments are preserved from iatrogenic damage during exposure in the lumbar pedicular dynamic stabilization systems. Hemilaminectomy, laminectomy, and/or discectomy are performed according to the indications of each patient before pedicle screw insertion. Dynamic screws, Cosmic or Saphinaz, are placed under lateral and anterior-posterior image fluoroscopic visualization by specific holders, which are designed to carry screw caps. The pedicle screws are first implanted. A bicortical position of the screw in the sacrum is desirable to avoid screw loosening in osteoporotic patients.

To achieve as great a press-fit as possible of the screw in the pedicle and vertebral body, the pedicle is drilled with a 3.2 mm drill, and the screw is then implanted. In very hard cancellous bone and in the sacrum, the thread tap is used first. Before the rods are implanted, the patient is checked for a good lordosis position. Straight rods are implanted in the case of one-segment use, and lordotically curved rods with bi- and three-segment use. More than three segments are not instrumented. No correction is performed, nor any reduction. If necessary, adequate decompression is performed, which may involve laminectomy with medial facetectomy. In the case of only lumbar pain, caused by no root nerve compressive black disc or painful facet joint arthritis, stabilization only is carried out. Moderate distraction of up to 3 mm is possible to expand the neural foramina. When there is marked decompression, a transverse stabilizer can be mounted in addition. After copious irrigation, a 12 mm suction drain is inserted, and the wound is closed in layers. Mobilization commences on the first or second postoperative day after removal of the wound drain. An external support, such as a lower back brace, is not prescribed.

The other surgical approach is named percutaneous transpedicular via the Wiltse paramedian approach [17]. The intramuscular access is approximately 3 cm lateral to the median line on both sides. The instrumentation is applied via a transmuscular approach. Following blunt dissection, the screws were placed with the C-arm fluoroscopy control as per routine transpedicular instrumentation (Fig. 11.5). In recent years, the instrumentation was performed via a midline incision (Fig. 11.6).

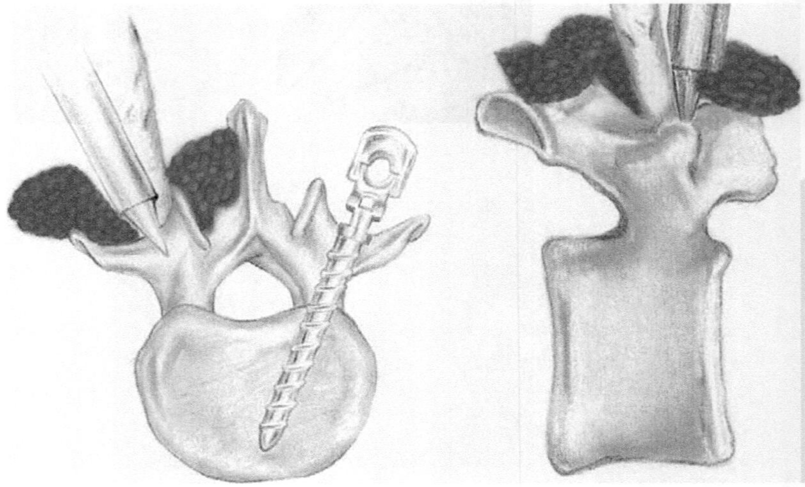

Fig. 11.5 The screws are placed through blunt muscle dissection. The junction of the transverse process and the lateral wall of the facet joint is found via finger palpation, and an awl is placed. (**a**) Axial, (**b**) sagittal views

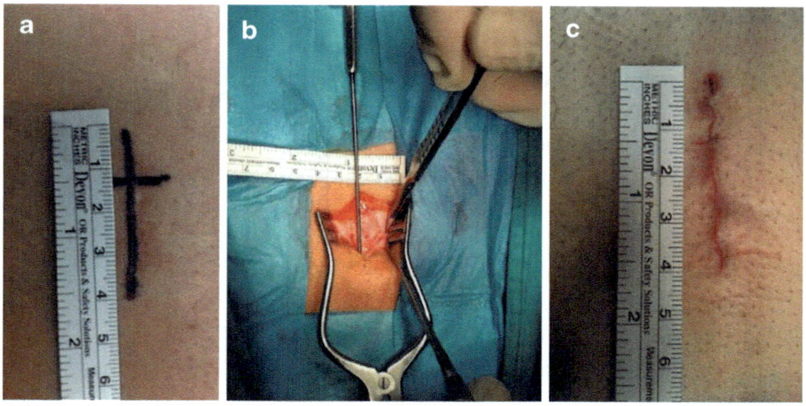

Fig. 11.6 (**a**) A 4- or 5-cm incision is performed on the midline. (**b**) The fascia is cut 2–3 cm lateral to the midline on both sides. (**c**) The incision is closed subcutaneously

11.6 Causes Affecting Spinal Instrument Failure

The junctions of the spine are important. Biomechanically, all the load from the top is on the screw, and the screw loosens, or if osteointegration has developed, this time it breaks due to metal fatigue. The other cause of inadequate bone quality: In osteoporosis, ankylosing spondylitis, and rheumatoid arthritis, bone quality is deteriorated, and the screws loosen or break easily, and instrument failure develops. Moreover, long-segment stabilizations may be insufficient if they end in L5-S1. It is correct to extend the system to the iliac bones. Instrument application is a crucial parameter to the error of instrument failure, as a screw malposition, a short and thin screw, or an improper screw can cause the system to be weak. Adjacent segment disease can be observed in both rigid as well as dynamic lumbar instrumentation. It may be present as a disc herniation, scoliosis, kyphosis deformity, or Modic degeneration.

11.7 The Challenges of Posterior Dynamic Spinal Stabilization

A. It is not enough to maintain the movement: In dynamic stabilizations in painful degenerated disc disease, the system remained mobile, and fusion developed in very few of the patients.

But the patients' VAS and Oswestry scores were satisfactory. It means that the degree of degeneration of the segment you support is important, and regardless of the result, we go to surgery to relieve pain, not to preserve movement. In a clinical study we conducted, disc degeneration returned and rehydration was observed in only one-third of the cases. In the remaining two-thirds, it either fused or remained intact, and this is in line with the literature [18]. In conclusion, when the dynamic system is applied, the degree of degeneration of the disc, which is the most important structure of the motion segment, is the main factor that plays a role in the continuation of the mobility of the motion segment.

If there is advanced disc degeneration, the probability of disc fusion is very high, and the results will not differ from fusion.

B. Screw or rod breakage or screw loosening: As the level increases, the loosening of the screw increases, and there are also breakage problems in screws and rods.

The negative aspect of this technology from fusion is that the screw systems used for fusion are sufficient to last for 4–6 months, and their task ends after the fusion develops [19]. The vast majority of chronic instability patients, especially those with multiple levels of instability and osteoporotic individuals who constitute the elderly group, are a major factor for loosening of the screw. Regardless of the system applied, loss of screws is at reasonable levels in patients in whom we applied the posterior dynamic system. In our 71 patients who underwent posterior dynamic instrumentation, we found screw loosening in two patients as well as screw breakage in one patient [11].

C. Adjacent segment disease: Changes in the biomechanics of the spine after arthrodesis include increased mobility of adjacent segments, increased facet loading, and increased discal pressure, leading to adjacent segment disorders in spinal posterior instrumentation. If the motion segment with the dynamic system can maintain its motion and the patient's bone quality is good, dynamic systems are more advantageous than rigid systems in terms of instrument failure. The system provides movement close to a normal spine. The adjacent segment ratio is 12.2–18.5% in fusion, whereas it is 9.8% in the dynamic system [20, 21]. Risk factors for adjunct segment disorders may include age, fusion length, decompression adjacent to the fusion, termination of a fusion at the apex of the deformity, and preexisting degenerative changes in the adjacent segment. One of the ultimate goals of dynamic technologies, either Cosmic or Saphinaz technologies, is to reduce the incidence of adjacent segment disease.

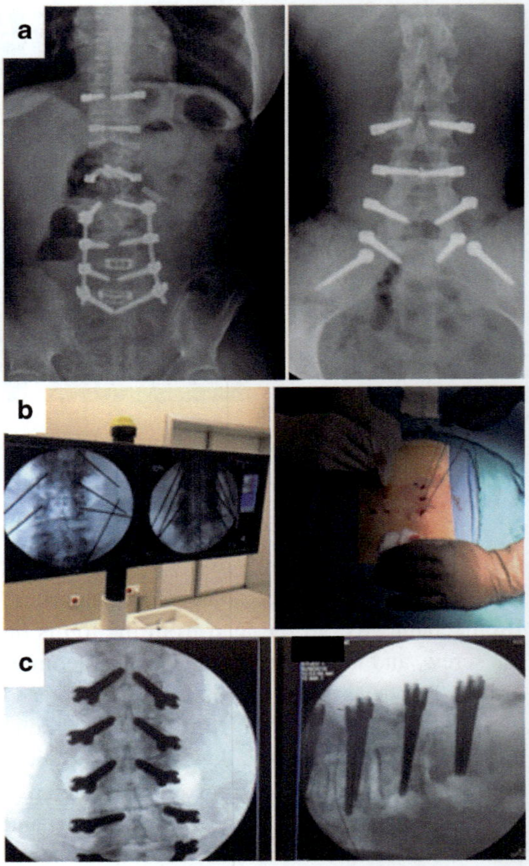

Fig. 11.7 (**a**) A hybrid system. The Rijid system was extended by a dynamic system. (**b**) To reduce the stress in S1 and transfer the load to the pelvis iliac wings. (**c**) Two-stage posterior dynamic instrumentation was performed

Results from biomechanical studies suggest that the difference in biomechanical effect between dynamic and rigid stabilization may not be as high as reported [22].

D. There are problems in long-segment stabilization: Whether the long-segment spinal posterior instrumentation is rigid or dynamic, the rate of screw loosening is high, especially in osteoporotic patients and in long-segment spinal instrumentation extended to S1. In summary, this is what we did to overcome loosening and long-segment problems. We applied the hybrid system as well (Fig. 11.7a). In patients with poor bone quality, distributing the load by placing screws in the iliac bones is another suggestion in terms of instrument failure [23]. Reaching the iliac bones, we tried to reduce the stress in S1 and transfer the load to the pelvis, as in fusion surgery (Fig. 11.7b). Two-stage posterior dynamic instrumentation was performed [24]. To begin with, screws were applied via percutaneous or mini-open skin incision under general or spinal anesthesia. Placement of rods in the second stage was performed 4 months after the first-stage surgery (Fig. 11.7c).

E. Pseudoarthrosis: Pseudoarthrosis is defined as the absence of solid bone fusion one year after the first lumbar instrument stabilization. It occurs in at least 15% of patients after primary lumbar fusions. Pseudoarthrosis is typically associated with lower back pain or radicular pain as a result of continued movement. However, pseudoarthrosis may also be asymptomatic, or symptoms may be atypical in a significant proportion of patients. Spinal revision surgery is performed for those with persistent or recurrent pain. Therefore, it is essential to objectively correlate pain symptoms with the degree of pseudoarthrosis. Pseudoarthrosis is most common in rigid dynamic lumbar instrumentation. Because the main purpose of this type of surgery is to create a fusion. However, whether lumbar dynamics is Cosmic or Saphinaz is not seen, because the surgical aim is not to create fusion. Some lumbar dynamic instrumentation patients may develop pseudoarthrosis due to reactive fusion.

11.8 Posterior Dynamic Systems: Polyaxial Dynamic Screw and Hinged Screw (Cosmic and Saphinaz)

There are two main systems currently in use: the "dynamic rod" and the "dynamic screw" [25]. Dynamic stabilization devices are a recent technological development. Theoretical success is based on immobilization of the injured spine segment to protect it from further injury and sharing of load across the bridged segment.

The extent of the challenges, such as loosened screws and breakage after lumbar instrumentation, will be proportional to how well the designed system assimilates into the spine biomechanics. Thus, the system that shows the most respect for the biological behavior of the spine will be the most successful. Therefore, the first generation of dynamic stabilization and the second generation of dynamic stabilization systems, which use rods as the dynamic part of the system and hinged heads of the screws, are consecutively chosen.

Dynamic systems, particularly posterior dynamic systems, are mostly used to treat degenerative disc disease. The first cause of degenerative disc disease is segmental instability. It is known that rigid fixation (fusion) systems have been introduced as the gold standard surgery to treat degenerative lumbar disc disease up to now. Whereas there are numerous disadvantages such as pseudoarthrosis (15–96%), facet and disc degeneration, adjacent segment disease because of the stress-shielding (2–3% per year after stabilization), device-related osteopenia, worsened biomechanical properties of the spinal ligaments, morbidity and mortality risk because of severe surgery, donor area pain, and loss of motion in treated spinal segments. Additionally, the absence of controlled motion makes the rigid system tend to fracture at the bone-implant interface because of increased surface stress [18]. On the other hand, if a fixation system that will provide vertical loads and segmental instability is used as a part of the movement of the lower back, it will be appropriate for the biodynamics of the lower back. For this reason, the posterior dynamic system, namely, the Cosmic and Saphinaz systems, has taken its place in degenerative disc disease day by day.

Load-sharing between the anterior and posterior spinal columns is the basic philosophy of dynamic systems [10]. The dynamic posterior stabilization technique offers load-sharing and load-bearing features. The system also preserves some motion but eliminates the risk of abnormal translational movement. These particular biomechanical properties can unload the disc and also prevent instability, thus helping to eliminate the pain originating from either degenerative disc disease or segmental instability [26].

Dynamic stabilization in the treatment of degenerative instability by using the Cosmic system [10, 27, 28]. In dynamic stabilization, the father of rendering dynamicity to a screw with the installation of a joint. We believed that the dynamic posterior system is a product of an ingenious idea because it is a simple and effective way to replace a facet joint. The biomechanics of the Cosmic system have been conducted and proven to work successfully in vitro analysis [29].

The system was not initially dynamic; rather, it was used to study and develop a better way to increase the weight on a fusion bone graft placed between vertebrae. However, although the

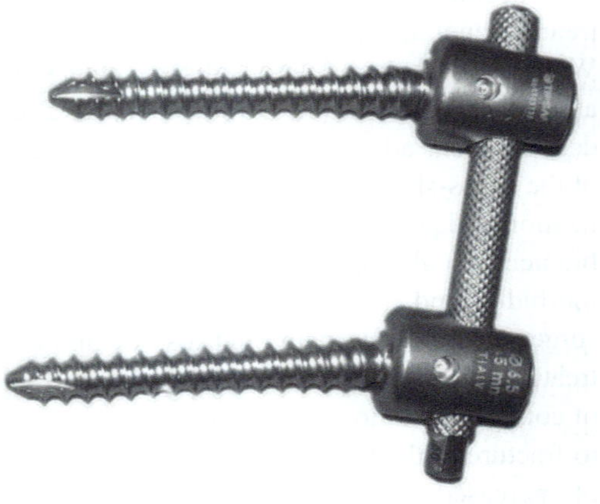

Fig. 11.8 In our biomechanical studies, the biomechanical results closest to a normal motion segment were obtained when the Saphinaz screw was used together with the dynamic Talin rod we designed for the study

Cosmic system did contribute to fusion development, due to the good results obtained from patients without fusion development, it began to be used as a non-fusion technology. The biomechanical properties of the Cosmic and Safinaz systems as stabilizing forces have been analyzed using human cadavers, and the results have been published [1]. Studies of both systems have revealed that the stabilizing effects of dynamic screws are similar to the rigid system [15]. Dynamic screws have also been used with movable rods, and successful results have been published. However, in these systems, there is no dynamic rod system other than the peak rod on the market at the moment [30] (Fig. 11.8).

Recently, in patients, long-level stabilization to generate a motile posterior tension band that could maintain the pace of the moving screws, as well as the entire moving rod with moving screws, was used. However, the use of this system with a dynamic rod was not applicable in younger patients because it is not flexible enough and is susceptible to breaking, so it was subsequently stopped. In addition, in long-segment dynamic instrumentation, double-headed screws Orthrus (Fig. 11.9) are used to reduce loosening between the bone and long-term side effects such as adjacent segment disorders. The main purpose of this system is to create multiple short segments by converting the long-segment dynamic instrumentation into a single short-segment unit. In this way, the system becomes more dynamic than a semi-rigid system [31].

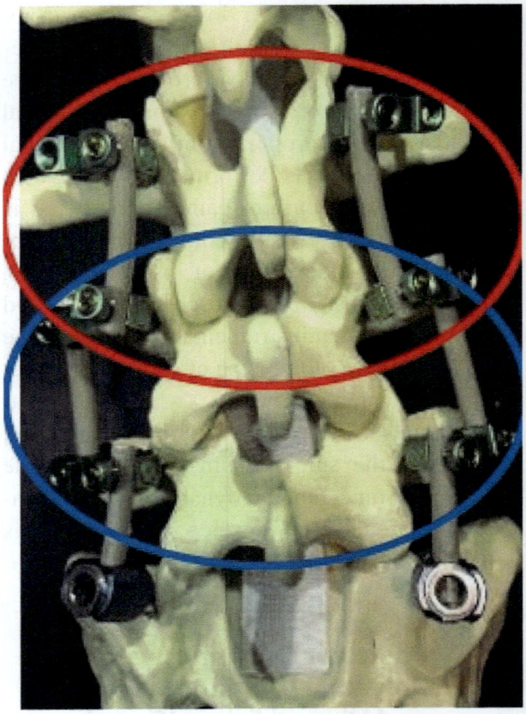

Fig. 11.9 The low incidence of side effects in short lumbar segment instrumentation led to the thought of dividing the screw caps into two or more, stabilizing each level as a single level in itself

Technological developments in lumbar dynamic instrumentation will undoubtedly change the fate of disc surgery procedures. One of the largest problems associated with lumbar degenerative disc disease is the side effects of the challenging dynamic instrumentation, which is mentioned in this chapter.

From this perspective, posterior dynamic instrumentation has taken its place in the surgery procedure in the treatment of degenerative lumbar spinal diseases, but new designs of screw and rod are needed to adapt it to the biodynamics and physiological movements of the lower back. We think that the closer these designs are to the biodynamics of the facet joint, the more realistic they will be.

References

1. Ozer AF, Crawford NR, Sasani M, Oktenoglu T, Bozkus H, Kaner T, Aydin S. Dynamic lumbar pedicle screw-rod stabilization: two-year follow-up and comparison with fusion. Open Orthop J. 2010;4:137–41. https://doi.org/10.2174/1874325001004010137.
2. Sengupta DK, Mulholland RC. Fulcrum assisted soft stabilization system: a new concept in the surgical treatment of degenerative low back pain. Spine (Phila Pa 1976). 2005;30(9):1019–29; discussion 1030. https://doi.org/10.1097/01.brs.0000160986.39171.4d.
3. Bogduk N. The innervation of the lumbar spine. Spine (Phila Pa 1976). 1983;8(3):286–93. https://doi.org/10.1097/00007632-198304000-00009.
4. Boos N, Webb JK. Pedicle screw fixation in spinal disorders: a European view. Eur Spine J. 1997;6(1):2–18. https://doi.org/10.1007/BF01676569.
5. Cunningham BW, Kotani Y, McNulty PS, Cappuccino A, McAfee PC. The effect of spinal destabilization and instrumentation on lumbar intradiscal pressure: an in vitro biomechanical analysis. Spine (Phila Pa 1976). 1997;22(22):2655–63.
6. McNally DS. Rationale for dynamic stabilization. In: Kim DH, Cammisa FP, Fessler RG, editors. Dynamic reconstruction of the spine. 1st ed. New York: Thieme; 2006. p. 237–43.
7. Graf H. Lumbar instability: surgical treatment without fusion. Rachis. 1992;412:123–37.
8. Beastall J, Karadimas E, Siddiqui M, Nicol M, Hughes J, Smith F, Wardlaw D. The Dynesys lumbar spinal stabilization system: a preliminary report on positional magnetic resonance imaging findings. Spine (Phila Pa 1976). 2007;32(6):685–90. https://doi.org/10.1097/01.brs.0000257578.44134.fb.
9. Grob D, Benini A, Junge A, Mannion AF. Clinical experience with the Dynesys semirigid fixation system for the lumbar spine: surgical and patient-oriented outcome in 50 cases after an average of 2 years. Spine (Phila Pa 1976). 2005;30(3):324–31. https://doi.org/10.1097/01.brs.0000152584.46266.25.
10. Strempel A. Nonfusion stabilization of the degenerated lumbar spine with Cosmic. In: Kim DH, Cammisa FP, Fessler RG, editors. Dynamic reconstruction of the spine. 1st ed. New York: Thieme; 2006. p. 330–9.
11. Ozer AF, Oktenoglu T, Egemen E, Sasani M, Yilmaz A, Erbulut DU, Yaman O, Suzer T. Lumbar single-level dynamic stabilization with semi-rigid and full dynamic systems: a retrospective clinical and radiological analysis of 71 patients. Clin Orthop Surg. 2017;9(3):310–6. https://doi.org/10.4055/cios.2017.9.3.310.
12. Liu C, Kamara A, Yan Y. Investigation into the biomechanics of lumbar spine micro-dynamic pedicle screw. BMC Musculoskelet Disord. 2018;19(1):231. https://doi.org/10.1186/s12891-018-2132-5.
13. Keller TS, Holm SH, Hansson TH, Spengler DM. Volvo award in experimental studies. The dependence of intervertebral disc mechanical properties on physiologic conditions. Spine (Phila Pa 1976). 1990;15(8):751–61. https://doi.org/10.1097/00007632-199008010-00004.
14. Ray CD, Hale JE, Norton BK. Minimally invasive posterior dynamic stabilization system. In: Kim DH, Cammisa FP, Fessler RG, editors. Dynamic reconstruction of the spine. 1st ed. New York: Thieme; 2006. p. 99–104.
15. Bozkuş H, Senoğlu M, Baek S, Sawa AG, Ozer AF, Sonntag VK, Crawford NR. Dynamic lumbar pedicle screw-rod stabilization: in vitro biomechanical comparison with standard rigid pedicle screw-rod stabilization. J Neurosurg Spine. 2010;12(2):183–9. https://doi.org/10.3171/2009.9.SPINE0951.
16. Goel VK, Konz RJ, Chang HT, Grosland NM, Grobler LJ, Chesmel KD. Hinged dynamic posterior device permits greater loads on the graft and similar stability as compared with its equivalent rigid device: a three-dimensional finite element assessment. JPO. 2001;13(1):17–20.
17. Wiltse LL, Bateman JG, Hutchinson RH, et al. The paraspinal sacrospinalis-splitting approach to the lumbar spine[J]. J Bone Joint Surg Am. 1968;50(5):919–26.
18. Yilmaz A, Senturk S, Sasani M, Oktenoglu T, Yaman O, Yildirim H, Suzer T, Ozer AF. Disc rehydration after dynamic stabilization: a report of 59 cases. Asian Spine J. 2017;11(3):348–55.
19. Ciplak NM, Suzer T, Senturk S, Yaman O, Sasani M, Oktenoglu T, Yilmaz A, Erbulut DU, Özer AF. Complications of 2-level dynamic stabilization: a correlative clinical and radiological analysis at two-year follow-up on 103 patients. Turk Neurosurg. 2018;28(5):756–62.
20. Park P, Garton HJ, Gala VC, Hoff JT, McGillicuddy JE. Adjacent segment disease after lumbar or lumbosacral fusion: review of the literature. Spine (Phila Pa 1976). 2004;29(17):1938–44. https://doi.org/10.1097/01.brs.0000137069.88904.03.
21. Kanayama M, Togawa D, Hashimoto T, Shigenobu K, Oha F. Motion-preserving surgery can prevent early breakdown of adjacent segments: comparison of posterior dynamic stabilization with spinal fusion. J Spinal Disord Tech. 2009;22(7):463–7.
22. Schmoelz W, Huber JF, Nydegger T, Claes L, Wilke HJ. Influence of a dynamic stabilization system on load bearing of a bridged disc: an in vitro study of intradiscal pressure. Eur Spine J. 2006;15:1276–85.
23. Özer AF, Aydın AL, Hekimoğlu M, Çerezci Ö, Başak AT, Ates O, Oktenoglu T, Sasani M. Should iliac wing screws be included in long segment dynamic stabilization? Cureus. 2021;13(2):e13543.
24. Özer AF, Başak AT, Özbek MA, Hekimoğlu M, Aydın AL, Ateş Ö, Günerbüyük C, Akgül T, Sasani M, Öktenoğlu T. Lumbar dynamic stabilization with 2-stage surgery: early results. Int J Spine Surg. 2022;16(4):638–45.

25. Kaner T, Sasani M, Oktenoglu T, Ozer AF. Dynamic stabilization of the spine: a new classification system. Turk Neurosurg. 2010;20(2):205–15.
26. Oktenoglu T, Ozer AF, Sasani M, Kaner T, Canbulat N, Ercelen O, Sarioglu AC. Posterior dynamic stabilization in the treatment of lumbar degenerative disc disease: 2-year follow-up. Minim Invasive Neurosurg. 2010;53(3):112–6. https://doi.org/10.1055/s-0030-1262810.
27. von Strempel A, Neckritz A, Mualenaere P, du Toit G. Dynamic versus rigid spinal implants. In: Gunzburg R, Szpalski M, editors. Lumbar spinal stenosis. Philadelphia: Lippincott-Williams and Wilkins; 2000. p. 275–85.
28. von Strempel A. Dynamische dorsale Stabilisierung mit dem Cosmic-System [Dynamic posterior stabilization with the cosmic system]. Oper Orthop Traumatol. 2010;22(5–6):561–72. German. https://doi.org/10.1007/s00064-010-9016-7.
29. Schmoelz W, Onder U, Martin A, von Strempel A. Non-fusion instrumentation of the lumbar spine with a hinged pedicle screw rod system: an in vitro experiment. Eur Spine J. 2009;18(10):1478–85. https://doi.org/10.1007/s00586-009-1052-3.
30. Kaner T, Sasani M, Oktenoglu T, Cosar M, Ozer AF. Utilizing dynamic rods with dynamic screws in the surgical treatment of chronic instability: a prospective clinical study. Turk Neurosurg. 2009;19(4):319–26.
31. Ozer AF, Cevik OM, Erbulut DU, Yaman O, Senturk S, Oktenoglu T, Sasani M, Suzer T, Goel V. A novel modular dynamic stabilization system for the treatment of degenerative spinal pathologies. Turk Neurosurg. 2019;29(1):115–20.

Combination of Dynamic Rods and Screws

12

Ali Fahir Özer and Caner Günerbüyük

Dynamic systems were developed long after fusion surgery. First, a structure that can replace the deteriorated disc and provide stabilization while the segment is in motion was considered. To stabilize instead of destroying the motion, natural motion preservation was another emerging approach. Although many patents were indicated for the protection-of-motion designs, they remained only at the design stage. However, Fernstrom tried to ensure the continuation of motion in the motion segment by placing a steel ball inside the disc after discectomy in 1966 [1] but failed as the steel ball fractured the cartilage end plates and became embedded in the vertebral bodies. Karin Buttner-Janz and Schellnack made the first modern artificial Charite prosthesis, named after the hospital where they worked, in 1984, after conducting intensive studies and many patient trials [2]. Later, other prostheses entered the market and started to be used in the USA with the Food and Drug Administration's approval. However, their use rapidly declined when insurance companies stopped the payments due to the consecutive emergence of serious complications. Although some centers still use it today, several companies stopped their R&D studies on disc prostheses due to their impractical use, and most of them have been withdrawn from the market. As a result, they lost their popularity due to complications and revision surgeries involving serious mortality and morbidity, not being able to demonstrate superiority over fusion surgery, and insurance companies stopping payments [3].

Before using posterior dynamic systems, the evolution of instrumentation in fusion surgery should be elucidated. Before going too far into history, some important points should be reviewed [4–6]. Hibbs and Albe [7, 8] started to use fusion surgery in spinal surgery in 1911, unaware of each other, in the treatment of tuberculosis, a very common disease at that time. Stabilization using only the posterior column was performed much later with Harrington rods. Harrington corrected the deformity by distracting the posterior column with hooks attached to the rods in 1953 [9, 10]. In the early 1970s, Eduardo Luque tried to achieve a tighter and more stable fixation using his eponymous "Luque" implant. He placed the rods at each level that should be stabilized and connected the vertebrae to these rods with wires [11]. The Luque implant was unique because it did not require patients to wear a corrective corset postoperatively; however, a risk of neurological damage existed due to wires running through the spinal canal.

This system was not abandoned as a concept in later years and was redeveloped and expanded

A. F. Özer (✉)
Department of Neurosurgery, Koc University School of Medicine, Istanbul, Turkey

C. Günerbüyük
Koc University Hospital, Istanbul, Turkey
e-mail: cgunerbuyuk@kuh.ku.edu.tr

A. F. Özer et al. (eds.), *Dynamic Lumbar Spine Stabilization*,
https://doi.org/10.1007/978-3-032-12122-6_12

by Mazda [12], known as a Universal Clamp instead of a wire (consisting of three components: a woven polyester tape [Dacron], a titanium (Ti) alloy [or stainless steel] clamp, and a locking screw [Ti alloy or stainless steel]) bands, just like in the Luque implant. Universal Clamp system is used to correct the deformity by passing through the laminae and is connected to the rods using strong reduction tools.

Luque primarily conceived of posterior column stabilization and achieved this with rods and wires. Harrington developed the instruments used in posterior stabilization with hook and rod systems. He added distraction capability to the instrument system. He pioneered the theory and practice of pedicular screw systems in which stabilization is predominantly performed from the posterior column. In 1984, two French orthopedic surgeons, Dr. Yves Cotrel and Dr. Jean Dubousset [13, 14], introduced a system that fixes the rods bilaterally to the vertebrae using hooks and screws and can be manipulated to provide the desired spine profile. This is a formable rod system consisting of multiple hooks and screws, which first provides derotation of the spine while allowing the preservation of lordosis and resulting in the development of various similar fixation systems used in clinical practice today.

Naturally, this development has led to the emergence of pedicular dynamic systems. Although the first experiences for stronger stabilization were presented by Cotrel and Dubousset in 1984, Graf [15, 16] presented dynamic stabilization without fusion using a pedicular screw and a flexible rod bearing his name at the second EUROSPINE congress in Rome and published his results afterward. Only 7 years had passed between the pedicular fusion system and the pedicular dynamic system developed by Cotrel and Dubousset. The common point of Graf's initial stabilization concept using the Graf ligament and von Strempel's [17] hinged screwhead concept is that they do not maintain the motion in the spine. They defined the dynamic pedicular screw system as a simple stabilization system that can only be used in minor instability. They also made no claims to protect the motion. Therefore, the concept of maintaining motion emerged with Fernstrom [1].

73 years after the introduction of pedicular screws and their use to achieve good fusion, the concept of the pedicular screw dynamic system emerged. Regardless of the concept, the recent emergence of modern designs and applications of dynamic systems is no paradox. This has evolved alongside the development of functional concepts, the stability and instability of the spine, and the growth of surgical knowledge and experience. With the development of function concepts, the stability and instability of the spine and the increase in surgical knowledge and experience have been parallel [17–22].

12.1 Pedicular Dynamic System

Some researchers have thought that if there is constant pressure on the graft, fusion should be developed because, based on Wolf's law, the graft must be under pressure to allow the occurrence of fusion. They reported that in rigid systems, since the incoming load is transmitted directly down by the rigid system, graft loading is prevented, and the rigid construction causes the "stress-shielding" problem. Even if the graft is under pressure at first, the load gradually decreases due to the occurrence of subsidence. Due to the non-stretchable rigid system and the decreased load on the graft, the risk of developing pseudoarthrosis increases. Therefore, dynamic pedicular systems have been developed to solve the problem of decreasing load on the graft in the rigid system and ensure continuous graft loading. Since the load transfer from instrumentation will be shared with the anterior column, a constant load transfer occurs on the graft, thereby increasing the possibility of fusion development [23–25].

In a functional lumbar unit with an intact disc and anterior and posterior columns, the facet joints are exposed to 17% of the axial load, and 90% of the axial load passes through the vertebral body and disc. However, there may also be load transfer between the columns. When this occurs, a column may be subject to a greater load than normal (Fig. 12.1) [26–28].

When support is placed on the anterior column, for example, the placement of a cage after discectomy, 80% of the axial force passes through the anterior column.

When the posterior column is stabilized with a flexible posterior rod, there is linear axial loading through the rod, which recreates normal spinal biomechanics.

When posterior instrumentation is placed in distraction or there is a gap in the anterior column, the posterior implant is overloaded, and almost 90% of the incoming load passes through the posterior rod (Fig. 12.2) [29].

In cadavers with spinal instability, there is enlargement of the neutral zone (NZ) that mimics the NZ of an intact spine after DYNESYS® implantation. The DYNESYS® (Zimmer Biomet, Warsaw, IN, USA) dynamic stabilization system controls motion across three planes, with a particular focus on axial rotation (AR). Therefore, it can be used in deformity and instability surgery. Since the system provides partial control of horizontal translation, it is appropriate for use in degenerative spondylolisthesis patients [30–32].

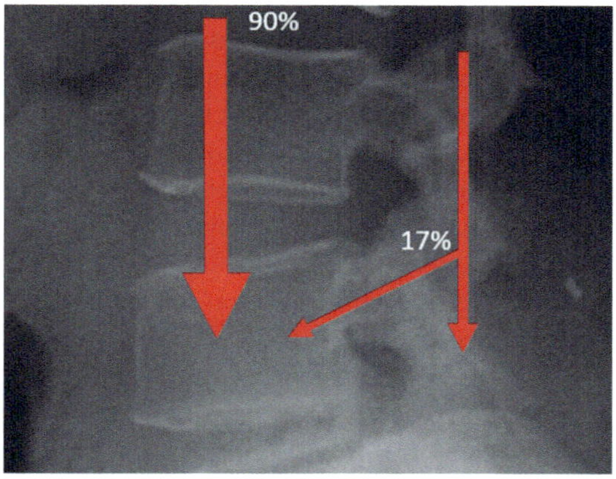

Fig. 12.1 Load distribution in the lumbar spine. The facet joints are exposed to 17% of the axial load, and 90% of the axial load passes through the vertebral body and disc. However, there may also be load transfers between columns

In this respect, dynamic systems have also been used in fusion surgery, and publications have reported that they play a positive role in fusion formation [33, 34]. Finally, satisfactory results were obtained in a meta-analysis of 17 articles with the DYNESYS® system in 2020 [35].

As a result, developers of the hinged screwhead system aimed to achieve better fusion as opposed to developing a non-fusion stabilization system. Adopting this idea and aiming to achieve better results in fusion, von Strempel made it movable by placing a hinge between the screwhead and the body. Thus, he developed the concept of a dynamic screw instead of a dynamic rod. Based on the same idea, its primary goal is to increase the load on the bone graft. However, while observing his cases, he made a very important observation; i.e., patients who had no problem with screw osteosynthesis to the bone did not have any clinical complaints even if pseudoarthrosis developed. During this observation, von Strempel started to apply the hinged screw system without fusion. Therefore, this application has led to the emergence of a new concept in dynamic systems [36, 37].

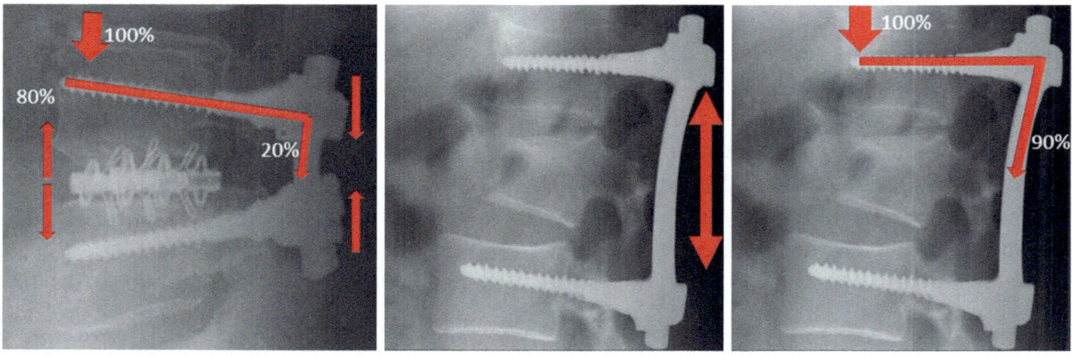

Fig. 12.2 When posterior instrumentation is placed in distraction or there is a gap in the anterior column, the posterior implant is overloaded, and almost 90% of the incoming load passes through the posterior rod

von Strempel developed spinal fusion surgery and a corresponding dynamic screw system. The efficacy of this has been confirmed by numerous studies. Liu et al. have demonstrated that micro-dynamic pedicle screws provide a better flexion (Flex)–extension (Ext) range of motion (ROM) than conventional pedicle screws without sacrificing stabilization. They also have the potential to normalize the load transfer behavior of the fused segments and reduce the stress values of the pedicle screws [38]. However, as most systems are designed for single-level use, the Orthrus system has been developed for multilevel application [39].

Graf's ligaments build on the advantages of dynamic systems by enabling fusionless stabilization. Later, von Strempel suggested that his dynamic screw system should be used without fusion, and his non-fusion dynamic stabilization system is now widely used in clinical practice.

In 2005, an important biomechanical study was conducted, in which the load distributions of semirigid, dynamic, and rigid systems were compared in cadavers. The study showed that dynamic systems result in load distribution closer to that of normal functional units than rigid and semirigid systems. The load transfer in semirigid and rigid systems was similar and was found to be transmitted from the predominantly used system.

Thus, dynamic systems are the optimal choice for spinal correction. The closer the behavior of an instrumentation system is to that of a functional anatomical unit, the more successfully it can maintain the range of motion. However, for the preservation of motion, it is also vital to ensure that there is no further disc degeneration. Such ongoing disc degeneration leads to the fusion of the functional unit, and the dynamic system will not maintain movement but will serve only as stabilization. Nevertheless, if degenerative processes cannot prevent functional unit fusion, dynamic systems should still be used for stabilization.

12.2 Dynamic Rod System

There are three basic biomechanical requirements for an ideal posterior dynamic stabilization system. First, it must ensure even loading of the intervertebral discs with predictable load distribution. Second, it must provide physiological movement control across three planes. Third, it must preserve sagittal balance and anatomical alignment (Fig. 12.3) [25].

After this important determination, according to our own experience, dynamic screws and rigid rods have been used in our department for many years. The results are extremely satisfactory, especially when stabilizing a single motion segment. When the dynamic screw is used with a rigid rod, significant restrictions have developed on the interspinous ligaments and posterior facet joints. Considering the biomechanical study of this system, including a dynamic screw and a rigid rod, the concept of semirigid rather than full dynamics has been more accurate for this and similar systems [40–43].

Deficiencies such as the Graf ligament weakness in hyperextension and decreased foramen volume were corrected using the DYNESYS® system. The developed rope-shaped rods and spacers have been used with rigid screws as a more advanced dynamic system. However, in the meantime, the Medtronic company has released a dynamic rod called the "Agile rod" (Fig. 12.4) to primarily stabilize the fusion-developed segment, using a dynamic rod instead of fusion, and keep the adjacent segment mobile when segment degeneration occurs.

We thought that if a dynamic screw could be used on this rod, we could make the system more mobile. Our goal was to address the following question: "Can we maintain motion while providing stabilization?" In cases where stabilization was required in a single motion segment, this rod was used instead of a rigid rod with a dynamic screw. If the stabilization of two mobile segments was required, using the mobile part in the less degenerative segment, our 19-month results were evaluated to be quite satisfactory [44].

In clinical follow-ups, patients did not have any complaints, although some of these rods

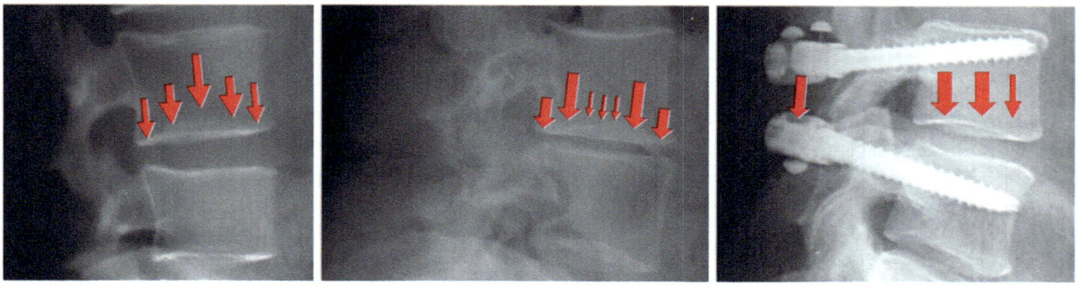

Fig. 12.3 The three basic biomechanical requirements for an ideal posterior dynamic stabilization system. The ideal spinal stabilization system ensures even loading of the intervertebral discs with predictable load distribution, allows physiological movement control across three planes, and preserves sagittal balance and anatomical alignment

Fig. 12.4 Dynamic Agile rod (Medtronic)

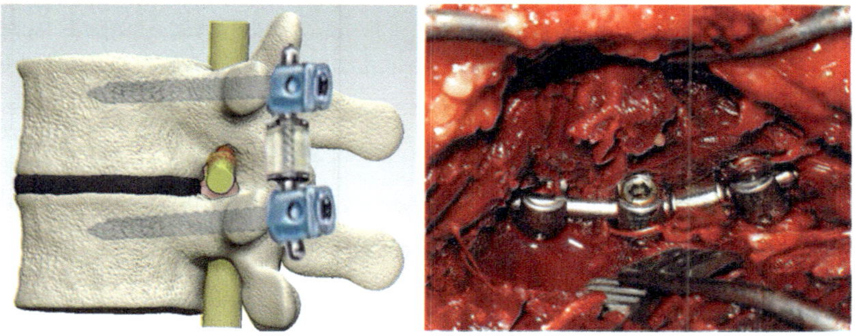

Fig. 12.5 Broken Agile rod

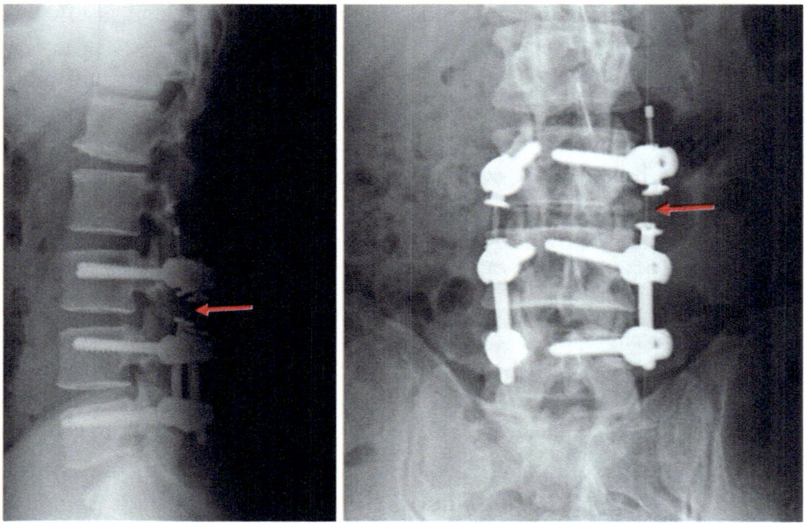

broke and had to be revised in the third and fourth years. Patients also reported that their quality of life was good until the Agile rods broke (Fig. 12.5). Therefore, we believe that our reasoning is correct, but we did not have a usable, safe rod. The good clinical results we obtained

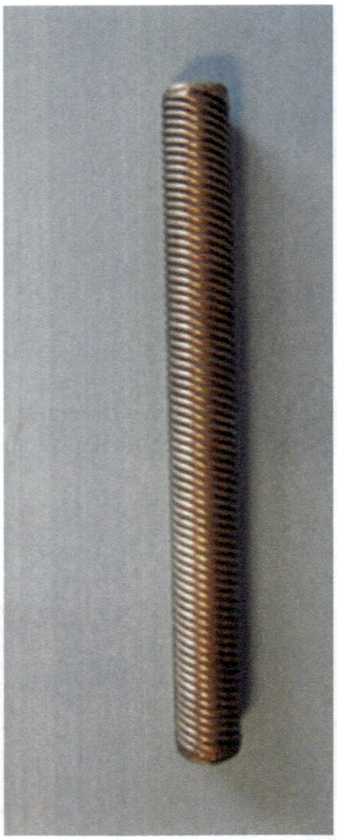

Fig. 12.6 The dynamic Talin rod was produced and used in our experimental study

led us to biomechanically investigate the effects of the dynamic screw–dynamic rod system on a disturbed motion segment.

While performing tests of the dynamic rod and screw implants in spine stabilization with finite element (FE) and cadaver studies at the University of Toledo (OH), we had the opportunity to try the dynamic screw and rod system. We used the rod that we produced as the dynamic rod and named it the Talin rod (Fig. 12.6).

12.3 Intact L1–S1 Finite Element Model

In this study, an experimentally validated nonlinear finite element model of the lumbar spine (L1–S1) was used [11–16]. To compose the mesh model, 1.5-mm-thick transverse sections were taken with computed tomography. The mesh was symmetrical along the midsagittal line. The material properties of the FE model components were selected from the literature, including our experimental data (Table 12.1).

The model included all major physiological characteristics of the true spine, including the seven major ligaments, intervertebral discs, and apophyseal (facet) joints. The FE spine was modified to simulate the following five surgical scenarios: (1) stabilized, (2) stabilized dynamic screw and dynamic rod (DSDR), (3) destabilized rigid screw and dynamic rod (RSDR), (4) destabilized dynamic screw and rigid rod (DSRR), and (5) stabilized rigid screw and rigid rod (RSRR).

The FE study aimed to simulate the biomechanical effects of a new posterior dynamic stabilization system consisting of a helical spring-based dynamic rod (DSDR) connecting dynamic (hinged) screws and compare it with semirigid (DSRR and RSRR) and rigid stabilization (RSRR) systems. The FE model of L1–S1 after single-level instrumentation with different posterior stabilization systems was used to measure the biomechanical parameters of the spine, such as the range of motion (ROM), intra-discal pressure, stresses, and facet loads. Experimentally obtained results from intact and instrumented spines in vitro were used to validate the FE model, and the model was used to compare the biomechanical effects of various fusion and stabilization constructs under a hybrid loading protocol. Segmental motion increased by 9.5% in L4–L5 and 16.3% in flexion and left rotation but decreased by 6.4% and 10.9% in extension and left-bending loads, respectively.

Intra-discal pressure at L3–L4 and L5–S1 induced by instrumentation in the adjacent segments was lower than that in the intact model of dynamic rod structures (DSDR and RSDR), except in the RSDR model. The movement in the RSDR model was 9.7% lower than the intact model at L3–L4 but was found to be 11.3% higher in L5–S1. Facet loads that did not exceed 12 N in any of the flexed instrumented cases were found to be insignificant. Furthermore, the facet load in the DSDR case was similar to that in the intact spine. Dynamic rod structures (DSDR and RSDR) resulted in less peak stress on screws compared to rigid rod structures (DSRR and RSRR) in all loading conditions. A dynamic

Table 12.1 Material properties for the spine FE model components

Part	Element type	Young's modulus (MPa)	Poisson ratio
Bony structures			
Cortical bone	Isotropic, elastic eight-node elements	12,000	0.3
Cancellous bone	Isotropic, elastic eight-node elements	100	0.2
Posterior bone	Isotropic, elastic eight-node elements	3500	0.25
Intervertebral disc			
Annulus (ground)	Neo-Hookean, hex elements	C10 ¼ 0.3448, D1 ¼ 0.3	–
Annulus (fiber)	REBAR	357–550	0.3
Nucleus pulposus	Incompressible fluid, cavity elements	1	0.499
Ligaments			
Anterior ligaments	Tension only, truss elements	7.8 (12%), 20 (0.12%)	0.3
Posterior ligaments	Tension only, truss elements	10 (11%), 20 (0.11%)	0.3
Ligamentum flavum	Tension only, truss elements	15.0 (6.2%), 19.5 (0.6.2%)	0.3
Transverse ligament	Tension only, truss elements	10.0 (18%), 58.7 (0.18%)	0.3
Capsular ligament	Tension only, truss elements	7.5 (25%), 32.90 (0.25%)	0.3
Interspinous ligament	Tension only, truss elements	10.0 (14%), 11.6 (0.14%)	0.3
Supraspinous ligament	Tension only, truss elements	8.0 (20%), 15.0 (0.20%)	0.3
Joint			
Apophyseal joints	Nonlinear soft contact, GAPUNI elements	–	–

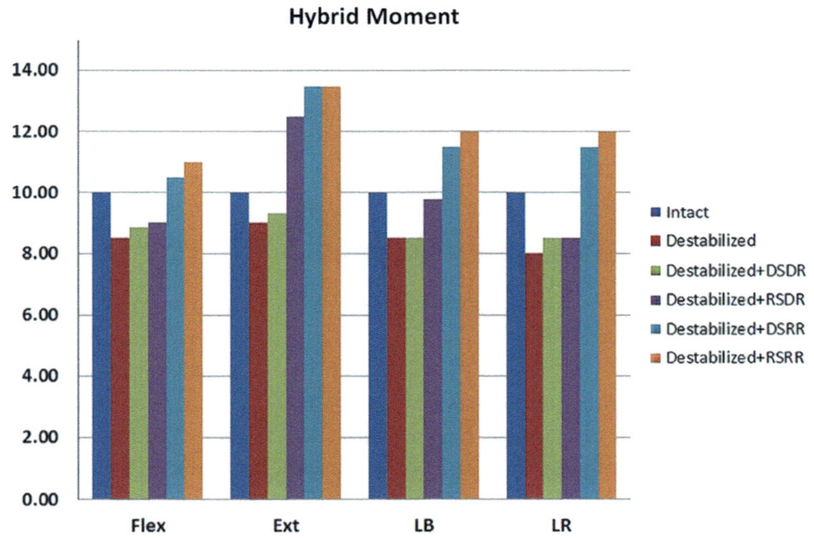

Fig. 12.7 When considering the results, in hybrid moment flexion, extension, and right and left lateral bending, we obtain the results closest to the intact spine with the dynamic screw–dynamic rod combination

structure consisting of a dynamic rod and a dynamic screw protected the adjacent level from excessive movement [40].

When considering the results, those closest to the intact spine were obtained with the dynamic screw combined with a dynamic rod in hybrid moment flexion, extension, and right and left lateral bending (LB) (Fig. 12.7).

Furthermore, when the mean ROM values in the L4–L5 spine are examined, the dynamic combination provides results close to the intact spine [40] (Fig. 12.8).

The outcome of this study reported the biomechanical effects of dynamic, semirigid, and rigid posterior stabilization systems on the lumbar spine. Ultimately, ROM, facet joint loads, intradisc pressures, and stresses on pedicle screws were observed and compared. The biomechanical results of this study support the hypothesis that DSDR structures provide a stabilizing function

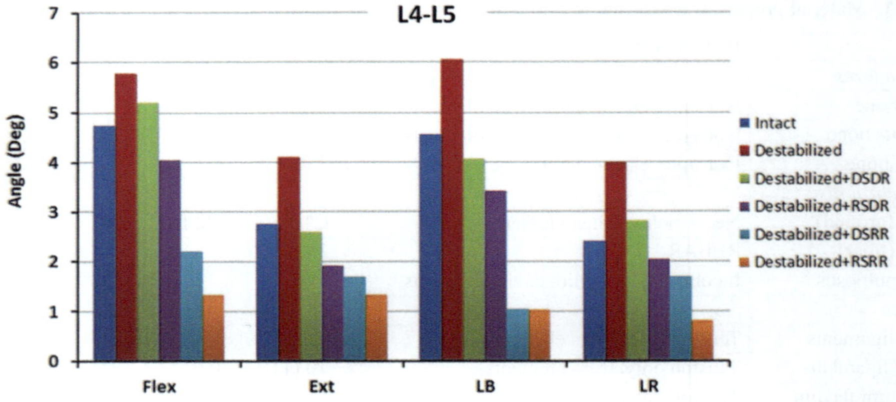

Fig. 12.8 When the average range of motion (ROM) values are examined at the L4–L5 spine, the dynamic combination gives results close to the intact spine compared to the others

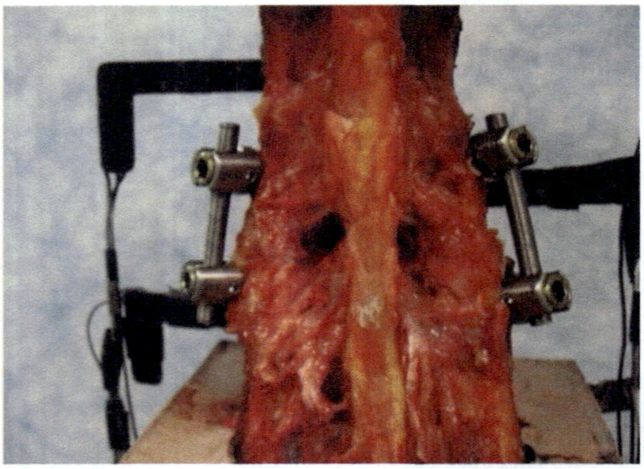

Fig. 12.9 Six fresh-frozen lumbar spine specimens, L2–S1, were used for the current study

as a posterior stabilization system and may better address the adjacent segment degeneration and implant failure problems than rigid or semirigid structures.

Based on the results of this study, we also performed studies on cadavers using the FE model [41]. Six fresh-frozen lumbar spine specimens, L2–S1, were used (Fig. 12.9).

Each sample was subjected to a pure bending force at a maximum of 10 Nm, obtained in increments of 1.5, 3.0, 4.5, 7.0, and 10 Nm, to simulate physiological flexion (Flex), extension (Ext), lateral bending (LB), and axial rotation (AR). Before sampling the data, each sample was preconditioned for three cycles for each loading plane (Flex, Ext, LB, and AR) to eliminate any viscoelastic effects. Each specimen was tested under the following conditions: (1) intact; (2) destabilized; (3) destabilized, followed by DSDR instrumentation; (4) destabilized, followed by DSDR and DSRR instrumentation; and (5) destabilized, followed by RSRR instrumentation. The dynamic rod used in this study has three concentric layers consisting of Ti6Al4 V alloy springs (Fig. 12.10a). The same alloy material was used for the springs and the rigid rod. The outer diameter of the dynamic and rigid rods was 6 mm in all structures. All screws were 50 mm long. Ti6Al4 V alloy dynamic screw (Safinaz and Medikon AS) and rigid screw (Medikon AS) were 6.5 mm in diameter (Fig. 12.10b). Details can be examined in our previous study [41].

When interpreting the results of this study (Fig. 12.11), we concluded that the results obtained with flexion, extension, and right and left bending of the dynamic rod and screw combination are very close to the intact motion segment. Based on our literature review, no concurrent FE and cadaver studies were similar to our study.

As is already known, dynamic systems are used in fusion surgery, as explained in detail above, and these systems are known as "semirigid systems." When evaluating the results of our and other biomechanical studies, stabilization close to the rigid system has been reportedly achieved and remains widely used for fusion purposes in spine surgery [23–25, 35, 41, 42, 45–48].

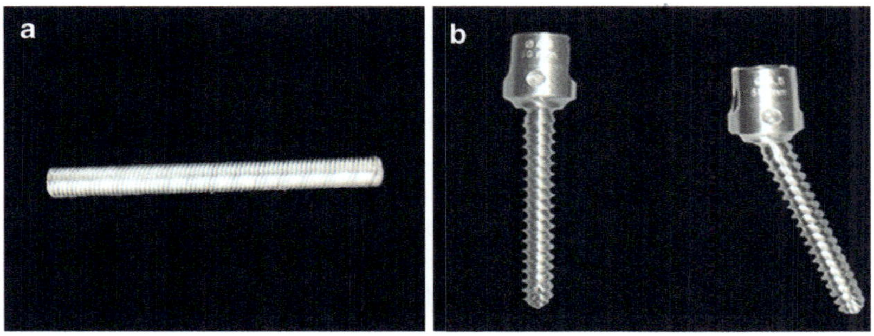

Fig. 12.10 (**a**) The dynamic rod used in our study and (**b**) a Safinaz screw

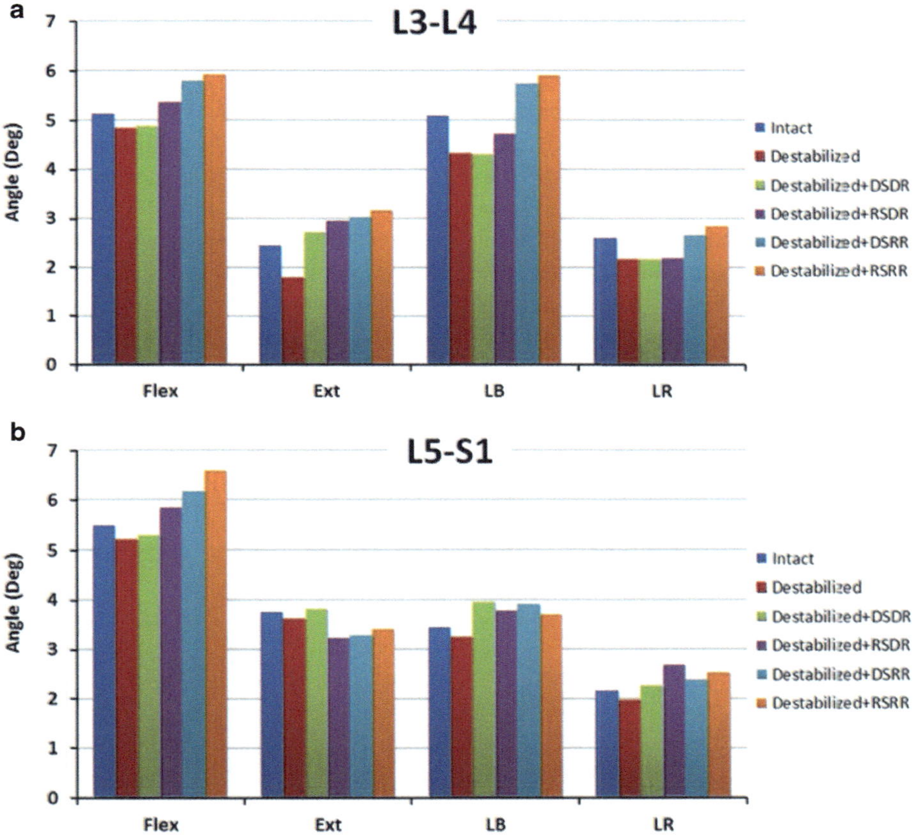

Fig. 12.11 Dynamic rod and screw combination results in flexion, extension, and right and left bending that are very close to the intact motion segment

If it is intended to maintain motion in the pedicular dynamic system, the dynamic system can be considered ideal if the neutral zone that is disturbed in the motion segment at or close to normal can be stabilized so that the motion segment can function normally. However, such a standard system may be impossible. Motion segments of people may differ for many reasons, including structural differences. The degree of structure degeneration that makes up the motion segment is also very important. Aiming for an ideal system for a motion segment with a severely degenerated disc may be useless because no matter what you do, the segment will gradually fuse.

Even in a series of patients with painful degenerative disc disease stabilized with a Polyetheretherketone (PEEK) rod and a dynamic screw, only one-third of the motion segments remained mobile post-procedure, and two-thirds lost motion. However, significant improvement in the Oswestry index and visual analog scales in all patients was reported in all groups compared to the preoperative scores. One-third benefited from the dynamic system, and the pain was relieved due to the dynamic system functionality, whereas the remaining two-thirds benefited from fusion development [49].

The questions to be investigated here are as follows: "Should we look at dynamic systems as a system trying to preserve motion?" or "Is it a stabilization method that should be used primarily in chronic instability, whether it keeps the movement or not?" Should we consider it? When we evaluate the disc in the motion segment to be stabilized following the Pfirrmann criteria preoperatively, we can decide whether the motion will be preserved or not. If we stabilize a disc with a dynamic rod and a dynamic screw at the early stages of degeneration, we can say that motion can be preserved.

However, it is notably slightly different from total disc prosthesis (TDR) indications. TDR can be used in advanced degeneration if the facet joints are intact and you can bring the motion segment to more physiological limits. Although complete integrity has not been achieved in TDR indications, at least the posterior colon remains healthy. Thus, TDR may not be appropriate for advanced degenerative disc diseases [50]. With TDR, however, the patient may have a chance to preserve motion, but when a degenerated disc is dynamically stabilized, it is more likely to be fused under the stabilizing influence of the dynamic system [49] (Fig. 12.12).

An ideal dynamic system should allow the movement provided by a normal movement segment. In other words, the movement capability of the dynamic exercise should be within physiological limits. Does moving in all directions within the normal physiological limits have anything to do with age, height, and muscle volume? Or do ethnic reasons play a role? The hypermobility of motion segments does not mean that they are unstable [51, 52]. "Do Olympic gymnasts perform their exercises in pain?" Who among us would dare to do what they do? In this case, it's impossible to expect

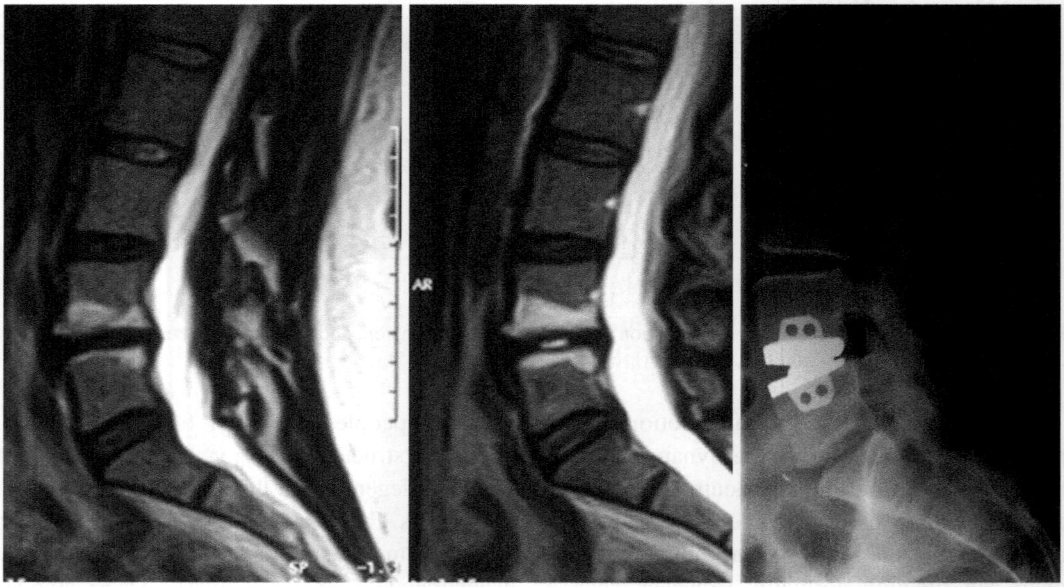

Fig. 12.12 TDR was performed on the patient with severe lower back pain with Modic degeneration. The patient is satisfied with her life postoperatively, and the motion segment is mobile

a single rod to provide the characteristics of a movement segment that varies from person to person. Perhaps in the future, rod systems will be custom-made or standardized based on factors like weight, age, and height. Maybe in the future, rod systems will be made individually or standardized based on a person's weight, age, and height. Therefore, the exact answer to the question "On what data do you actuate the rod or screw?" remains unclear. When we discovered the biomechanically dynamic rod–dynamic screw system to restore the deteriorated neutral zone and its clinical results were satisfactory, we thought that a new classification should be made. In pedicular dynamic systems, we made a new classification by including the dynamic screw–dynamic rod combination in a separate group [52].

In lumbar canal stenosis, the spine may become unstable after decompression; hence, should we do fusion in this case? Although we tried to preserve the anatomy in order to not increase instability when performing a laminectomy, we removed the medial edges of the facet joints, which are part of the canal stenosis, and performed a discectomy on the protruded disc to effectively widen the canal. In these patients, the possibility of increased minor instability preoperatively and becoming more overt postoperatively is observed. In these patients, we can consider fusion surgery, together with a rigid instrument system. However, the ideal treatment is to remove parts of the ipsilateral and contralateral facets that protrude into the canal with a unilateral approach so that the anatomy during decompression will not be disturbed. We think that it would be more appropriate to use the pedicular dynamic system to prevent the increasingly limited instability that may develop in the future [53].

We observed that for the surgical treatment of disc herniation, stabilization with a pedicular dynamic system by performing limited discectomy instead of subtotal discectomy would be a more suitable physiological operation. This issue is discussed in detail in a separate chapter in the book. We used dynamic stabilization without considering the degenerative disc disease that progresses with pain, with insufficient medical treatment, and does not respond to physical therapy and rehabilitation (PTR) and algological interventions [54].

We used it in painful disc degenerations with Modic degeneration and obtained very positive results [55]. We showed that the radiological "high-intensity zone" due to the tear in the posterior annulus will disappear over time after stabilizing with the pedicular dynamic system [56].

In degenerated disc disease, based on the indications, our clinical results were found to be quite satisfactory in the TDR applications but with only a small number of patients for spinal stabilization [57]. However, the pedicular dynamic system can be primarily used because it is a simpler applicable method [58].

We thought that the "prosthetic disc nucleus" (PDN), which is produced to fulfill the functions of degenerated discs and is recommended to be used alone, could be used more safely with posterior dynamic systems. The Prosthetic Disc Nucleus (PDN) was not successful because the cartilage broke the end plates and the PDN embedded itself into the vertebral bodies above and below (Fig. 12.13) [59].

To better evaluate the clinical results, a controlled study was conducted on patients who underwent single-level fusion surgery and reported excellent results. The point that should be kept in mind is that pedicular dynamic systems are so simple that they cannot be compared with fusion surgery, and revision is easier based on mortality/morbidity rates [60]. Thus, results should be compared with pedicular dynamic systems rather than fusion surgery.

We used a dynamic rod and a dynamic screw, combined with an agile rod. No complications were encountered until the agile rods broke. Later, the CD HORIZON BalanC™ dynamic rod was introduced to the market by the same company (Fig. 12.14) to increase the load on the graft at a single level and reduce the stress on the adjacent segment.

From our previous dynamic rod experience, we thought that the new dynamic rod, Balance C, was built based on Agile rod experiences, as our clinical results were good in some patients until the Agile rods broke. In our clinical study, which included 71 patients who underwent single-level

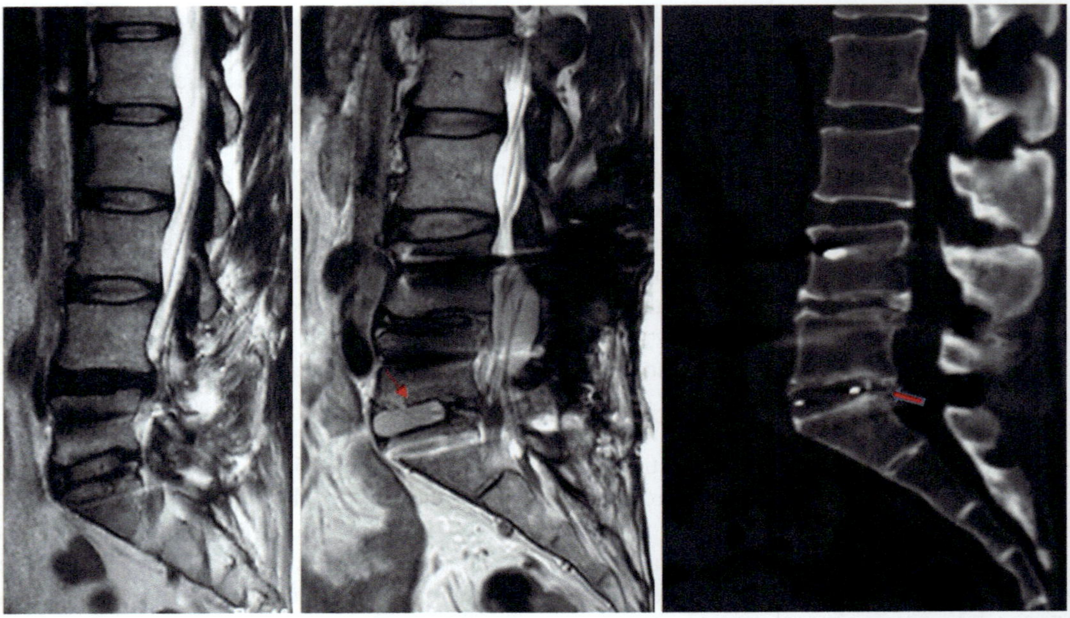

Fig. 12.13 "Prosthetic disc nucleus" was not successful because it broke the cartilage end plates and fused the vertebral bodies around the PDN

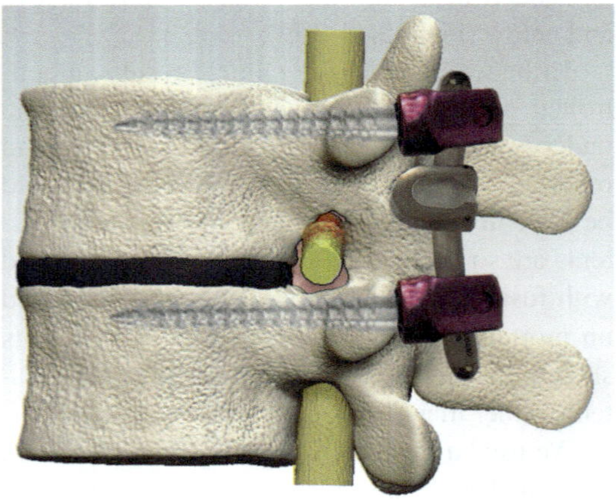

Fig. 12.14 CD HORIZON BalanC™. (Courtesy of Ali Fahir Özer)

stabilization using different dynamic instruments, we used a combination of "dynamic screw and Balance C rod" in 17 patients [61]. We did not encounter any complications of this combination in our mean follow-up of 30 months. However, the company withdrew it from the market after these rods broke. We were worried that these rods, which we used as non-fusion in our patients, would break. We found that the rods were broken in four patients who presented with recurrent lower back pain after an average of 4 years. As with the Agile rod, no problem was reported in the Balance C rod until it broke in all four patients [61].

We currently use a FLEX +2 system rod for single-level stabilizations, and after >1 year of stabilizations, only one out of 15 patients had broken rods (unpublished data). We noticed that the patient's body mass index was higher than normal, and he was larger than his peers. As is already known, the FLEX +2 system rod provides rod movement with a multifilament wire, as in the Agile rod. A polyurethane ring is placed around this wire that prevents excessive flexing and elongation movements of the rod (Fig. 12.15).

A multifilament wire is not a suitable material for a dynamic rod (Fig. 12.16). Different designs and materials are required for an ideal and long-lasting, powerful dynamic rod. Clinical findings related to the FLEX +2 system rod will be described in a separate section in this book.

Moreover, the facet replacement systems should also be considered. Despite intensive studies on this subject and a large amount of budget allocated by companies, no product has entered the market. Systems with pedicular dynamic screws and dynamic rods act as facet replacement systems that support the facets. It can be used unilaterally when removal of the facet joint is required in the surgical treatment of unilateral foraminal stenosis (Fig. 12.17). Thus, surgery can become minimally invasive [62].

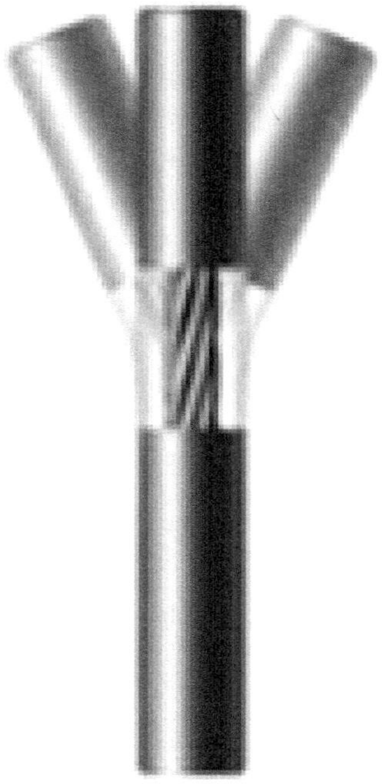

Fig. 12.15 FLEX +2 system, a multifilament wire like the Agile rod, provides the mobile part of the rod

However, the problem stems from the absence of an ideal dynamic rod. In dynamic systems, the instrument should be planned to last for a very long time, as in knee and hip prostheses. Since it is faced with continuous loading, it should be designed using biocompatible materials that withstand long-term loads. Our problem is not that the concept is wrong but that the material is insufficient.

Although there is no clinical problem in patient stabilization, we think that instability caused by more than one motion segment can be eliminated with rods made of a biocompatible material. However, since we could not overcome the material problem at the moment, we changed the screw design and created the Orthrus system. We started using it in the clinic because it was biomechanically sufficient [39]. Clinical findings related to Orthrus will be discussed as a separate chapter in this book.

In conclusion, no problem in fusion-free stabilization was encountered with pedicular dynamic systems, regardless of a single motion segment.

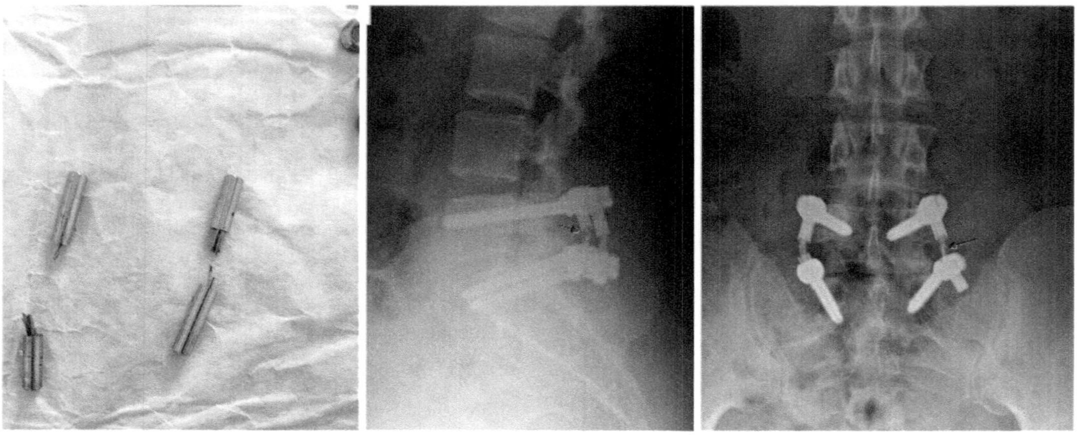

Fig. 12.16 Flex-2 rod, a multifilament wire, is not a suitable material for dynamic rods

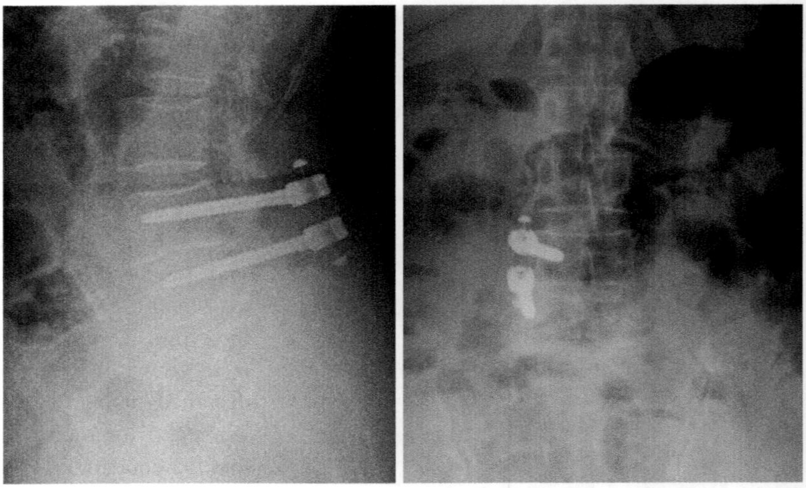

Fig. 12.17 A dynamic system can even be used unilaterally

However, systems using DSDRs, in order to protect the motion, restore the disturbed motion segment and bring the motion segment closer to physiological limits. However, the dynamic rod must be sufficiently rigid not to cause abnormal movement. Thus, the rod should be at least softer than the PEEK rod being used dynamically at the moment.

References

1. Fernström U. Arthroplasty with intercorporal endoprothesis in herniated disc and in painful disc. Acta Chir Scand Suppl. 1966;357:154–9.
2. Büttner-Janz K, Schellnack K, Zippel H. An alternative treatment strategy in lumbar intervertebral disk damage using an SB Charité modular type intervertebral disk endoprosthesis. Z Orthop Ihre Grenzgeb. 1987;125(1):1–6. https://doi.org/10.1055/s-2008-1039666.
3. Vital JM, Boissière L. Total disc replacement. Orthop Traumatol Surg Res. 2014;100(1 Suppl):S1–14. https://doi.org/10.1016/j.otsr.2013.06.018.
4. Cui XD, Li HT, Zhang W, Zhang LL, Luo ZP, Yang HL. Mid- to long-term results of total disc replacement for lumbar degenerative disc disease: a systematic review. J Orthop Surg Res. 2018;13(1):326. https://doi.org/10.1186/s13018-018-1032-6.
5. Kitzen J, Vercoulen TFG, van Kuijk SMJ, Schotanus MGM, Kort NP, van Rhijn LW, Willems PCPH. Long-term clinical outcome of two revision strategies for failed total disc replacements. Eur Spine J. 2020;29(7):1536–43. https://doi.org/10.1007/s00586-019-06184-x.
6. Gomleksiz C, Sasani M, Oktenoglu T, Ozer AF. A short history of posterior dynamic stabilization. Adv Orthop. 2012;2012:629698. https://doi.org/10.1155/2012/629698.
7. Hibbs RA. An operation for progressive spinal deformities: a preliminary report of three cases from the service of the orthopaedic hospital. 1911. Clin Orthop Relat Res. 2007;460:17–20. https://doi.org/10.1097/BLO.0b013e3180686b30.
8. Albee F. Transplantation of a portion of the tibia into the spine for Pott's disease: a preliminary report. JAMA. 1911;57:885.
9. Harrington PR. Treatment of scoliosis. Correction and internal fixation by spine instrumentation. J Bone Joint Surg Am. 1962;44-A:591–610.
10. Harrington PR. Present status of spine instrumentation in scoliosis. Am J Orthop. 1963;5:228–31.
11. Luque ER. Interpeduncular segmental fixation. Clin Orthop Relat Res. 1986;203:54–7.
12. Mazda K, Ilharreborde B, Even J, Lefevre Y, Fitoussi F, Penneçot GF. Efficacy and safety of posteromedial translation for correction of thoracic curves in adolescent idiopathic scoliosis using a new connection to the spine: the Universal Clamp. Eur Spine J. 2009;18(2):158–69. https://doi.org/10.1007/s00586-008-0839-y.
13. Hopf CG, Eysel P, Dubousset J. Operative treatment of scoliosis with Cotrel-Dubousset-Hopf instrumentation. New anterior spinal device. Spine (Phila Pa 1976). 1997;22(6):618–27. https://doi.org/10.1097/00007632-199703150-00008.
14. Cotrel Y, Dubousset J. A new technic for segmental spinal osteosynthesis using the posterior approach. Rev Chir Orthop Reparatrice Appar Mot. 1984;70:489–94.
15. Graf H. Second meeting. Rome: European Spine Society; 1991.
16. Graf H. Lumbar instability: surgical treatment without fusion. Rachis. 1992;412:123–37.
17. Panjabi MM. The stabilizing system of the spine. Part II. Neutral zone and instability hypothesis.

J Spinal Disord. 1992;5(4):390–6. https://doi.org/10.1097/00002517-199212000-00002.
18. Dupuis PR, Yong-Hing K, Cassidy JD, Kirkaldy-Willis WH. Radiologic diagnosis of degenerative lumbar spinal instability. Spine (Phila Pa 1976). 1985;10(3):262–76. https://doi.org/10.1097/00007632-198504000-00015.
19. Pope MH, Panjabi M. Biomechanical definitions of spinal instability. Spine (Phila Pa 1976). 1985;10(3):255–6. https://doi.org/10.1097/00007632-198504000-00013.
20. Panjabi MM. The stabilizing system of the spine. Part I. Function, dysfunction, adaptation, and enhancement. J Spinal Disord. 1992;5(4):383–9. https://doi.org/10.1097/00002517-199212000-00001.
21. Gertzbein SD, Seligman J, Holtby R, Chan KH, Kapasouri A, Tile M, Cruickshank B. Centrode patterns and segmental instability in degenerative disc disease. Spine (Phila Pa 1976). 1985;10(3):257–61. https://doi.org/10.1097/00007632-198504000-00014.
22. Paris SV. Physical signs of instability. Spine (Phila Pa 1976). 1985;10(3):277–9. https://doi.org/10.1097/00007632-198504000-00016.
23. Duffield RC, Carson WL, Chen LY, Voth B. Longitudinal element size effect on load sharing, internal loads, and fatigue life of tri-level spinal implant constructs. Spine (Phila Pa 1976). 1993;18(12):1695–703. https://doi.org/10.1097/00007632-199309000-00019.
24. Goel VK, Konz RJ, Chang HT, Grosland NM, Grobler LJ, Chesmel KD. Hinged-dynamic posterior device permits greater loads on the graft and similar stability as compared with its equivalent rigid device: a three-dimensional finite element assessment. J Prosthet Orthot. 2001;13(1):17–20.
25. Goel VK, Gilbertson LG. Basic science of spinal instrumentation. Clin Orthop Relat Res. 1997;335:10–31.
26. Kummer B. Biomechanische Aspekte der Instabilität der Wirbelsäule. In: Fuchs GA, editor. Die instabile Wirbelsäule. Stuttgart/New York: Georg Thieme; 1991. p. S 8–14.
27. Bergmark A. Stability of the lumbar spine. A study in mechanical engineering. Acta Orthop Scand Suppl. 1989;230:1–54.
28. Lowery GL, Harms J. In: Bridwell KH, DeWald RL, editors. Principles of load sharing in the textbook of spinal surgery. 2nd ed. Lippincott-Raven Publishers; 1997. p. 155–65.
29. Biedermann L. Biomechanics of pedicle fixation as related to implant design. Presented at the American-European meeting on pedicle fixation of the spine and other advanced Tehniques. Munich, Germany; 1994.
30. Niosi CA, Zhu QA, Wilson DC, Keynan O, Wilson DR, Oxland TR. Biomechanical characterization of the three-dimensional kinematic behaviour of the Dynesys dynamic stabilization system: an in vitro study. Eur Spine J. 2006;15(6):913–22. https://doi.org/10.1007/s00586-005-0948-9.
31. Barrey C, Freitas E, Perrin G. Pedicle screw-based dynamic stabilization devices in the lumbar spine: biomechanical concepts, technologies, classification, and clinical results. In: Advanced concepts in lumbar degenerative disk disease. Springer; 2016.
32. Freudiger S, Dubois G, Lorrain M. Dynamic neutralization of the lumbar spine confirmed on a new lumbar spine simulator in vitro. Arch Orthop Trauma Surg. 1999;119:127–32.
33. Barrey C, Perrin G, Champain S. Pedicle-screw-based dynamic systems and degenerative lumbar diseases: biomechanical and clinical experiences of dynamic fusion with isobar TTL. ISRN Orthop. 2013;2013:183702. https://doi.org/10.1155/2013/183702.
34. Templier A, Denninger L, Mazel C, et al. Comparison between two different concepts of lumbar posterior osteosynthesis implants a finite-element analysis. Eur J Orthop Surg Traumatol. 1998;8:27–36. https://doi.org/10.1007/BF01782894.
35. Wang H, Peng J, Zeng Q, Zhong Y, Xiao C, Ye Y, Huang W, Liu W, Luo J. Dynesys system vs posterior decompression and fusion for the treatment of lumbar degenerative diseases. Medicine (Baltimore). 2020;99(21):e19784. https://doi.org/10.1097/MD.0000000000019784.
36. von Strempel A. Dynamic stabilisation: cosmic system. Interact Surg. 2008;3(4):229–36.
37. Maleci A, Sambale RD, Schiavone M, Lamp F, Özer F, von Strempel A. Nonfusion stabilization of the degenerative lumbar spine. J Neurosurg Spine. 2011;15(2):151–8. https://doi.org/10.3171/2011.3.SPINE0969.
38. Liu C, Kamara A, Yan Y. Investigation into the biomechanics of lumbar spine micro-dynamic pedicle screw. BMC Musculoskelet Disord. 2018;19:231.
39. Ozer AF, Cevik OM, Erbulut DU, Yaman O, Senturk S, Oktenoglu T, Sasani M, Suzer T, Goel V. A novel modular dynamic stabilization system for the treatment of degenerative spinal pathologies. Turk Neurosurg. 2019;29(1):115–20. https://doi.org/10.5137/1019-5149.JTN.23227-18.1.
40. Erbulut DU, Kiapour A, Oktenoglu T, Ozer AF, Goel VK. A computational biomechanical investigation of posterior dynamic instrumentation: combination of dynamic rod and hinged (dynamic) screw. J Biomech Eng. 2014;136(5):051007. https://doi.org/10.1115/1.4027060.
41. Oktenoglu T, Erbulut DU, Kiapour A, Ozer AF, Lazoglu I, Kaner T, Sasani M, Goel VK. Pedicle screw-based posterior dynamic stabilisation of the lumbar spine: in vitro cadaver investigation and a finite element study. Comput Methods Biomech Biomed Engin. 2015;18(11):1252–61. https://doi.org/10.1080/10255842.2014.890187.
42. Bozkuş H, Senoğlu M, Baek S, Sawa AG, Ozer AF, Sonntag VK, Crawford NR. Dynamic lumbar pedicle screw-rod stabilization: in vitro biomechanical comparison with standard rigid pedicle screw-rod stabili-

zation. J Neurosurg Spine. 2010;12(2):183–9. https://doi.org/10.3171/2009.9.SPINE0951.

43. Schmoelz W, Onder U, Martin A, von Strempel A. Non-fusion instrumentation of the lumbar spine with a hinged pedicle screw rod system: an in vitro experiment. Eur Spine J. 2009;18(10):1478–85. https://doi.org/10.1007/s00586-009-1052-3.
44. Kaner T, Sasani M, Oktenoglu T, Cosar M, Ozer AF. Utilizing dynamic rods with dynamic screws in the surgical treatment of chronic instability: a prospective clinical study. Turk Neurosurg. 2009;19(4):319–26.
45. Jahng TA, Kim YE, Moon KY. Comparison of the biomechanical effect of pedicle-based dynamic stabilization: a study using finite element analysis. Spine J. 2013;13(1):85–94. https://doi.org/10.1016/j.spinee.2012.11.014.
46. Schmoelz W, Huber JF, Nydegger T, Dipl-Ing, Claes L, Wilke HJ. Dynamic stabilization of the lumbar spine and its effects on adjacent segments: an in vitro experiment. J Spinal Disord Tech. 2003;16(4):418–23. https://doi.org/10.1097/00024720-200308000-00015.
47. Cook DJ, Yeager MS, Thampi SS, Whiting DM, Cheng BC. Stability and load sharing characteristics of a posterior dynamic stabilization device. Int J Spine Surg. 2015;9:9. https://doi.org/10.14444/2009.
48. Liu CL, Zhong ZC, Shih SL, Hung C, Lee YE, Chen CS. Influence of Dynesys system screw profile on adjacent segment and screw. J Spinal Disord Tech. 2010;23(6):410–7. https://doi.org/10.1097/BSD.0b013e3181b63d89.
49. Yilmaz A, Senturk S, Sasani M, Oktenoglu T, Yaman O, Yildirim H, Suzer T, Ozer AF. Disc rehydration after dynamic stabilization: a report of 59 cases. Asian Spine J. 2017;11(3):348–55. https://doi.org/10.4184/asj.2017.11.3.348.
50. Büttner-Janz K, Guyer RD, Ohnmeiss DD. Indications for lumbar total disc replacement: selecting the right patient with the right indication for the right total disc. Int J Spine Surg. 2014;8:12. https://doi.org/10.14444/1012.
51. Beazell JR, Mullins M, Grindstaff TL. Lumbar instability: an evolving and challenging concept. J Man Manip Ther. 2010;18(1):9–14. https://doi.org/10.1179/106698110X12595770849443.
52. Kaner T, Sasani M, Oktenoglu T, Ozer AF. Dynamic stabilization of the spine: a new classification system. Turk Neurosurg. 2010;20(2):205–15. https://doi.org/10.5137/1019-5149.JTN.2358-09.2.
53. Kaner T, Sasani M, Oktenoglu T, Aydin AL, Ozer AF. Clinical outcomes of degenerative lumbar spinal stenosis treated with lumbar decompression and the Cosmic "semi-rigid" posterior system. SAS J. 2010;4(4):99–106.
54. Oktenoglu T, Ozer AF, Sasani M, Kaner T, Canbulat N, Ercelen O, Sarioglu AC. Posterior dynamic stabilization in the treatment of lumbar degenerative disc disease: 2-year follow-up. Minim Invasive Neurosurg. 2010;53(3):112–6. https://doi.org/10.1055/s-0030-1262810.
55. Eser O, Gomleksiz C, Sasani M, Oktenoglu T, Aydin AL, Ataker Y, Suzer T, Ozer AF. Dynamic stabilisation in the treatment of degenerative disc disease with modic changes. Adv Orthop. 2013;2013:806267. https://doi.org/10.1155/2013/806267.
56. Canbay S, Ataker Y, Canbulat N, Kabaoglu ZU, Oktenoglu T, Sasani M, Ozer AF. Effect of posterior dynamic instrumentation on high-intensity zone in lumbar degenerative disc disease. Turk Neurosurg. 2015;25(4):578–85. https://doi.org/10.5137/1019-5149.JTN.12350-14.1.
57. Sasani M, Oktenoğlu T, Tuncay K, Canbulat N, Carilli S, Ozer FA. Total disc replacement in the treatment of lumbar discogenic pain with disc herniation: a prospective clinical study. Turk Neurosurg. 2009;19(2):127–34.
58. Oktenoglu T, Ozer AF, Sasani M, Ataker Y, Gomleksiz C, Celebi I. Posterior transpedicular dynamic stabilization versus total disc replacement in the treatment of lumbar painful degenerative disc disease: a comparison of clinical results. Adv Orthop. 2013;2013:874090. https://doi.org/10.1155/2013/874090.
59. Sasani M, Aydin AL, Oktenoglu T, Cosar M, Ataker Y, Kaner T, Ozer AF. The combined use of a posterior dynamic transpedicular stabilization system and a prosthetic disc nucleus device in treating lumbar degenerative disc disease with disc herniations. SAS J. 2008;2(3):130–6. https://doi.org/10.1016/SASJ-2008-0008-NT.
60. Kaner T, Dalbayrak S, Oktenoglu T, Sasani M, Aydin AL, Ozer AF. Comparison of posterior dynamic and posterior rigid transpedicular stabilization with fusion to treat degenerative spondylolisthesis. Orthopedics. 2010;33(5) https://doi.org/10.3928/01477447-20100329-09.
61. Ozer AF, Oktenoglu T, Egemen E, Sasani M, Yilmaz A, Erbulut DU, Yaman O, Suzer T. Lumbar single-level dynamic stabilization with semi-rigid and full dynamic systems: a retrospective clinical and radiological analysis of 71 patients. Clin Orthop Surg. 2017;9(3):310–6. https://doi.org/10.4055/cios.2017.9.3.310.
62. Ozer AF, Suzer T, Sasani M, Oktenoglu T, Cezayirli P, Marandi HJ, Erbulut DU. Simple facet joint repair with dynamic pedicular system: technical note and case series. J Craniovertebr Junction Spine. 2015;6(2):65–8. https://doi.org/10.4103/0974-8237.156049.

Indications of Dynamic Stabilization Without Fusion

13

Mario Di Silvestre

13.1 Introduction

Different dynamic neutralization systems have been introduced as alternatives to lumbar rigid fixation to permit restricted motion across a functional spinal unit and reduce adjacent disc degeneration [1–3]. The theory is to reduce loading of the facet joints and preserve the operated segment kinematics. The goal is to preserve lumbar motion, achieving lumbar stability in patients who have lumbar spinal problems.

In the category of dynamic neutralization systems, the DYNESYS® (Zimmer, Switzerland) is the most popular [1, 4]. This system is a bilateral posterior device, which consists of titanium alloy pedicle screws and polycarbonate urethane (PCU) spacers that surround tensioned polyethylene terephthalate (PET) cords. The PCU spacers are placed bilaterally between the pedicle screwheads. Tensile forces, which act during flexion movements, are stabilized by the pretensioned PET cords, which run through the hollow core of the PCU spacers. A standardized preload of 300 N is applied to the cord during implantation; however, the length of the spacer, which must be adjusted to match each patient, directly influences lordosis, the intersegmental motion, and loading [5].

M. Di Silvestre (✉)
Chief of Spinal Deformity Department, Ospedale Santa Corona, Pietra Ligure, Italy

The research toward dynamic neutralization systems required in the past an evolution of implants design. For example, Gedet et al. [6] performed an in vitro study to compare the properties of a modular dynamic lumbar stabilization system (Synthes, Switzerland) with those of DYNESYS®, under the influence of an axial preload. In contrast to DYNESYS®, this different system consisted of a metallic rod with an integrated polymeric (PCU) damping unit, joined to a second metallic rod, which could be trimmed to length. The two rod components were assembled via a form-fitting, locking connection at the damper unit to form a single continuous element of variable length but with a predefined bending stiffness. Segmental range of motion (ROM) was significantly reduced for flexion–extension and lateral bending with both DYNESYS® and the modular implant ($P < 0.001$). On average, motion in flexion was reduced to less than 20% of the intact level and, in extension, to approximately 40% of the intact level. In lateral bending, a motion reduction to less than 40% of the intact level was measured. In torsion, the total ROM was not significantly different than that of the intact level. No significant differences were found between the two implant types for total ROM (flexion–extension: $P = 0.89$, lateral bending: $P = 0.98$, and torsion: $P = 0.56$). The degree of stabilization observed in the study of Gedet et al. [6] exceeds that measured in previous in vitro testing of dynamic stabilization systems

A. F. Özer et al. (eds.), *Dynamic Lumbar Spine Stabilization*,
https://doi.org/10.1007/978-3-032-12122-6_13

by Schmoelz et al. [7] (Fig. 13.1). However, it should also be noted that when one summarizes in vitro and in vivo results to date for DYNESYS® [1, 5, 7], the measured stabilization is in the range of 20–40% of the intact motion, which is similar to the results obtained in the study of Gedet et al. [6]. Tawackoli et al. [8] have shown that a compressive axial preload reduces segmental motion, most substantially for loads in the order of 300 N, with a much less substantial increase in stiffness for a further increase in preload to 1000 N. The finding of a substantial stabilizing effect of DYNESYS® is also in agreement with the results of Jensen et al. [9], who were not able to show the expected flexibility of the implant in their in vitro test. In that study, DYNESYS® performed identically to a normal metallic fixator, and it was also observed that a compressive preload decreased the segmental ROM even further (Table 13.1).

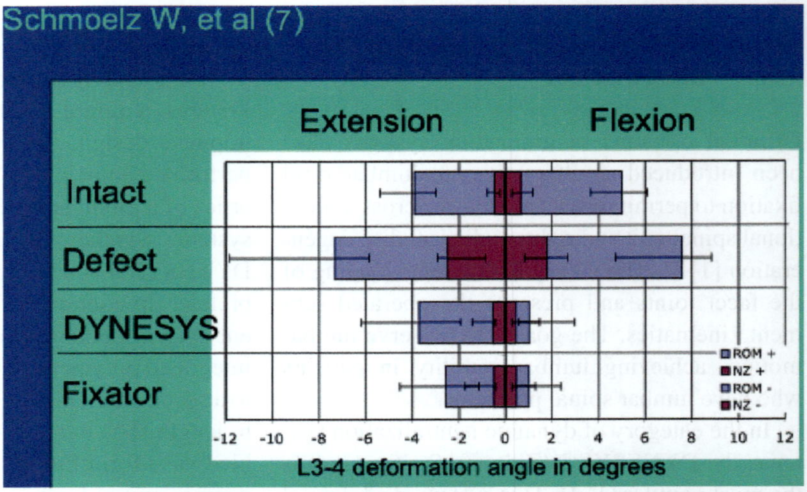

Fig. 13.1 Results of in vitro kinematics. (From Schmoelz et al. [7])

Table 13.1 Range of motion (ROM) comparison for intact specimen in different studies about DYNESYS®

	Flexion	Extension	Lateral bending	Axial rotation
Panjabi et al. 7.5 Nm	6.5	2.0	5.0/4.5	1.8/2.0
Fujiwara et al. 6.6 Nm (Male)	3.0	2.4	7.3	2.3
Mimura et al. 10 Nm	12.8	→	11.0 (2.5)	2.5 (2.0)
Schmoelz et al. 10 Nm	4.5	4.0	4.0/5.0	1.0/1.0
Yamamoto et al. 10 Nm	7.5 (0.8)	3.7 (0.3)	5.8 (0.5)/5.7 (0.3)	2.7 (0.4)/2.5 (0.4)
Freudiger et al. 18.3 Nm	9.6 (1.7)	2.1 (1.0)		
Niosi et al. [5] 7.5 Nm	3.7 (1.5)	3.3 (1.5)	3.5 (1.4)/4.1 (1.5)	2.2 (0.9)/1.2 (0.6)

From Niosi et al. [5]

13.2 Indications

According to Kaner et al. [10], indications of posterior dynamic stabilization devices are represented by degenerative spinal instability (disc degeneration, facet degeneration, and degenerative spondylolisthesis). In particular, DYNESYS® is indicated in the treatment of spinal degenerative pathologies, such as lumbar stenosis, disc degeneration with or without spondylolisthesis, or herniated discs. Moreover, the indication is lumbar disc degeneration, from mild discopathy up to stenosis with fixed deformation, restoring a better physiology of the disc: a certain degree of movement results preserved by the spacers of DYNESYS®.

There is still discussion about the advantages of dynamic stabilization in stopping the progression of spondylolisthesis. The advantages include a shorter operative time and hospital stay, less blood loss, and avoidance of morbidity due to bone graft harvesting. Kaner et al. [10] and Yu et al. [11] had similar clinical and radiological outcomes, which were not inferior to those of posterior fusion with instrumentation. Previous reports also found that DYNESYS® provides similar radiographic stability and clinical effects regardless of preoperative spondylolisthesis. These previous studies usually dealt with Grade I spondylolisthesis and achieved results comparable to those that dealt with no spondylolisthesis. Some investigators included Grade II spondylolisthesis and found favorable outcomes; however, an argument against the DYNESYS® system in this spinal disease pertains to its poor outcomes compared with those of fusion in patients with spondylolisthesis and concomitant spinal stenosis.

In conclusion, the main indication for DYNESYS® is represented by instability, i.e., dynamic instability in the early stages of disc degeneration; in this disease, the consequences are represented by dynamic stenosis or stenosis with degenerative olisthesis.

Another indication for DYNESYS® is represented by mono- or multi-segmental degenerative disc disease, as well as iatrogenic instability following decompression.

Expanded indications, as we experienced in the past years, are represented by multilevel decompression for stenoinstability of the lumbar spine or by elderly scoliotic deformities, often combined with multi-segmental disc degeneration of the lumbar spine. A severe contraindication for DYNESYS® instrumentation is the presence of a kyphotic lumbar spine or, in general, a sagittal imbalance of the spine.

13.3 Efficacy of DYNESYS®

Concerning the efficacy of the DYNESYS® system, Chang Hyun et al. [12] performed a meta-analysis of clinical studies: There were seven studies involving patients with a mean age of 50.3 years; treatment with dynamic stabilization using the DYNESYS® system was compared with conventional posterior lumbar interbody fusion (PLIF); the result was a similar clinical outcome at 2 years of follow-up and better perioperative outcomes in patients in the DYNESYS® group. Moreover, the ROM at the treated segment decreased by 42.0% in the DYNESYS® group and by 88.0% in the PLIF group. The DYNESYS® group maintained partial segmental motion and achieved clinical and functional outcomes comparable with those of the PLIF group. Regarding the protective effect against adjacent segment degeneration (ASD), previous studies have had conflicting results. This meta-analysis shows that the DYNESYS® group had no competitive advantage. The reasons for these contradictory results are unclear. One reason might be the difference in the pretension of the polyethylene terephthalate cord by surgeons. The DYNESYS® implantation guide recommends that a 300-N preload be applied to the cords to distract the disc during the implantation procedure. The use of a 300-N cord pretension causes a much higher stiffness at the implanted level than the intact lumbar spine. Because the effects of spacer length and cord tension on segmental flexibility and rigidity are still debated in the literature, in our experience, it is better to adjust the pretension below 300 N depending on the patient's condition. Other advantages of the DYNESYS® system are that the procedure to implant it is less invasive than PLIF, and it results in earlier recovery. The proponents of dynamic stabilization claim that, compared with conventional rigid spinal fusion, dynamic stabilization results in less morbidity by being less invasive. In short-term outcomes, this meta-analysis reveals that PDS provides a substantial advantage over PLIF in terms of recovery time. The DYNESYS® group showed a substantially reduced length of hospital stay and operative duration. The authors concluded that "both PDS and PLIF provide similar clinical outcomes in relatively adult patients (in their 5th to 6th decade of life) who undergo surgery for degenerative disc disease or spinal stenosis with or without spondylolisthesis." The DYNESYS® system reduces instability at the treated segment; the level of ASD prevention by DYNESYS® is unclear. Fusion remains the method of choice for advanced degeneration and severe instability. However, "degenerative spinal disease with or without Grade I spondylolisthesis, particularly in patients who require a quicker recovery after surgery, will likely constitute the indication for PDS using the DYNESYS® system" [12].

Considering the literature, now, the question of whether the DYNESYS® system is superior to posterior lumbar fusion in the treatment of lumbar degenerative diseases remains with no clear answer. Bao-Gan Peng and Chun-Hua Gao [13] compared clinical and radiological outcomes of patients who underwent dynamic stabilization with the DYNESYS® system with those who underwent posterior lumbar fusion to see if the application of the DYNESYS® system is superior to the traditional lumbar fusion surgery. The short-term effects of the DYNESYS® dynamic stabilization system are similar to those of traditional lumbar fusion surgery. Three comparative studies of DYNESYS® dynamic stabilization and fusion surgery with medium-term follow-up are encouraging. However, the results at long-term follow-up were not so encouraging. Actually, it is not possible to conclude that the DYNESYS® dynamic stabilization system is superior to fusion surgery for lumbar degenerative diseases [13]. A meta-analysis [14] showed that the ROM of the treatment segment in the DYNESYS® group and the PLIF group decreased by 42.0% and 88.0%, respectively. In the DYNESYS® group, partial segmental motion was maintained, and the clinical and functional results were comparable to those in the PLIF group [15–17].

Concerning the midterm results, the efficacy is still an object of different opinions. Wu et al. [18] compared the midterm clinical and imaging results of the DYNESYS® system and PLIF in the treatment of multi-segmental lumbar degenerative diseases. The visual analogue scale (VAS) score and oswestry disability index (ODI) of the two groups improved significantly at 3 months and the final follow-up, but there was no significant difference between the two groups. ROM decreased from 6.20° to 2.76° in the DYNESYS® group and from 6.56° to 0.00° in the PLIF group at the final follow-up. The ROM of the proximal adjacent segment in the PLIF group was significantly larger than that in the DYNESYS® group. Compared with PLIF, DYNESYS® stabilization maintained the mobility of the stabilized segments and had little effect on the adjacent segments, which helped prevent the degeneration of the adjacent segments. The authors considered the DYNESYS® system a feasible surgical procedure for the treatment of multilevel lumbar degenerative diseases in the midterm of follow-up.

In a retrospective study, Bredin et al. [19] compared 25 cases of lumbar posterolateral fusion with 32 cases of DYNESYS® dynamic stabilization for recurrent lumbar disc herniation or lumbar spinal canal stenosis and followed up for at least 5.5 years. The results showed that VAS and ODI were significantly lower in the DYNESYS® group than the fusion group, the SF-12 is a clear and international evaluation scale after spine surgery physical sub-score was significantly higher in the DYNESYS® group than the fusion group, and ROM in the treated segment was significantly greater in the DYNESYS® group than the fusion group (4.1 ± 2.0° vs 0.7 ± 0.5°). Imaging of adjacent disc degeneration of the fusion group was significantly higher than that of the DYNESYS® group (36.0% vs. 12.1%). Zhang et al. [20] retrospectively compared the clinical and imaging results of 96 cases of lumbar degenerative diseases treated by DYNESYS® and PLIF, including 46 cases in the DYNESYS® group and 50 cases in the PLIF group, with an average follow-up period of more than 50 months. At the final follow-up, the ODI and VAS scores were significantly improved in both groups. ROM of stabilized segments in the DYNESYS® group decreased from an average of 7.1° to 4.9° ($P < 0.05$), while the ROM of the stabilized segment of the PLIF group decreased from an average of 7.3° to 0°. At the last follow-up, the ROM of the proximal adjacent segments in both groups increased significantly, but the ROM of the PLIF group was higher than that of the DYNESYS® group. The incidence of ASD in the PLIF group was significantly higher than that in the DYNESYS® group. This study showed that the DYNESYS® system retained the ROM of the treated segment to a certain extent, limited the hypermobility of the proximal adjacent segment, and prevented the occurrence of ASD.

At present, the literature on long-term outcomes of dynamic stabilizers is represented by few studies, and the results of DYNESYS® are not encouraging. Only four long-term studies of the DYNESYS® system have been published. A comparative study of dynamic stabilization and fusion surgery with long-term follow-up is still lacking. Hoppe et al. [21] reported 39 consecutive patients who had symptomatic degenerative lumbar spondylolisthesis and were treated with decompression bilaterally and the DYNESYS® dynamic stabilization system at the L4/5 level, with an average follow-up period of 7.2 years, ranging from 5.0 to 11.2 yrs. At the final follow-up, 86% of the patients obtained improvement in back pain, and 89% obtained improvement in leg pain. Eighty-three percent of patients reported overall subjective improvement. Eight cases (21%) needed further surgical treatment due to symptomatic adjacent segment disease. In nine cases, imaging progress in spondylolisthesis was found. Adjacent segment pathology, though not clinically relevant, was diagnosed at 17.9% in the L5/S1 and 28.2% in the L3/4 segments. Zhang et al. [22] reported 38 patients with lumbar spinal stenosis, who were treated with the DYNESYS® system, with an average follow-up of 6.6 years (72–96 mo.). At the final follow-up, both lumbar spine function and lower back pain were significantly improved. The incidence of radiological and symptomatic ASD was 16% (6/38) and 3% (1/38), respectively. Veresciagina et al. [23] followed up 36 patients with degenerative spondylolisthesis and stenosis for at least 10 years, who were treated with decompression and DYNESYS® dynamic stabilization. Despite good clinical results, 17 cases and eight cases of progressive degenerative osteochondrosis and spondylolisthesis, respectively, were found in the adjacent segments, indicating that the DYNESYS® system did not prevent adjacent segment disease. St-Pierre et al. [24] followed up 52 patients with lumbar degenerative disease who underwent DYNESYS® dynamic stabilization for at least 5 years. The study showed that the DYNESYS® system was associated with a high incidence of ASD (15/52, 29%).

13.4 Conclusions

Dynamic stabilization with DYNESYS® is indicated for mobile and self-reducible lesions when they occur during disc degeneration. The suppression of movements enables improvement of the pain symptoms and the appearance of healing at both the posterior and nuclear annular ligament level and at the level of the end plates and articular processes. Due to the preservation of a certain degree of freedom in an area that functions normally from the anatomical point of view, this facilitates a return to local conditions that foster healing of the cartilaginous structures. Achieving this moderate postoperative intervertebral mobility is, moreover, the most important problem because it means that the primary fixation of the pedicle implants must be perfect, with no technical error whatsoever and no screw back-out during implantation because of the conical shape of the screw.

The pedicle screw-based system acts as a tension band, reducing the load on the disc and thus improving disc function. The DYNESYS® system is still the most widely implanted posterior unfused pedicle screw system. The primary biomechanical objective of the pedicle screw-based system is to reduce spinal instability while maintaining as much movement as possible to achieve uniform load transfer. Numerous clinical studies have shown that the DYNESYS® system can maintain partial segmental motion and prevent the degeneration of adjacent segments.

According to published clinical reports, the short-term effects of the posterior dynamic stabilization system are similar to those of traditional lumbar fusion surgery. The curative outcomes mainly come from the roles of lumbar decompression and temporary stabilization. Adjacent disc degeneration happened more frequently in the fusion group than in the DYNESYS® group. DYNESYS® stabilization can indeed maintain the mobility of the stabilized segments, which has little impact on adjacent segments and helps prevent ASD. However, comparative clinical studies with long-term follow-up are lacking so far. The results from four single-treatment-arm and small-sample studies of case series with long-term follow-up were not encouraging. These studies showed that although DYNESYS® maintains a good clinical effect, it is still associated with a high incidence of ASD in long-term follow-up.

Fixation of L5–S1 requires attention and presents problems. It is better to use adequate sacral screws for effective stabilization of this level (i.e., a screw that is 40 mm long, with a diameter of 7 mm) to avoid screw loosening at the S1 level.

References

1. Freudiger S, Dubois G, Lorrain M. Dynamic neutralization of the lumbar spine confirmed on a new lumbar spine simulator in vitro. Arch Orthop Trauma Surg. 1999;119:127–32.
2. Putzier M, Schneider SV, Funk JF, Tohtz SW, Perka C. The surgical treatment of the lumbar disc prolapse: nucleotomy with additional transpedicular dynamic stabilization versus nucleotomy alone. Spine. 2005;30(5):109–14.
3. Sengupta DK. Point of view: dynamic stabilization in addition to decompression for lumbar spinal stenosis with degenerative spondylolisthesis. Spine. 2006;31:450.
4. Stoll TM, Dubois G, Schwarzenbach O. The dynamic neutralization system for the spine: a multi-center study of a novel non fusion system. Eur Spine J. 2002;11(Suppl 2):170–8.
5. Niosi CA, Zhu QA, Wilson DC, et al. Biomechanical characterization of the three-dimensional kinematic behaviour of the Dynesys dynamic stabilization system: an in vitro study. Eur Spine J. 2006;15:913–22.
6. Gedet P, Haschtmann D, Thistlethwaite PA, Ferguson S. Comparative biomechanical investigation of a modular dynamic lumbar stabilization system and the Dynesys system. Eur Spine J. 2009;18(10):1504–11.
7. Schmoelz W, Huber JF, Nydegger T, et al. Dynamic stabilization of the lumbar spine and its effects on adjacent segments: an in vitro experiment. J Spinal Disord Tech. 2003;16(4):418–23.
8. Tawackoli A, Marco R, Liebschner MA. The effect of compressive axial preload on the flexibility of the thoracolumbar spine. Spine. 2004;29(9):988–93.
9. Jensen LM, Dawson JM, Springer S, et al. Kinematic evaluation of non-rigid posterior stabilization. Proceedings of the 50th annual meeting of the Orthopaedic Research Society, San Francisco, 2004.
10. Kaner T, Sassani M, Oktenoglu, Ozer AF. Dynamic stabilization of the spine: a new classification system. Turk Neurosurg. 2010;20(2):205–15.
11. Yu SW, Yang SC, Ma CH, Wu CH, Yen CY, Tu YK. Comparison of Dynesys posterior stabilization and posterior lumbar interbody fusion for spinal stenosis L4L5. Acta Orthop Belg. 2012;78:230–9.
12. Lee C-H, Jahng T-A, Hyun S-J, et al. Dynamic stabilization using the Dynesys system versus posterior lumbar interbody fusion for the treatment of degenerative lumbar spinal disease: a clinical and radiological outcomes-based meta-analysis. Neurosurg Focus. 2016;40(1):E7.
13. Peng B-G, Gao C-H. Is Dynesys dynamic stabilization system superior to posterior lumbar fusion in the treatment of lumbar degenerative diseases? World J Clin Cases. 2020;8(22):5496–500.
14. Lee CH, Jahng TA, Hyun SJ, Kim CH, Park SB, Kim KJ, Chung CK, Kim HJ, Lee SE. Dynamic stabilization using the Dynesys system *vs* posterior lumbar interbody fusion for the treatment of degenerative lumbar spinal disease: a clinical and radiological outcomes-based meta-analysis. Neurosurg Focus. 2016;40:E7.
15. Cakir B, Carazzo C, Schmidt R, Mattes T, Reichel H, Käfer W. Adjacent segment mobility after rigid and semirigid instrumentation of the lumbar spine. Spine. 2009;34:1287–91.

16. Kumar A, Beastall J, Hughes J, Karadimas EJ, Nicol M, Smith F, Wardlaw D. Disc changes in the bridged and adjacent segments after Dynesys dynamic stabilization system after two years. Spine. 2008;33:2909–14.
17. Stoll TM, Dubois G, Schwarzenbach O. The dynamic neutralization system for the spine: a multi-center study of a novel non-fusion system. Eur Spine J. 2002;11(Suppl 2):S170–8.
18. Wu H, Pang Q, Jiang G. Medium-term effects of Dynesys dynamic stabilization *vs* posterior lumbar interbody fusion for treatment of multisegmental lumbar degenerative disease. J Int Med Res. 2017;45:1562–73.
19. Bredin S, Demay O, Mensa C, Madi K, Ohl X. Posterolateral fusion *vs* Dynesys dynamic stabilization: retrospective study at a minimum 5.5years' follow-up. Orthop Traumatol Surg Res. 2017;103:1241–4.
20. Zhang Y, Shan JL, Liu XM, Li F, Guan K, Sun TS. Comparison of the Dynesys dynamic stabilization system and posterior lumbar Interbody fusion for lumbar degenerative disease. PLoS One. 2016;1:e0148071.
21. Hoppe S, Schwarzenbach O, Aghayev E, Bonel H, Berlemann U. Long-term outcome after Monosegmental L4/5 stabilization for degenerative spondylolisthesis with the Dynesys device. Clin Spine Surg. 2016;29:72–7.
22. Zhang Y, Zhang ZC, Li F, Sun TS, Shan JL, Guan K, Zhao GM, Zhang LZ. Long-term outcome of Dynesys dynamic stabilization for lumbar spinal stenosis. Chin Med J. 2018;131:2537–43.
23. Veresciagina K, Mehrkens A, Schären S, Jeanneret B. Minimum ten-year follow-up of spinal stenosis with degenerative spondylolisthesis treated with decompression and dynamic stabilization. J Spine Surg. 2018;4:93–101.
24. St-Pierre GH, Jack A, Siddiqui MM, Henderson RL, Nataraj A. Nonfusion does not prevent adjacent segment disease: Dynesys long-term outcomes with minimum five-year follow-up. Spine. 2016;41:265–73. 1976

14 The Orthrus Pedicular Dynamic Stabilization System

Ali Fahir Özer and Mehdi Hekimoğlu

The concept of dynamically stabilizing the spine emerged almost 50 years after the introduction of fusion surgery. Fusion surgery is built on arresting movement in the discs, the basic structure that provides motion in the spine. Although it has significant benefits, its use in the clinical setting has brought to the surface its limitations, as with all other implants. Due to the side effects of fusion surgery, researchers have been pushed to find other solutions. Basically, two views began to emerge. The first of these views was "let's stabilize the spine but keep the motion," and the other was "to stabilize the spine in a simpler way." Those who support the first view hold that the spine must be stabilized in such a way that abnormal motion is eliminated while preserving disc movement. First, the development of the dynamic stabilization system was based on replacing the disc with a mobile artificial structure rather than preserving its motion. Fernström, the pioneer of this concept, tried to provide movement to the motion segment by placing a steel ball in the disc after the discectomy. Thus, Fernström started a surgical journey for the dynamic stabilization of the motion segment [1]. German Karin Büttner-Janz and Kurt Schellnack performed this surgery in 1984 by removing the entire disc and replacing it with an artificial disc [2, 3].

The second concept, also known as the simple stabilization system, should be examined under two headings: supporting the motion of the existing disc, a pedicular dynamic system; and attempting to improve the deteriorated disc structure, biological repair. Although both clinical and experimental studies on these subjects are still intense, it has not been widely used yet. The disc, the cornerstone of motion in a functional unit, is of utmost importance to the second concept. Barr, who defined discectomy surgery, said in his article, "Once we remove the disc, we can no longer say that the ratio is anatomically and mechanically normal" [4]. Therefore, the statement "disc surgery is not a physiological surgery, it is a destructive surgery" is valid. It has been established that degeneration in the disc, whether after surgery or after an injury, causes some other problems in the process. From this point of view, it should be emphasized that our aim is to preserve the disc in its current state rather than destroy it and, if necessary, plan the surgery to preserve the disc. Disc preservation, that is, the preservation of the motion of the motion segment, is closely related to the degree of degeneration of the disc. Consequently, if the load on the disc at the beginning of the degeneration process can be shared with the dynamic system, it will be possible to protect the disc close to a healthy

A. F. Özer (✉)
Department of Neurosurgery, Koc University School of Medicine, Istanbul, Turkey

M. Hekimoğlu
American Hospital, Istanbul, Turkey
e-mail: mehdih@amerikanhastanesi.org

A. F. Özer et al. (eds.), *Dynamic Lumbar Spine Stabilization*,
https://doi.org/10.1007/978-3-032-12122-6_14

state. It has been established that even if a dynamic system is applied to the motion segment of a disc at an advanced stage of degeneration, that motion segment goes into fusion in the process. There is clinical improvement in these patients, but radiological motion disappears. Therefore, in a motion segment with an advanced degenerative disc, a fusion will be made using a dynamic system [5]. Researchers working on the concept of the pedicular dynamic system have not come forward with the claim of protecting motion. They argue that instead of applying exaggerated fusion surgery in every pathology, a simpler stabilization system could exist. However, even if fusion develops after dynamic system application, considering the complication rates of fusion surgery, fusion is achieved through a simpler method, even if it cannot preserve motion. This reality proves that the pedicular dynamic system is the primary surgery that should be preferred in the surgical treatment of chronic instability.

14.1 Posterior Dynamic Systems

After the initiation of fusion surgery in the treatment of spinal diseases, it began to be viewed as a panacea and was applied in the treatment of almost every pathology. Today, fusion surgery is seen as the gold standard by many surgeons. However, this generalization is not justified, and it has been reported that fusion surgery is an overtreatment, especially in the surgery of pathologies with chronic instability. For the first time, in 1991, Henry Graf presented his artificial ligament, which is named after him, at the second meeting of the European Spine Society in Rome and published it a year later [6, 7]. He stated that rotational forces cause lower back pain in chronic instability. Therefore, this pain will disappear when rotation is restricted, and he stabilized the spine by using Graf's artificial ligament with transpedicular screws instead of rods. This method has been used by many surgeons in Europe and the Far East [8–11]. However, since the ligament compresses the vertebrae, it has been claimed that the foramen narrows during compression and the artificial ligament loosens in hyperextension [12–14]. Later, the DYNESYS® system was developed by Dubois in order to eliminate the deficiencies of this system [15]. A spacer was placed in between the vertebrae to prevent the narrowing of the foramen and the damage to the bone while the screws were tightened; the screws are tightened with an artificial thread-shaped rod by exerting a standard force. However, this system has received criticism due to the associated deterioration of the preexisting lumbar lordosis, loosening, and high infection rate [16–19].

As concerns posterior dynamic systems, von Strempel was the first to put a hinge between the screwhead and body [20–22]. It was originally conceived and designed to increase the likelihood of the development of fusion. However, during the follow-up of the patients, they found that although some patients had pseudoarthrosis, they were clinically well. Despite the pseudoarthrosis, it was noticed that the motion segment was also mobile in this patient group, with good osteointegration of the screws into the bone. In addition, this observation has led to the rise of a new concept with the hinge on the screwhead in dynamic systems. There have also been very important improvements in the development of dynamic systems. A multicenter study using hinged screws was conducted and positive results were published [23].

14.2 Criticisms About Posterior Dynamic Systems

Today, there are two groups of systems in the spinal market: rigid screws used with a dynamic rod and systems containing dynamic screws used with a rigid rod. In our biomechanical studies at the University of Toledo biomechanics laboratory, we developed the "Talin dynamic rod" for these studies (Fig. 14.1).

When we used the "Talin dynamic rod" together with the dynamic screws in the stiff motion segments of cadavers, we found that this system restored the stiff motion segment. In addition, we determined that the dynamic rod–hinged screw cou-

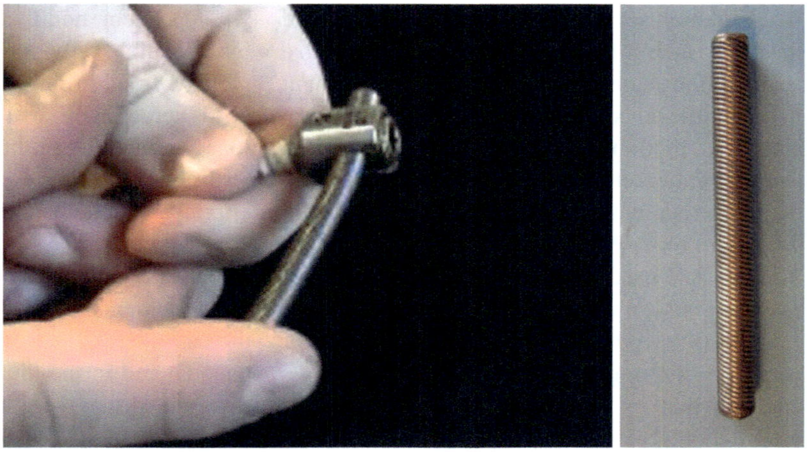

Fig. 14.1 Talin dynamic rod

ple gave the most appropriate results for the physiological motion segment. Following the guidance of this finding in our patient practices, we used Agile rods and Balan-C dynamic rods, developed by the Medtronic company but are now withdrawn from the market, together with dynamic screws for single motion segment stabilizations. We achieved good results until these rods broke [24–26]. Not considering the breaking of the rods, we realized that the clinical process will be good and long-lasting in patients with a well-functioning rod and that the concept is applicable even if the rods are insufficient at the moment of implementation. Presently, we continue to use FLEX +2 system rods in some patients for single-level stabilizations. Clinical results will be given in a separate chapter in this book. The most important result is the existence of a third system that includes dynamic screws used together with a dynamic rod in dynamic systems.

We see that the results are successful, no matter the system used, in patients for whom we have to stabilize a single motion segment. It has been seen both in our own studies and in the literature that the results are not different when compared with the clinical results of patients who underwent fusion surgery [25–31]. However, a problem arises in patients for whom more than single motion segment has to be stabilized. Di Silvestre was the first to stabilize more than single motion segment and also apply this method to deformity. He published successful results and revealed that dynamic systems can also be used in long-segment instability [32–34]. However, a meta-analysis examining publications using 21 DYNESYS® systems, conducted in 2016, found a surgical-site infection rate of 4.3%, a pedicle screw loosening rate of 11.7%, a pedicle screw fracture rate of 1.6%, and an adjacent segment disease (ASD) rate of 7.0%. In studies reporting revision surgeries, 11.3% of patients underwent a reoperation. Of patients who developed ASD, 40.6% underwent a reoperation for treatment. Compared with the published literature on lumbar fusion, the DYNESYS® dynamic stabilization system appears to have a fairly similar complication rate profile and is associated with a slightly lower incidence of ASD [16].

Although the stabilization of a single motion segment can be tolerated in systems with hinged screws and rigid rods, it is not recommended to use more than two-motion segments, as the system will become rigid as the number of stabilized levels increases. In our two-motion segment stabilization results, the complication rates for the instrument were much higher than those obtained at a single level [35]. Therefore, we realized that a durable dynamic rod or a new design to use with dynamic screws are required. Polyurethane rods, which are now on the market, may meet this need, but clinical results have not yet emerged.

14.3 The Orthrus System

We designed a new screw system for use in multilevel instability. The conception of this design was inspired by the successful clinical results in single motion segment stabilizations. We wanted to create such a system that we could stabilize each motion segment as a single motion segment in a multilevel stabilization. In stabilizing the single motion segment, we used Polyetheretherketone (PEEK) rods with a more flexible structure since we did not have a problem with rigid rods. We also divided the screwheads into two and used each head to stabilize a separate motion segment (Fig. 14.2).

When it becomes necessary to stabilize two or more motion segments with this method, we envision that by stabilizing each segment one after the other, our clinical results would be better, and the complication rate would be less (Fig. 14.3).

As explained, the system is actually a modular system, and it was designed accordingly. A very important advantage of this system is that when there is a problem in one of the modules for any reason, there is no need to remove the whole system, and the problem can be resolved by revealing only the affected module in the patient. In addition, the Orthrus system can be used very easily with fusion systems. If the fused segment is in the middle of the spine, the Orthrus system can easily be extended to the cranial and caudal sides by adding it to the rigid construction.

Biomechanical tests of the Orthrus system on finite elements and cadavers were carried out at the University of Toledo. Since no problems were encountered in the finite element studies, it was determined that there was no material deterioration in the mechanical loading tests performed on the screws (Fig. 14.4).

In cadaver studies, it was determined that the screws stabilized the segments individually (modularly) when 700–1200-N vectorial forces were applied to the screws in standard tests. Thus, it was determined that the screws gave the expected results functionally. After the results

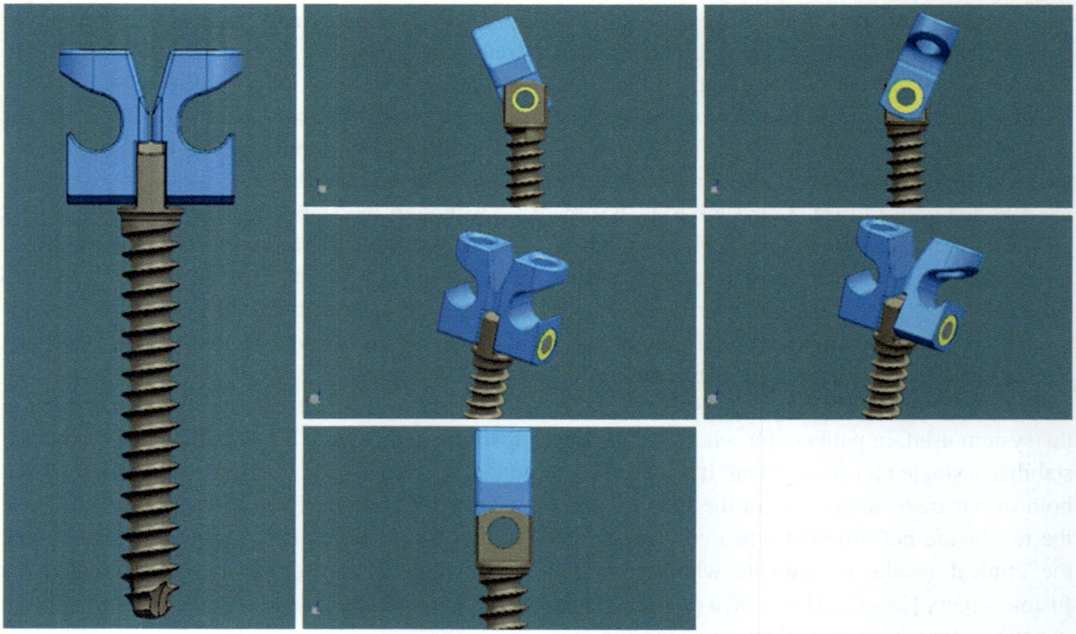

Fig. 14.2 Each head was used to stabilize a separate motion segment by dividing the screwheads into two

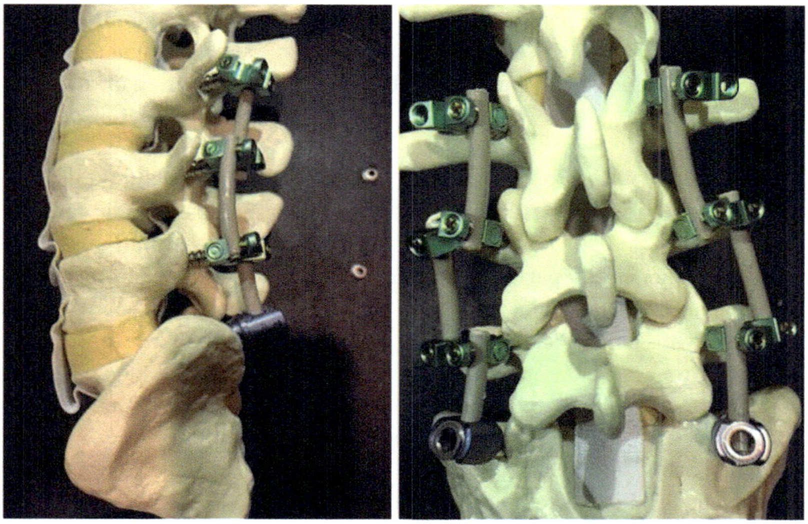

Fig. 14.3 The Orthrus spinal system

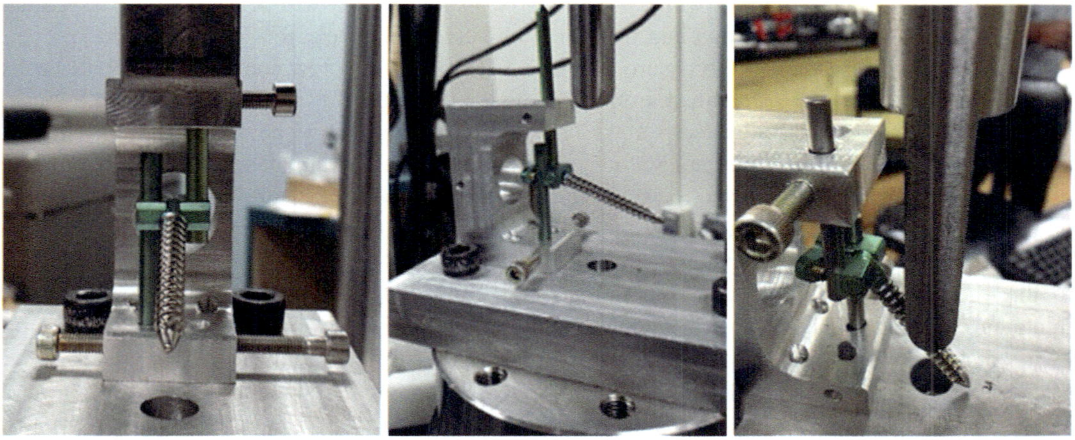

Fig. 14.4 It was determined that there was no material deterioration in the mechanical loading tests performed on the screws

were satisfactory, it was decided that the system could be used in patients as well.

14.4 Indications for the Use of the Orthrus System

Dynamic systems are designed for use in cases of degenerative instability. Patients have progressive instability, and more than one functional unit is usually affected. Benzel [36, 37] named this type of instability chronic instability and divided it into subgroups: glacial instability and dysmotion segment movements. In this group of patients, the patient continues his/her daily life with pain, but since the degenerative process progresses slowly, the patient is pushed toward a more painful and restricted mobility process. This is the ideal patient group for dynamic systems and Orthrus. Pathologies in this patient group include painful multilevel black discs due to disc degeneration, antero- and retro-degenerative spondylolisthesis involving more than single motion segment, multilevel canal stenosis, diffuse degenerative disc disease, and related scoliotic or kyphotic deterioration. In the patient group in which we applied Orthrus, the patients had the aforementioned pathologies involving more than single motion segment.

14.5 Surgical Technique

Surgery is generally performed under general anesthesia. However, spinal anesthesia is used for patients who are older and have additional medical problems. Patients with advanced osteoporosis are operated on in two stages. Currently, in cases where we apply Orthrus or any dynamic system, great attention is paid to the degree of bone density. In our clinic, the surgeries of patients with a T-score of −1.5 and above are performed in a single stage. In cases with a T-score below −1.5, screws are placed first and rods are placed at least 4–8 months later to ensure osteointegration. Thus, a good osteointegration with the bone is provided in unloaded screws. If decompression is required in patients with signs of neurological irritation, only one rod is placed on the decompressed side, and all screws are left unloaded. In the meantime, the patient is referred to the endocrine department, and osteoporosis treatment is initiated. When the patient comes for the second stage, if there is any loosening in the screws on which the rod is attached, only these screws are revised since the system is designed modularly. However, so far, no revision has been required in patients in whom the Orthrus system has been applied. In the second stage, since the screws that are attached to the spine are relatively stronger than a normal bone, interventions are performed for pathologies in the motion segments if necessary. These may be due to degenerative spondylolisthesis or isolated spinal canal stenosis, foraminal stenosis, or a degenerative disc herniation. Degenerative spondylolisthesis may be isolated and may not be associated with canal stenosis. Consequently, in the first or second stage, the problems related to the canal are resolved, the compression on the nervous system is relieved, and the rods are placed on the screws that are firmly attached to the bone. In the published series, this approach was used as a guide, and there were no complications in construction for the patients who were operated upon [38]. Two-stage surgery will be described in a separate chapter in this book.

The Orthrus screw consists of two half-heads that move cranially and caudally around a hinge. Each half-head must be attached with a rod to either the ipsilateral half-head of an upper screw or the half-head of the lower screw because it is designed for the stabilization of two or more segments (Fig. 14.5).

The standard rods are 5-mm-diameter PEEK rods, but we are working on a more mobile rod design for a more mobile spine.

The bottom screw or the top screw can be a dynamic polyaxial normal screw (Safinaz, Medikon, Turkey) (Fig. 14.6).

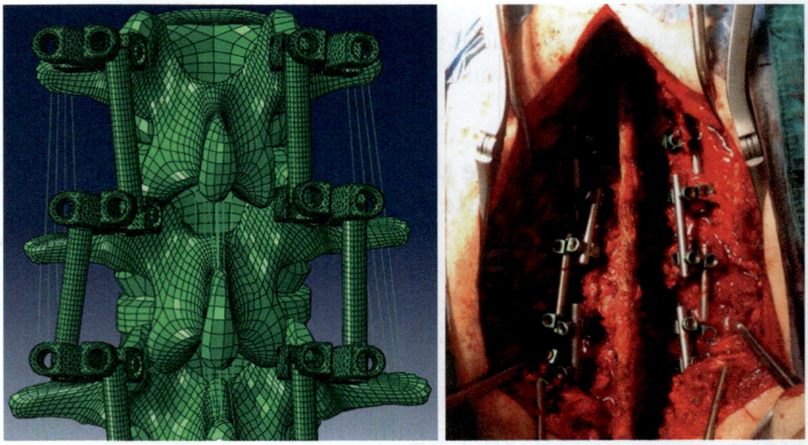

Fig. 14.5 Each half-head must be attached with a rod either to the ipsilateral half-head of an upper screw or to the half-head of the lower screw because it is designed for the stabilization of two or more motion segments

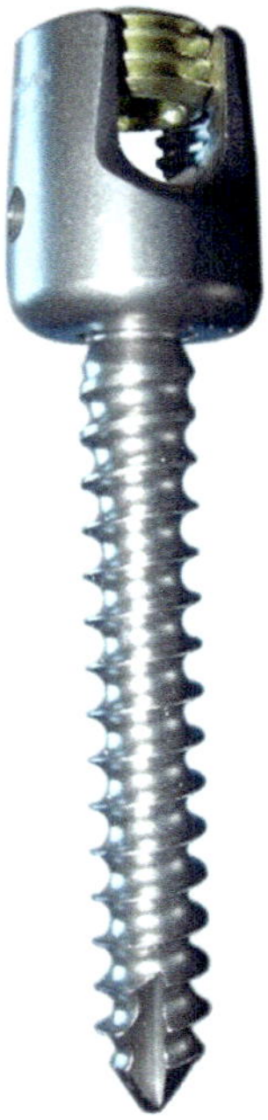

Fig. 14.6 The bottom screw or the top screw can be a dynamic polyaxial normal screw

For the sacrum, another craniocaudal screw was added to the upper part of the polyaxial dynamic screw to make the system more mobile and tested in biomechanical experiments. The use of this screw is optional.

If there is a complication that requires decompression from the midline surgically, this is resolved by opening it, and the midline fascia is closed. Subsequently, a separate fascial incision is made on both sides of the midline, approximately two fingers outward. Screws are placed in accordance with the Wiltse technique. After the fascia is removed, the transverse process is reached by following the thin fibrous structure between the multifidus and longissimus muscles [39]. By following the upper part of the transverse process, the side wall of the facet joint and the corner made by the transverse process are found, and with the help of a C-arm X-ray, it is placed on the spine by crossing the pedicle from this corner, from the midpoint of the pedicle. Navigation can be used in patients

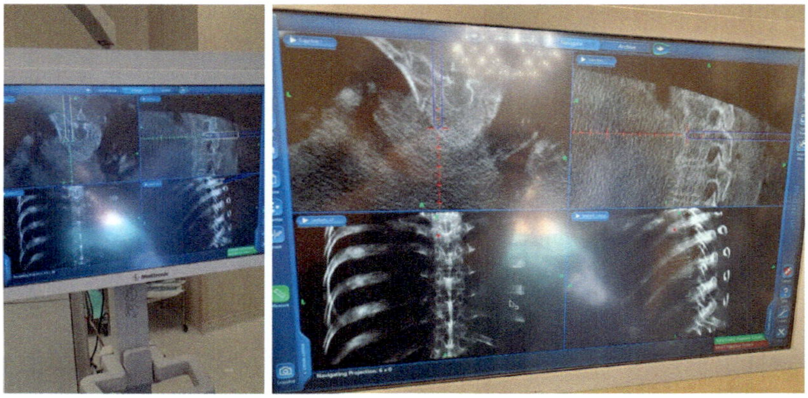

Fig. 14.7 Navigation can be used in patients with multilevel instability and deformity

with deformities. In this way, since the screw crosses the pedicle, it travels further in the pedicle, which is a solid bone structure, creating more contact area with the bone (Fig. 14.7).

After the screws are placed, the rods are placed on the two-headed screws. Both medial and lateral heads are used for single motion segment. The outer head of a screw is connected to the outer head of the lower screw, while its inner head is connected to the inner head of the upper screw. Thus, the half-heads of the two screws facing the same side stabilize a motion segment. Then, the fasciae are also closed, and the surgery is completed with a skin incision.

14.6 Clinical Trial Results

The Orthrus system is a useful system developed for long-segment stabilization. Dynamic systems neutralize motion segments that are impaired as a result of degeneration and that begin to move abnormally. The application phase is very important for degenerative disc disease. If the motion segment is not in an advanced degenerative process, signs of improvement in the motion segment are seen in control examinations [5]. It has been observed that the capsule of the disc and its hydration are recovered, although cases exist where early-stage Modic degenerations become reversible. The motion segment with a neutralized abnormal motion will bring about clinical improvement. The advantage of this system is that if there is multilevel instability, there is a chance to protect them all. In this case, it further increases the probability of clinical improvement.

In addition, if the patient can correct himself by using his muscles in mobile deformities, it can also be used in deformity surgery. In this group of patients, if X-rays taken in the supine position can show the correction of the deformity, this would be the ideal indication for the application of the system. The system is applied by giving the patient the final position on the table. This does not contribute to active correction; the deformity must therefore be mobile. As the deformity improves, the abnormal movement in the unstable segments is eliminated, and the patient improves both radiologically and clinically (Fig. 14.8).

In the patient series we published, ten patients had multilevel degenerative disc disease, as well as canal stenosis requiring decompression in only single motion segment. Eight of the patients had canal stenosis requiring decompression in two-motion segments. In another group of eight patients, there was canal stenosis or foraminal stenosis that required decompression in three or more motion segments. Additionally, a discectomy was performed in six of these patients. In ten patients, there was multilevel segmental instability due to reasons such as degenerative disc and degenerative spondylolisthesis; hence, stabilization was performed. There was no pathology requiring decompression in these ten

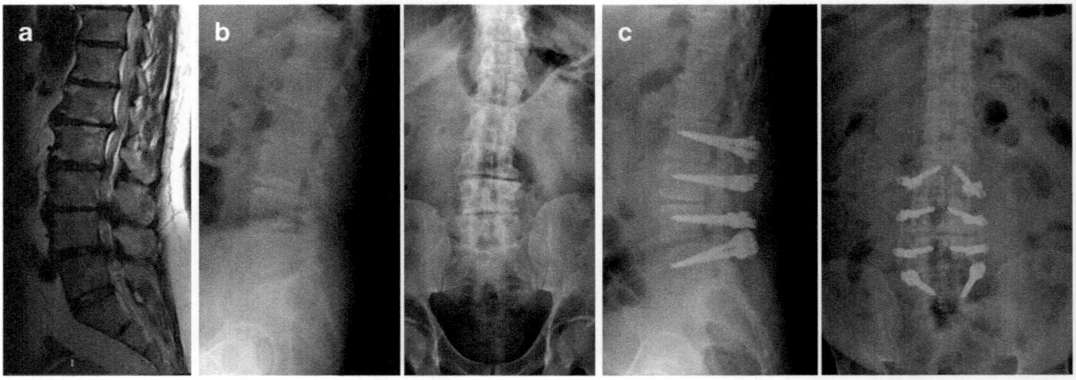

Fig. 14.8 A 65-year-old male patient. (**a**) On MRI, there is multilevel degenerative disc disease and lumbar canal stenosis in the MR T2 sagittal section. (**b**) Sagittal and coronal balance is preserved, and there is enough lumbar lordosis. (**c**) The decompression anterior-posterior (AP) and lateral X-ray are shown after surgery

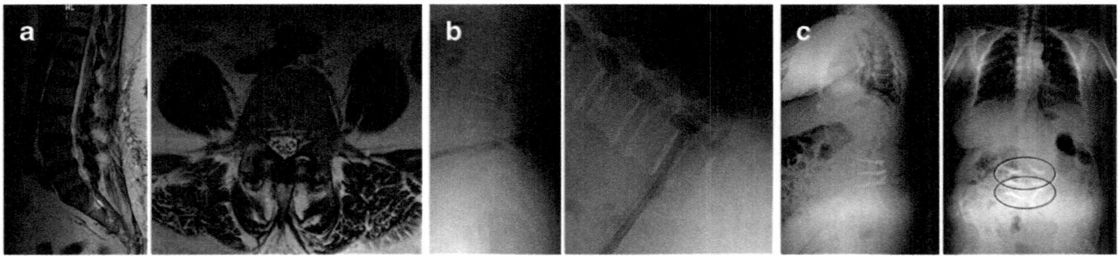

Fig. 14.9 A 61-year-old female with severe back pain upon walking or standing. (**a**) There is no severe pathology visible on MRI but for fatty degeneration. (**b**) No other pathology visible except for sacralization. (**c**) In dynamic graphics, L3 slips anteriorly over L4, and L4 slips anteriorly over L5 in hyperflexion X-ray. Notice that there is no remarkable pathology on standard X-rays and MRI. The Orthrus system was used in surgery, and the patient satisfaction is outstanding at 3 years postoperatively

patients. In a series of 36 cases we published, the clinical findings were quite good in the one-year early results, and we did not have any serious complications [38] (Fig. 14.9).

14.7 Conclusion

The Orthrus system can be used safely in patients requiring the stabilization of two or more motion segments. In cases requiring revision due to its modular structure, reexploration of the problematic functional unit alone will be sufficient. Therefore, it is a very easy system to use. In addition, its modular structure makes its neighboring segments very easily accessible. As a hybrid of fusion, both distal and proximal extensions of the spine can be easily achieved.

References

1. Fernström U. Arthroplasty with intercorporal endoprothesis in herniated disc and in painful disc. Acta Chir Scand Suppl. 1966;357:154–9.
2. Büttner-Janz K, Schellnack K, Zippel H. An alternative treatment strategy in lumbar intervertebral disk damage using an SB Charité modular type intervertebral disk endoprosthesis. Z Orthop Ihre Grenzgeb. 1987;125(1):1–6. https://doi.org/10.1055/s-2008-1039666.
3. Büttner-Janz K, Schelnack K, Zippel H, et al. Experience and results with the SB Charité lumbar intervertebral endoprosthesis. Zeitschrift fur Klinische Medizin. 1988;43:1785–9.
4. Barr JS, Mixter WJ. Posterior protrution of the lumbar intervertebral disk. J Bone Joint Surg. 1941;23:444–56.
5. Yilmaz A, Senturk S, Sasani M, et al. Disc rehydration after dynamic stabilization: a report of 59 cases. Asian Spine J. 2017;11(3):348–55. https://doi.org/10.4184/asj.2017.11.3.348.
6. Graf H. Second meeting. Rome: European Spine Society; 1991.
7. Graf H. Lumbar instability: surgical treatment without fusion. Rachis. 1992;412:123–37.
8. Madan S, Boeree NR. Outcome of the Graf ligamentoplasty procedure compared with anterior lumbar interbody fusion with the Hartshill horseshoe cage. Eur Spine J. 2003;12(4):361–8. https://doi.org/10.1007/s00586-002-0488-5.
9. Gardner A, Pande KC. Graf ligamentoplasty: a 7-year follow-up. Eur Spine J. 2002;11(Suppl 2):S157–63. https://doi.org/10.1007/s00586-002-0436-4.
10. Hasegawa K, Hirata Y, Morita T, Kobayashi H. Stabilization effects of Graf ligamentoplasty. J Musculoskelet Res. 1999;03(03):217–32.
11. Kanayama M, Hashimoto T, Shigenobu K. Rationale, biomechanics, and surgical indications for Graf ligamentoplasty. Orthop Clin North Am. 2005;36(3):373–7. https://doi.org/10.1016/j.ocl.2005.02.013.
12. Wild A, Jaeger M, Bushe C, Raab P, Krauspe R. Biomechanical Analysis of Graf's Dynamic Spine Stabilisation System ex vivo – Biomechanische Analyse des dynamischen Wirbelsäulenstabilisationssystems nach Graf ex vivo. Biomed Tech (Berl). 2001;46(10):290–4.
13. Grevitt MP, Gardner AD, Spilsbury J, Shackleford IM, Baskerville R, Pursell LM, Hassaan A, Mulholland RC. The Graf stabilisation system: early results in 50 patients. Eur Spine J. 1995;4(3):169–75.; discussion 135. https://doi.org/10.1007/BF00298241.
14. Sengupta DK. Dynamic stabilization devices in the treatment of low back pain. Coluna/Columna. 2005;4(1):31–41.
15. Dubois G, de Germay B, Schaerer NS, Fennema P. Dynamic neutralization: a new concept for restabilization of the spine. In: Szpalski M, Gunzburg R, Pope MH, editors. Lumbar segmental instability.

Philadelphia: Lippincott Williams and Wilkins; 1999. p. 233–40.

16. Pham MH, Mehta VA, Patel NN, Jakoi AM, Hsieh PC, Liu JC, Wang JC, Acosta FL. Complications associated with the Dynesys dynamic stabilization system: a comprehensive review of the literature. Neurosurg Focus. 2016 Jan;40(1):E2. https://doi.org/10.3171/2015.10.FOCUS15432.
17. Ko CC, Tsai HW, Huang WC, Wu JC, Chen YC, Yang-Hsin Shih YH, et al. Screw loosening in the Dynesys stabilization system: radiographic evidence and effect on outcomes. J Neurosurg Spine. 2010;28(6):E10. https://doi.org/10.3171/2010.3.FOCUS1052.
18. Lutz JA, Otten P, Maestretti G. Late infections after dynamic stabilization of the lumbar spine with Dynesys. Eur Spine J. 2012;21(12):2573–9. https://doi.org/10.1007/s00586-012-2366-0.
19. Akyoldas G, Cevik OM, Suzer T, Sasani M, Oktenoglu T, Ozer AF. Dynamic stabilization of the lumbar spine using the Dynesys® system. Turk Neurosurg. 2020;30(2):190–3. https://doi.org/10.5137/1019-5149.JTN.26475-19.2.
20. von Strempel A, Neckritz A, de Muelenaere P, du Toit G. Dynamic versus rigid spinal implants. In: Gunzberg R, Spalski M, editors. Lumbar Spinal Stenosis. Philadelphia: Lippincott Williams & Wilkins; 2000. p. 275–85.
21. Von Strempel A, Moosmann D, Stoss C, Martin A. Stabilization of the degenerated lumbar spine in the nonfusion technique with cosmic posterior dynamic system. WSJ. 2006;1:40–7.
22. Von Strempel A. Dynamic stabilisation: cosmic system. Interact Surg. 2008;3:229–36.
23. Maleci A, Sambale RD, Schiavone M, Lamp F, Özer F, von Strempel A. Nonfusion stabilization of the degenerative lumbar spine. J Neurosurg Spine. 2011;15(2):151–8. https://doi.org/10.3171/2011.3.SPINE0969.
24. Kaner T, Sasani M, Oktenoglu T, Cosar M, Ozer AF. Utilizing dynamic rods with dynamic screws in the surgical treatment of chronic instability: a prospective clinical study. Turk Neurosurg. 2009;19(4):319–26.
25. Ozer AF, Oktenoglu T, Egemen E, Sasani M, Yilmaz A, Erbulut DU, Yaman O, Suzer T. Lumbar single-level dynamic stabilization with semi-rigid and full dynamic systems: a retrospective clinical and radiological analysis of 71 patients. Clin Orthop Surg. 2017;9(3):310–6. https://doi.org/10.4055/cios.2017.9.3.310.
26. Zhang Y, Zhang ZC, Li F, et al. Long-term outcome of Dynesys dynamic stabilization for lumbar spinal stenosis. Chin Med J. 2018;131(21):2537–43. https://doi.org/10.4103/0366-6999.244107.
27. Guigui P, Ferrero E. Surgical treatment of degenerative spondylolisthesis. Orthop Traumatol Surg Res. 2017;103(1S):S11–20. https://doi.org/10.1016/j.otsr.2016.06.022.
28. Hoppe S, Schwarzenbach O, Aghayev E, Bonel H, Berlemann U. Long-term outcome after monosegmental L4/5 stabilization for degenerative spondylolisthesis with the Dynesys device. Clin Spine Surg. 2016 Mar;29(2):72–7. https://doi.org/10.1097/BSD.0b013e318277ca7a.
29. Lee CH, Jahng TA, Hyun SJ, Kim CH, Park SB, Kim KJ, Chung CK, Kim HJ, Lee SE. Dynamic stabilization using the Dynesys system versus posterior lumbar interbody fusion for the treatment of degenerative lumbar spinal disease: a clinical and radiological outcomes-based meta-analysis. Neurosurg Focus. 2016 Jan;40(1):E7. https://doi.org/10.3171/2015.10.FOCUS15426.
30. Kuo CH, Chang PY, Wu JC, Chang HK, Fay LY, Tu TH, Cheng H, Huang WC. Dynamic stabilization for L4-5 spondylolisthesis: comparison with minimally invasive transforaminal lumbar interbody fusion with more than 2 years of follow-up. Neurosurg Focus. 2016 Jan;40(1):E3. https://doi.org/10.3171/2015.10.FOCUS15441.
31. Gille O, Challier V, Parent H, Cavagna R, Poignard A, Faline A, Fuentes S, Ricart O, Ferrero E, Ould Slimane M, French Society of Spine Surgery (SFCR). Degenerative lumbar spondylolisthesis: cohort of 670 patients, and proposal of a new classification. Orthop Traumatol Surg Res. 2014;100(6 Suppl):S311–5. https://doi.org/10.1016/j.otsr.2014.07.006.
32. Di Silvestre M, Lolli F, Bakaloudis G, Parisini P. Dynamic stabilization for degenerative lumbar scoliosis in elderly patients. Spine (Phila Pa 1976). 2010 Jan 15;35(2):227–34. https://doi.org/10.1097/BRS.0b013e3181bd3be6.
33. Di Silvestre M, Lolli F, Bakaloudis G. Degenerative lumbar scoliosis in elderly patients: dynamic stabilization without fusion versus posterior instrumented fusion. Spine J. 2014 Jan;14(1):1–10. https://doi.org/10.1016/j.spinee.2012.10.023.
34. Di Silvestre M, Lolli F, Greggi T, Vommaro F, Baioni A. Adult's degenerative scoliosis: midterm results of dynamic stabilization without fusion in elderly patients-is it effective? Adv Orthop. 2013;2013:365059. https://doi.org/10.1155/2013/365059.
35. Ciplak NM, Suzer T, Senturk S, Yaman O, Sasani M, Oktenoglu T, Yilmaz A, Erbulut DU, Özer AF. Complications of 2-level dynamic stabilization: a correlative clinical and radiological analysis at two-year follow-up on 103 patients. Turk Neurosurg. 2018;28(5):756–62. https://doi.org/10.5137/1019-5149.JTN.21036-17.1.
36. Benzel EC. Biomechanics of spine stabilization principles and clinical practice. In: Benzel EC, editor. . McGraw-Hill; 1995. p. 25–41.
37. Benzel EC. The anatomic basis of spinal instability. In: Clinical neurosurgery. Baltimore: Williams and Wilkins; 1993. p. 224–41.
38. Ozer AF, Cevik OM, Erbulut DU, Yaman O, Senturk S, Oktenoglu T, Sasani M, Suzer T, Goel V. A novel modular dynamic stabilization system for the treatment of degenerative spinal pathologies. Turk Neurosurg. 2019;29(1):115–20. https://doi.org/10.5137/1019-5149.JTN.23227-18.1.
39. Wiltse LL, Bateman JG, Hutchinson RH, Nelson WE. The paraspinal sacrospinalis-splitting approach to the lumbar spine. J Bone Joint Surg Am. 1968 Jul;50(5):919–26.

Dynamic Rod

15

Ahmet Levent Aydın and Ali Fahir Özer

According to our experiences, one of the most compromising problems of the dynamic system is the dynamic rod. In order to give flexibility to the spine, it is necessary to combine the dynamic pedicle screws with flexible rods to maintain the movement feature of a vertebral segment. It is a fundamentally correct concept and so very popular, and in this perspective, it is a reality for the concept of "motion preservation."

However, on the other hand, in order to achieve a good fusion, a constant load is necessary on the intervertebral graft. For the constructs with rigid screws, subsidence of the graft in the vertebral corpus leads to pseudoarthrosis because the necessary load on the graft according to Wolff's law is not enough. The solution for this problem is to use a flexible rod. Thus, the load on the graft becomes continuous, and the likelihood of fusion is better, and the incidence of pseudoarthrosis decreases. Finally, in terms of fusion, this is an admissible concept.

The key point here is that if you use a dynamic rod to achieve a good fusion, the substance of the rod exhausts within 2–4 months after fusion. But if you are using it for "motion preservation" purposes, the duration of motion should theoretically be infinite. From this perspective, the composition of the rod should be from a material that is biocompatible and resistant to lifelong movement. Unfortunately, there is currently no such rod on the market.

In this chapter, we want to review both the rods currently used on the market and those taken off the market.

15.1 Graf Ligament

The Graf ligament is very important in terms of the history of motion preservation. It was the first example of the pedicular dynamic rod system and was also the beginning of the concept of dynamic stabilization. In 1992, Graf described the use of the Graf ligamentoplasty system to treat lower back pain without fusion. According to his theory, abnormal rotational motion was the primary source of mechanical lower back pain. He later improved this system by placing titanium pedicle screws into the vertebrae, both above and below the symptomatic level, and used braided polypropylene tension tape to connect the titanium pedicle screws together. Six- or seven-millimeter titanium pedicle screws are used bilaterally, and 8-mm braided polyester tapes are placed over the screws protruding posteriorly. The bands are protected from adjacent bone prominences by cylindrical diabolos and are prevented from slipping from the pedicle screws by caps on the screws [1, 2] (Fig. 15.1).

A. L. Aydın (✉)
Medicana Bahçelievler, Istanbul, Turkey

A. F. Özer
Department of Neurosurgery, Koc University School of Medicine, Istanbul, Turkey

A. F. Özer et al. (eds.), *Dynamic Lumbar Spine Stabilization*,
https://doi.org/10.1007/978-3-032-12122-6_15

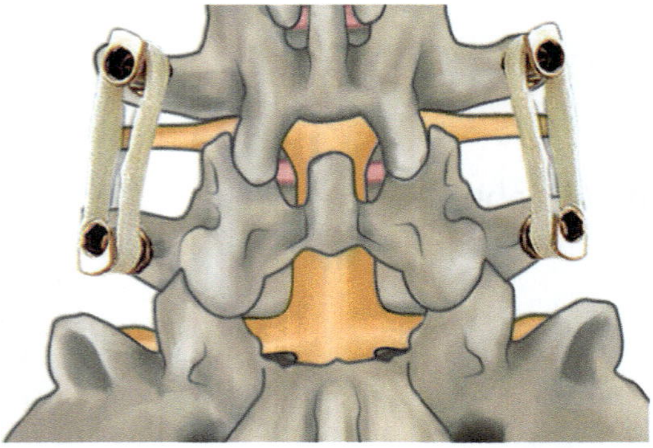

Fig. 15.1 Graf screws and artificial bands. (Courtesy of Ali Fahir Özer)

Kirkaldy-Willis described three stages of disc degeneration. The first stage is dysfunction [3, 4]. It is characterized by circumferential and radial tears in the disc annulus and the degeneration and hypermobility of the facet joints. The second stage is instability. There is degeneration of the facet joints, together with internal degradation of the disc, progressive disc resorption, capsular laxity, subluxation, and erosion of the facet joint. The final stage is stabilization. This stage includes the formation of osteophytosis and, sometimes, spinal stenosis. It is assumed that Graf ligaments will stabilize the spine in stages 1 and 2.

In the literature, there are case series supporting the affirmative results of cases where the Graf ligament was used [2, 5, 6].

As a rare complication, the Graf ligamentoplasty system leads to symptomatic lateral canal stenosis by forcing a marked lordosis of the instrumented segment. This was observed mostly in patients exhibiting preexisting degenerative changes in the facet joints or inward folding of the ligamentum flavum. Early clinical failures were mostly associated with this surgical complication [7]. However, besides this discouraging complication, when good results were obtained in most of the cases, the Graf system became popular. Besides, it led to the emergence of the idea of development and provided the first step in the development of the DYNESYS® system.

15.2 Talin Rod

We designed this rod for experimental studies. It never entered the market, but due to the economic difficulties of a young patient, we used this rod in his operation, with approval from his family (Fig. 15.2).

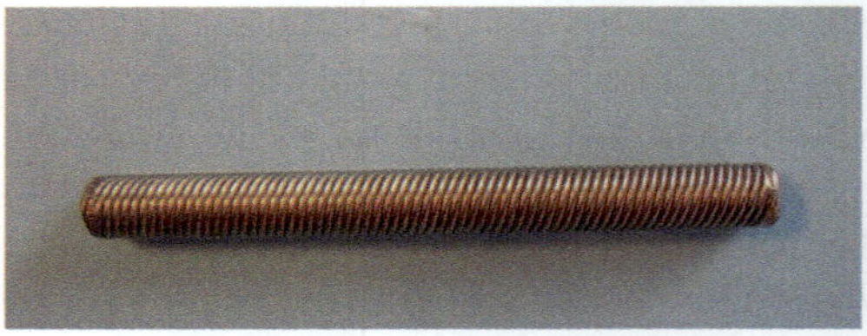

Fig. 15.2 Spring shaped titanium Talin rod

The patient was pain-free after the surgery. He came for routine follow-up 7 years after the surgery, and on investigation, we realized that the rod had broken. The patient mentioned pain in his lower back for the past few months. But surprisingly, the patient's discs remained reasonably healthy. This situation gave us motivation and showed that the concept of "dynamic stabilization" was correct. We wanted to share this experience as well.

15.3 Agile Rod

It was promoted by the Medtronic company in 2007 (CD HORIZON® AGILE™).

The floating cable design allows for an axial compressive load while retaining a constant stiffness without buckling the cable. This provides better fatigue properties and axial compressive capability of the spacer. Predetermined stiffness options are available to match individual patient anatomy and clinical needs. The stiffness of the rod correlates with the spacer size (e.g., increasing stiffness with shorter spacers). The 15 mm spacer size allows the most axial compression, while the 10 mm spacer offers a slightly stiffer option (Fig. 15.3).

The flexible part of the rod is composed of two components; one inner titanium cable and an outer silicone coat, at a length of 10–15 mm. The purpose of using this rod is primarily for non-fusion expectances. If the disc height has not decreased by more than 50% and there is no defect such as lysis, the appropriate rod is placed and slightly distracted in between the vertebrae.

If there is a degenerated disc in the neighborhood level, adjacent to the fusion, the part to be fused is connected with a polyetheretherketone (PEEK) rod, and the adjacent segment is connected with the mobile part of this hybrid rod system (Fig. 15.4).

However, these rods were withdrawn from the market in a short time due to the breakage of the multifilament buckling cable. Although we used these rods with dynamic screws in our own clinic, they failed too, although they lasted a little longer than when used with rigid screws (Fig. 15.5).

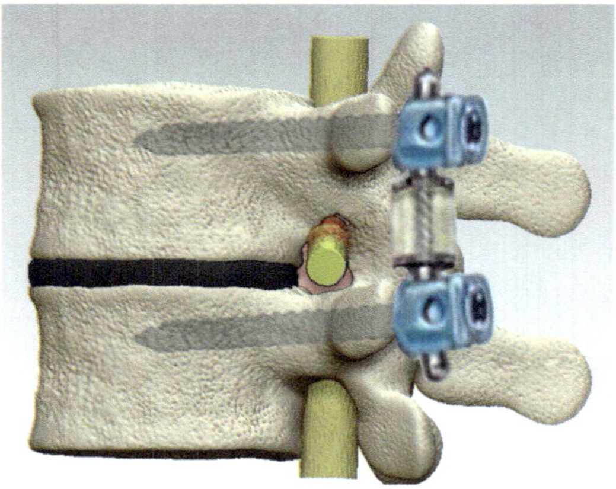

Fig. 15.3 Agile rod. (Courtesy of Ali Fahir Özer)

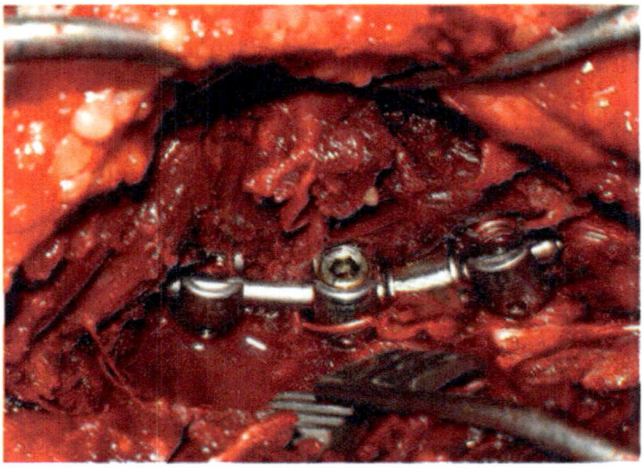

Fig. 15.4 Agile rod: To prevent adjacent segment degeneration (ASD), the moving part is placed at the end of the PEEK rod

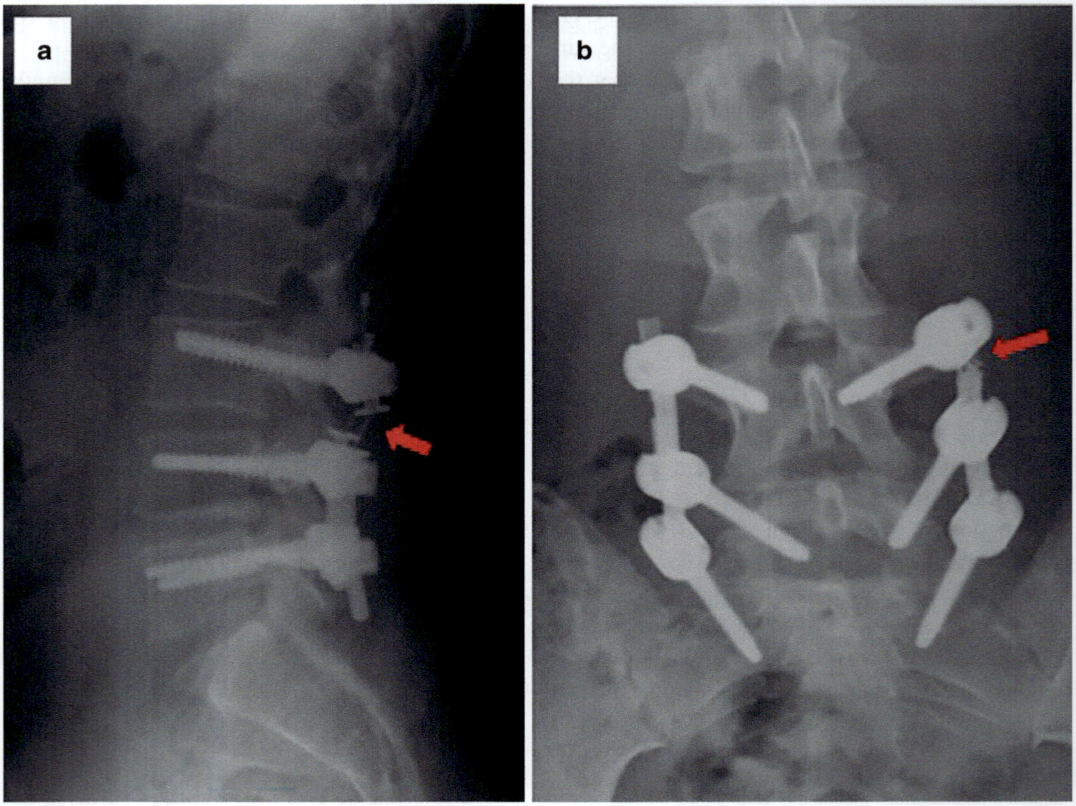

Fig. 15.5 (**a**) The dynamic part of the Agile rod was ruptured (**b**) ruptured Talin rod

15.4 Dream Rod

It was presented to the market by obtaining a Europian Conformity certificate (EC) certificate from a Korean company. The rod consisted of a multifilament wire encased in a stretched titanium shield. The multifilament wire was tautly attached to the ends of the rod. We can say that this rod was almost an extended form of the flexible part of the Agile rod. But unfortunately, in cases where we planned motion preservation, this rod did not last long either, like the Agile rod, so we suspended it (Fig. 15.6). This rod was an important touchstone in the dynamic rod history of our clinic [8].

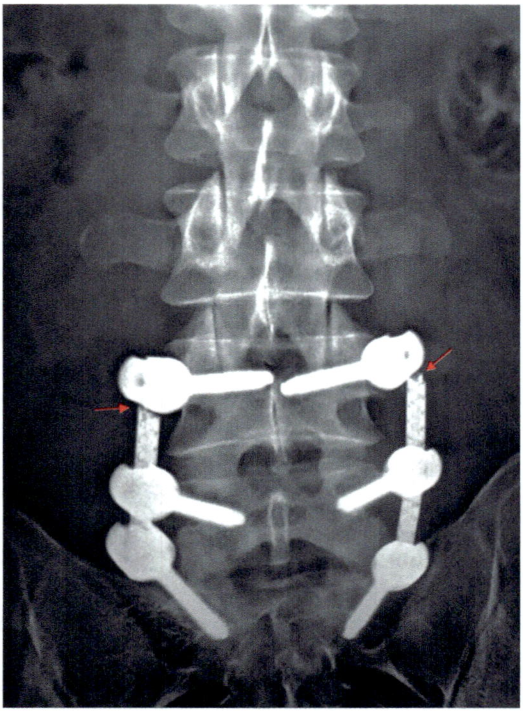

Fig. 15.6 Dream rod rupture at the end point

15.5 CD HORIZON BalanC™ Rod

It was brought into the market by Medtronic after the failure of Agile. CD HORIZON BalanC™ rod is made of two separate parts. Its dynamic part is made of silicone and polyetheretherketone (PEEK), and its fusion part is made entirely of PEEK. The dynamic part is designed to sustain movement by creating a transition zone between fused and moving segments. In the CD HORIZON BalanC™ Spinal System brochures, it is stated that, when used in a single-level procedure, only the dynamic part will provide stabilization, even without the long PEEK part for fusion.

The indications of this rod overlap with Agile, and it has been used all over the world. Due to our own perspective and our previous studies on dynamic rods, which are discussed in detail in the relevant chapters of this book, we used this rod, together with dynamic screws, within the framework of the "motion preservation" concept. Unfortunately, in our country, as in the rest of the world, the rods ruptured within an average of 2 years after use and were withdrawn from use by the company (Fig. 15.7).

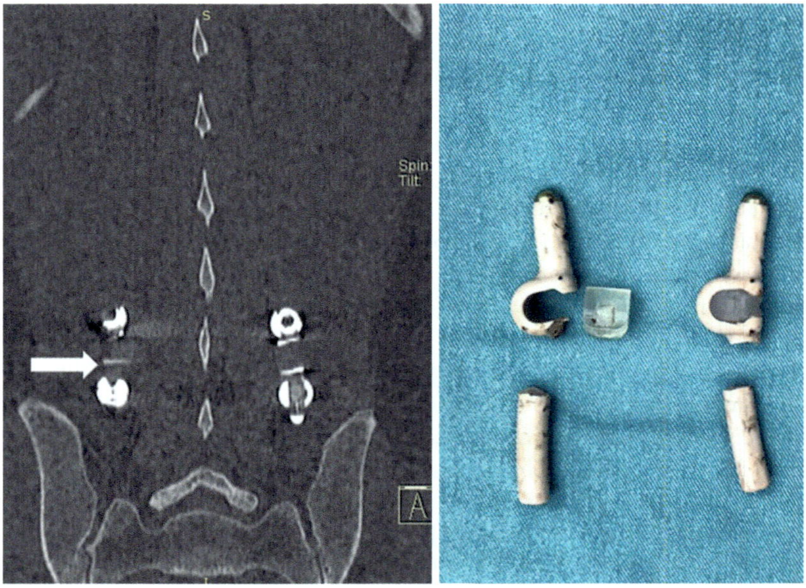

Fig. 15.7 Broken BalanC™ rod

15.6 Tether Systems

The most widely used of these systems around the world is the DYNESYS® (Zimmer Spine, Minneapolis, MN, USA) system. It was developed entirely by compensating for the vulnerabilities of the Graf system. It is a spinal fixation technique developed by the French scientist Gilles G. Dubois in 1991 and was clinically introduced in 1994.

In the procedure, rigid titanium alloy screws are placed in the pedicles. The screws are attached to each other with a polyethylene terephthalate (PET) cord (tether). After the tether is passed through the hole at the head of the first screw, it is compressed, and thereafter, it is passed through a polyurethane spacer and passed through the hole at the head of the second screw. The tether is stretched under a certain standard tension, with a spacer in between, and compressed onto the last screwhead. In this way, the screwheads do not come close to each other, and loosening in hyperextension or a decrease in foraminal volume is prevented.

Biomechanical studies have shown that this system neutralizes the functions of an impaired segment of motion [9–11].

It is one of the new fusion-free, dynamic stabilization instruments for lumbar degeneration and instability and is defined as a dynamic neutralization system. It reduces the load on the intervertebral disc and zygapophysial joint. It shares the load transfer in the movement segment and protects or restores the function of the movement segments for which it is responsible, without adversely affecting them. These are all factors that ensure the physiological stability of the spine [12–15].

On the contrary, numerous recent studies declare that this dynamic system is acceptable in reducing complications associated with fusion and rigid stabilization procedures, including screw loosening, rod breakage, post junctional kyphosis, and pseudoarthrosis [16].

Although there are many articles for and against it, it is a surgical method on which we have a lot of experience. Frankly, although we have experienced many complications, ranging from screw breakage to infection, when compared to fusion, it has become our priority option in the treatment of minor instabilities due to degeneration because the patient can participate in daily life after surgery, complications are less and milder, and the surgery is simpler and more effective than fusion surgery. However, we observed that the tether broke during multilevel use, especially in patients with deformities, and although the long-term results are not yet clear, we used two rods, especially in multilevel instabilities with deformities. It is discussed in related chapters in this book [16–19].

15.7 Flex-2 Rod

It is a CE-certified dynamic rod system launched by the SpineVision company. In the brochure promotion of the system, the Flex-2 rod is introduced as an innovative sterile rod designed for degenerative lumbar dynamic stabilization or topping off assembly. It is accepted to keep the intervertebral height and provide durable stabilization without fusion. Its percutaneous application system is patented for low-profile dynamic rods (6-mm-diameter rods). One or two levels of hybrid rods for topping off constructs are available in this system. It has been reported that it has a true 3D dynamic range of motion (ROM) and preserves motion in the frontal, sagittal, and transverse planes. The rod consists of a multifilament wire, whose two ends are attached to a titanium alloy rod and surrounded by a polyurethane material.

Although it is recommended for use with the company's products, we used it with dynamic screws in a limited number of cases to alleviate the stress on the rod. However, we found that the rod broke in the moving area in the majority of cases within approximately 2 years, and we abolished this rod (Fig. 15.8). Eventually, we determined that dynamic rods made of multifilament wires do not last long.

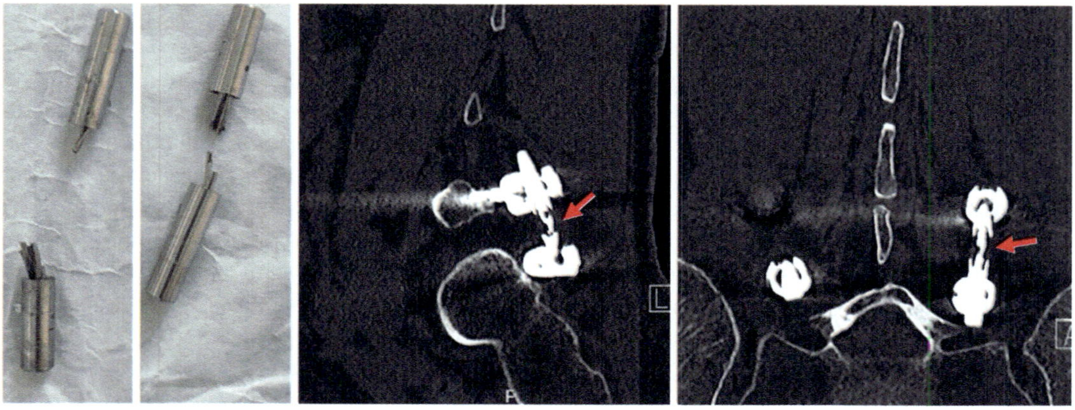

Fig. 15.8 Ruptured Flex-2 rod

15.8 BioFlex System

The BioFlex system is a flexible pedicle screw-based dynamic stabilization system, which has been used to treat degenerative lumbar conditions, with the goal of preserving motion in the area of implantation. This system is a pedicle screw-based instrument with a semirigid metallic rod, enabling dynamic stabilization and, less likely, influencing adjacent segments adversely than rigid fusion. So expectably, adjacent system degeneration would be less with this system [20].

The semirigid metallic dynamic rod of this device is made of a class of metals known as shape memory alloys, such as "nitinol." Nitinol is an alloy of nickel and titanium that belongs to a class of materials called shape memory alloys. Nitinol spring rods preserve the normal movement of implantation segments through their elasticity. This system was introduced as a dynamic rod–rigid screw device (BioSpine Corp., Seoul, Korea) (Food and Drug Administration (FDA) approval: K072321). It was developed in Korea in 2005 and was approved by the Food and Drug Administration (FDA) as a semirigid fixation system. Its stability is assured by a titanium pedicle screw, similar to conventional screws, and a coiled-shaped nitinol rod. As a semirigid stabilization system, it theoretically preserves the motion of the involved spinal segment, allowing physiological stability during flexion, extension, and lateral bending and is thought to provide physiological mobility after a decompressive laminectomy (Fig. 15.9) [21–24].

According to Heo et al., the nitinol spring rods may be more rigid during extension than flexion. Therefore, at the moment of extension, the BioFlex system may not have a load-sharing effect, and the additional load may be transferred to the adjacent levels [25].

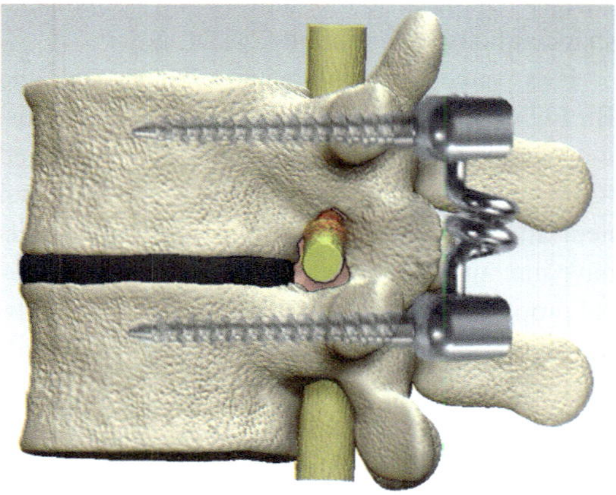

Fig. 15.9 BioFlex system with nitinol rod. (Courtesy of Ali Fahir Özer)

Biomechanical tests conducted on the BioFlex system revealed that no particular strains were imposed on the device during the fatigue strength test (American Society for Testing and Materials F1717) of 9-mm displacement with 20 million vibrations at 5 Hz, and the compression, torsion, and tension tests did not transmit much strain to the device. A test of the biocompatibility of the BioFlex rod was also performed. A nickel extraction test using inductively coupled plasma–atomic emission spectroscopy was conducted for 9 days with no signs of extraction. A galvanic corrosion test performed to assess the interaction between other metal contacts revealed no noticeable effects, which led to the conclusion that the BioFlex rod is safe for the body.

The diameter of the BioFlex rod is 4 mm, and the coiled shapes allow physiological stability during flexion, extension, and lateral bending. A design-specific advantage also allows ease in implantation and modularity for each segment.

Nitinol rods are available for the left and right sides, with appropriate left- and right-sided coils. There are two grooves in the screwhead (one groove for each rod); the set screw must be secured in the set housing after rod insertion. If rod insertion is hard, it is immersed in cold saline (below 10 °C), which makes the rod flexible and easy to handle. The rod subsequently regains its shape at body temperature [20, 24, 26].

It is stated that, unlike the Graf system, the BioFlex system prevents excessive lordosis during extension and, thereby, maintains a controlled ROM and allows the modification of segmental neutral angle and disc height. The rod's coils have one and two turns, and due to the mechanical properties of nitinol and the shape of the rods, these components have super-elasticity and rigidity, and thus, the rod acts as a tension band at the posterior spinal columns.

The BioFlex dynamic stabilization system allows the modification of the segmental neutral angle and disc height because it is a pedicle screw–based system. Thus, modification is possible through the compression or distraction of the two screws after inserting the rods and before final fixation. Also, the BioFlex screwhead has two grooves (modular system), which enable insertion of two rods per segment, and this is a strong point of this system. The system is designed to use one rod per segment, so if the surgeon needs to operate on multiple segments, the number of rods to be used increases accordingly. Due to this design and the flexibility and elasticity of the rod, there is no need to contour the device to fit the natural sagittal curve of the spine. The system can realign the normal sagittal balance even if the patient's preoperative lumbosacral angle was kyphotic or hyperlordotic (flat back syndrome).

If ASD is encountered with the BioFlex system, an easy repeat operation and extension of BioFlex soft fixation can be achieved without a long incision by including the whole scar from the previous operation because of the advantage of the modular design of the system.

BioFlex allows physiological mobility in both flexion and extension. In the study of Park et al., early postoperative clinical results were good regarding the preventive effect on ASD. The range of motion of the instrumented levels and the whole lumbar lordosis angle changed postoperatively, but they were statistically insignificant. However, the system may not prevent ASD completely in long-term follow-up studies [20, 21, 25].

15.9 Conclusion

A dynamic rod is one of the basic structures of the motion preservation concept. As mentioned here, an ideal dynamic rod system is not yet available on the market. We believe that new rod systems will emerge with the development of technology and the introduction of new biocompatible materials. Semirigid rods such as PEEK rod and BioFlex may be ideal to use for fusion, but they act as a rigid system for motion preservation, so their use in this way is not appropriate, in our opinion. But we believe that it would be more appropriate to use dynamic screws in the stabilization of a single motion segment. There seem to be fewer problems in the stabilization of a single motion segment, but there are more serious problems encountered in multilevel stabilization, especially in patients with sagittal imbalance, and the importance of the dynamic rod for multilevel stabilization will gradually develop.

References

1. Graf H. Lumbar instability: surgical treatment without fusion. Rachis. 1992;412:123–37.
2. Kanayama M, Hashimoto T, Shigenobu K, Togawa D, Oha F. A minimum 10-year follow-up of posterior dynamic stabilization using Graf artificial ligament. Spine (Phila Pa 1976). 2007;32(18):1992–7. https://doi.org/10.1097/BRS.0b013e318133faae.
3. Kirkaldy-Willis WH. Managing low back pain. Churchill Livingstone New York, 1983.
4. Kirkaldy-Willis WH, Hill RJ. A more precise diagnosis for low back pain. Spine. 1979;4:102.
5. Kanayama M, Hashimoto T, Shigenobu K. Rationale, biomechanics, and surgical indications for Graf ligamentoplasty. Orthop Clin North Am. 2005;36(3):373–7.
6. Markwalder TM, Wenger M. Dynamic stabilization of lumbar motion segments by use of Graf's ligaments: results with an average follow-up of 7.4 years in 39 highly selected, consecutive patients. Acta Neurochir (Wien). 2003;145(3):209–14. https://doi.org/10.1007/s00701-002-1056-9.
7. Grevitt MP, Gardner AD, Spilsbury J, Shackleford IM, Baskerville R, Pursell LM, Hassaan A, Mulholland RC. The Graf stabilisation system: early results in 50 patients. Eur Spine J. 1995;4(3):169–35. https://doi.org/10.1007/BF00298241.
8. Akgün MY, Ateş Ö, Günerbüyük C, Karadağ MK, Özer AF. Long-term failure of dynamic rods used in full dynamic stabilization. J Turk Spinal Surg. 2023;34:137–42.
9. Niosi CA, Zhu QA, Wilson DC, Keynan O, Wilson DR, Oxland TR. Biomechanical characterization of the three-dimensional kinematic behaviour of the Dynesys dynamic stabilization system: an in vitro study. Eur Spine J. 2006;15(6):913–22.
10. Barrey C, Freitas E, Perrin G. Pedicle screw-based dynamic stabilization devices in the lumbar spine: biomechanical concepts, technologies, classification, and clinical results. In: Advanced concepts in lumbar degenerative disk disease. Berlin, Heidelberg: Springer Berlin Heidelberg; 2016. p. 633–64.
11. Freudiger S, Dubois G, Lorrain M. Dynamic neutralization of the lumbar spine confirmed on a new lumbar spine simulator in vitro. Arch Orthop Trauma Surg. 1999;119:127–32.
12. Schwarzenbach O, Berlemann U, Stoll TM, Dubois G. Posterior dynamic stabilization systems: DYNESYS. Orthop Clin North Am. 2005;36(3):363–72.
13. Stoll TM, Dubois G, Schwarzenbach O. The dynamic neutralization system for the spine: a multi-center study of a novel non-fusion system. Eur Spine J. 2002;11:170–8.
14. Huang RC, Wright TM, Panjabi MM, Lipman JD. Biomechanics of nonfusion implants. Orthop Clin North Am. 2005;36(3):271–80.
15. Sengupta DK. Dynamic stabilization devices in the treatment of low back pain. Orthop Clin North Am. 2004;35:43–56.
16. Akgun MY, Ucar EA, Gedik CC, Gunerbuyuk C, Hekimoglu M, Cerezci O, Oktenoglu T, Sasani M, Ates O, Ozer AF. Use of dynamic spinal instruments (Dynesys) in adult spinal deformities according to Silva-Lenke and Berjano-Lamartina classifications. Diagnostics (Basel). 2024;14(5):549.
17. Akyoldaş G, Cevik OM, Suzer TM, Sasani M, Oktenoğlu T, Ozer AF. Dynamic stabilization of the lumbar spine using the Dynesys® system. Turk Neurosurg. 2020;30(2):190–3.
18. Akyoldas G, Yilmaz A, Aydin AL, Oktenoglu T, Sasani M, Suzer T, Akiz C, Ozer AF. High infection rates in patients with long-segment Dynesys system. World Neurosurg. 2018;119:403–6.
19. Karadağ MK, Akıncı AT, Başak AT, Hekimoğlu M, Yıldırım H, Akyoldaş G, Aydın AL, Ateş Ö, Öktenoğlu T, Sasani M, Akgün MY, Günerbüyük C, Özer AF. Preoperative magnetic resonance imaging abnormalities predictive of lumbar herniation recurrence after surgical repair. World Neurosurg. 2022;165:e750–6.
20. Zhang HY, Park JY, Cho BY. The BioFlex system as a dynamic stabilization device: does it preserve lumbar motion? J Korean Neurosurg Soc. 2009;46:431–6.
21. Yang JS, Cho YJ, Kang SH, Choi HJ. Dynamic radiographic results of different semi-rigid fusion devices for degenerative lumbar spondylolisthesis: "dynamic rod" vs. "dynamic screw head". Turk Neurosurg. 2016;26(2):268–73.
22. Würgler-Hauri CC, Kalbarczyk A, Wiesli M, Landolt H, Fandino J. Dynamic neutralization of the lumbar spine after microsurgical decompression in acquired lumbar spinal stenosis and segmental instability. Spine (Phila Pa 1976). 2008;33(3):66–72.
23. Cho BY, Murovic J, Park KW, Park J. Lumbar disc rehydration postimplantation of a posterior dynamic stabilization system. J Neurosurg Spine. 2010;13(5):576–80.
24. Kim YS, Zhang HY, Moon BJ, Park KW, Ji KY, Lee WC, Oh KS, Ryu GU, Kim DH. Nitinol spring rod dynamic stabilization system and Nitinol memory loops in surgical treatment for lumbar disc disorders: short-term follow up. Neurosurg Focus. 2007;22(1):E10.
25. Heo DH, Cho YJ, Cho SM, Choi HC, Kang SH. Adjacent segment degeneration after lumbar dynamic stabilization using pedicle screws and a nitinol spring rod system with 2-year minimum follow-up. J Spinal Disord Tech. 2012;25(8):409–14.
26. Kim YS, Moon BJ. Bioflex spring rod pedicle screw system. In: Kim DH, Cammisa Jr FP, Fessler RG, editors. Dynamic reconstruction of the spine. New York: Thieme; 2006. p. 340–6.

16 Biomechanical Analysis of Different Dynamic Rods Used with Rigid Screws

Freudiger Stefan, Cathrein Philipp, Abramovic Sarah, Lorrain Michel, and Dubois Gilles

16.1 Introduction

Dynamic stabilization, or neutralization ("neutralize," to suppress abnormal movements), by means of an internal bracing, restores near-normal rigidity, returning the patient to the natural course of disco-vertebral degeneration, which is usually silent up to its completion [1].

The aim of dynamic stabilization (or neutralization) is to provide sufficient additional segmental rigidity to eliminate parasitic intervertebral movements while maintaining a certain degree of intervertebral freedom.

The ability to modulate the "elasticity" of the rod to suit the local failure of the intervertebral segment concerned is an undeniable advance on the previous device, DYNESYS (Zimmer Biomet, Warsaw, IN, USA); it enables the surgeon, specialized in spinal surgery, to choose the modulus of elasticity and, therefore, the rigidity required to correct the segmental defect to be treated.

Therefore, spineshape S-IV is considered an evolution of DYNESYS. DYNESYS had one unique stiffness given by its cord (polyethylene terephthalate (PET)), its spacer (polycarbonate urethane (PCU)), and the cord's pretension in order to prevent any dislocation of the assembly. Spineshape S-IV provides rods (PCU) with three different stiffnesses (soft, medium, and hard), achieved by varying the ratio of the same polymeric components. With the rod as a single structure simply clamped in the head of the pedicle screws, dislocation is no longer an issue, and pretension is no longer required.

The flowchart followed for this development is given in Fig. 16.1.

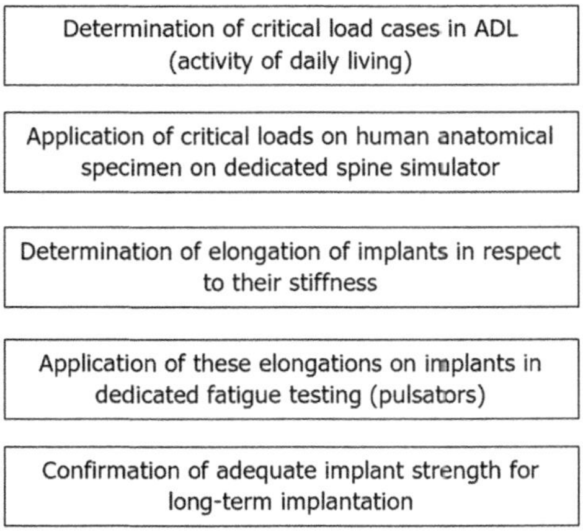

Fig. 16.1 Flowchart of development

F. Stefan (✉) · A. Sarah
Research & Development, SpineSave, Embrach, Switzerland
e-mail: stefan.freudiger@spinesave.com; sarah.abramovic@spinesave.com

C. Philipp
Dorsomed, Biel, Switzerland
e-mail: cathrein@dorsomed.ch

L. Michel · D. Gilles
Toulouse, France

A. F. Özer et al. (eds.), *Dynamic Lumbar Spine Stabilization*,
https://doi.org/10.1007/978-3-032-12122-6_16

16.2 Critical Load Cases

In order to design implants and ascertain that their strength and stiffness are appropriate, critical load cases need to be determined. Flexion and extension load cases are thus derived from [2] and shown in Figs. 16.2 and 16.3.

The resulting loads of Figs. 16.2 and 16.3 represent the nominal worst-case loads acting on a functional spinal unit (FSU) in forward (inclination) and backward (reclination) bending.

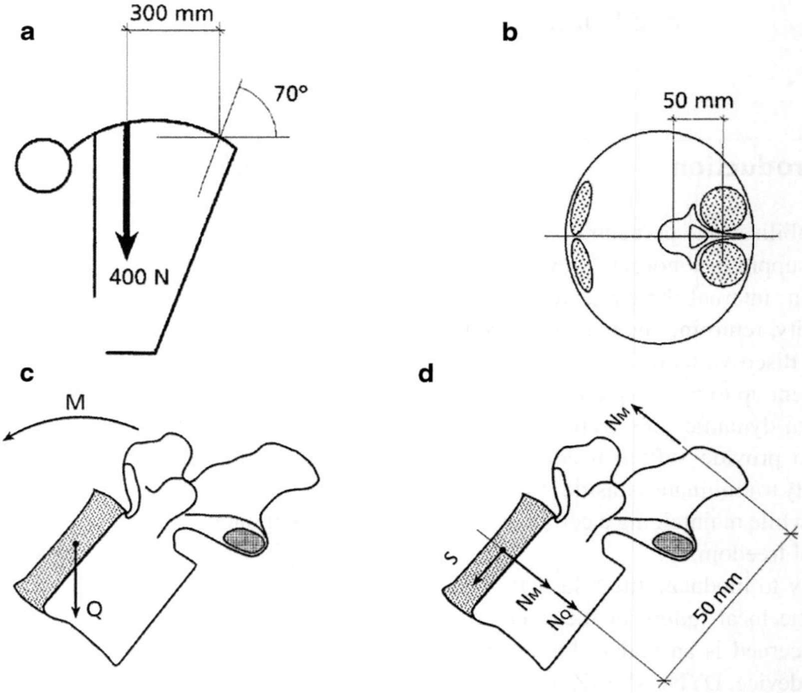

Fig. 16.2 (**a**) Schematic person bent forward. (**b**) Assumed geometry of a transverse trunk section. (**c**) $M = 400 \times 0.3 = 120$ Nm and $Q = 400$ N. (**d**) $N_M = 120/0.05 = 2400$ N, $N_Q = Q \cdot \cos 70° \approx 140$ N, $N = N_M + N_Q =$ **2540 N**, and $S = Q \cdot \sin 70° \approx$ **380 N**

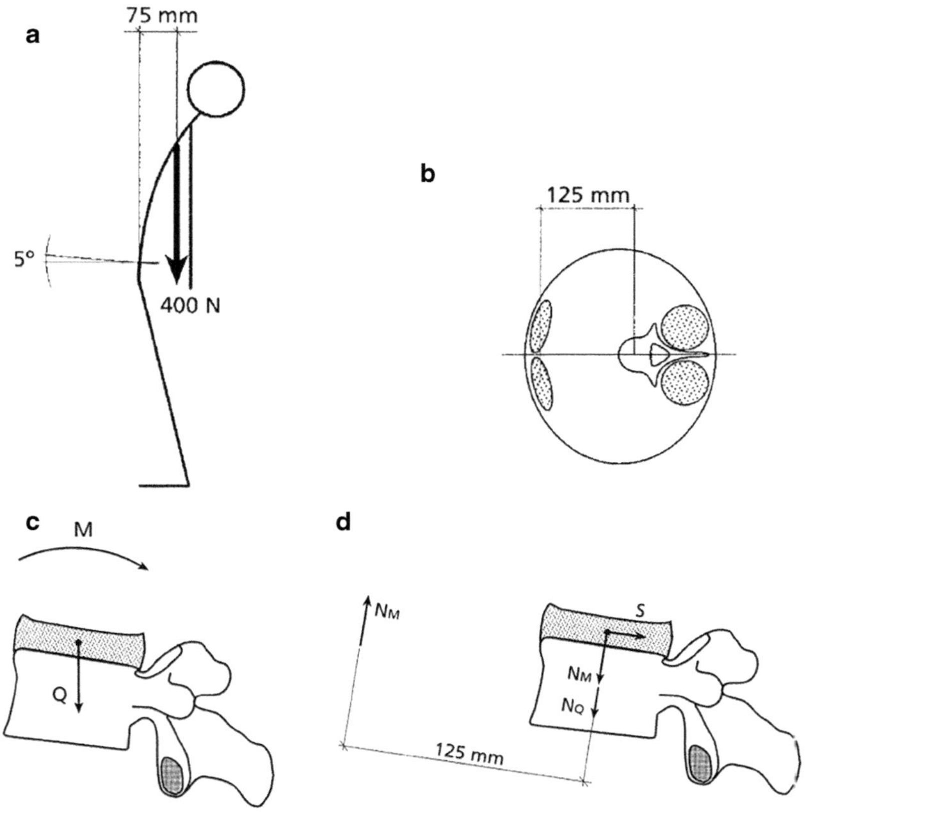

Fig. 16.3 (**a**) Schematic person bent backward. (**b**) Assumed geometry of a transverse trunk section. (**c**) $M = 400 \times 0.075 = 30$ Nm and $Q = 400$ N. (**d**) $N_M = 30/0.125 = 240$ N, $N_Q = Q \cdot \cos 5° \approx 400$ N, $N = N_M + N_Q = \mathbf{640\ N}$, and $S = Q \cdot \sin 5° \approx \mathbf{30\ N}$

16.3 Simulator

At the time of development of this system, no satisfactory load setups were available. Panjabi et al. [3] limited the loads to an FSU to a pure moment of 10 Nm, and Patwardhan et al. [4] simply added a so-called follower load of 1200 N. Also, American Society for Testing and Materials (ASTM) F2624-07 [5] was not considered satisfactory for the real-life worst-case testing of the given system.

Therefore, the above determined loads were applied to human anatomical specimens using a specially dedicated spine simulator [2]. The average loads, which were finally acting on the specimen, were, in flexion, 2420 N compression, 570 N anterior shear, and 27 Nm residual forward-bending moment and, in extension, 630 N compression, 60 N rearward shear, and 11 Nm residual extension moment (Figs. 16.4 and 16.5).

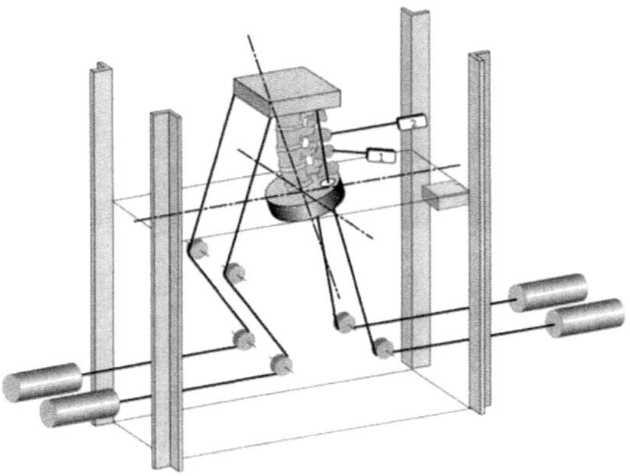

Fig. 16.4 Schematized spine simulator

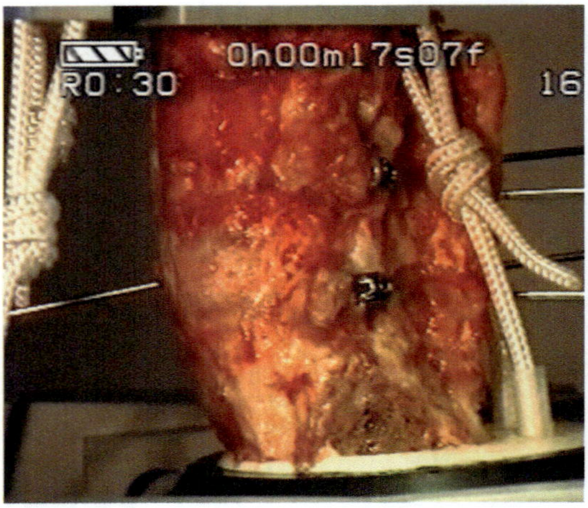

Fig. 16.5 Anatomical specimen in the simulator

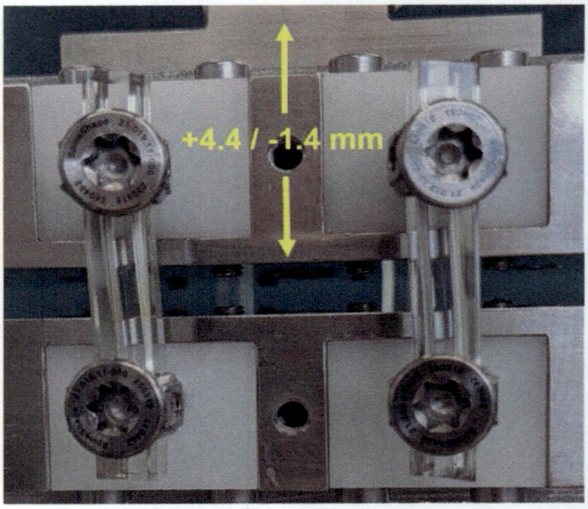

Fig. 16.6 Test setup: longitudinal

Table 16.1 Rod length changes

Rod type	Elongation/shortening	Total
Soft	+4.40/−1.40 mm	5.80 mm
Medium	+2.20/−0.70 mm	2.90 mm
Hard	+1.10/−0.35 mm	1.45 mm

Table 16.2 Rod displacements

Rod type	Displacement
Soft	+6.0/−0.0 mm
Medium	+5.0/−0.0 mm
Hard	+4.0/−0.0 mm

By inserting rods of different stiffnesses, corresponding rod elongation and shortening could be determined as follows (Table 16.1).

These numbers represent the average measured length changes and were multiplied by a safety factor of 1.5 to also cover the extreme values (scattering while measuring the anatomical specimen).

16.4 Cyclic Testing (Fatigue Testing)

The different rods are then subjected to the related length changes in a fatigue testing machine, i.e., a pulsator (Fig. 16.6).

Regarding the transversal loads, a more pragmatic approach is chosen. Transversal loads occur in spondylolisthesis movements. Naturally, polymeric rods are not as efficient as metal rods in regard to shear stiffness. Consequently, indications for dynamic stabilization are limited to rather low spondylolisthesis, e.g., Meyerding grade 1. The goal of a polymeric rod is therefore not primarily the reduction of slipping movement but the support of any residual slipping.

Based on clinical observations, the following transversal displacements are derived based on the different rod stiffnesses (Table 16.2).

The different rods are then subjected to the related lateral displacements in a fatigue testing machine, i.e., a pulsator (Fig. 16.7).

The following considerations have to be made when it comes to the appropriate number of testing cycles, which need to be related to a corresponding load level. Typical loads occur more often in activities of daily living (ADLs) than maximum loads. Maximum loads on the lumbar spine happen when a person bends forward until the fingertips touch the ground, e.g., for washing one's feet or for putting on socks and shoes. Typical loads happen during the more frequent sitting down or standing up. Typical loads are estimated to achieve one-third of the maximum loads.

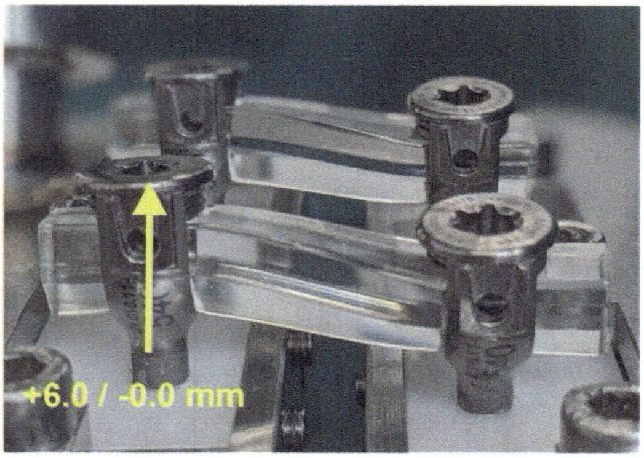

Fig. 16.7 Test setup: transversal

To put these loads and frequencies in numbers of years during implantation time, two approaches are considered, i.e., a bottom-up approach and a top-down approach, with the following results (Table 16.3).

Table 16.3 Number of cycles versus years in situ

	Cycles (laboratory)	Load-case	Per day	Years (patient)
Bottom-up	1 Mio	Max	22 times →	124
Top-down	1 Mio 9 Mio	Max Typ	91 times 822 times	30 30 ←

16.5 Hystereses

Since we are dealing with polymeric rods and polymers underlie the rules of viscoelasticity, the results of these tests cannot simply be presented on stress/strain curves but need to be plotted as force versus displacement curves after one million cycles at maximum load. Tests are carried out at 3 Hz, the maximum speed without load reduction due to internal heat. All probes are tested in water at 37° ± 0.2 °C using the so-called vertebrectomy model [6]. In order to respect viscoelastic properties, the results are given as hysteresis. Green is the zone of true dynamic stabilization, red is the zone of fusion implants, and yellow is the transition zone. A stiffness threshold of 200 N/mm has also been confirmed by Schmidt et al. [7]. Figure 16.7 shows hysteresis for longitudinal and Fig. 16.8 for transversal loadings. Figure 16.7 also includes curves for titanium and Polyethetetherketone (PEEK) rods, as well as for the DYNESYS system (Fig. 16.9).

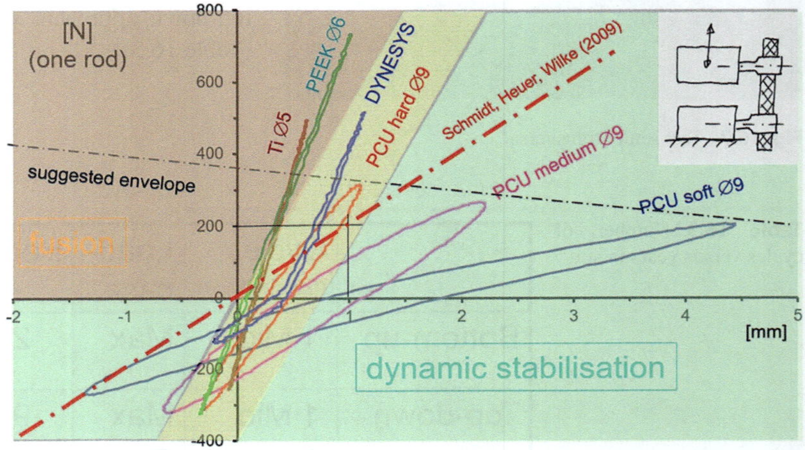

Fig. 16.8 Hysteresis of longitudinal loading

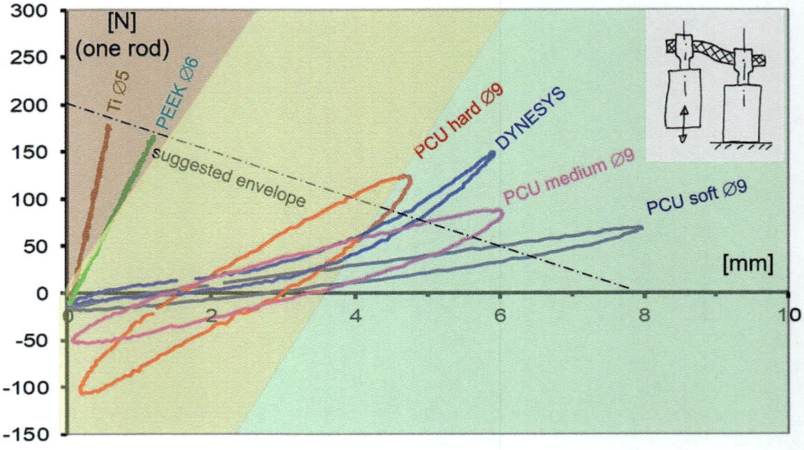

Fig. 16.9 Hysteresis of transversal loading

16.6 Design Feature

Since polymeric rods have viscoelastic properties, they have the disadvantage of flowing out through any gap and thus reducing their clamping force. In order to maintain the clamping force for a long time, the clamping plane should not have any gaps but must rather be designed as a so-called cage fit. Refer to Fig. 16.10 for a patented cross section.

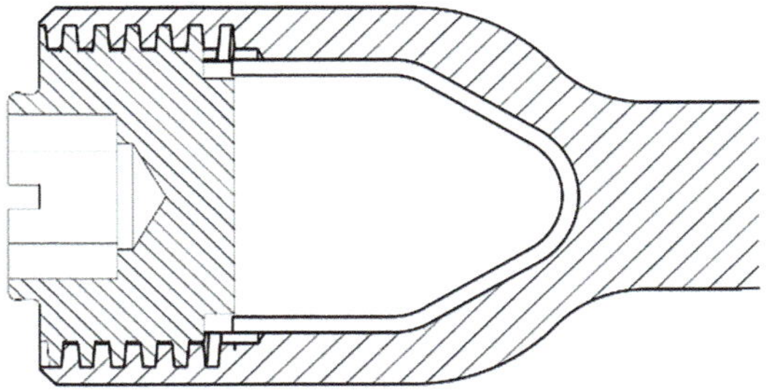

Fig. 16.10 Cage fit

16.7 Indications

With different rod stiffnesses, the indications also have to address different pathologies. However, the different indications cannot be strictly distinguished since overlaps are possible (Table 16.4).

The major reason for overlaps is the functional length of the connection rod between its anchorage in the pedicle screw heads. Doubling the functional length also doubles the elasticity of the connection, thus corresponding to the rod with the next higher elasticity. Likewise, halving the functional length doubles the stiffness of the connection, thus corresponding to the rod of the next higher stiffness (Fig. 16.11). Where two rod types are possible, also consider the rod's length and take higher elasticity for shorter rods.

Table 16.4 Indication scheme

	Soft	Medium	Hard
(Dynamic) stenosis	x	x	
Facet joint syndrome/spondyloarthrosis	x	x	
Osteochondrosis Modic type I or III	x	x	
Discopathy (recurrent disc prolapse/herniation)		x	
Late adjacent segment disease (ASD)		x	
Complement to disc prosthesis		(x)	
Osteochondrosis Modic type II		x	x
Degenerative spondylolisthesis (Meyerding <1)		x	x
(Degenerative) scoliosis (early stage: nonrigid)		x	x
Instability[a]		x	x
Complement to cage		(x)	(x)

(x) Not a preferred indication
[a]Hypermobility with antelisthesis/hypomobility with retrolisthesis when decompressed

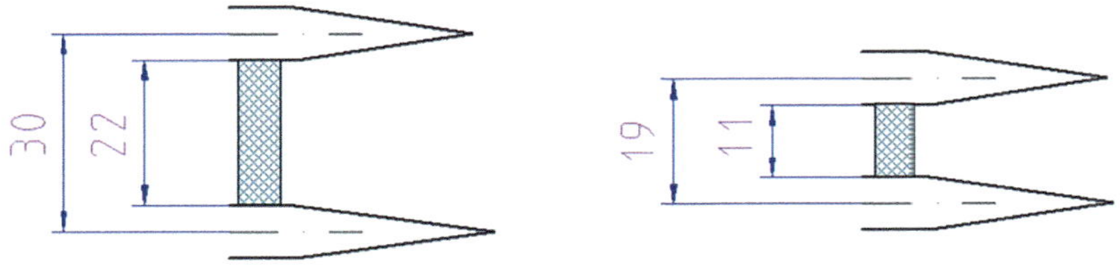

Fig. 16.11 Functional length

16.8 Load Sharing

It is obvious that a stiff connection rod takes more load than an elastic rod and that a stiff rod reduces the mobility of the treated spinal segment more than an elastic rod. Roughly, it can be assumed that hard, medium, and soft rods reduce the normal mobility by approximately 75%, 50%, and 25%, respectively. The load on the relevant soft tissues as structural elements of the spinal segment is then shared by the implant with the approximate ratios shown in Fig. 16.12.

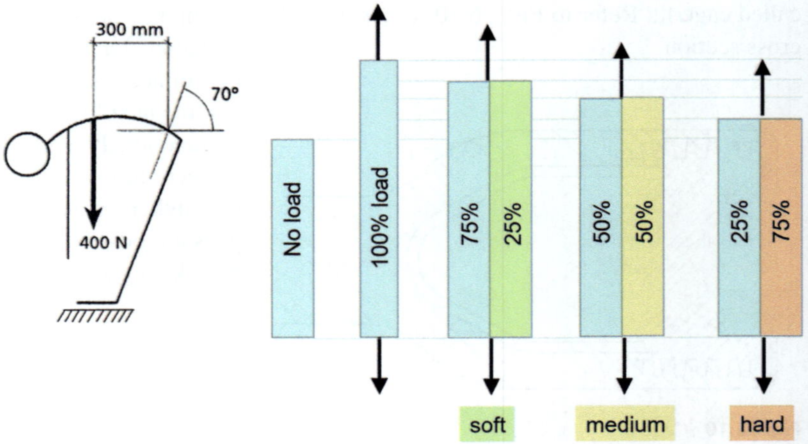

Fig. 16.12 Load sharing

16.9 Biocompatibility

The material polycarbonate urethane (PCU) is well-known to be highly biocompatible, bio-inert is an enhancement of highly biocompatible if not even means depending on the point of view [8]. Furthermore, this material also has an extraordinary stability with regard to the long-term mechanical performance. On several occasions (e.g., lengthening procedures), explanted rods could be subjected to the same fatigue test as new rods, where the resulting hysteresis lay amazingly close to each other (Fig. 16.13).

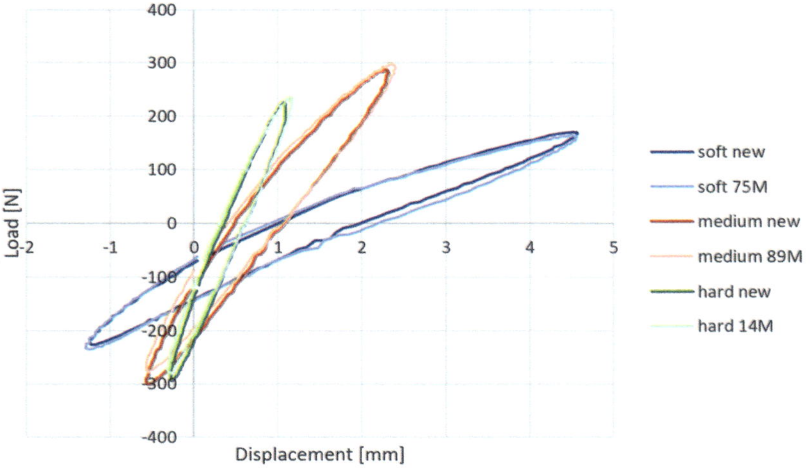

Fig. 16.13 Comparison of hysteresis

16.10 High Demand on the Ideal Path of the Rod (Mono-axial Screw)

Since a pedicle screw for a dynamic stabilization must last for the lifetime of the implant to preserve motion as many years as possible, its strength requirements are much more demanding than for a pedicle screw for a fusion procedure. As soon as a fusion is successfully accomplished (i.e., bone consolidation), a pedicle screw is no longer subjected to important loads, in contrast to a pedicle screw for dynamic stabilization. For this reason, slender necks, as used for poly-axial screws, are seldom seen on screws for dynamic stabilization, which are mostly mono-axial. This is to ascertain a fatigue strength high enough for long-term usage.

Consequently, the correct placement of mono-axial pedicle screws is of great importance in order to achieve a rod curvature suitable for a gentle loading of polymeric rods (Figs. 16.14 and 16.15).

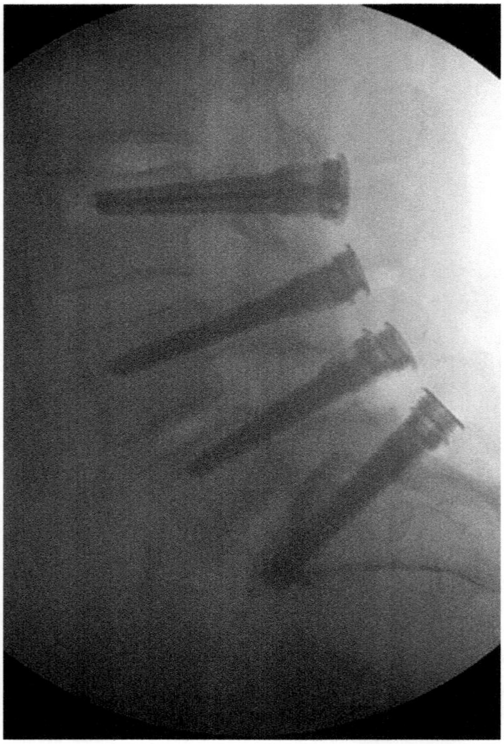

Fig. 16.14 Side view of a perfect curvature

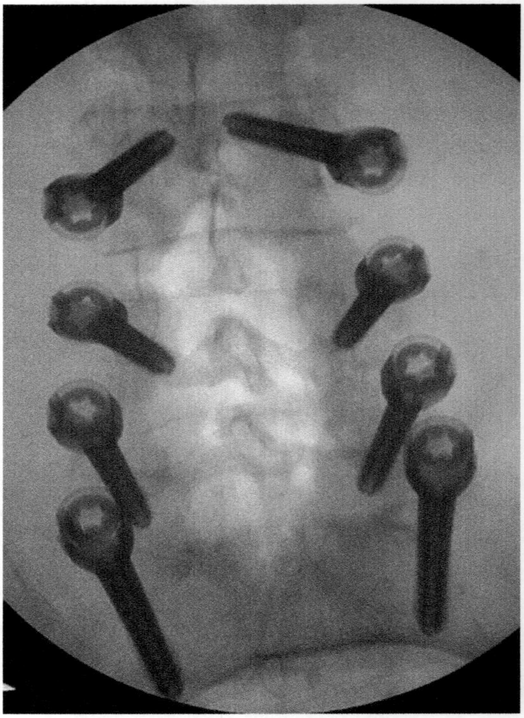

Fig. 16.15 Anterior-posterior (AP) view of a perfect curvature

16.11 Postoperative Mobility

An interim evaluation of the postoperative mobility (standard deviation in brackets), i.e., the segmental range of motion (ROM) between inclination and reclination, yields the following values (Table 16.5).

At the time of evaluation, no data for patients who received hard rods were available. For medium rods, 294, 86, and 39 patients were available for analysis at 3, 12, and 36 months, respectively. For soft rods, 81, 30, and 24 patients were available for analysis at 3, 12, and 36 months, respectively.

These numbers are well in line with the findings in the literature [9–11]. Approximately 3° is considered by treating surgeons to be an appropriate amount of mobility in the treated lumbar segments. A higher ROM might be critical for persisting pain due to pathological movements, and a lower ROM may lead to prematurely spontaneous fusion.

Table 16.5 Range of motion

	3 months	12 months	36 months
Hard rod	–	–	–
Medium rod	2.3° (±1.4°)	2.6° (±1.6°)	2.2° (±1.6°)
Soft rod	2.9° (±1.8°)	2.9° (±2.7°)	2.9° (±2.0°)

16.12 Conclusion

The residual mobility is considered rather small. Patients with degenerated discs can no longer reach the mobility of intact spines despite repeated, occasionally reported observations of disc regeneration and disc rehydration after the implantation of dynamic stabilization systems [12–14]. There is no statistically significant difference in ROM between a soft and a medium rod. Many overlaying factors influence the outcome of the selected rod's stiffness, such as the remaining disc height, previous surgeries, functional length of the rod, patient's weight, intraoperative mobility, patient's age, etc.

The dynamic stabilization of the degenerative lumbar spine has been shown to have comparable functional improvement to that of fusion for the same indications [9, 15, 16]. However, the shorter duration of surgery and less intraoperative blood loss for dynamic stabilization result in lower hospital treatment costs compared to fusion [10, 16]. The other advantage of dynamic stabilization with DYNESYS or spineshape S-IV over fusion is the reversibility of the instrumentation and makes it a valuable procedure in the rather early phase of lumbar spine degeneration. The rod stiffness of spineshape S-IV can be chosen according to the indications, and in case of further progression, the patient can still be fused at a later point of time. Our results with spineshape S-IV and the literature show that the segmental ROM can be preserved with dynamic stabilization even after 5 years postoperatively [9–11]. However, the focus of spine surgeons and the spine research community has shifted. Today, the goal is not only to preserve mobility in the instrumented segments but, even more, to show that adjacent segment disease (ASD) occurs at a far later stage with dynamic stabilization than fusion. The published rates of revision surgeries due to ASD in fused patients go up to 29.4% 5 years postoperatively [17–19], whereas in dynamic stabilization with DYNESYS, the rates go up to 15.4% [20, 21]. In comparison, being on the market for over 10 years, of all patients treated for degenerative lumbar spine diseases with spineshape S-IV, 5.5% of the patients were documented to have received revision surgery due to ASD.

References

1. Kirkaldy Willis WH, Farfan HF. Instability of the lumbar spine. Clin Orthop. 1982;165:110–23.
2. Freudiger S, Dubois G, Lorrain M. Dynamic neutralisation of the lumbar spine confirmed on a new lumbar spine simulator in vitro. Arch Orthop Trauma Surg. 1999;119:127–32.
3. Panjabi MM, Oxland TR, Yamamoto I, Crisco JJ. Mechanical behaviour of the human lumbar and lumbosacral spine as shown by three-dimensional load-displacement curves. J Bone Joint Surg Am. 1994;76:413–24.
4. Patwardhan AG, Havey RM, Carandang G, Simonds J, Voronov LI, Ghanayem AJ, Meade KP, Gavin TM, Paxinos O. Effect of compressive follower preload on the flexion-extension response of the human lumbar spine. J Orthop Res. 2003;21:540–6.
5. ASTM F2624-07 standard test method for static, dynamic, and wear assessment of extra-discal spinal motion preserving implants. Copyright © ASTM International, West Conshohocken.
6. ASTM F1717-21 standard test methods for spinal implant constructs in a vertebrectomy model. Copyright © ASTM International, West Conshohocken.
7. Schmidt H, Heuer F, Wilke HJ. Which axial and bending stiffnesses of posterior implants are required to design a flexible lumbar stabilization system ? J Biomech. 2009;42:48–54.
8. Shan-hui H, Zu-Chang L. Biocompatibility and biostability of a series of poly(carbonate)urethanes. Colloids Surf B Biointerfaces. 2004;36:1–12.
9. Bredin S, et al. Posterolateral fusion versus Dynesys dynamic stabilization: retrospective study at a minimum 5.5years' follow-up. Orthop Traumatol Surg Res. 2017;103:1241–4.
10. Luo L, et al. Comparison between dynamic stabiliaztion and instrumented fusion in the treatment of spinal stenosis with degenerative lumbar scoliosis. Pain Res Manag. 2022;2022:9367106.
11. Wu H, et al. Medium-term effects of Dynesys dynamic stabilizatio nversus posterior lumbar interbody fusion

for tretament of multisegmental lumbar degenerative disease. J Int Med Res. 2017;45(5):1562–73.
12. Schnake KJ, Putzier M, Haas NP, Kandziora F. Mechanical concepts for disc regeneration. Eur Spine J. 2006;15(Suppl. 3):S354–60.
13. Bordes-Monmeneu M, Bordes-García V, Rodrigo-Baeza F, Sáez D. A dynamic neutralisation system for the spine. DYNESYS SYSTEM experience in 94 cases. Neurocirurgia. 2005;16:499–506.
14. Yilmaz A, Senturk S, Sasani M, Oktenoglu T, Yaman O, Yildirim H, Suzer T, Ozer OF. Disc rehydration after dynamic stabilization: a report of 59 cases. Asian Spine J. 2017;11(3):348–55.
15. Prud'homme M, et al. Clinical outcomes and complications after pedicle-anchored dynamic or hybrid lumbar spine stabilization: a systematic literature review. J Spinal Disord Tech. 2015;28(8):E439–48.
16. Meyer BT, et al. Lumbar dynamic pedicle-based stabilization versus fusion in degenerative disease: a multicenter, double-blind, prospective, randomized controlled trial. J Neurosurg Spine. 2022;37:515–24.
17. Koban O, et al. Radiological and clinical comparisons of the patients with rheumatoid arthritis operated with rigid and dynamic instrumentation systems due to lumbar degenerative spinal diseases. J Orthop Sci. 2021;26:369–74.
18. Sears WR, et al. Risk of adjacent segment disease after 'topping-off' multi-level lumbar fusions with posterior dynamic stabilisers: an observational cohort study. Eur Spine J. 2021;30:181–90.
19. Yuan W, et al. Evaluation of Coflex interspinous stabilization following decompression compared with decompression and posterior lumbar interbody fusion for the treatment of lumbar degenerative disease: a minimum 5-year follow-up study. J Clin Neurosci. 2017;35:24–9.
20. Khalifé M, et al. Dynesys dynamic stabilization outcomes in degenerative spine surgery. Acta Orthop Belg. 2021;87(4):795–803.
21. Hoppe S, et al. Long-term outcome after monosegmental L4/5 stabilization for degenerative spondylolisthesis with the Dynesys device. Clin Spine Surg. 2016;29:72–7.

Long-Segment Pedicular Stabilization in Multilevel Steno-instability Using Hybrid Fixation

17

Mario Di Silvestre

17.1 Introduction

Multi-segmental lumbar spinal stenosis represents a frequent condition that worsens with aging. The pain and intermittent neurogenic claudication caused by spinal stenosis have a severe impact on the daily life of patients and, therefore, necessitate surgical treatment. For the treatment of multilevel stenosis, posterior fusion with rigid instrumentation has been largely used [1]. However, successful fusion has not always been accompanied by clinical improvement [2]. This apparent lack of correlation between surgical and clinical outcomes raises important questions about secondary, delayed phenomena that could adversely affect the final clinical outcome. Achievement of fusion may, in fact, have long-term effects on the immediately adjacent motion segments [3, 4]. At the junction with adjacent mobile segments, the rigidity of the fused segments induces increased constraints that can constitute a clinical concern [5–7]. The primary junctional complications can be facet degeneration, ligament hypertrophy, disc degeneration, and spinal stenosis [5, 8]. This adjacent level degeneration is typically seen rostral to a fused segment but may also occur caudal to a fusion, especially when it is performed until the L4–L5 level. The phenomenon is thought to be due to the altered biomechanics of the fused spine, wherein abnormal forces acting upon the intervertebral discs and facet joints adjacent to the fused segment precipitate the accelerated failure of these stabilizing elements [9].

From this evidence emerged the choice of using a "dynamic" long stabilization of the lumbar spine [10–12]. So DYNESYS® instrumentation has been used in our department for multi-segmental steno-instability of the lumbar spine, often combined with multi-segmental disc degeneration (Fig. 17.1). However, this long construct of DYNESYS® instrumentation (from T11/T12 to S1) presented a weak point at the lumbosacral fixation, with loosening of the S1 screws. Therefore, we preferred to adopt hybrid fixation for multi-segmental stenosis, i.e., a posterior dynamic stabilization, in which pedicle screw fixation is coupled with a flexible longitudinal connecting system, to allow for the normalization of intersegmental motion. An example of a hybrid construct is the DTO system: This implant combines the DYNESYS® Neutralization System with the Optima Spinal System, i.e., a dynamic fixation combined with a rigid one. This stands in contrast to traditional fusion surgery, in which the goal is complete and immediate elimination of motion and, ultimately, arthrodesis. These hybrid systems present dynamic stabiliza-

M. Di Silvestre (✉)
Chief of Spinal Deformity Department,
Ospedale Santa Corona, Pietra Ligure, Italy

A. F. Özer et al. (eds.), *Dynamic Lumbar Spine Stabilization*,
https://doi.org/10.1007/978-3-032-12122-6_17

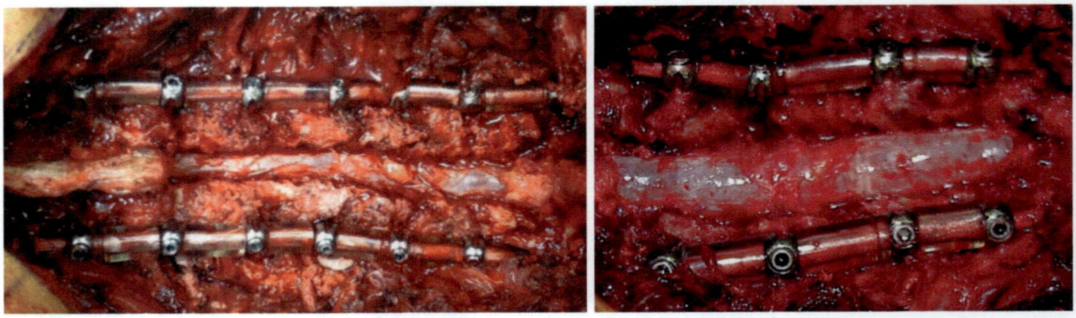

Fig. 17.1 An example of wide and long decompression in a multi-segmental stenosis using a long DYNESYS® fixation

tion, associated with a rigid fixation and a lumbosacral fusion. These systems are intended for use in patients in whom fusion is desired to treat severe instability or advanced degeneration at one or more lumbosacral levels and in whom many adjacent segments exhibit degenerative changes (that are thought to be contributing to the patient's symptoms but are not of a severe-enough degree to warrant arthrodesis). So the unstable degenerative segments are instrumented with the static fixator, and the adjacent segments are protected by the dynamic fixator [13]. From a biomechanical viewpoint, mobility of the transition disc can be preserved to some extent, and thus, the mechanical load can be partially shared by the dynamic fixator [14, 15]. However, at least two problems are inherent to hybrid fixation. First is whether hybrid fixators simply transfer the junctional constraints to the next adjacent segments. Second is regarding which degenerative grade of the transition disc indicates the use of a hybrid fixator. No follow-up study has previously been dedicated to the detailed investigation of these two questions [14, 16].

17.2 Technique

The patients were treated under general anesthesia in the prone position.

1. The first step was the implantation of screws. The DTO implant combines the DYNESYS® Neutralization System and the Optima Spinal System. The DYNESYS® (Zimmer) system was always placed cranially to the Optima system. The DTO implant is made of a combined 100 mm polyethylene terephthalate DYNESYS® cord and a standard titanium 6 mm rod. DYNESYS® implants were used for dynamic fixation. DYNESYS® implants consist of titanium alloy pedicle screws, polyethylene terephthalate cords, and polycarbonate urethane spacers, which fit between the pedicle screwheads. Optima implants were used for rigid fixation and consist of titanium alloy pedicle screws. The pedicle screws used in lumbar vertebrae and in the sacrum were 7 mm in diameter and 40 or 45 mm in length. Between DYNESYS® pedicle screws and Optima pedicle screws, there were poly-axial Optima Transition screws.
2. After the insertion of screws, the second step was the treatment of stenosis by laminectomy: The patients' hips were flexed at an angle of 90° to facilitate decompression of the stenotic levels. The decompression was extended to the lateral recess, and foraminotomy was performed without interrupting the isthmus. After decompression, the patients' position was modified to obtain the maximum lumbar lordosis. For reducing surgery time, during a laminectomy, another surgeon prepared the spacers of DYNESYS® system by cutting them according to the length measured previously between adjacent screws. Each of the polycarbonate urethane spacers was cut to the desired length and threaded with a polyester cord, which was stretched between and fixed to two adjacent screwheads. The length of fixation could be very long, of about six levels, from T12 to the sacrum, in general (Fig. 17.2).

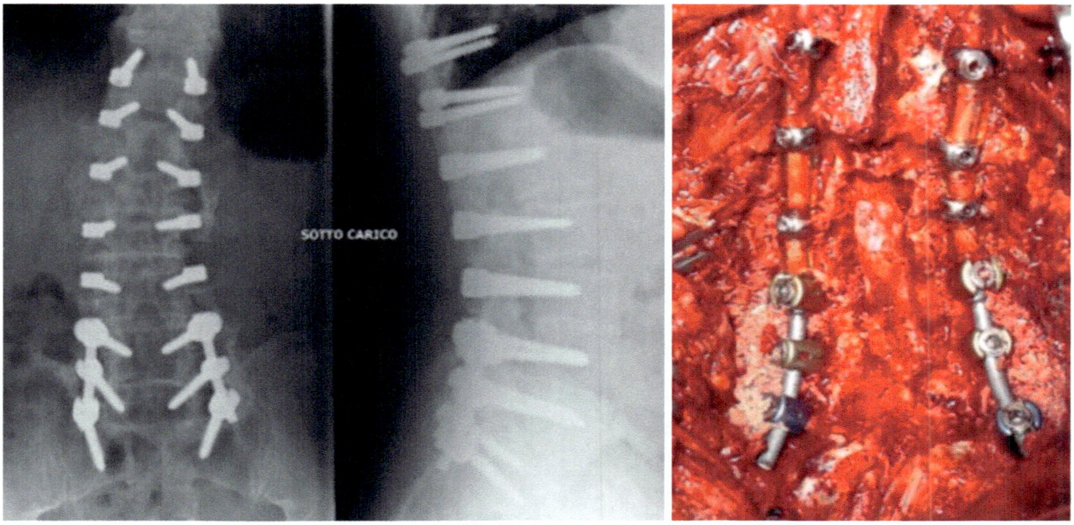

Fig. 17.2 Example of hybrid fixation from T11 to S1, with wide L4–S1 laminectomy and rigid fixation L4–S1

3. After decompression, the patients' position was modified to obtain the maximum lumbar lordosis, and the instrumentation was completed. Iliac screws were not used in any of the patients. Circumferential lumbosacral fusion was not performed in these patients to reduce the impact of surgery, considering that the great part of patients were elderly. Allograft bank bone (one femur head for every patient) and autograft bone (spinous processes and laminae obtained from decompression procedure) were used at the posterolateral fusion levels (L5–S1 or L4–S1). The mean operating time was about 130 min (range: 10–160 min), the mean hospital stay was 5.9 days (range: 4–8 days), and the mean blood loss was 950 cc (range: 200–1.600 cc).

17.3 Discussion

The problems of a long instrumentation for the treatment of multi-segmental stenosis are represented by the L5–S1 fixation and the disc degeneration in the upper junction of the instrumented spine. The experience with DTO instrumentation resulted in a resolution of the problems of L5–S1 fixation. The other problem, i.e., adjacent segment disease (ASD), is still a subject of discussion [17, 18]. Degenerative changes at the adjacent segments must be considered to exist when there are at least two of the following criteria: (1) On standing X-rays, the height of the adjacent disc was reduced by more than 70%, (2) displacement of more than 3 mm on the X-ray of the sagittal plane of the closest upper or lower segment, (3) segmental instability of more than 15° on the lateral X-rays in flexion and extension [3, 19], and (4) segmental stenosis and/or disc degeneration (grade III according to the Pfirmann classification [20]) at the adjacent level on the follow-up MRI. We reviewed the patients treated with hybrid fixation for multi-segmental stenosis: Degenerative changes at adjacent segments were observed in three patients (10.0%), whose mean age at index operation was 75.0 (range: 60–82) years. Two of them presented symptoms, whereas the other one was asymptomatic. Only the two symptomatic patients underwent another surgery (Fig. 17.3).

The phenomenon of adjacent segment disease (ASD), referring to accelerated degenerative changes occurring at the extremities of a posterior fusion, has received increasing attention, as more spinal fusions are being performed and long-term follow-up data have become available [3, 11]. While the evolution and prevalence of ASD are not fully known, there is increasing evi-

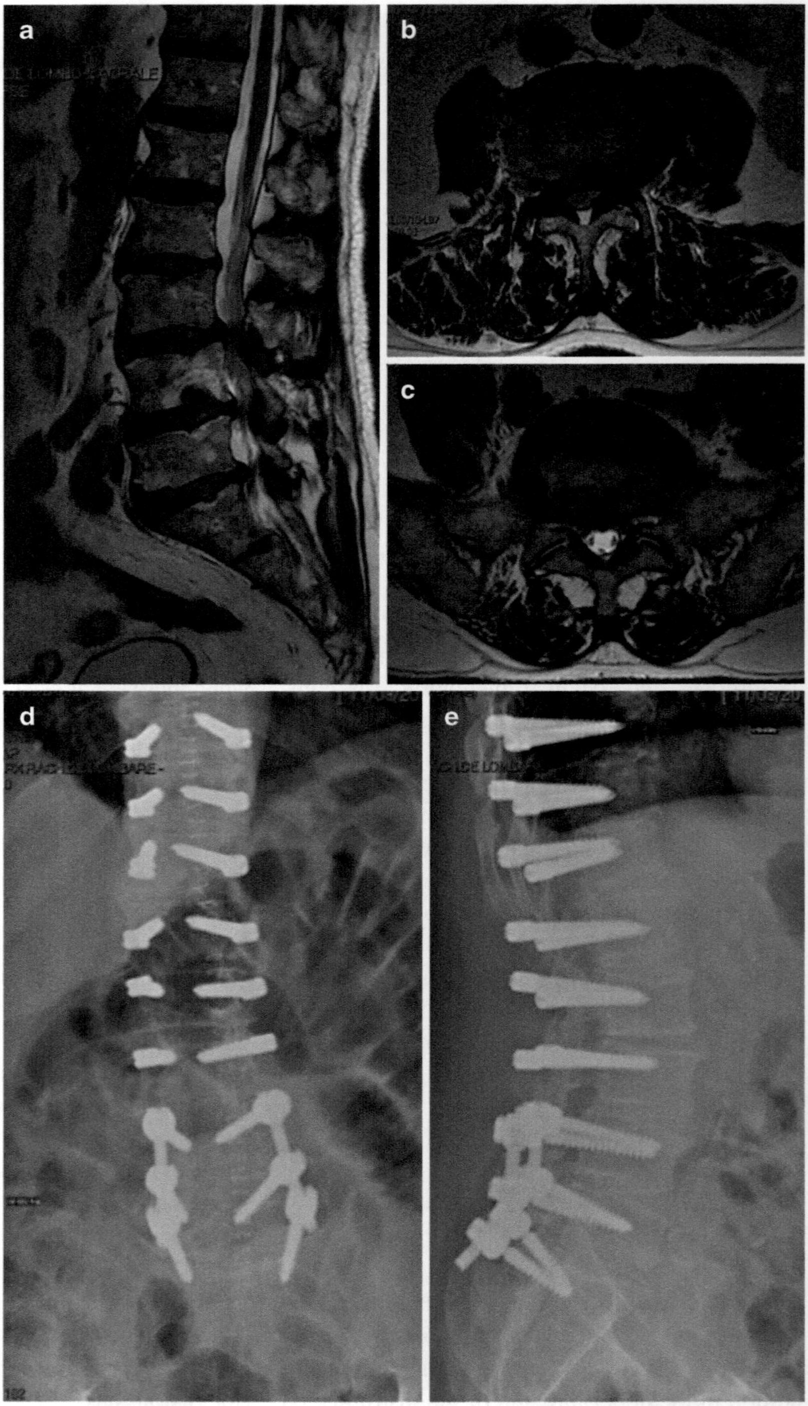

Fig. 17.3 Male, 76 years old, persistent pain in the legs and neurological disturbances (intermittent claudication). Multi-segmental stenosis, as evident in MRI (a, b, c), treated with a hybrid long construct from T10 to S1 (d, e)

dence in the literature that its effects may be seen soon after fusion surgery and in as many as 30% of patients [3, 4]. Cheh et al. [3] reported a rate of clinical ASD of 30.3% and showed that patients in whom adjacent level disease developed had significantly worse Oswestry Disability Index scores than those without adjacent segment disease. They further identified age > 50 years at the time of surgery, increasing length of fusion, and extension of the fusion to L1–L3 as significant risk factors for the development of adjacent segment disease. No significant difference was identified between posterior and circumferential fusion [3].

Over the past 20 years, an array of posterior pedicle fixation–based motion preservation systems has been introduced, as many in the spine community have sought to decrease the incidence of ASD [21]. One of these systems, the dynamic neutralization system (DYNESYS®), has been in use at our department for the past 20 years [18]. The dynamic stabilization approach promises to do it in a more physiological manner. By "restoring" normal motion, mobility is theoretically preserved rather than eliminated, and the forces acting above and below the construct are altered to a lesser extent, reducing the potential undesirable effects of fusion. Compared with static fixation, numerous types of dynamic fixators have been developed to preserve the mobility of the transition segments and reduce the occurrence of the junctional problem [21–23]. Among them, the dynamic neutralization system (DYNESYS®) is one of the commonly used dynamic fixators [12, 24]. Similar to static fixation, the DYNESYS® system uses pedicle screws for anchorage in the vertebral bodies via the pedicles. Subsequently, the flexible cords in spacers of adequate length are extended between and connected to the screwheads.

The use of hybrid systems has spread in the treatment of patients in whom decompression and fusion are required at many levels but in whom there is also the potential for symptomatic degenerative changes at one or more adjacent levels. One of these is the DTO implant (DYNESYS® transition option), in which a DYNESYS®-like extension is added above the Optima fusion instrumentation. Published studies about hybrid pedicle screw constructs are few, and long-term follow-up data are even more scarce. Maserati et al. reported that three (12.0%) of their 24 patients developed symptomatic degenerative changes at or above the dynamically stabilized levels, but the mean follow-up was only 8 months [25]. In our review of patients treated with DTO, at a minimum of 5 years of follow-up, evidence of radiographic ASD was noted in three (10.0%) of the original 30 patients, an incidence similar to that in the preliminary report of Maserati et al. [25] but after much longer follow-up in our patients. The present incidence of 10% radiographic ASD was four times lower than the incidence of radiographic ASD reported during the first 5 years after fusion surgery by Cheh et al. [3], suggesting that hybrid fixation may indeed delay the development of ASD above lumbar fusion. More importantly, the present incidence of symptomatic ASD (6.7%) was also four times lower than the incidence of ASD after fusion alone (30%) [3]. The clinical presentation was the development of lower back pain in both of our patients, with cruralgia without neurological deficit, who required additional surgery at adjacent levels. The third patient was asymptomatic, and another surgery was not necessary. The reason that we did not observe ASD in the caudal segment was that the last instrumented vertebra was S1. Finally, in our series, the two patients who developed ASD had a high pelvic incidence (PI) (>60°) or a moderate PI (46° < PI <60°), with insufficient lordosis correction. The third patient had a low PI, with an acceptable lordosis correction, and he was asymptomatic. Despite this, we did not observe any mechanical complication [26]. Because we had no case of implant breakage or screw loosening, the present series supports the safety and reliability of the hybrid posterior fixation system. Clinical improvement, as measured by changes in the ODI score, Roland-Morris Disability Questionnaire (RMDQ) score, and Visual Analog Scale (VAS) score (both back and leg pain), was better in patients without radiographic ASD than in the three patients who developed ASD.

17.4 Conclusions

The hybrid posterior fixation system represents a technology that allows for the coupling of arthrodesis with dynamic stabilization at adjacent levels in the lumbar spine. This fixation proved to be particularly effective in multi-segmental steno-instability cases of the lumbar spine.

The prevalence of radiographic ASD was 10.0%. Patients over the age of 50 could be at a higher risk of developing ASD than those who were 50 years old or younger. The number of instrumented segments was not a risk factor for the development of ASD in the lumbar degenerative spine. Because the observed clinical outcomes were good and there was no case of implant breakage or screw loosening, our experience supports the efficacy, safety, and reliability of the hybrid posterior fixation system.

References

1. Weinstein JN, Lurie JD, Olson PR, et al. United States' trends and regional variations in lumbar spine surgery: 1992–2003. Spine (Phila Pa 1976). 2006;31:2707–14.
2. Bono CM, Lee CK. Critical analysis of trends in fusion for degenerative disc disease over the past 20 years: influence of technique on fusion rate and clinical outcome. Spine (Phila Pa 1976). 2004;29:455–63.
3. Cheh G, Bridwell KH, Lenke LG, et al. Adjacent segment disease following lumbar/thoracolumbar fusion with pedicle screw instrumentation: a minimum 5-year follow-up. Spine (Phila Pa 1976). 2007;32:2253–7.
4. Chou WY, Hsu CJ, Chang WN, et al. Adjacent segment degeneration after lumbar spinal posterolateral fusion with instrumentation in elderly patients. Arch Orthop Trauma Surg. 2002;122:39–43.
5. Chen WJ, Lai PL, Tai CL, et al. The effect of sagittal alignment on adjacent joint mobility after lumbar instrumentation—a biomechanical study of lumbar vertebrae in a porcine model. Clin Biomech (Bristol, Avon). 2004;19:763–8.
6. Heini PF. Non rigid stabilization of the spine—problems observed: screw loosening/breakage/implant failure/adjacent segment degeneration. In: Szpalski M, Gunzburg R, Rydevik BL, et al., editors. Surgery for low Back pain. Heidelberg: Springer; 2010. p. 233–9.
7. Hudson RS, Gee JE, Billys JB, et al. Hybrid dynamic stabilization with posterior spinal fusion in the lumbar spine. SAS J. 2011;5:36–43.
8. Morishita Y, Ohta H, Naito M, et al. Kinematic evaluation of the adjacent segments after lumbar instrumented surgery: a comparison between rigid fusion and dynamic non-fusion stabilization. Eur Spine J. 2011;20:1480–5.
9. Lee CK, Langrana NA. Lumbosacral spinal fusion. A biomechanical study. Spine (Phila Pa 1976). 1984;9:574–81.
10. Nockels RP. Dynamic stabilization in the surgical management of painful lumbar spinal disorders. Spine (Phila Pa 1976). 2005;30:S68–72.
11. Schmoelz W, Huber JF, Nydegger T, et al. Dynamic stabilization of the lumbar spine and its effects on adjacent segments: an in vitro experiment. J Spinal Disord Tech. 2003;16:418–23.
12. Schnake KJ, Schaeren S, Jeanneret B. Dynamic stabilization in addition to decompression for lumbar spinal stenosis with degenerative spondylolisthesis. Spine (Phila Pa 1976). 2006;31:442–9.
13. Schwarzenbach O, Rohrbach N, Berlemann U. Segment-by-segment stabilization for degenerative disc disease: a hybrid technique. Eur Spine J. 2010;19:1010–20.
14. Galbusera F, Bellini CM, Anasetti F, et al. Rigid and flexible spinal stabilization devices: a biomechanical comparison. Med Eng Phys. 2011;33:490–6.
15. Zander T, Rohlmann A, Burra NK, et al. Effect of a posterior dynamic implant adjacent to a rigid spinal fixator. Clin Biomech (Bristol, Avon). 2006;21:767–74.
16. Rohlmann A, Zander T, Bergmann G, et al. Optimal stiffness of a pedicle-screw-based motion preservation implant for the lumbar spine. Eur Spine J. 2012;21:666–73.
17. Aebi M. The adult scoliosis. Eur Spine J. 2005;14:925–48.
18. Di Silvestre M, Lolli F, Bakaloudis G, et al. Dynamic stabilization for degenerative lumbar scoliosis in elderly patients. Spine. 2010;35(227):34.
19. Soh J, Lee JC, Shin BJ. Analysis of risk factors for adjacent segment degeneration occurring more than 5 years after fusion with pedicle screw fixation for degenerative lumbar spine. Asian Spine J. 2013;7:273–81.
20. Pfirrmann CW, Metzdorf A, Zanetti M, et al. Magnetic resonance classification of lumbar intervertebral disc degeneration. Spine (Phila Pa 1976). 2001;26:1873–8.
21. Bono CM, Kadaba M, Vaccaro AR. Posterior pedicle fixation-based dynamic stabilization devices for the treatment of degenerative diseases of the lumbar spine. J Spinal Disord Tech. 2009;22:376–83.
22. Barrey CY, Ponnappan RK, Song J, et al. Biomechanical evaluation of pedicle screw-based dynamic stabilization devices for the lumbar spine: a systematic review. SAS J. 2008;2:159–70.
23. Sangiorgio SN, Sheikh H, Borkowski SL, et al. Comparison of three posterior dynamic stabilization devices. Spine (Phila Pa 1976). 2011;36:E1251–8.
24. Putzier M, Hoff E, Tohtz S, et al. Dynamic stabilization adjacent to single-level fusion: part II. No clinical

benefit for asymptomatic, initially degenerated adjacent segments after 6 years follow-up. Eur Spine J. 2010;19:2181–9.
25. Maserati MB, Tormenti MJ, Panczykowski DM, et al. The use of a hybrid dynamic stabilization and fusion system in the lumbar spine: preliminary experience. Neurosurg Focus. 2010;28:E2.
26. Le Huec JC, Cogniet A, Demezon H, et al. Insufficient restoration of lumbar lordosis and FBI index following pedicle subtraction osteotomy is an indicator of likely mechanical complication. Eur Spine J. 2015;24(Suppl 1):S112–20.

Dynamic Stabilization in Scoliosis Deformity

18

Mario Di Silvestre

18.1 Introduction

The use of DYNESYS® in scoliosis treatment represented, in the past, an expanded indication for this dynamic system [1]: We started using DYNESYS® fixation in elderly scoliosis about 20 years ago, obtaining satisfying results. Degenerative lumbar scoliosis, also described as de novo or primary degenerative scoliosis, is a frequent disease in the elderly population. Its incidence is reported to be from 6% to 68% [2–5] and increases with age [6]. Two different studies [3, 7] followed adults without previous scoliosis and reported 7 [7] and 12 years [3] later, respectively, the development of de novo scoliosis; the incidence was quite similar in both series: 36.7% [7] vs. 34.4% [3]. Degenerative curves are located at the thoracolumbar or lumbar levels and must be distinguished from degenerated preexisting idiopathic scoliosis. The degenerative curves in question develop de novo after skeletal maturity, with no history of scoliosis. Decreased bone density was initially considered to be the cause of de novo lumbar scoliosis [2]. At present, asymmetric degenerative changes of the disc, vertebral body wedging, and facet joint arthritis are held to be the predominant causes [1, 3, 8, 9], with disc degeneration appearing to be the starting point [3, 8]. In the adult population, lateral end plate osteophytes longer than 5 mm and an asymmetric tilt of the disc space are risk factors for the development of de novo scoliosis [3].

Lumbar de novo scoliosis is frequently associated with degenerative spondylolisthesis and stenosis [6, 10–12]. Moreover, the progression of degenerative scoliosis can lead to decreased lumbar lordosis [6, 8, 13].

In elderly patients, medication for painful symptoms associated with degenerative scoliosis should be limited to short-term use [11]. Although nonsurgical procedures have unproven long-term efficacy in these patients [14], surgical treatment should be considered only after their failure. The most frequent indication for surgical treatment is neurogenic claudication, followed by severe pain refractory to nonoperative procedures and progressive neurologic deficit [11, 15]. Moreover, the progression of scoliosis alone, without other symptoms, rarely warrants surgery in elderly patients [10].

Decompression alone has been proposed: It obtained satisfying results in patients with mild degenerative scoliosis and in stabilizing osteophytes [16]. However, different authors [10, 17, 18] presented poor results, related to the progression of deformity.

Posterior fusion with pedicle screw instrumentation, in addition to decompression, represented the most widely accepted technique [10, 11, 19–21]. However, the incidence of complica-

M. Di Silvestre (✉)
Chief of Spinal Deformity Department,
Ospedale Santa Corona, Pietra Ligure, Italy

A. F. Özer et al. (eds.), *Dynamic Lumbar Spine Stabilization*,
https://doi.org/10.1007/978-3-032-12122-6_18

tions was high, ranging from 20% to 80% [1, 17, 20, 21]: Factors appearing to play important roles include age more than 65 years, medical comorbidities, blood loss, and the number of levels fused. In one study, excessive intraoperative blood loss was found to be the most significant risk factor for early postoperative complications [20]. Arthrodesis can increase the operative time and blood loss and, consequently, the incidence of complications, especially in elderly patients [19, 22, 23]. In patients older than 75 years undergoing spinal fusion, one large cohort study reported a complication rate 1.9 times greater than that of age-matched patients who had surgery without fusion [22].

Our strategy was to consider dynamic stabilization without fusion, using DYNESYS® as an alternative to fusion in elderly patients with degenerative lumbar scoliosis, as reported previously [1, 24]. The DYNESYS® device was introduced by Dubois et al. [25] in 1994. An in vitro study demonstrated that DYNESYS® stabilized unstable spine segments sufficiently to be considered a potential option to replace fusion [26]. This was confirmed in patients with degenerative spondylolisthesis treated by decompression and DYNESYS® instrumentation instead of arthrodesis; the dynamic stabilization device remained stable in most patients and prevented the progression of spondylolisthesis [27, 28]. Our purpose was especially to reduce the incidence of complications after posterior fusion, such as adjacent segment degeneration, which generally occurs proximal to posterior instrumentation and has been reported primarily after short lumbar fusion [20, 21]. Cahill et al. [29] suggested that the adjacent problems at the proximal end of a scoliosis construct may be completely eliminated with the use of a transition rod at the most proximal level. Our hypothesis was that the choice of a dynamic system could lead to similar results, permitting us to perform a short stabilization with a decreased risk of junctional problems. In instrumented patients, using DYNESYS® preserved some kind of motion at the lumbar levels (Table 18.1) [24].

Table 18.1 The range of motion at different levels after DYNESYS® instrumentation [24]

Level	Number of cases	Pre-op	Follow-up
T12–L1	5	1.3° (0–3)	0.6° (0–1)
L1–L2	12	3.9° (2–6)	1.9° (1–4)
L2–L3	24	4.2° (3–6)	2.3° (1–4)
L3–L4	29	3.3° (2–5)	1.5° (1–3)
L4–L5	6	4.8° (3–7)	2.7° (2–4)
L5–S1	12	1.8° (0–3)	0.8° (0–2)

18.2 Technique

For DYNESYS® instrumentation in scoliosis treatment, the patient was treated under general anesthesia in the prone position. The first step was the implantation of DYNESYS® screws. The pedicle screws used in the lumbar vertebrae, the thoracolumbar vertebrae, and in the sacrum were 7.2-mm-diameter screws: long enough to reach the anterior cortex of the vertebra (Fig. 18.1). The pedicle entry point was more lateral, in comparison with rigid fixation at the basis of the transverse process. The screws were inserted as deep as possible. So as not to compromise the bone purchase of the screws, given their conical core, we avoided removing and reinserting them in the same hole.

After that, in cases with associated stenosis of the vertebral canal, patients' hips were flexed at an angle of 90° to facilitate decompression of the stenotic levels. Stenosis was treated by laminectomy: The decompression was extended to the lateral recess, and a foraminotomy was performed without interrupting the isthmus.

After decompression, the patient's position was modified to obtain the maximum lumbar lordosis, and screws were inserted.

During laminectomy, another surgeon prepared the spacers, cutting them according to the length measured previously between adjacent screws. Each of the polycarbonate urethane spacers was cut to the desired length and threaded with a polyester cord, which was stretched between and fixed to two adjacent screwheads (Fig. 18.2). Larger spacers were used on the concave side and shorter ones on the

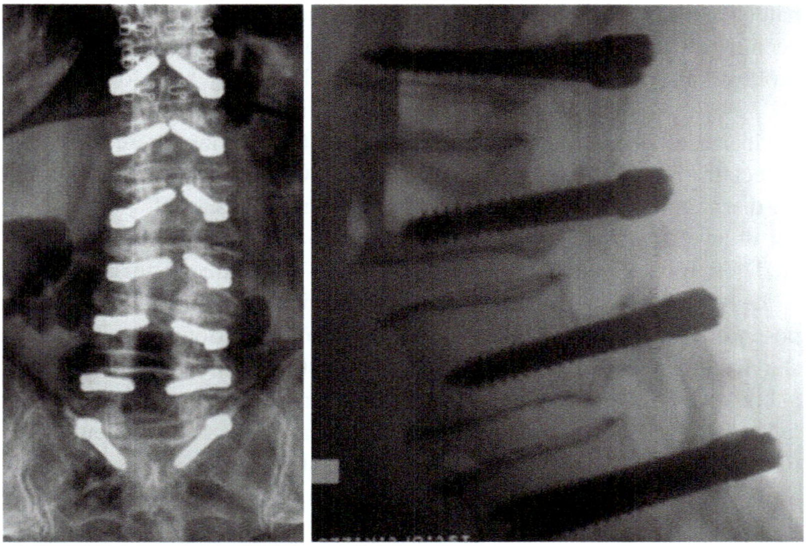

Fig. 18.1 Pedicle screws of a diameter of 7.2 mm, long enough to reach the anterior cortex of the vertebra

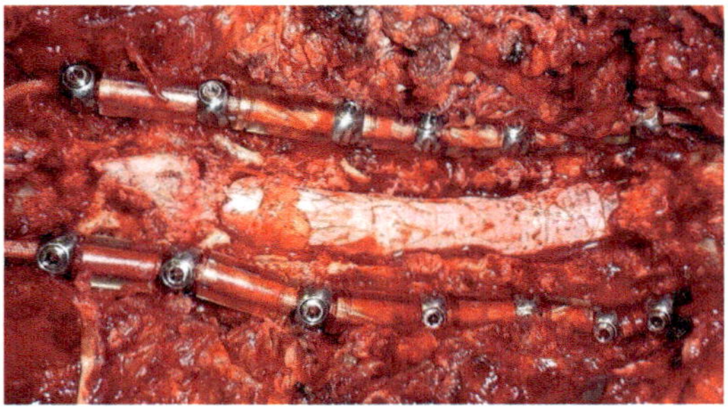

Fig. 18.2 DYNESYS® system instrumentation from L2 to S1 and combined laminectomy

convex side of the scoliosis curve, obtaining a reduction of the mild scoliosis. The length of fixation could be very long, about six levels, from T12 to the sacrum, in general. The weak point of this long construct is represented by the S1 fixation: It is necessary to use a longer screw with a diameter of 7.2 mm to avoid sacral screw loosening.

18.3 Discussion

The surgical treatment of degenerative lumbar scoliosis in elderly patients presents demanding aspects. Important concerns include the older age of patients, their frequent medical comorbidities, and senile osteoporosis. Most patients with degenerative scoliosis are women, in whom osteoporosis may be severe after menopause. The main goals of surgery in these cases are pain relief and improvement in the quality of life. Some correction of the deformity is desirable, but this is not the most important issue. In contrast, it is essential to limit the aggressiveness of the surgical procedure as much as possible [10, 11]. Posterior fusion with pedicle screw instrumentation, in addition to laminectomy [10, 11, 19–21], is one of the most commonly used procedures, achieving both decompression and stabilization of the spine. Short posterior fusion extended within the deformity has been proposed for cases with a small Cobb angle or minimal lateral vertebral listhesis [21], as well as for patients with no coronal and sagittal imbalance. Longer posterior fusion has been proposed for patients with a large Cobb angle [21]. Posterior lumbar interbody fusion has been combined with posterior fusion [20]. In any event, as the posterior elements are removed for decompressive laminectomy and the pedicles represent the strongest points of anchorage in elderly patients, especially those who have osteopenia, the use of pedicle screw fixation is recommended by many authors [10]. Unfortunately, a high incidence of complications has been reported in older patients with degenerative scoliosis after posterior fusion procedures [19, 20, 30–32]. Notably, age has been correlated with an increased incidence of complications [30], especially in patients older than 80 years [30]. Furthermore, excessive blood loss and the number of levels fused have been found to be associated with higher complication rates [20].

Less invasive than posterolateral fusion with posterior fixation, pedicle screw–based dynamic stabilization without fusion might be a useful alternative in elderly patients with degenerative lumbar scoliosis. A previous series of degenerative scoliosis patients with associated lumbar stenosis had shown that it can prevent progression of scoliosis and postoperative instability, even after a wide laminectomy [24]. In that report, the operative duration was short, blood loss was low, and there was no screw loosening or breakage at follow-up (Fig. 18.3). Another study [33] confirmed the impression of a shorter procedure, with limited blood loss. Compared with the control arthrodesis procedure [24], the mean operating time proved to be shorter using dynamic fixation (190 vs. 240 minutes; $p = 0.05$), and blood loss was reduced (950 vs. 1400 cc; $p = 0.05$). The overall complication rate was lower in the dynamic fixation group, reflecting both a lower incidence of minor complications (18.7% vs. 28%) and an even markedly lower incidence of major complications (6.2% vs. 16%).

A frequent complication observed in elderly patients after posterior fusion is adjacent segment disease, which generally occurs proximal to posterior instrumentation and has been reported primarily after short lumbar fusion [20, 21]. Proximal adjacent segment disease appears to develop more frequently when stopping fusion from T11 to L1 compared with extending it to T10 [20, 34]. In older patients, the advantage of a short posterior fusion is obvious, even if the instrumentation should not stop at a junctional zone or adjacent to a rotatory subluxation, spondylolisthesis, or a segment with significant spinal stenosis because this may lead to spinal instability. In a study, Cho et al. [21] compared the results of short posterior fusion, within the deformity, vs. long fusion, extended above the upper-end vertebra, for degenerative lumbar scoliosis in patients whose mean age was 65.5 years. In that series, there was a trade-off in complications between short and long fusions. Whereas all cases of proximal adjacent segment disease developed in the short fusion group, long fusion induced excessive intraoperative blood loss, which was closely related to the development of perioperative complications [21]. In our previous experience [24], comparing DYNESYS® vs. instrumented fusion, elderly patients received a short instrumentation in both groups, extending up to T11 at the most. In the fusion group, three patients (12%) were reoperated after a mean of 18 months for adjacent segment disease. In the dynamic group, only one patient (3.1%) required subsequent surgery for adjacent segment disease, for a distal junctional disc degeneration 32 months after surgery. At present, there is no consensus on whether dynamic instrumentation protects adjacent levels more than fusion. A study concluded that dynamic stabilization can prevent degeneration of the adjacent segment [35]. However, the results of the study of Schnake et al. [27] after DYNESYS® instrumentation in cases with degenerative spondylolisthesis did not support this theory: The authors found signs of adjacent degeneration in 29% of the patients after 2 years. Although longer follow-up studies are necessary for definitive conclusions, the theoretical protective effect of dynamic stabilization against adjacent segment degeneration is consistent with our findings, with a minimum of a 5-year follow-up [24]. In our series, dynamic fixation provided substantial stability by preventing further scoliosis progression or the translation of associated spondylolisthesis despite the use of decompressive laminectomy. By applying asymmetric spacers, larger on the concave side and shorter on the convex side of scoliosis, it was possible to obtain some reduction of the scoliosis Cobb angle, albeit lesser than with fusion constructs. There was no case of screw loosening or breakage during follow-up. In five of the patients (15.6%), asymptomatic radiolucent lines up to

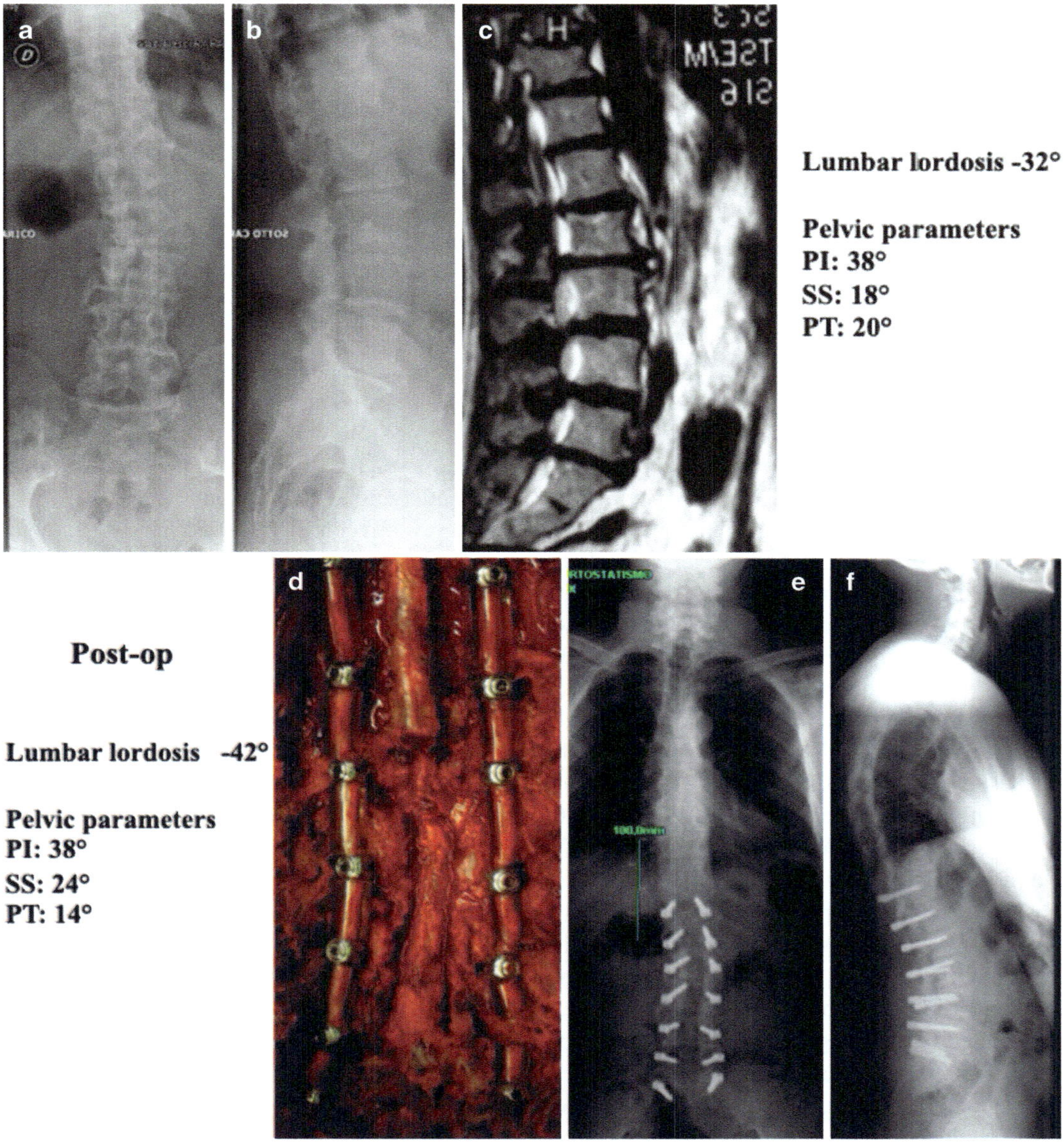

Fig. 18.3 Male, 77 years old. Lumbar de novo scoliosis with multi-segmental stenosis and satisfying preoperative lumbar lordosis (**a**–**c**). Treatment: T12–S1 DYNESYS® instrumentation with L2–S1 laminectomy (**d**). The follow-up X-rays at the control after 5.4 years (**e**–**f**)

2 mm did appear around the thread of pedicle screws in S1 at the last follow-up; however, a screw mobilization or a loss of scoliosis correction was not observed, and the patients were asymptomatic, so we did not classify these cases as unstable. In this series, posterior fusion corrected scoliosis better than dynamic fixation (56.9% vs. 37.3%). However, in de novo scoliosis patients, the goal of treatment is less the amount of correction of the curve and more its stability over time. The same could be said for final lumbar lordosis. Although the value of final

lordosis tended to be better in the fusion group, in elderly patients with degenerative scoliosis, pedicle screw-based dynamic stabilization was less invasive, with a shorter operative duration, lesser blood loss, and lower adverse event rates than instrumented posterior fusion, obtaining similar results in terms of functional clinical outcomes at the last follow-up.

18.4 Future of DYNESYS® in Scoliosis Correction

In our studies [1, 24], patients presented with moderate lumbar scoliosis and a preoperatively satisfying sagittal balance. Recently, the indication for DYNESYS® instrumentation has been extended by Ozer et al. [36] to degenerative scoliosis with sagittal imbalance. A total of 25 patients with a mean age of 62.9 ± 10.8 (range: 41–79 years) were included in this study. Spinal, sagittal, and coronal deformities were corrected with dynamic stabilization performed in a single session in patients with good bone quality (without osteopenia and osteoporosis), while two-stage surgery was performed in patients with poor bone quality. The first stage consisted of a percutaneous placement of screws, and the second stage was for the placement of dynamic rods and the correction of spinal deformity 4–6 months after the first stage. At the 2-year follow-up, no significant loss was observed in the instrumentation system, and no significant loss of correction was observed in sagittal and coronal deformities. The correction of scoliosis was obtained by adequate supine position of the patient and by cutting the spacers shorter than normal and providing greater torque than normal in the concave part of the deformity. The procedure was completed with foraminal or canal decompression when indicated. Since cortical bone is formed around the loosened screw when the screw is replaced in the second surgery with a larger screw, the screw clings to the more stable bone, greatly reducing the possibility of loosening. Patients are evaluated with CT after an average of 16–20 weeks to determine the osteointegration of the screws.

18.5 Conclusions

In elderly patients with degenerative scoliosis, pedicle screw–based dynamic stabilization can be less invasive, with a shorter operative duration, lesser blood loss, and lower adverse event rates than instrumented posterior fusion, obtaining similar results in terms of functional clinical outcomes at the last follow-up. In elderly patients without sagittal imbalance, pedicle screw-based dynamic stabilization permitted to maintain a satisfying balanced spine at follow-up. Dynamic fixation achieved scoliosis curve stabilization at an average follow-up of more than 7 years. Furthermore, the functional outcomes resulted were satisfying at the last control.

However, recently, DYNESYS® instrumentation has been employed in more complex cases of scoliosis, characterized by sagittal imbalance, obtaining good results, and such use can open new avenues for the treatment of adult scoliosis.

References

1. Di Silvestre M, Lolli F, Bakaloudis G, et al. Dynamic stabilization for degenerative lumbar scoliosis in elderly patients. Spine. 2010;35:227–34.
2. Vanderpool DW, James JI, Wynne-Davies R. Scoliosis in the elderly. J Bone Joint Surg Am. 1969;51:446–55.
3. Kobayashi T, Atsuta Y, Takemitsu M, et al. A prospective study of de novo scoliosis in a community based cohort. Spine. 2006;31:178–82.
4. Schwab F, Dubey A, Gamez L, et al. Adult scoliosis: prevalence, SF-36, and nutritional parameters in an elderly volunteer population. Spine. 2005;30:1082–5.
5. Weinstein SL, Ponseti IV. Curve progression in idiopathic scoliosis. J Bone Joint Surg Am. 1983;65:447–55.
6. Prichett JW, Bortel DT. Degenerative symptomatic lumbar scoliosis. Spine. 1993;18:700–3.
7. Robin GC, Span Y, Steinberg R, et al. Scoliosis in the elderly: a follow-up study. Spine. 1982;7:355–9.
8. Murata Y, Takahashi K, Hanaoka E, et al. Changes in scoliotic curvature and lordotic angle during the early phase of degenerative lumbar scoliosis. Spine. 2002;27:2268–73.
9. Benoist M. Natural history of the aging spine. Eur Spine J. 2003;12(suppl 2):S86.
10. Simmons ED. Surgical treatment of patients with lumbar spinal stenosis with associated scoliosis. Clin Orthop Relat Res. 2001;384:45–53.

11. Ploumis A, Transfledt EE, Denis F. Degenerative lumbar scoliosis associated with spinal stenosis. Spine J. 2007;7:428–36.
12. Liu H, Ishihara H, Kanamori M, et al. Characteristics of nerve root compression caused by degenerative lumbar spinal stenosis with scoliosis. Spine J. 2003;3:524–9.
13. Ploumis A, Transfeldt EE, Gilbert TJ, et al. Degenerative lumbar lordosis: radiographic correlation of lateral rotator olisthesis with neural canal dimensions. Spine. 2006;31:2353–8.
14. Oskouian RJ Jr, Shaffrey CI. Degenerative lumbar scoliosis. Neurosurg Clin N Am. 2006;17:299–315.
15. Kostuik JP, Israel J, Hall JE. Scoliosis surgery in adults. Clin Orthop Relat Res. 1973;93:225–34.
16. Gupta MC. Degenerative scoliosis. Options for surgical treatment. Orthop Clin North Am. 2003;34:269–79.
17. Hanley EN Jr. The indications for lumbar spinal fusion with and without instrumentation. Spine. 1995;20:143S–53S.
18. Vaccaro AR, Ball ST. Indications for instrumentation in degenerative lumbar spinal disorders. Orthopedics. 2000;23:260–71.
19. Carreon LY, Puno RM, Dimar JR, et al. Perioperative complications of posterior lumbar decompression and arthrodesis in older adults. J Bone Joint Surg Am. 2003;85A:2089–92.
20. Cho KJ, Suk SI, Park SR, et al. Complications in posterior fusion and instrumentation for degenerative lumbar scoliosis. Spine. 2007;32:2232–7.
21. Cho KJ, Suk SI, Park SR, et al. Short fusion versus long fusion for degenerative lumbar scoliosis. Eur Spine J. 2008;17:650–6.
22. Deyo RA, Ciol MA, Cherkin DC, et al. Lumbar spinal fusion. A cohort study of complications, reoperations, and resource use in the Medicare population. Spine. 1993;18:1463–70.
23. Benz RJ, Ibrahim ZG, Afshar P, et al. Predicting complications in elderly patients undergoing lumbar decompression. Clin Orthop Relat Res. 2001;384:116–21.
24. Di Silvestre M, Lolli F, Bakaloudis G. Degenerative lumbar scoliosis in elderly patients: dynamic stabilization without fusion versus posterior instrumented fusion. Spine J. 2014;14:1–10.
25. Dubois B, de Germay B, Schaerer NS, et al. Dynamic neutralization: a new concept for restabilization of the spine. In: Szpalski M, Gunzburg R, Pope MH, editors. Lumbar segmental instability. Philadelphia: Lippincott Williams & Wilkins; 1999. p. 233–40.
26. Schmoelz W, Huber JF, Nydegger T, et al. Dynamic stabilization of the lumbar spine and its effects on adjacent segments: an in vitro experiment. J Spinal Disord Tech. 2003;16:418–23.
27. Schnake KJ, Schaeren S, Jeanneret B. Dynamic stabilization in addition to decompression for lumbar spinal stenosis with degenerative spondylolisthesis. Spine. 2006;31:442–9.
28. Schaeren S, Broger I, Jeanneret B. Minimum four-year follow-up of spinal stenosis with degenerative spondylolisthesis treated with decompression and dynamic stabilization. Spine. 2008;33:E636–42.
29. Cahill PJ, Wang W, Asghar J, et al. The use of a transition rod may prevent proximal junctional kyphosis in the thoracic spine following scoliosis surgery: a finite element analysis. Spine. 2012;37:E687–95.
30. Raffo CS, Lauerman WC. Predicting morbidity and mortality of lumbar spine arthrodesis in patients in their ninth decade. Spine. 2006;31:99–103.
31. Daubs MD, Lenke LG, Cheh G, et al. Adult spinal deformity surgery: complications and outcomes in patients over age 60. Spine. 2007;32:2238–44.
32. Wang MY, Green BA, Shah S, et al. Complications associated with lumbar stenosis surgery in patients older than 75 years of age. Neurosurg Focus. 2003;14:e7.
33. Tribus CB. Degenerative lumbar scoliosis: evaluation and management. J Am Acad Orthop Surg. 2003;11:174–83.
34. Shufflebarger H, Suk S-I, Mardjetko S. Debate: determining the upper instrumented vertebra in the management of adult degenerative scoliosis: stopping at T10 versus L1. Spine. 2006;31:S185–94.
35. Stoll TM, Dubois G, Schwarzenbach O. The dynamic neutralization system for the spine: a multi-center study of a novel non-fusion system. Eur Spine J. 2002;11(suppl 2):S170–8.
36. Ozer AF, Akgun AM, Ucar EA, et al. Can dynamic spinal stabilization be an alternative to fusion surgery in adult spinal deformity cases? Int J Spine Surg. 2024;18(2):152–63.

19 Pedicular Dynamic Stabilization in Kyphotic Deformities

Ali Fahir Özer and Turgut Akgül

One of the most important problems in spine surgeries is deformity. While the spine functions in harmony with the nervous system, it is a special structure that simultaneously protects the brain, spinal cord, and nerves. From the C1 vertebra to the L1 vertebra, a part of the medulla and the spinal cord are covered by the spine. The remaining lumbar spine is filled with nerve fibers formed by the nerve roots coming out of the spinal cord, and each pair of these fibers leaves the spine from the related segment and, subsequently, continues to decrease until the end of the sacral spine. The spine has a natural curve. Although it shows some minor changes from person to person, the cervical and lumbar regions are lordotic, and the thoracic and sacral regions are kyphotic. Each naturally occurring and normal gentle slope dissipates the mechanical stress that occurs when the body is stationary and in motion.

Preserving the anatomical integrity of this structure is extremely important for maintaining a healthy and high-quality human life. Various pathologies decrease the integrity of this structure, which decreases the quality of life. Besides, other pathologies develop slowly, and if recognized in time, preventing or correcting them is possible using simpler surgical or nonsurgical methods.

The classical approach for deformity surgery is to correct the deformity using instruments, sometimes performing osteotomies in more severe deformities, and correct the patient's spine using rigid instrumentation systems and fusion. The dissatisfaction and complication rates are high in these patients [1–6]. In a recent study, one of every five patients regrets undergoing such a surgery [7].

19.1 Sagittal Plane Deformity (Kyphosis)

Leaving aside the congenital vertebral anomalies, ankylosing spondylitis, or Scheuermann's disease, kyphotic deformities are predominantly diseases of advanced age. Thoracic kyphosis is observed at advanced ages after osteoporotic fractures of the thoracic vertebrae. Kyphotic deformity of the entire spine occurs as a result of the loss of lordosis in the lumbar region following the degenerative process in the elderly. Lenke's classification for idiopathic adolescent scoliosis of the spine could not fully guide the treatment of adult deformities. Furthermore, it could also not be used for guiding the treatment of sagittal deformities. For this rea-

A. F. Özer (✉)
Department of Neurosurgery, Koc University School of Medicine, Istanbul, Turkey

T. Akgül
Faculty of Medicine, Department of Orthopaedics and Traumatology, Koç University Hospital Spine Center, Istanbul, Turkey
e-mail: takgul@kuh.ku.edu.tr

A. F. Özer et al. (eds.), *Dynamic Lumbar Spine Stabilization*,
https://doi.org/10.1007/978-3-032-12122-6_19

son, although there are many classifications and guidelines for treatment, the Scoliosis Research Society (SRS)–Schwab classification is more instructive in terms of revealing the pathology. Schwab and SRS made a new classification for adult spinal deformities in 2012. With this classification, it also brought a solution for sagittal deformities, which are predominantly an adult age problem (Fig. 19.1).

The sagittal modifiers in this classification provide essential information for evaluating a patient's sagittal balance. The development of deformity in the sagittal plane occurs because of an increase or decrease in the natural curves of the spine. Normally, the projection of the head falls into the pelvis. With the development of deformity in the sagittal plane, this balance is disturbed; however, the organism tries to compensate for it. The most common cause of deformity in the sagittal plane is the anterior or posterior shift of the projection of the head. A backward shift of the head is a much rarer pathology and mostly occurs in cases where lumbar hyperlordosis develops. The most common pathology is the increase in kyphosis in the thoracic region of the spine or the disappearance of lordosis in the lumbar region, and the projection of the head begins to move anteriorly from the pelvis.

It is at least as important as coronal deformity in evaluating sagittal balance. If we look briefly at the main points related to sagittal balance, a person who is on the ground with both feet can stand with extraordinarily little energy expenditure. This corresponds to a small circle around both feet. This circle is the most economical in terms of energy saving. Considering three dimensions, including the body, an economical cone is obtained in terms of energy saving. If the person draws wider circles by going out of this circle or cone with back and head movements, they must expend more energy. Disrupting the ideal sagittal balance and leaving the economical circle of the person will cause excessive energy use. After individuals started walking on two legs, their pelvis also expanded, according to bipedalism. Particularly with this evolutionary development in human anatomy, due to the expansion of the anteroposterior diameter of the pelvis, the continuity of the projection of the head in the pelvis has been ensured, and individuals have been provided with the opportunity to move by using less energy (Fig. 19.2).

Sagittal measurements of a standing person were defined based on the vertical line through the femoral head. In a standing, healthy person, the spine rises above the pelvis. For the spine to stand upright, some changes occur in the pelvic orientation; therefore, the deterioration of its

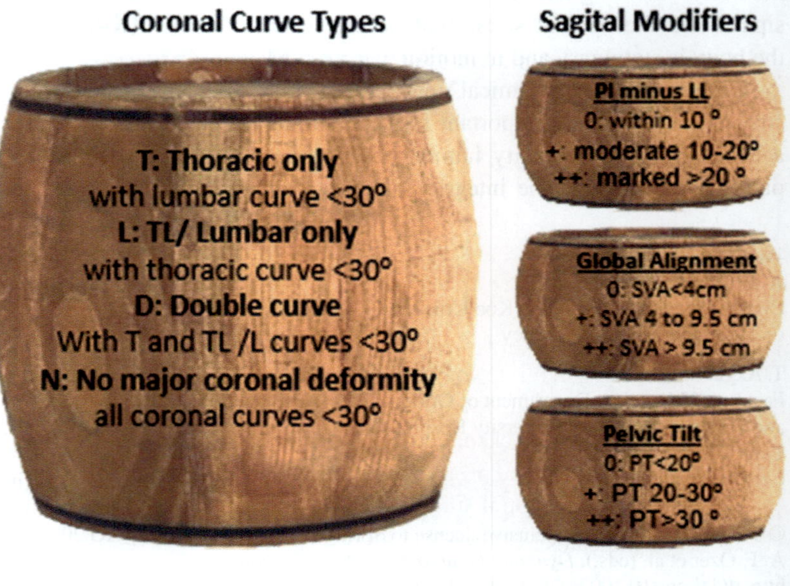

Fig. 19.1 SRS–Schwab classification

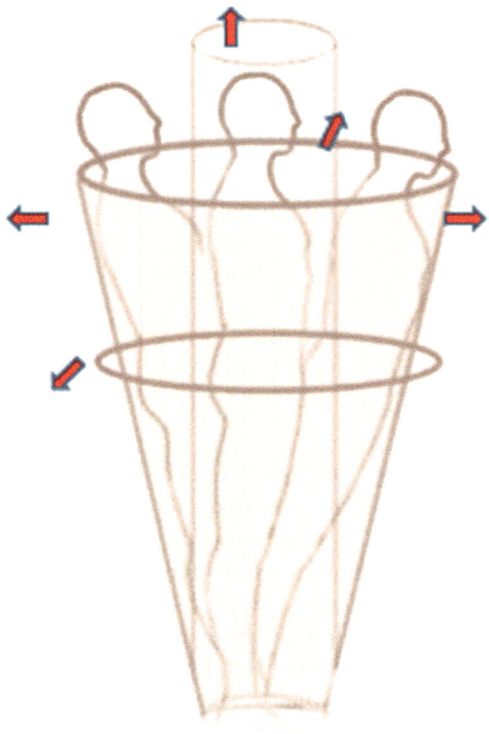

Fig. 19.2 The cone formed by the circle on which the person stands is the standing position with the least energy expenditure. If the person moves outside this cone, they will consume more energy

relationship with the pelvis affects the normal inclinations of the entire spine [8].

19.2 Spinopelvic Parameters

The first pelvic parameter to consider is the pelvic incidence (PI). The PI corresponds to the angle between the line perpendicular to the midpoint of the line passing through the upper end plate of S1 and the line connecting it to the axis of the femoral heads, as described by Legaye and Duval-Beaupère [9, 10]. One characteristic of PI is that it remains constant from childhood to adolescence.

The sacral tilt (SS) angle is described as the angle between a line tangential to the upper S1 end plate and the horizontal line. A vertical pelvis indicates a low angle of the SS, whereas a horizontal pelvis indicates a high angle of the SS.

The pelvic tilt (PT) is described as the angle between the vertical line and the line connecting the center of the sacral end plate to the axis of the femoral heads. These two angles are positional and related to the pelvic orientation because the pelvis can rotate around the axis of the femoral heads (Fig. 19.3).

This movement can be forward (anteversion) or backward (retroversion). The PT angle increases during pelvic retroversion (Fig. 19.4).

There is a relationship between these three parameters: PI is equal to the arithmetic sum of the SS and PT (PI = PT + SS) [9]. This indicates that a patient with a high PI angle has a greater potential for pelvic retroversion. This is one of the important compensation mechanisms and is also important for the patient. Disruption of the spinopelvic relationship affects the entire spine. It is necessary to start with the lumbar parameters.

Sacral inclination is strongly correlated with lumbar lordosis. The relationship between the sacral slope and PI explains the link between PI and lumbar lordosis. For example, it has been stated that there is a mathematical relationship between lumbar lordosis and PI. For example, Schwab [11] suggested that PI=LL ± 9° can be formulated. Similar mathematical calculations have been made; however, Roussouly [12] defined four types of vertebrae with different spinal and pelvic parameters, particularly in terms of the transition from lumbar lordosis to thoracic kyphosis, in a prospective study involving individuals without spinal problems (Fig. 19.5).

Types 1 and 2 are characterized by a small sacral slope (less than 35°).

Type 1 has a small lower lordosis arc with a lower lordosis apex (approximately L5). Therefore, the lordosis is short, and the kyphosis is thoracolumbar.

Type 2 has a flattened lower arch with extraordinarily little curvature, and the back is straight.

Type 3 corresponds to the lordotic apex at L4 and the mean sacral inclination (between 35° and 45°). The lordosis is almost evenly distributed over the two arches. This is the most balanced type.

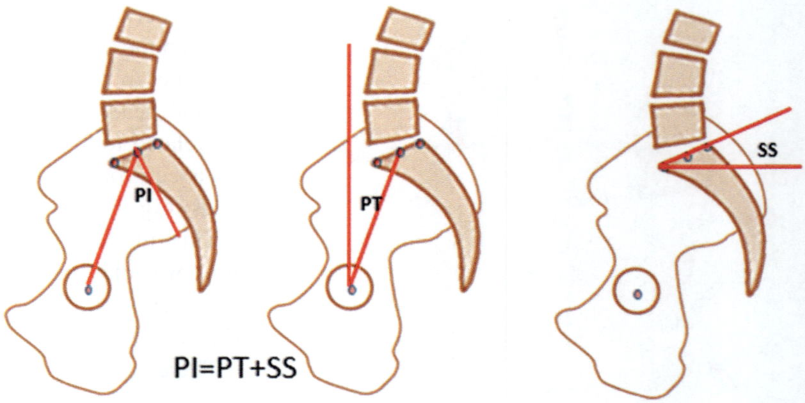

Fig. 19.3 Pelvic parameters. Definition of different pelvic angles. PI pelvic incidence angle, PT pelvic tilt, SS sacral tilt. These last two parameters reflect the spatial orientation of the pelvis

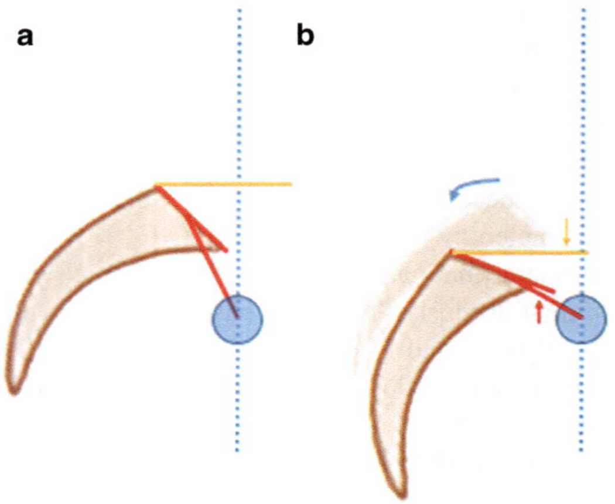

Fig. 19.4 (**a**) Normal pelvic version. With more vertical sacrum, (**b**) the pelvic tilt (PT) increases, the sacral tilt (SS) decreases, and the pelvic incidence (PI) remains constant. This corresponds to the retroversion of the pelvis

Type 4 corresponds to a steep sacral slope (>45°) with a lordotic apex at the anterior–bottom corner of L3. The global lordosis angle (LL) is larger and contains more vertebrae than other types. Thoracic kyphosis is shorter.

According to Roussouly's definition, when the studies by Barrey [13] and Le Huec [14] are added, in general, the LL tends to increase for PIs below the mean value (50°), whereas when the PI is approximately 50°, we can conclude that lordosis tends to equal the PI (LL = PI), and when the PI is above 65°, the LL tends to be less than the PI. Therefore, the frequently used formula PI= LL + 9° is only valid for small PI angles, which leads to more estimation errors when the PI is greater than 50° [11].

The most important measurement in the thoracic region is the thoracic kyphosis angle (TK). We have already mentioned enough about how the lumbar region affects the thoracic region while describing the lumbar region above. Thoracic kyphosis is the angle between the lines tangent to the upper T1 end plate and the lower T12 end plate. The theoretical value of thoracic kyphosis has been shown to be equal to 0.75 times the global lumbar LL, L1 to S1: T1T12 lordosis = 0.75 × L1S1 lordosis [14].

However, it has been stated that the measurement of the thoracic kyphosis angle between T4 and T12 would be more appropriate for ease of measurement because the humeral heads are superimposed and normal radiographs are often of poor quality. In a study involving 403 patients, the thoracic kyphosis angle (TK) was found to be 43.55° ± 6.44° [15].

It is one of the most affected areas in the cervical region. Although various parameters are used in the cervical region, three parameters are important for us [16].

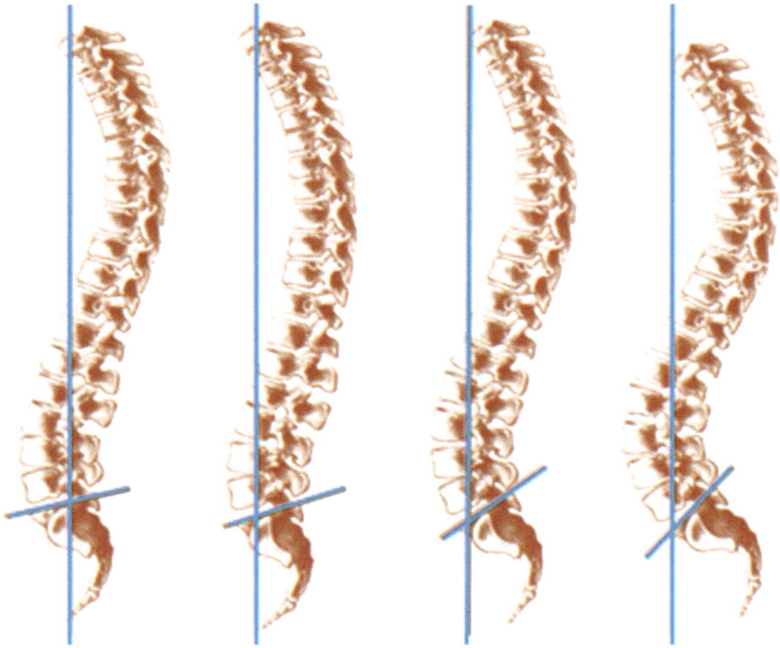

Fig. 19.5 Types of spine, according to Roussouly

1. High cervical angle occipito-C2 (O-C2): It is the angle between the McGregor line and the tangential line passing through the lower C2 end plate. The McGregor line connects the posterior edge of the hard palate to the lower point of the occipital bone. Between the ages of 20 and 39 years, the mean value of this angle is 15.81° ±7.15°, and this angle is always lordotic.
2. C2–C7 angle: It is the angle between the tangential line passing through the C2 end plate and the tangential lines on the lower C7 end plate, ranging from kyphosis to lordosis among the normal population. It is normally lordotic, with an average value of 17.15° ± 12.33°. It changes markedly with age.

   The O-C2 angle is inversely proportional to the C2–C7 angle: As one increases, the other decreases.
3. C7 slope angle (slope): It is a key parameter for statically examining the cervical spine [16] (Fig. 19.6).

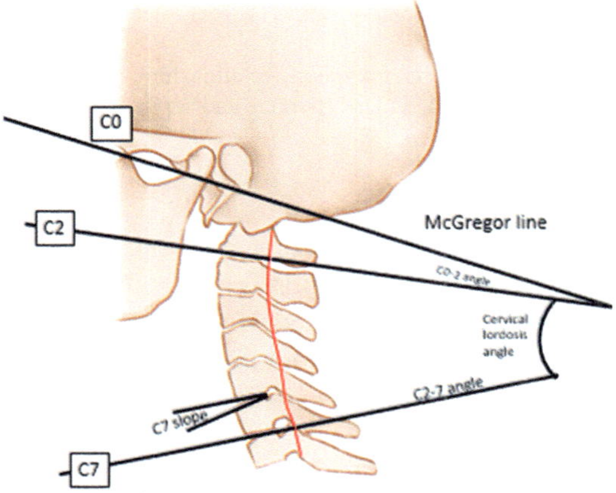

Fig. 19.6 O-C2 angle and C7 slope angle

The mean value is 20°. Patients with a C7 inclination >20° have a lordotic cervical spine (between C2 and C7). Patients with a C7 slope <20° have a neutral or kyphotic cervical spine (between C2 and C7).

As a result, if pathology in the lumbar region cannot be corrected with compensation mecha-

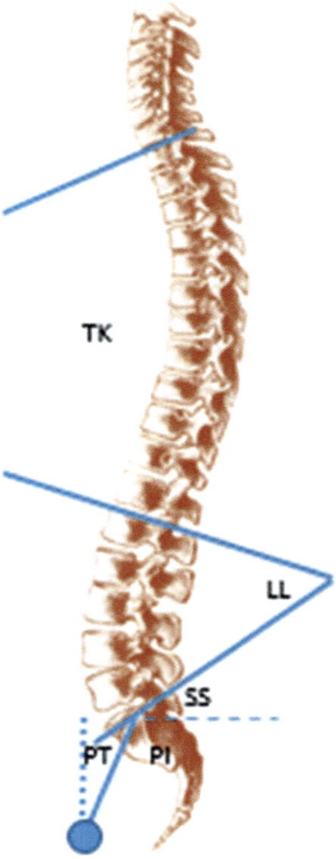

Fig. 19.7 Lordotic or kyphotic relationship of the pelvis, the lumbar region, and the thoracic and cervical regions in a normal spine

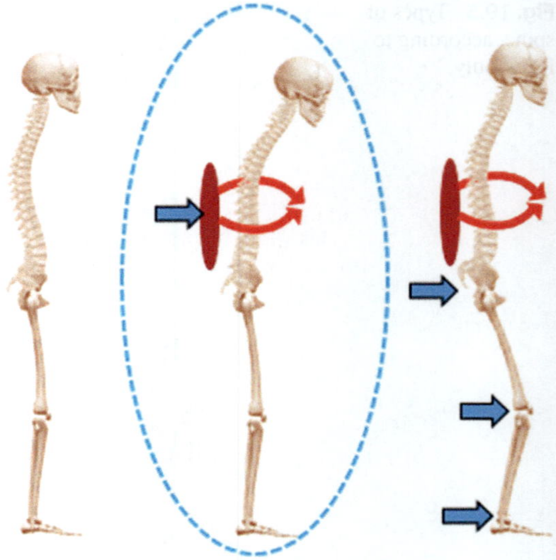

Fig. 19.8 The dynamic system is the most ideal method for patients whose deformity can be corrected using their muscles

nisms, it will affect the thoracic region. However, because the thoracic region is attached to the rib cage, it will be less affected. However, everything from kyphosis to hyperlordosis can be observed in the very mobile cervical region (Fig. 19.7).

19.3 Compensation Mechanisms

Because of the changes in the spine with age, the body uses compensation mechanisms and attempts to stand upright to look ahead in the horizontal plane. This compensation in the spine occurs in three anatomical structures: the spine, the pelvis, and the lower extremities. Evaluating these data enables better planning of the surgical management of patients. Fusion surgery alone should not be considered. Revealing the final shape that the entire spine can take is important. Measuring and evaluating spinopelvic parameters will help in deciding between dynamic or fusion surgery and hybrid surgery for intraoperative correction.

Ankylosing spondylitis, osteoporotic fractures, or degeneration and fusion developing in the lower lumbar spines occur together with an increase in segmental lordosis in the adjacent spine and in the anteroposterior opening of the disk. When the spinous processes touch each other, retrolisthesis develops. Meanwhile, the patient attempts to pull back the recovered lumbar spine using the lumbar muscles. However, this does not provide long-term relief. As the pelvis is retroverted, the SS angle decreases, while the PT angle increases, and the patient attempts to keep the spine upright. TK is reduced and becomes limited; however, cervical hyperlordosis develops, and when all these mechanisms are insufficient, the patient attempts to maintain the horizontal gaze by flexing the knee joints and extending the feet from the heel (Fig. 19.8).

19.4 Indications for the Use of the Dynamic System in Sagittal Deformities

Using the dynamic system in patients who can no longer restore their sagittal balance is impossible, even if they use the aforementioned compensation mechanisms. The most comfortable usage time of the dynamic system is when the patient can correct their sagittal balance using their muscles. There is no discussion about the treatment of fixed sagittal imbalance with osteotomy and instrumentation. However, fusion and rigid instrumentation surgery in a mobile sagittal deformity is debatable. "I start walking normally, but after a while I bend over" is the best expression of mobile deformity. Here, instead of fixing the spine using a rigid instrument, providing some support to the muscle compartment that attempts to keep the spine upright for a while will be sufficient.

We classified adult deformities using the SRS–Schwab classification in 2012 because sagittal modifiers also explain the condition of sagittal balance very well. However, there have been two other excellent studies classifying adult deformities [17, 18]. We have revised both the SRS–Schwab classification and other Lenke–Silva and LaMartine–Berjano classifications by changing the indications according to groups, in a way that the dynamic system will be used [19]. Because the surgeons who made these classifications were advocates of fusion surgery, they did not include dynamic stabilization in the treatment. These two classifications of deformities are important to us because the purpose of classification is to provide a common definition of the deformity and to standardize surgery. Those who developed and perform these classifications are dedicated to fusion surgery. However, with current knowledge and technology, it has become clear that it is now possible to perform surgery without fusion in some cases classified as such. In the early stages of these two studies, the scoliotic spine was mobile. In these stages, dynamic stabilization can be used instead of fusion surgery. Similarly, sagittal deformities as well as scoliotic deformities can be corrected with dynamic stabilization in the early stages in patients with mobile sagittal deformity (Fig. 19.9).

Note that in adult deformities, the spine must be adequately corrected for the patient, regardless of its plane. Recovering as much as possible from the deformity is sufficient for the patient; moreover, being able to stand upright without effort is essential. It is also an important gain in stopping the progression of the deformity.

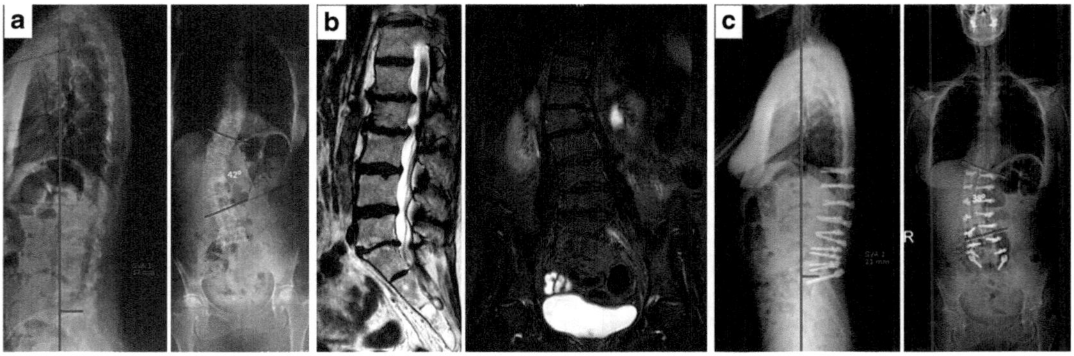

Fig. 19.9 61-year-old female patient. There is severe pain when standing and bending forward while walking. No neurological deficit. (**a**) The patient has lost her lumbar lordosis, the sagittal vertical axis has started to protrude out of the pelvis, and she has a 42° scoliotic deformity. (**b**) In T2-weighted sections, the L5–S1 disks have fused, there is advanced degenerative disk disease in the L1–2 and L2–3 distances, and it constitutes the dome of the deformity. (**c**) In the 1st-year postoperative radiographs of the patient, improvement in the sagittal and coronal balance is observed

Adult deformities should not be considered idiopathic adolescent spondylolisthesis. Most patients are happy to live with their deformity. The reason that brings them to the doctor is that they are slowly falling forward or experience minor nerve root irritations. It may not be correct to try to bring the spine into its ideal shape in an elderly person. Naturally, regardless of the posture of the spine, it must be corrected appropriately for the patient, but exaggerated surgeries should be avoided. The patient's deformity should be corrected as much as possible. It is very important for the patient to be able to stand upright and look straight ahead. It is also an important gain in terms of stopping the progression of the deformity with a simpler surgical intervention.

19.5 Dynamic Stabilization in Kyphotic Deformity Surgery

19.5.1 Surgical Technique

Fusion is not necessary in patients with mobile deformities. However, fusion may be essential in cases that need to be completed in the first stage. These patients may have root irritation, foraminal stenosis, or advanced canal stenosis and may not be able to wait 4–6 months. In that case, performing the surgery in one operation is possible, including the iliac bones [20].

If the bone quality of the patient is insufficient, surgery can be performed in two stages. In patients with T-scores below −1.5, screws are placed first, and rods are placed 3–6 months after osteosynthesis of the screws.

The patient is operated under general anesthesia in the prone position [21]. Preoperative neuromonitoring is performed on the patient. The most important step is controlling the C-Arm by making the operating table concave within the limits where the person can correct themselves before the surgery. Then, the table is brought to a flat position, and the screws are placed using the aforementioned method. Decompression is performed if necessary, and the table is brought to the position where the lordosis of the patient's spine is given; if the DYNESYS® system is used, the screws are connected to each other using the system's rod in this position, or if the Orthrus system is used, the rods are placed and tightened to the screws (Fig. 19.10).

Depending on the bone quality, this surgery can be performed in two stages. Two-stage surgery can be performed in patients with osteoporosis and a T-score of −1.5. If there is a local pathology that needs to be corrected at the initial stage, intervention can be performed at this stage. After the necessary decompression process, by placing a temporary rod only on the screws of that distance, it is expected that osteointegration will occur after 3–6 weeks. After the waiting period has elapsed, osteointegration is confirmed using computed tomography, and the second step of the surgery, rod insertion, is completed at this time (Fig. 19.11).

In adult sagittal deformity, the patient begins to find themself leaning forward when they walk. For clinicians, the biggest mistake at this stage is to sub-

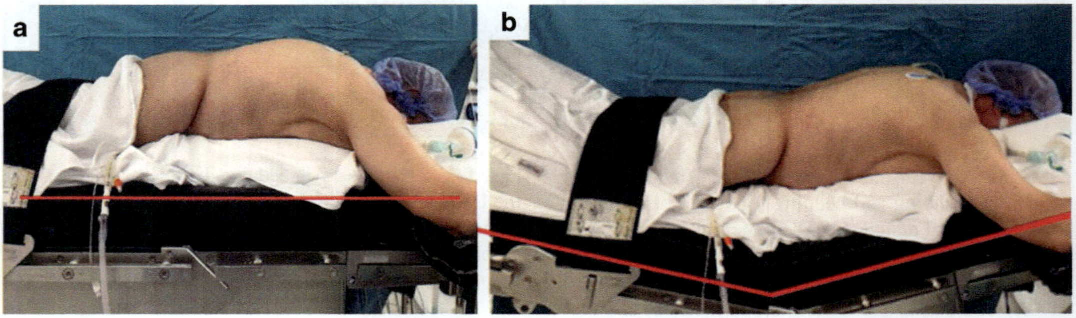

Fig. 19.10 (**a**) In the first stage, screws are placed. (**b**) In the second stage, approximately 4-6 months later, the table is brought into a concave position and the deformity is corrected, and then the rodkar is placeds

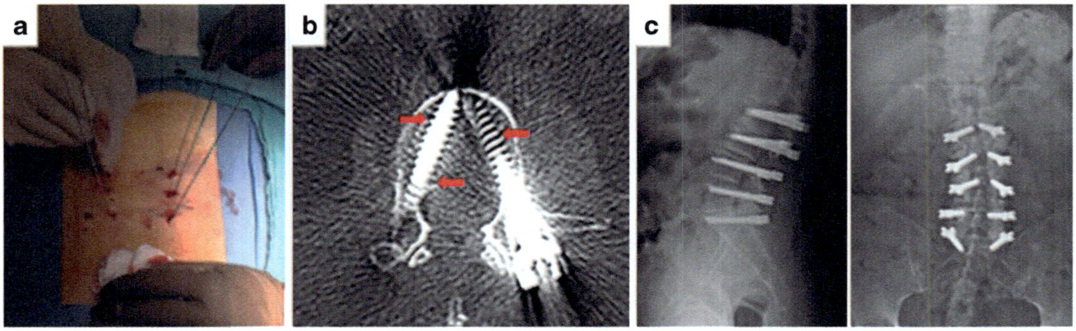

Fig. 19.11 (**a**) Percutaneous placement of screws. (**b**) After at least 4 months of waiting, computed tomography confirms that the osteointegration process of the screws is complete. (**c**) The screws are tightened using a spacer and rods, the table is brought to the concave position, and the rods are tied in this position

mit the patient to control examinations or send them to physical therapy for muscle-strengthening exercises. Attempting to control the condition with anti-inflammatory or analgesic drugs and trying to strengthen the lumbar muscles through exercise are both futile in such patients. Fatty degeneration in the muscles, loss of collagen in the ligaments connecting the spine, and pain caused by degenerative changes mean that the patient will not obtain positive results from an exercise program. This early stage in the disease is the golden period, during which the deformity can be corrected with a simple surgical procedure. In untreated patients and those whose condition has progressed further, positive sagittal balance develops, and more severe procedures such as osteotomy and fusion surgery become necessary. At this later stage, there are significantly higher mortality and morbidity rates, particularly since the majority of this patient population is advanced in age, with poor bone quality and additional medical problems. However, sagittal deformity can be resolved relatively easily if addressed with sufficient alacrity.

If there is a loosening of the screws placed on the temporary rod or if we detect it during surgery, only these screws are replaced with larger-diameter screws, and the second stage of the operation is completed [22].

Two-stage surgery can also be applied to patients with serious additional medical problems. The risk of general anesthesia is eliminated, and the surgical procedure is terminated by performing spinal anesthesia twice.

Both the DYNESYS® and Orthrus systems are effective in correcting mobile sagittal deformities. Multiaxial dynamic tulip screws form a system that can be used safely in deformity surgery. We use the Safinaz system, which is a multiaxial dynamic screw of our own design (Safinaz screw; Tipsan, Izmir, Turkey). Considering the complication rates of fusion surgery or considering that numerous patients do not have pain despite their excellent radiographs, these systems with low complication rates should be preferred primarily (Fig. 19.12).

When the DYNESYS® system is used in kyphotic deformity surgery, the retraction of the entire body is loaded on the DYNESYS® rope-shaped rod. This situation is different from the stabilization of multiple degenerative disk diseases with normal sagittal balance. The rod is likely to break during the process. For this reason, a double-rod-bearing screw system would be more appropriate for correcting patients with impaired balance. In sagittal deformity, the spine is different from a balanced spine and tends to move forward. The function of the DYNESYS® tether is to stabilize the spine and keep the body balanced. Thus, the tether has an additional serious responsibility, and a single tether is insufficient. Therefore, two tethers should be used on each side to ensure sagittal balance. For this reason, we designed and used screws with two holes so that two tethers can be tightened in sagittal or coronal deformities. In order to avoid removing the screws in cases where the tether came loose,

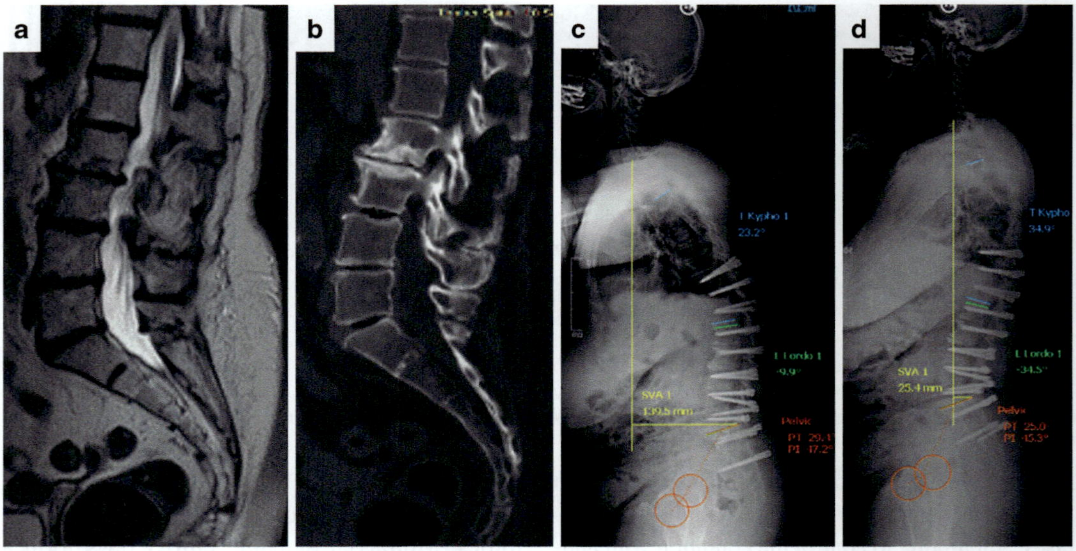

Fig. 19.12 A 66-year-old female patient has had lower back pain for a long time but has been slowly bending forward while walking or standing for the past year. (**a**) Diffuse degenerative disk disease is observed in a T2-weighted magnetic resonance scan. (**b**) Modic degeneration, osteophyte, and gas appearance in the disk are observed on computed tomography. (**c**) Two-stage surgery was considered for the patient with a T-score of −2.5, and in the control X-ray taken 4 months after the screws were placed in the first stage, the sagittal vertical axis was obviously outside of the pelvis. (**d**) After the rods were placed, a significant improvement in the spinopelvic parameters was observed

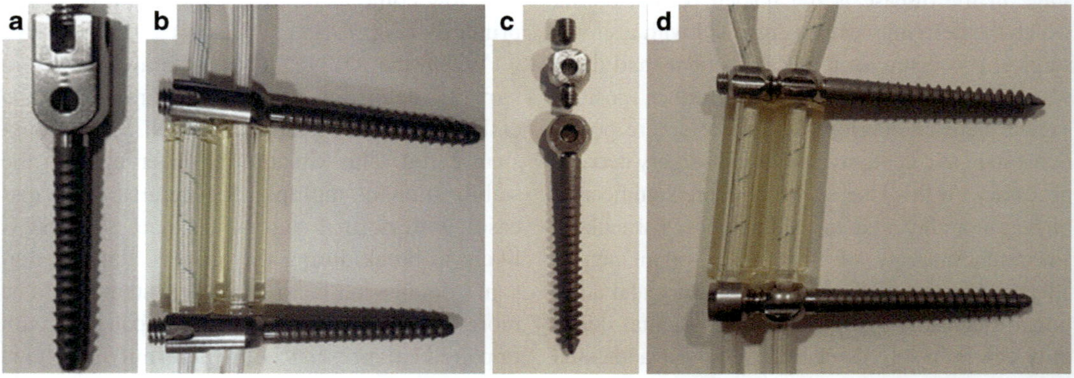

Fig. 19.13 (**a**) Double hole screws. (**b**) Tether stretched over double hole screws and two spacers. (**c**) The cap is designed to allow the tether to pass through it. (**d**) The caps were attached to the DYNESYS® screws, allowing the second tether to be tensioned

we designed the screw cap as a second head, through which the second tether would pass, and used it by passing the second tether through it and tightening it (Fig. 19.13).

Spinal stabilization in patients with kyphotic deformity is different from spinal stabilization in those without a balance problem. Because of the deformity, the rod must be heavily loaded in the lum-

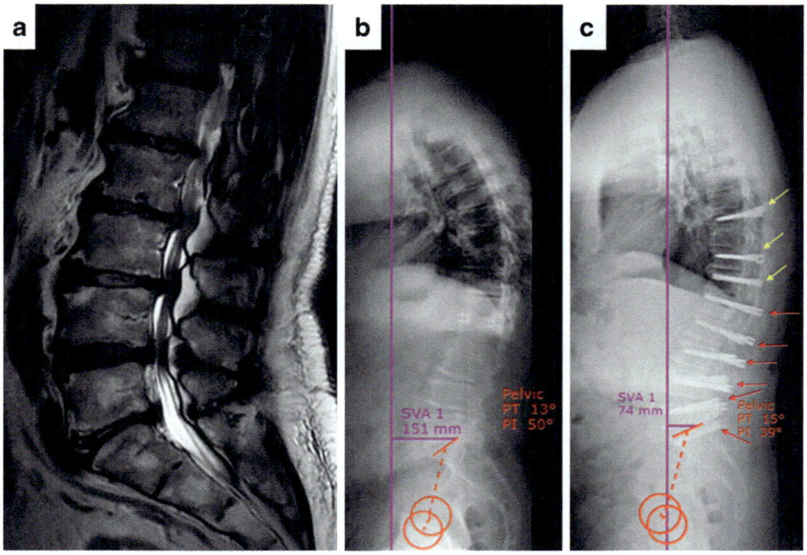

Fig. 19.14 A 65-year-old male with kyphotic deformity. The patient had suffered from progressive lower back pain for a long period and had begun to lean forward while walking. Long walks led to tingling and numbness in both feet. Neurological examinations were normal. (**a**) Magnetic resonance imaging showed extensive degenerative disk disease and a narrow spinal canal. (**b**) Positive sagittal balance was observed. The patient stated that this increased when he was walking. (**c**) The patient's sagittal balance improved after two-stage surgery. This comprised a first stage in which the screws were placed and a second for rod placement 4 months later. Yellow arrows: DYNESYS® screws and red arrows: double hole screws

bar region due to the tendency of the body to lean forward and the possibility of the rods breaking. This is especially true when using rope-shaped rods, which are subject to greater loads over time. For this reason, we developed a two-hole screw system. This allows the load on the lumbar region to be spread across a two-rope rod system. The problem with this approach is that, in vertebrae with poor bone quality, stretching the two rods over the screwheads causes the screw bodies to move more easily within the bone. Biomechanically, this may weaken the system. Therefore, we recommend two-rod tensioning with two-hole screws in two-stage surgeries (Fig. 19.14) [22].

We use the Orthrus system with Polyetheretherketone (PEEK) rods on the balanced spine. However, if the spine is out of balance and moves forward, controlling the forward bending of the trunk will put additional load on the system. Therefore, it is more suitable to be used with titanium rods. The biggest advantage of this system is that it is modular, and when a problem occurs, instead of removing the entire system, it will be sufficient to open only the problematic module. It is an effective system as a dynamic system in deformity surgery (Fig. 19.15).

It is another method used in deformity surgery with poly-axial dynamic screws (Safinaz screw). If this system is preferred, it is safer to perform the surgery in two stages. Since the forward bending problem of the body will cause additional load on the rods and screws, the screws should be placed first to prevent the screw from loosening. When the screws are mobile, they absorb the load on them. However, there is a possibility that the single PEEK rod body will become weak and deformed due to the additional load caused by the body bending forward. For this reason, it would be appropriate to attach an additional rod to the rods on both sides with intermediate connections (Fig. 19.16).

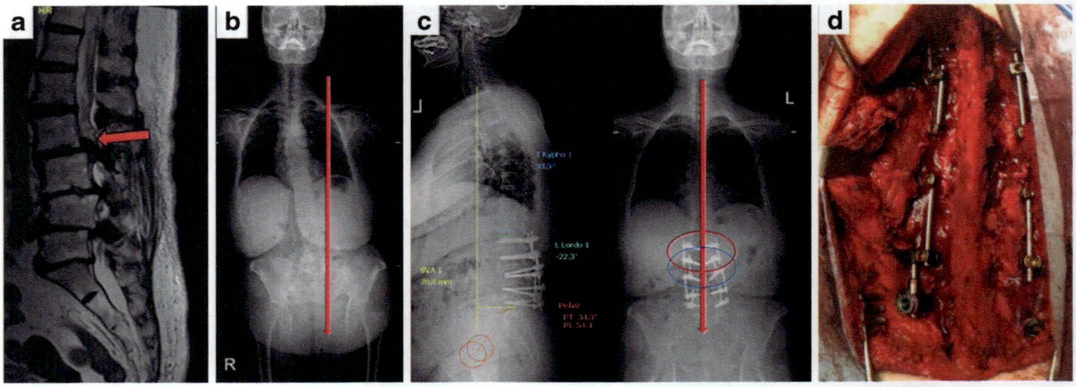

Fig. 19.15 70-year-old female. Severe femoralgia in the left leg for the past 10 days. Severe quadriceps weakness. (**a**) Widespread degenerative changes, with lumbar disk herniation, on MRI. (**b**) The patient's sagittal balance as well as coronal balance is impaired. (**c**) It is seen that the sagittal and coronal balance have recovered in the postoperative period. (**d**) The Orthrus system was used with a titanium rod

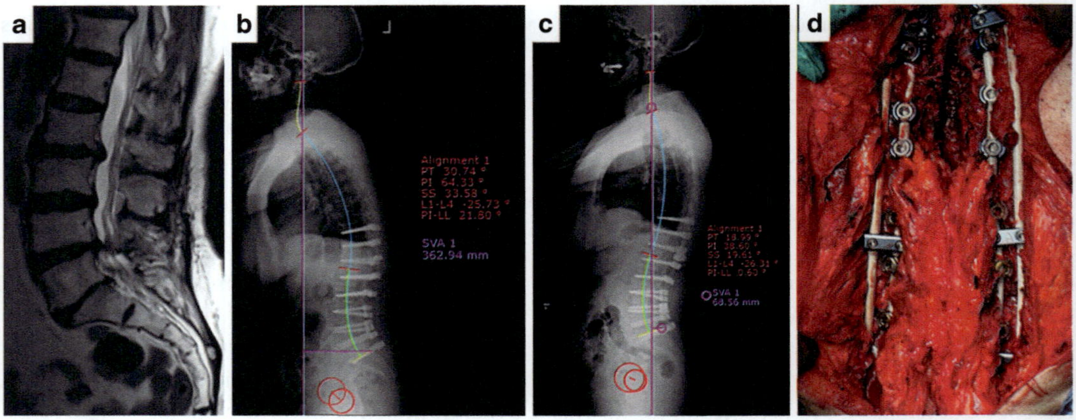

Fig. 19.16 55-year-old female. She has back pain and an inability to walk long distances, and she bends forward while walking. She states that her range of motion is narrowing day by day. Neurologic examination is normal. (**a**) Widespread degenerative changes in the lumbar region are observed in the patient's MRI. (**b**) Significant sagittal imbalance is observed in the patient's direct radiograph taken 4 months after the first stage. (**c**) It is seen that the patient's sagittal balance improved after the second stage, and the sagittal vertical axis (SVA) retreated to its normal line. (**d**) After lordosis was achieved with the operating table, the screws were attached with a PEEK rod, and a second PEEK rod was added for support

It should not be forgotten that the dynamic system is not essentially a movement preservation surgery. It provides easy stabilization and is more flexible than rigid stabilization. Since it can mostly be done in two stages and with spinal anesthesia if necessary, the risk of surgical complications is greatly reduced. Compared with rigid stabilization and fusion surgery, it is the most hassle-free way to achieve the goal.

19.5.2 Hybrid Surgery

If the patient has a fixed sagittal imbalance, stabilization with surgical osteotomy should be indisputably considered. However, after the osteotomy is performed to the rigid system and the necessary correction is achieved in the spine, the remaining parts of the spine can continue with the dynamic system (Fig. 19.17), or the entire

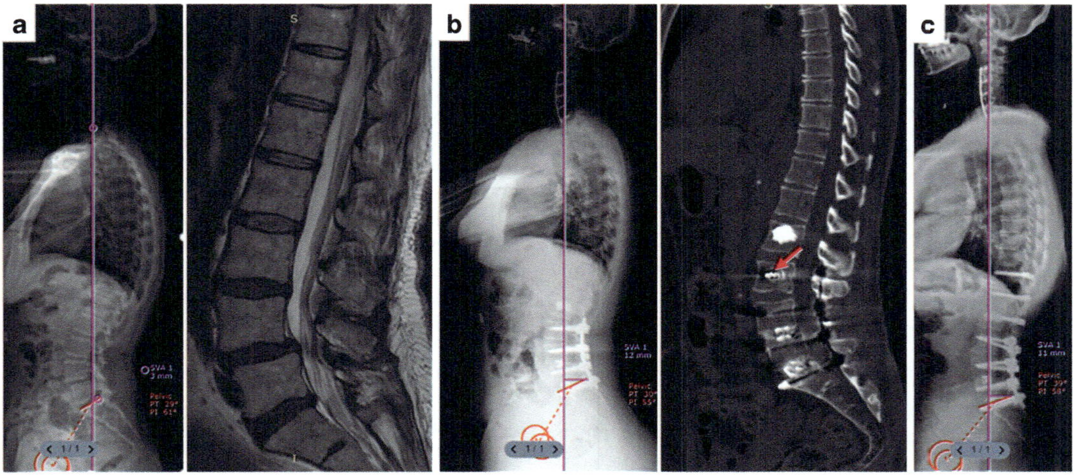

Fig. 19.17 A 60-year-old female patient presenting with untreatable back pain with medication and injection techniques. (**a**) Degenerative spondylolisthesis in L4–L5 on direct radiography and degenerative disk disease on L3–L4 and L5–S1 on T2-weighted magnetic resonance sections. (**b**) The patient has a degenerative disk disease. In another center, L4–L5 and L5–S1 interbody fusion was added to the L3 instrumentation system by placing only screws, and kyphoplasty was performed on L2. In the computed tomography images taken 1 year later, the L3 screw had loosened, and the patient had lower back pain, the same as preoperatively. (**c**) The loosened screw of the patient was replaced, and the upper part of the fusion was continued using a dynamic system until T12. In the 3rd postoperative year, the patient's visual analog scale and Oswestry scale scores improved significantly, and the patient had no complaints

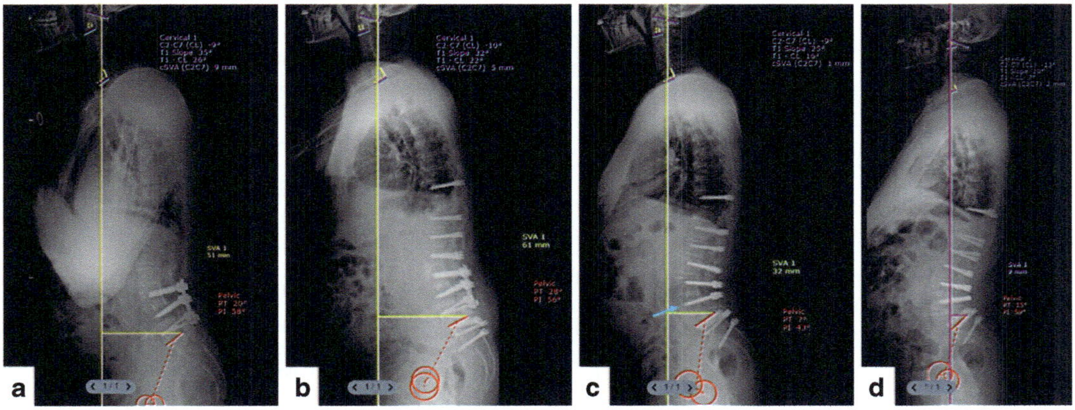

Fig. 19.18 The patient, who had undergone prior multiple back surgeries, started to lean forward over time. (**a**) The patient cannot correct himself in the dynamic radiographs taken, and there is a fixed sagittal balance. (**b**) Screws were placed in the patient in the first stage, considering a two-stage surgery. (**c**) L4 osteotomy (blue arrow) was performed, and the rod was placed. (**d**) In this way, soft stabilization was made to the other functional segments, while L4–L5 fused. The patient's spinopelvic parameters returned to normal limits

system can be stabilized using the dynamic system after the osteotomy is performed (Fig. 19.18).

I believe that these two systems will be used widely in the future.

19.5.3 Postoperative Care

The patient is mobilized immediately after surgery. If one-stage surgery is performed, staying at the hospital for 3 or 4 days after the surgery is sufficient. Moreover, there is no chain of possible complications awaiting the patient after fusion surgery for deformities.

In a one-stage surgery, performing the first control 4–6 months later for detecting osteointegration and the other controls once a year is sufficient. After two-stage surgery, the first control is performed after 4–6 months. When the osteointegration process is finished, the second operation is performed. Staying 3 or 4 days after this surgery is sufficient for the patient. Subsequent checks can be performed once a year.

As a result, surgery using a dynamic system is easier and more physiological for providing balance than spinal fusion surgery using a rigid system for patients with mobile deformities. Dynamic stabilization can also be used as a hybrid after osteotomies.

References

1. Formica M, Zanirato A, Cavagnaro L, Basso M, Divano S, Felli L, Formica C. Extreme lateral interbody fusion in spinal revision surgery: clinical results and complications. Eur Spine J. 2017;26(Suppl 4):464–70.
2. Kwon B, Kim DH. Lateral lumbar interbody fusion: indications, outcomes, and complications. J Am Acad Orthop Surg. 2016;24(2):96–105.
3. Katz JN. Lumbar spinal fusion. Surgical rates, costs, and complications. Spine (Phila Pa 1976). 1995;20(24 Suppl):78S–83S.
4. Coe JD, Arlet V, Donaldson W, Berven S, Hanson DS, Mudiyam R, Perra JH, Shaffrey CI. Complications in spinal fusion for adolescent idiopathic scoliosis in the new millennium. A report of the Scoliosis Research Society Morbidity and Mortality Committee. Spine (Phila Pa 1976). 2006;31(3):345–9.
5. Ratliff JK, Lebude B, Albert T, Anene-Maidoh T, Anderson G, Dagostino P, Maltenfort M, Hilibrand A, Sharan A, Vaccaro AR. Complications in spinal surgery: comparative survey of spine surgeons and patients who underwent spinal surgery. J Neurosurg Spine. 2009;10(6):578–84.
6. Saleh A, Thirukumaran C, Mesfin A, Molinari RW. Complications and readmission after lumbar spine surgery in elderly patients: an analysis of 2,320 patients. Spine J. 2017;17(8):1106–12.
7. Adogwa O, Caruso JP, Eldridge CM, Singh R, Chilakapati S, Deme P, Stutzman S, Aoun S, Naik AD, Bagley CA, Makris U. Decisional regret among older adults undergoing corrective surgery for adult spinal deformity: a single institutional study. Spine (Phila Pa 1976). 2022;47(8):E337–46.
8. Dubousset J. Three-dimensional analysis of the scoliotic deformity. In: Weinstein SL, editor. Pediatric spine: principles and practice. New York: Raven Press; 1994. p. 479–96.
9. Duval-Beaupère G, Schmidt C, Cosson P. A Barycentremetric study of the sagittal shape of spine and pelvis: the conditions required for an economic standing position. Ann Biomed Eng. 1992;20:451–62.
10. Legaye J, Duval-Beaupère G, Hecquet J, Marty C. Pelvic incidence: a fundamental pelvic parameter for three-dimensional regulation of spinal sagittal curves. Eur Spine J. 1998;7:99–103.
11. Schwab F, Lafage V, Patel A, Farcy J-P. Sagittal plane considerations and the pelvis in the adult patient. Spine. 2009;34:1828–33.
12. Roussouly P, Gollogly S, Berthonnaud E, Dimnet J. Classification of the normal variation in the sagittal alignment of the human lumbar spine and pelvis in the standing position. Spine. 2005;30:346–53.
13. Barrey C, Jund J, Noseda O, Roussouly P. Sagittal balance of the pelvis-spine complex and lumbar degenerative diseases. A comparative study about 85 cases. Eur Spine J. 2007;16:1459–67.
14. Le Huec JC, Hasegawa K. Normative values for the spine shape parameters using 3D standing analysis from a database of 268 asymptomatic Caucasian and Japanese subjects. Eur Spine J. 2016;25:3630–7.
15. Abrisham SMJ, Ardekani MRS, Mzarch MAB. Evaluation of the normal range of thoracic kyphosis and lumbar lordosis angles using EOS imaging. Maedica (Bucur). 2020;15(1):87–91.
16. Le Huec JC, Demezon H, Aunoble S. Sagittal parameters of global cervical balance using EOS imaging: normative values from a prospective cohort of asymptomatic volunteers. Eur Spine J. 2015;24:63–71.
17. Berjano P, Lamartina C. Classification of degenerative segment disease in adults with deformity of the lumbar or thoracolumbar spine. Eur Spine J. 2014;23(9):1815–24.
18. Silva FE, Lenke LG. Adult degenerative scoliosis: evaluation and management. Neurosurg Focus. 2010;28(3):E1. https://doi.org/10.3171/2010.1.FOCUS09271.
19. Akgun MY, Ucar EA, Gedik CC, Gunerbuyuk C, Hekimoglu M, Cerezci O, Oktenoglu T, Sasani M, Ates O, Ozer AF. Use of dynamic spinal instruments (Dynesys) in adult spinal deformities according to Silva-Lenke and Berjano-Lamartina classifications. Diagnostics (Basel). 2024;14(5):549.
20. Özer AF, Aydın AL, Hekimoğlu M, Çerezci Ö, Başak AT, Ates O, Oktenoglu T, Sasani M. Should iliac wing screws be included in long segment dynamic stabilization? Cureus. 2021;13(2):e13543. https://doi.org/10.7759/cureus.13543.
21. Ozer AF, Akgun MY, Ucar EA, Hekimoglu M, Basak AT, Gunerbuyuk C, Toklu S, Oktenoglu T, Sasani M, Akgul T, Ates O. Can dynamic spinal stabilization be an alternative to fusion surgery in adult spinal deformity cases? Int J Spine Surg. 2024;18:8588.
22. Özer AF, Başak AT, Özbek MA, Hekimoğlu M, Aydın AL, Ateş Ö, Günerbüyük C, Akgül T, Sasani M, Öktenoğlu T. Lumbar dynamic stabilization with 2-stage surgery: early results. Int J Spine Surg. 2022;16:8306. https://doi.org/10.14444/8306.

20 Complications of the DYNESYS® System

Mario Di Silvestre

20.1 Introduction

The use of the DYNESYS® system can present a variable number of complications that must be considered when planning the use of this particular construct. The complications reported are represented more often by screw loosening, infections (sometimes, later after the surgery), and junctional diseases. Reviewing recently, after 10 years on average, our series of 175 patients treated with DYNESYS®, the incidence of complications such as screw loosening was 10.3%, wound infection occurred in 1.7% of all patients, and junctional diseases occurred in 4% of the cases.

20.2 Screw Loosening (Fig. 20.1)

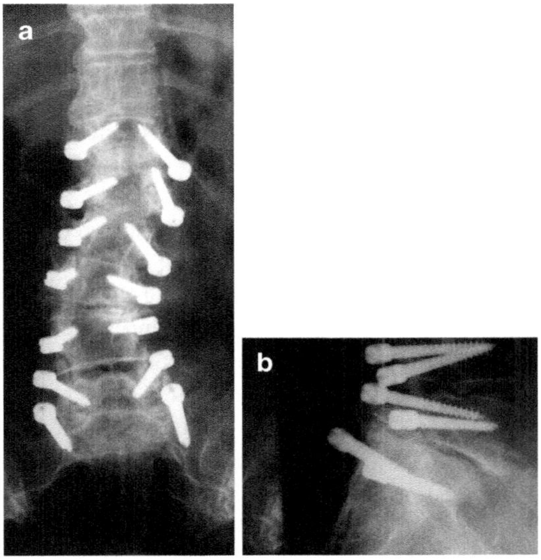

Fig. 20.1 (**a**, **b**) Long-DYNESYS® instrumentation (T12–S1) and laminectomy for degenerative scoliosis with multilevel stenosis in an elderly patient (79 years old). Monolateral screw loosening at S1. No clinical symptoms and no revision surgery at the last follow-up (63 months)

Considering that the DYNESYS® system does not reach a rigid fusion in the operated segment of the spine, the repetitive mechanical strain on this instrumentation can cause pedicle screw loosening or fracture, suggesting an abnormal range of motion in the stabilized lumbar spine segments that is higher than expected [1]. The reported screw loosening rate with DYNESYS® found in the literature [2] is 11.7%, while pedicle screw fracture has a reported rate from 1.3% to 21% but mostly within the 4%–6% range: This suggests a much bigger biomechanical flexibility of this system compared to rigid instrumented fusion constructs [1, 3], which can be at the base of the mechanism of screw loosening.

Screw loosening can be a problematic entity when radiographically found at follow-up X-rays, even though it does not always represent a clinical issue for the patient. There is no consensus in

M. Di Silvestre (✉)
Chief of Spinal Deformity Department, Ospedale Santa Corona, Pietra Ligure, Italy

A. F. Özer et al. (eds.), *Dynamic Lumbar Spine Stabilization*,
https://doi.org/10.1007/978-3-032-12122-6_20

the literature on whether or not this mechanical complication can be related to the onset of clinical symptoms such as back or leg pain. Different studies described pedicle screw loosening and pedicle screw fracture after the use of the DYNESYS® system. The group of Ko et al. [1] studied a pool of 71 patients treated with a dynamic stabilization system and found analogous results between the visual analog scale for lower back pain and the Oswestry Disability Index for functional disability, independent of screw loosening, concluding that loosening might not have a negative effect on the clinical improvement of the patients treated with this instrumentation. Similar results are described by Schaeren et al. [4], with no sign of back pain in patients with screw loosening or screw fracture. Other studies, on the contrary, correlated the persistence of back pain or leg symptoms with hardware-related complications, such as screw loosening or fracture, which ultimately required revision surgery [5–8]. Reviewing the literature, Pham et al. [2] concluded that 96 of 822 patients (11.7%) had pedicle screw loosening, and 13 of 822 patients (1.6%) had pedicle screw fracture over a mean follow-up period of 30.0 months (range: 16.4–54.0 months). The diagnosis of pedicle screw loosening was not uniform and was not always described in these articles. Wu et al. [9] observed an incidence of 4.7% of screw loosening, but no patient had to undergo another surgery.

Screw loosening is represented by a radiolucent zone around the screw on radiographs, which has been previously described as a "halo sign" or a "double-halo sign" [7, 10, 11]. The problem is that the diagnosis of screw loosening is a radiographic interpretation, whereas other studies did not explain their methods of diagnosis. Lutz et al. [7] reported the highest rate of screw loosening in 36 of their 49 patients (73.5%) compared with all other reporting studies, for which the average was 60 of 773 patients (7.8%). These authors diagnosed their loose screws using single or double-halo zones at a mean follow-up of 43 months. They hypothesized that the high rate of screw loosening was possibly due to poor integration at the bone–screw interface due to the biomechanical screw design. They stated that since their study was done, hydroxyapatite-coated screws have been developed to achieve better osseointegration, which may reduce the risk of screw loosening in future patients. Screw loosening occurs, in general, at the end of the construct, particularly at the distal level (Fig. 20.1), in our experience. According to Wang et al. [12], there are no differences between patients with and without screw loosening, but our experience is different, with an incidence of 10.3% of all screws implanted, more often at the sacral level, requiring another surgery in 2.1% of our series (Fig. 20.1) [13].

In conclusion, screw loosening can be a problematic entity when radiographically found at follow-up X-rays, even though it does not always represent a clinical issue for the patient. There is no consensus in the literature on whether it can be related to the onset of clinical symptoms. Ko et al. [1] concluded that loosening might not have a negative effect on the clinical improvement of the patients treated with this instrumentation. Similar results are described by Schaeren et al. [4], with no sign of back pain in patients with screw loosening or screw fracture. Other studies, on the contrary, correlated the persistence of back pain or leg symptoms with screw loosening or fracture, which ultimately required a revision surgery [5–8]. In our experience, according to Lutz et al. [7], another aspect to consider is that there is some kind of correlation between screw loosening and late infections: In the presence of new or increasing pain, every sign of screw loosening must be confirmed with a computed tomography (CT) study. In view of the frequency of signs of screw loosening observed [7] (73.5%, 36/49 patients), some authors hypothesize that there is a biomechanical lack of integration at the bone–screw interface, probably due to the screw design. This could eventually lead to a chronic inflammation with a "dead space" prone to opportunistic skin flora superinfection.

20.3 Adjacent Segment Disease

One of the main objectives of the DYNESYS® system is to avoid the onset of adjacent segment disease (ASD) [4, 14] (Fig. 20.2). ASD represents a significant complication of lumbar spine surgery that can occur due to the excessive overload on the segments adjacent to the stabilized area of the spine [15, 16]. The available data on ASD frequency after lumbar stabilization surgery are different in the literature. Pham et al. [2] experienced a 7% incidence of ASD over a mean follow-up of 33.5 months in their population of patients. Park et al. [17] found an incidence of radiographically diagnosed ASD to be from 8% to 100%, while a clinically symptomatic ASD ranged from 5.2% to 18.5% in their series of patients. Lawrence et al. [18] identified a mean clinical incidence of 0.6%–3.9% for clinically relevant ASD after lumbar fusion surgery. Although the DYNESYS® system allows us to reduce the biomechanical stress at the adjacent segments after lumbar stabilization, ASD still represents an eventuality after this kind of surgery. Several studies in the literature reported high rates of ASD after using the DYNESYS® stabilization system, with Yu et al. [19] identifying a 17.1% risk in their patients and Schaeren et al. [4] reporting an ASD incidence of 47% in their series; therefore, the DYNESYS® construct may have an intrinsic stability that acts similarly to a rigid fusion, overloading the adjacent segments of the instrumented spine [4]. It is not clear whether ASD is caused by the increased biomechanical stress on the instrumented spine levels or if it is a manifestation of the natural history of the degenerated lumbar spine. Reoperation rate for ASD, as described in the literature, was 40.6%, while the majority of other reoperations were for infections, hardware revision, or removal [19–24]. In conclusion, reviewing the literature [2], 12 studies were characterized by the development of ASD after the use of the

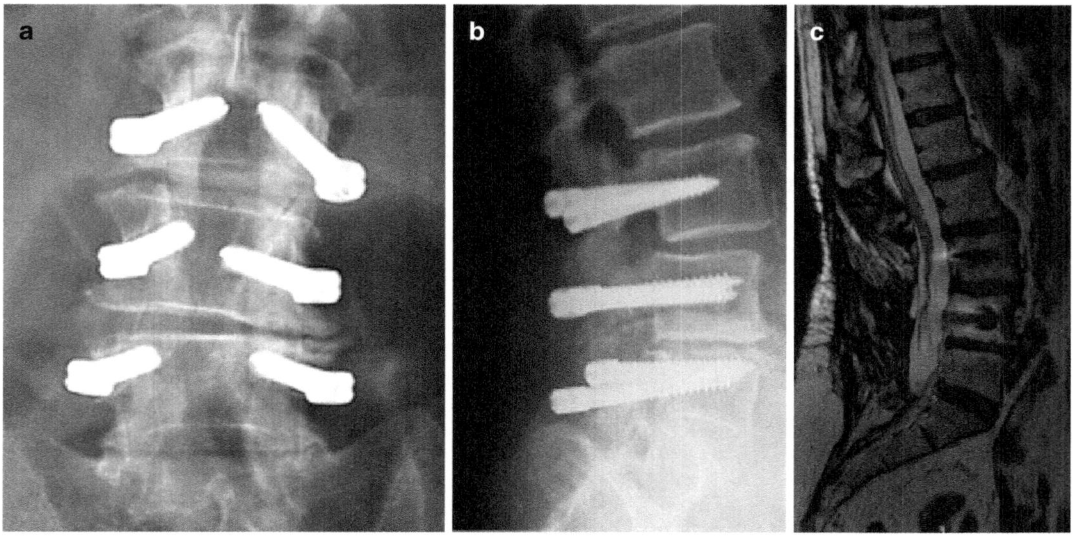

Fig. 20.2 (a–c) Adjacent segment disease at the L2–L3 level, well-evident in MRI (c), after 56 months from surgery: L3–L5 DYNESYS® instrumentation with laminectomy. No revision surgery

DYNESYS® dynamic stabilization system. Of a total of 456 patients, 32 (7.0%) subsequently developed ASD over a mean follow-up period of 33.5 months (range: 12–54 months).

20.4 Infection (Fig. 20.3)

The overall infection rate reported in the literature by Pham et al. [2] is 4.3% when the DYNESYS® dynamic stabilization system was used. Infections occurred in 40 of 923 patients (4.3%) over a mean follow-up period of 34.8 months (range: 16.0–81.6 months). These results are similar to the data reported in the literature on the infection rates for lumbar fusion, ranging from 1% to 5% [25–27]. These infections included superficial wound infections, managed with antibiotic care, as well as deep infections requiring reoperation, with irrigation and debridement. Risk factors for surgical site infections are well-described by Chaichana et al. [25]; they found that age greater than 70 years, diabetes, obesity, previous spinal surgery, and a hospital stay of more than 7 days were independently associated with an increased risk of infection. Lutz et al. [7] reported cases of late infections in their patients. *Propionibacterium* has been shown to cause infections; the authors observed a high incidence of infections (22%) and, especially, their late presentation with a median of 52 months, peaking at 77 months. The clinical experience was similar to that of Collins et al. [28]. In most cases, a combination of recurrent or persistent lumbar pain, with radiological signs of screw loosening or a broken screw, prompted the indication for revision surgery. Only one patient presented with classic symptoms of infection (night sweats, elevated white blood cell count, and C-reactive protein). The proportion of *Propionibacterium* infections was high (7/11 patients), but the spectrum of pathogens was still comparable to that in the study by Collins et al. [28]. Additionally, according to other authors [7], *Propionibacterium* is not only a contaminant but also a germ with a clear pathogenicity for spinal implants, as confirmed by gram-positive probe staining in this study. Some authors [29] found the same correlation between infection risk and the length of operation but not with smoking habits or the number of operated levels. Dakhil-Jerew et al. [30] suggested that the "double-halo sign" described screw loosening: They showed that this sign was associated

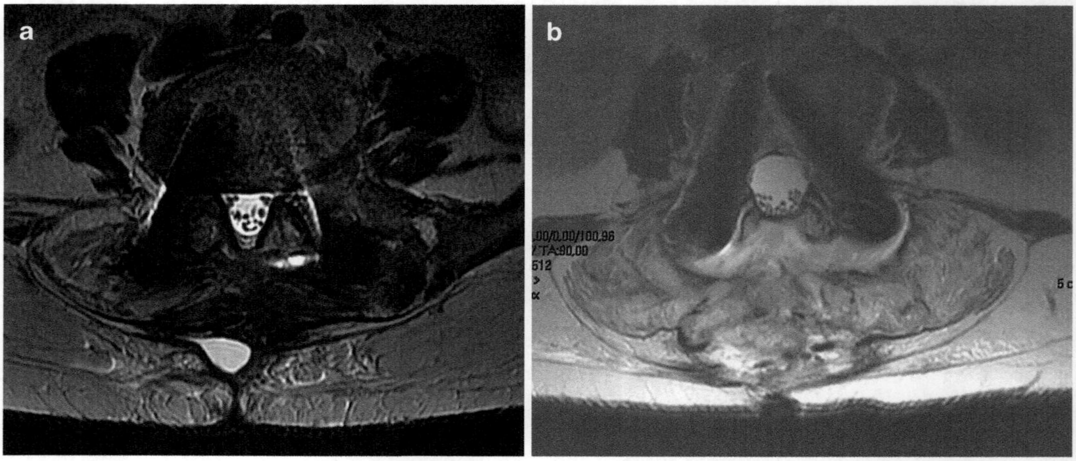

Fig. 20.3 (**a**, **b**) Deep infection after DYNESYS® instrumentation 5 weeks after surgery. Treatment: irrigation and debridement

with better interobserver reliability; in the presence of new or increasing pain, every sign of screw loosening must be scrutinized and confirmed with a computed tomography. The authors [7] do not have an explanation for the high rate of long-term infections observed.

20.5 Conclusions

Incidence of complications is not low after DYNESYS® instrumentation. It occurred in 21.7 of the patients of our series, quite similar to the incidence of rigid instrumentation. Considering the review of literature [2], 17 articles reported reoperations for various reasons. One hundred and seventeen of 1032 patients (11.3%) required a reoperation over a mean follow-up period of 35.9 months (range: 12.0–81.6 months). Indications for repeat surgery included infection, hardware revision, hardware removal, ASD, further decompression, vertebral body fracture, cerebrospinal fluid fistula (CSF) fistula, and epidural hematoma. Nine studies reported reoperation rates associated with the development of ASD after the use of the DYNESYS® system. In these studies [2], a total of 354 patients were followed up over a mean period of 35.7 months. Of the 32 patients who developed ASD, 13 (40.6%) required reoperations for treatment. These 13 revision surgeries constituted part of a total of 57 reported reoperations for any indication in this group.

References

1. Ko CC, Tsai HW, Huang WC, Wu JC, Chen YC, Shih YH, et al. Screw loosening in the Dynesys stabilization system: radiographic evidence and effect on outcomes. Neurosurg Focus. 2010;28(6):E10.
2. Pham MH, Mehta VA, Patel NN, Jakoi AM, Hsieh PC, Liu JC, Wang JC, Acosta FL. Complications associated with the Dynesys dynamic stabilization system: a comprehensive review of the literature. Neurosurg Focus. 2016;40(1):E2.
3. Schmoelz W, Huber JF, Nydegger T, Dipl-Ing, Claes L, Wilke HJ. Dynamic stabilization of the lumbar spine and its effects on adjacent segments: an in vitro experiment. J Spinal Disord Tech. 2003;16:418–23.
4. Schaeren S, Broger I, Jeanneret B. Minimum four-year follow-up of spinal stenosis with degenerative spondylolisthesis treated with decompression and dynamic stabilization. Spine (Phila Pa 1976). 2008;33:E636–42.
5. Bothmann M, Kast E, Boldt GJ, Oberle J. Dynesys fixation for lumbar spine degeneration. Neurosurg Rev. 2008;31:189–96.
6. Haddad B, Makki D, Konan S, Park D, Khan W, Okafor B. Dynesys dynamic stabilization: less good outcome than lumbar fusion at 4-year follow-up. Acta Orthop Belg. 2013;79:97–103.
7. Lutz JA, Otten P, Maestretti G. Late infections after dynamic stabilization of the lumbar spine with Dynesys. Eur Spine J. 2012;21:2573–9.
8. Sapkas G, Mavrogenis AF, Starantzis KA, Soultanis K, Kokkalis ZT, Papagelopoulos PJ. Outcome of a dynamic neutralization system for the spine. Orthopedics. 2012;35:e1497–502.
9. Wu H, Pang Q, Jiang G. Medium-term effects of Dynesys dynamic stabilization versus posterior lumbar interbody fusion for treatment of multisegmental lumbar degenerative disease. J Int Med Res. 2017;2017(45):1562–73.
10. Dakhil-Jerew F, Jadeja H, Cohen A, Shepperd JA. Interobserver reliability of detecting Dynesys pedicle screw using plain X-rays: a study on 50 post-operative patients. Eur Spine J. 2009;18:1486–93.
11. Sandén B, Olerud C, Petrén-Mallmin M, Johansson C, Larsson S. The significance of radiolucent zones surrounding pedicle screws. Definition of screw loosening in spinal instrumentation. J Bone Joint Surg Br. 2004;86:457–61.
12. Wang Q, Liu J, Shi Y, et al. Short-term effects of a dynamic neutralization system (Dynesys) for multi-segmental lumbar disc herniation. Eur Spine J. 2016;25:1409–16.
13. Di Silvestre M, Lolli F, Bakaloudis G. Degenerative lumbar scoliosis in the elderly patients: dynamic stabilization witout fusion versus posterior instrumented fusion. Spine J. 2014;14:1–10.
14. Freudiger S, Dubois G, Lorrain M. Dynamic neutralisation of the lumbar spine confirmed on a new lumbar spine simulator in vitro. Arch Orthop Trauma Surg. 1999;119:127–32.
15. Rahm MD, Hall BB. Adjacent-segment degeneration after lumbar fusion with instrumentation: a retrospective study. J Spinal Disord. 1996;9:392–400.
16. Aota Y, Kumano K, Hirabayashi S. Post fusion instability at the adjacent segments after rigid pedicle screw fixation for degenerative lumbar spinal disorders. J Spinal Disord. 1995;8:464–73.
17. Park P, Garton HJ, Gala VC, Hoff JT, McGillicuddy JE. Adjacent segment disease after lumbar or lumbosacral fusion: review of the literature. Spine (Phila Pa 1976). 2004;29:1938–44.

18. Lawrence BD, Wang J, Arnold PM, Hermsmeyer J, Norvell DC, Brodke DS. Predicting the risk of adjacent segment pathology after lumbar fusion: a systematic review. Spine (Phila Pa 1976). 2012;37(22 Suppl):S123–32.
19. Yu SW, Yang SC, Ma CH, Wu CH, Yen CY, Tu YK. Comparison of Dynesys posterior stabilization and posterior lumbar interbody fusion for spinal stenosis L4L5. Acta Orthop Belg. 2012;78:230–9.
20. Ciol MA, Deyo RA, Kreuter W, Bigos SJ. Characteristicsin Medicare beneficiaries associated with reoperation after lumbar spine surgery. Spine (Phila Pa 1976). 1994;19:1329–34.
21. Ghiselli G, Wang JC, Bhatia NN, Hsu WK, Dawson EG. Adjacent segment degeneration in the lumbar spine. J Bone Joint Surg Am. 2004;86-A:1497–503.
22. Hu RW, Jaglal S, Axcell T, Anderson G. A population-based study of reoperations after back surgery. Spine (Phila Pa 1976). 1997;22:2265–71.
23. Malter AD, McNeney B, Loeser JD, Deyo RA. 5-year reoperation rates after different types of lumbar spine surgery. Spine (Phila Pa 1976). 1998;23:814–20.
24. Martin BI, Mirza SK, Comstock BA, Gray DT, Kreuter W, Deyo RA. Reoperation rates following lumbar spine surgery and the influence of spinal fusion procedures. Spine (Phila Pa 1976). 2007;32:382–7.
25. Chaichana KL, Bydon M, Santiago-Dieppa DR, Hwang L, McLoughlin G, Sciubba DM, et al. Risk of infection following posterior instrumented lumbar fusion for degenerative spine disease in 817 consecutive cases. J Neurosurg Spine. 2014;20:45–52.
26. Olsen MA, Mayfield J, Lauryssen C, Polish LB, Jones M, Vest J, et al. Risk factors for surgical site infection in spinal surgery. J Neurosurg. 2003;98(2 Suppl):149–55.
27. Fang A, Hu SS, Endres N, Bradford DS. Risk factors for infection after spinal surgery. Spine (Phila Pa 1976). 2005;30:1460–5.
28. Collins I, Wilson-MacDonald J, Chami G, Burgoyne W, Vineyakam P, Berendt T, Fairbank J. The diagnosis and management of infection following instrumented spinal fusion. Eur Spine J. 2008;17:445–50.
29. Schimmel JJP, Horsting PP, Kleuver M, Wonders G, Limbeck J. Risk factors for deep surgical site infections after spinal fusion. Eur Spine J. 2010;19:1711–9.
30. Dakhil-Jerew F, Jadeja H, Cohen A, Shepperd JAN. Inter-observer reliability of detecting Dynesys pedicle screw using plain X-rays: a study on 50 post-operative patients. Eur Spine J. 2009;18:1486–93.

21 Two-Stage Surgery for Dynamic Stabilization of the Spine

Ali Fahir Özer and Alper Yeni

Every development in science arises from a need. Two-stage surgery was developed to increase the rates of surgical success. The method has been used in spinal surgery for some time, particularly in the correction of severe deformity, in which it can prevent excessive blood loss and long anesthesia duration. The two-stage surgery that will be discussed in this section is recommended for systematic use with high-risk patients of advanced age, with whom dynamic stabilization systems are predominantly used. In older patients, screw loosening due to poor bone quality is a common problem in spinal surgery. In addition, older patients often have additional medical problems affecting many organs, especially the lungs. Two-stage surgery is a simple approach to the treatment of such patients. When a single operation is performed, the patient is placed under general anesthesia, and instrumentation and decompression are performed. Using a two-stage approach, the same operation is performed by placing the screws in the first stage and, in the second stage, performing decompression and placing the rods in the screws. Both stages can be performed using a spinal anesthetic. This approach is not specific to dynamic systems but can also be adopted with fusion and instrumentation surgery. We have successfully used this method in our fusion surgery patients with additional medical problems (Fig. 21.1).

Fusion surgery on patients with poor bone quality carries a high risk of pseudoarthrosis, which can cause the screws to loosen. The loosening of screws is a common problem when dynamic systems are used in patients with poor bone quality, and loose screws prevent the instrumentation system from functioning. In instrumentation, the screws fuse with the bone to form a new solid structure. This causes loading stress on the screw to spread more widely so that it is shared by the merged screw and bone. This fusion also eliminates the possibility of screw vibration within the bone. The instrumentation system is well-protected and can maintain its function. An important criterion for good fusion is screw–bone osteosynthesis. Fusion begins around 8 weeks after surgery, and as the fused structure strengthens, the task of the instrumentation system ends. Good screw–bone osteointegration is much more important in dynamic systems, as the firm attachment of the instrumentation system to the bone is necessary for it to fulfill its function.

Before we discuss the reasoning behind two-stage surgery, we need to look at segmental instability and the evolution of dynamic systems. The causes of lower back pain are multifactorial. Radicular lower back pain may occur as a result

A. F. Özer (✉)
Department of Neurosurgery, Koc University School of Medicine, Istanbul, Turkey

A. Yeni
Department of Neurosurgery, Prof. Dr. Mazhar Osman Mental Health and Neurological Diseases Training and Research Hospital, Istanbul, Turkey

A. F. Özer et al. (eds.), *Dynamic Lumbar Spine Stabilization*,
https://doi.org/10.1007/978-3-032-12122-6_21

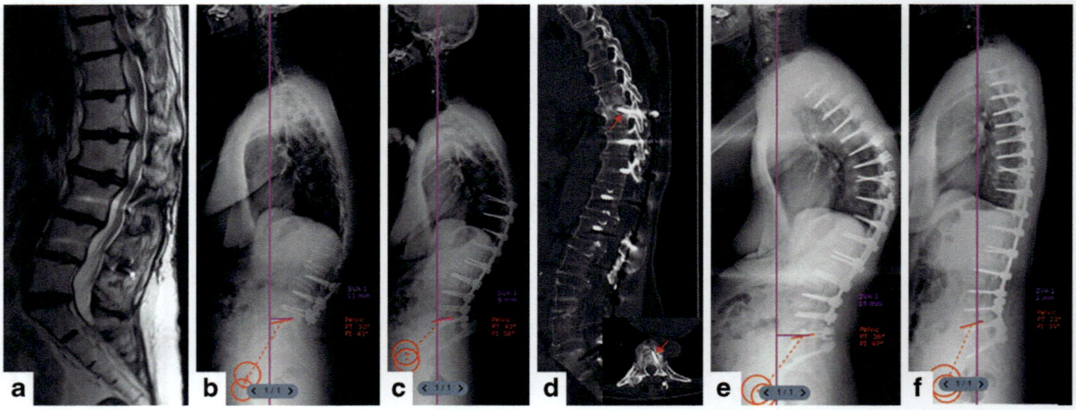

Fig. 21.1 Two-stage lower back surgery on a 60-year-old female patient with poor bone quality, who had failed to benefit from previous surgeries. The patient underwent a lumbar discectomy 15 years ago but did not benefit at all from this operation. A second surgery was then performed on her lower back, and a screw was placed, but the patient did not benefit from this surgery either. The patient's lower back pain did not go away, and she had been leaning forward when walking for the 2 years preceding our treatment. (**a**) Degenerative disc disease was prominent, particularly above the instrumentation. (**b**) After lumbar stabilization, kyphotic deformity developed. (**c**) T10-iliac dynamic stabilization was performed, but the patient's pain continued, and an examination detected loosening in the upper screws. (**d**) A bone density test found the patient's T-score to be −3, indicative of severe osteoporosis. Therefore, a two-stage surgery was performed. In the first stage, the instrumentation was extended to T3 by removing the loosened screws. (**e** and **f**) Examinations performed 6 months after the surgery determined complete osteointegration. The second stage of surgery was performed, in which rods were placed by placing the patient in lumbar lordosis on the operating table. In the second postoperative year, the general condition of the patient is good, and her quality of life is within normal limits

of compression or irritation of the nerve root, which may manifest as isolated degeneration of the disc, lumbar disc herniations, lateral recess, and degeneration-induced spinal canal stenosis. These conditions frequently co-occur. The fundamental cause of pain is the deterioration of the functional units that form the spine due to degenerative processes. As the most prominent structure in each functional segment of the spine, the disc is a common source of problems.

The decrease in disc height caused by the degenerative process reduces the space between the lumbar vertebral bodies, causing the disc to lose its ability to immediately transfer stress to the annulus. It also adds to the stress on the facet joints, which are the other main structures of the segmental unit. In the mid-stage of degeneration, the segments become hypermobile, but in the final stage, motion is lost [1]. This mid-stage increase in mobility causes ruptures in the annulus. The ruptures themselves or the changes induced by them over time are thought to be major contributors to the emergence of lower back pain [2–4]. The degeneration of the facet joints also contributes significantly to the onset of pain [5–7].

In the advanced stage of degeneration, the loss of segmental mobility means that there is nothing stimulating the pain receptors in the annulus, so in advanced degeneration that is not a symptom of a more complex condition, the patient's pain lessens or disappears. The onset of lower back pain most often occurs in the fourth and fifth decades of life, and its gradual disappearance with age is due to ankylosis in the functional segments. Spinal surgeons will sometimes use the last stage of the natural process of degeneration to treat lower back pain [8–10]. Control of abnormal motion in the hypermobile stage of degeneration is not generally considered a viable treatment option. Previously, many apparently healthy discs have been removed and the loss of motion left untreated during fusion surgery performed at a later stage of spinal degeneration.

The stabilization of mobile spinal units is an important aspect of treatment that was overlooked until Graf [11] presented this as the gold standard in the treatment of spinal degeneration.

The therapeutic value of exercise for the reduction of lower back pain has been known for some time. The first real study of spinal muscle function was by Farfan and Gracovetsky [12], who suggested that the lumbar spine and its passive structures, the ligaments and discs, are better designed to resist compression and much less resistant to segmental shear force. They showed that the joint contractions of the abdominal wall and back extensor muscles can provide lumbar spine stability when it is subjected to shear force. The study is an important work for physiotherapists, as it evidences the value of muscle strengthening to increase the stability of the lumbar spine. Healthily structured functional segments are controlled by musculotendinous, osteoligamentous, and neural systems, which provide strength and coordination. The strength of functional segments is derived from the muscular system [12].

In 1982, Kirkaldy-Willis [1] described the degenerative cascade of the spine. He stressed the need for consensus on the definition of instability, its diagnosis, and guidelines on the delivery of a treatment that allows for the severity of the instability. In 1985, Pope and Panjabi [13] interpreted instability as a biomechanical loss of spinal stiffness. They introduced the concepts of neutral and elastic zones. In a functional segment of a normal spine, the least energy-intensive component during motion is the posterior third of the spinal column, called the neutral zone (Fig. 21.2).

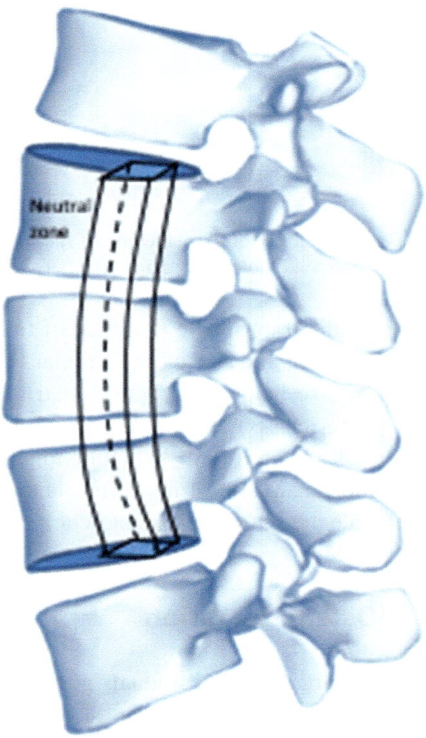

Fig. 21.2 The neutral zone of the spine. The least energy-intensive component of the spine during movement is the posterior third of the spinal column, called the neutral zone

They found that degenerative events disrupt spinal continuity, causing the neutral zone to widen. As a result, more energy is required to maintain the neutral zone. If the expansion of this zone cannot be compensated for, there will be scaling and hypermobility in the functional segment (Fig. 21.3). However, hypermobility is not necessarily synonymous with instability. Gymnasts have highly hypermobile spines but do not suffer from the pain or instability seen in those with degenerative spinal complaints. In these athletes, the muscles and functional segments have been trained to utilize the maximum range of motion, none of which is pathological [14, 15].

Benzel [15] identified two types of spinal instability: overt and chronic, with chronic instability subdivided into glacial instability and dysfunctional segmental movements. Dynamic systems are used to surgically address chronic instability, which develops gradually over many years. Unlike overt instability, there is no set of clinical characteristics that indicate chronic instability requiring immediate correction.

How to diagnose spinal instability is an important issue that is still under discussion. As yet, no consensus has been reached on the matter. The most commonly used parameters are the presence of angulation greater than 15° or a translational shift of more than 3 mm on flexion–

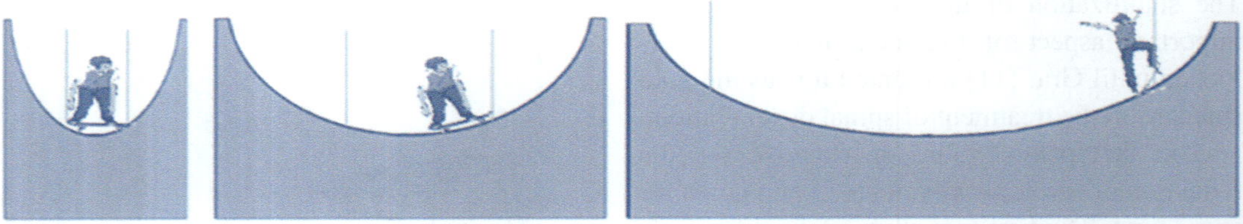

Fig. 21.3 An analogy for the widening of the neutral zone of the spinal column. On a steep, narrow track, a skateboarder must expend more energy traveling between the apexes on either side than on a wider, flatter track

extension radiographs. The presence of traction spurs in the spine, the size of any annular tears, a decrease in disc height, and a millimetric anterior or posterior spinal shift also support the existence of instability in the functional segment. The clearest sign of instability is the subjective pain experienced by the patient.

21.1 Osteointegration

Osteointegration is the gradual postoperative union of the screw and the bone. In both fusion and dynamic stabilization surgery, every surgeon must fully understand osteointegration. The surgeon must be aware of how organic matter responds to the presence of foreign objects, such as metal plates or screws. It is vital to know each phase of this process and its possible outcomes. These phases are very similar to the stages that a broken bone goes through as it heals and reintegrates.

For osteointegration to occur, the screw must be firmly attached to the bone. The implant and bone surface should be firmly and healthily attached to ensure the stability of the implant. However, during implant–bone healing, both metal-to-bone contact and, inevitably, a very small distance between them are very important for osteogenesis that occurs where the implant comes in contact. This is because, as the new bone is formed on the implant surface, it begins to be filled with bone tissue that grows appositionally from the surface of the old bone and toward the implant surface. If the surface of the implant and the bone surface have complementary surface topography, contact-induced osteogenesis can lead to the healthy attachment of the bone to the implant. The early stage of bone healing around the implant is very important, as it includes the body's initial response to a foreign substance, including protein adsorption, platelet activation, coagulation, and inflammation, which then lead to the formation of a stable fibrin clot, a reservoir for growth factors that permits osteoconduction. Osteoconduction is the evolution and differentiation of osteogenic cells such as pericytes into osteoblasts and is the first step in the development of new bone tissue at the implant surface through contact osteogenesis. The late stage of healing involves remodeling of the bone that has woven into this implant. In many ways, this process is similar to bone healing that occurs after a fracture [16], and these biological processes underlying bone attachment occur not only in normal human bone but also in all vertebrates, as part of physiological bone remodeling. During bone remodeling, osteoclasts remove old bone and, thereby, provide a surface with appropriate topography over the old bone to which the newly formed bone can attach. This bonding occurs when the implant line intersects the surface of the old bone. As the implant surface is the first matrix to be formed during de novo bone formation, pores in the surface topography of the implant will facilitate bone attachment [17]. Additionally, hydroxyapatite-coated screws are advantageous in osteointegration.

Healing at the surface where the implant contacts the bone begins during surgery, i.e., when the surgeon prepares to insert the screw into the bone, e.g., making a hole from the pedicle to insert a screw in a vertebra. This preparation of the bone is important for implant healing because it causes bleeding from the intact bone and subsequent hematoma formation within the hole. A fibrin clot is then formed, which allows osteoconduction [17].

21.2 Primary Implant Stability

Primary implant stability is a requirement for successful bone–implant healing [18]. The surgeon secures the implant to the bone, i.e., attaches the cervical plate to a vertebra with screws or inserts screws into the pedicle and connects these screws with a rod. This is similar to an implant that the dentist inserts with a screw into the jawbone, and it may or may not initially load. A stable implant has limited micromotion between the bone and the implant, which allows successful tissue growth (e.g., angiogenesis and osteogenesis) around the implant [19] and is analogous to a healing fracture. In a broken bone, movement at the microlevel between the broken bone ends is called a micro-instability, and this micromotion directs cartilage formation toward bone development [20, 21]. However, if movement between the broken bone ends is extreme, union between the bone ends is not possible, which leads to the development of pseudoarthrosis. This is true for implants as well because it has been shown that excessive movement between the bone and the implant promotes the growth of fibrous connective tissue rather than chondrocytes that subsequently evolve into bone tissue [22]. Further, as Pilliar et al. have suggested that a micromotion greater than 150 μm will cause fibrous tissue to adhere to the implant surface instead of evolving into bone tissue [23], it is recommended to limit early loading of the implants. Nevertheless, a micromotion of less than 25–50 μm is required to support bone formation during fracture and implant healing [24].

Thus, it is evident from the above that the distance between the bone and the implant is very important because ossification may slow down if there is no distance and micromotion between the implant and the bone or if the distance is more than 500 μm, as there is too much for cartilage tissue that has to evolve into bone tissue [19, 25].

21.3 Implant Contact with Blood

Blood is always the first tissue that the implant screw comes into contact with when it enters the bone, and this contact results in a series of biological processes such as protein deposition, coagulation, inflammation, and tissue formation. For the bone, these processes represent an evolutionary response to injury caused by the penetration of foreign material (i.e., the screw), and the surface chemistry and topography of the screw affect these processes. Just seconds after contact with blood, a single protein layer is formed on the surface of the screw, and platelets and mesenchymal cells interact with this monolayer. Blood contains more than 200 different proteins, but only certain proteins adhere appreciably to the implant surface. Additionally, this protein composition is largely determined by the surface properties of the implant, and the screw surface will determine the structure of the adsorbed proteins. The types of proteins adsorbed to the screw surface can also determine the bone response to the material and can, therefore, determine whether successful healing will occur around the implant. Fibrinogen, von Willebrand factor, complement, and IgG are also absorbed onto the screw surface and are important for platelet activation, coagulation, and inflammation [26].

21.4 Coagulation and Platelet Activation

Platelets are the first cells that come into contact with the implant surface and have been shown to be present on the implant surface 5 seconds after contact with blood [27]. Platelets are small cells composed of megakaryocytes and foreign matter (implant surface), damaged endothelium, subendothelium, or other platelets or factors released by cells (e.g., adenosine diphosphate [ADP], thromboxane A2, and thrombin). Platelet activation results in a number of important intracellular processes, including conformational changes in the receptor that allow it to bind to proteins adsorbed on the implant [28] and the release of bioactive molecules stored in granules into the surrounding environment. Platelet activation also causes a significant change in the shape of the cell, which leads to the expression of adhesion receptors and is important for coagulation. Platelets also contain membrane-bound adhesion receptors on their surface, and their adhesion to an implant surface is mediated by these receptors.

Platelet activation also causes them to clump together to form a clot, and fibrinogen is an important plasma protein in this process that supports the aggregation of platelets. Activated platelets catalyze the production of thrombin from prothrombin, and this occurs concurrently with coagulation. Thrombin then acts to stabilize the growing platelet thrombus by producing a stable fibrin polymer from fibrinogen [28]. The formation of a stable clot provides both the mechanical and biochemical components necessary for osteoconductivity, which is defined as the recruitment and migration of osteogenic cells [29]. The fibrin clot is a three-dimensional temporary matrix containing adherent plasma proteins that allows cell adhesion and migration from the capillary bed to the implant. This clot also contains many signaling molecules, such as cytokines, chemoattractants, mitogens, and growth factors, which induce the migration of osteoprogenitor cells via signaling pathways [30–33].

21.5 Inflammatory Response and Signaling Molecules

The inflammatory response is concurrent with coagulation and platelet activation and interacts with both processes as well [34]. Neutrophils and monocytes are important leukocytes in the inflammatory response, and they are the next set of cells to migrate into the space between the implant and the bone after the platelets. Moreover, neutrophils are the first to arrive, and their numbers reach peak levels between 24 and 48 hours. However, monocytes rapidly transform into macrophages, which are the predominant leukocytes after 48 hours [30]. Leukocytes circulating in the capillaries surrounding the implant are activated in response to the cytokines released by the platelets [34], and they release inflammatory mediators such as the macrophage colony-stimulating factor [30].

Bone–implant space hematoma is similar to a fracture hematoma, as they express similar signaling molecules. Inflammatory cytokines are the first signaling molecules to be expressed and appear to be necessary for initiating bone formation.

Similar to mediators of inflammation, members of the tissue growth factor family are expressed within 24 hours of injury [35], and these include bone morphogenic proteins (BMPs) and growth and differentiation factors that have been shown to promote bone formation at a fracture site. Currently, BMP-2 and BMP-7 are used to expedite the healing of non-unions after fracture [36–40].

Metabolically active osteogenic cells require a blood supply, and therefore, angiogenesis is essential. Angiogenic factors disrupt the extracellular matrix surrounding preexisting capillaries and allow new vessels to sprout, indicating that they may also modulate the osteoblast function [41–43].

Complex interactions among signaling molecules within the bone–implant space result in the recruitment, migration, and differentiation of mesenchymal cells, i.e., both osteoinduction and osteoconduction, and osteogenic cells participate in the formation of a woven bone.

21.6 Woven Bone Formation

Mesenchymal cells, which we will call pericytes, converge at the cambium layer of the periosteum from the bone marrow [44], are considered to be tissue-resident mesenchymal cells, and are brought to the wound site during angiogenesis [45]. Pericytes move toward the implant surface through the preliminary matrix formed by the fibrin clot, and this is probably mediated by numerous factors released by platelets and leukocytes [46], which also promote pericyte differentiation into osteoblastic cells, which will then colonize the implant surface and begin to secrete the matrix. Notably, the initial matrix laid down by these cells does not contain collagen [47]; rather, this matrix, secreted by the osteoprogenitor cells reaching the implant surface, forms the afibrillar interface region, and it has been reported that the thickness of this zone varies from 0.2 to 0.5 μm [22]. This afibrillar interface region forms a non-collagenous, calcified layer on the surface of the implant, beyond which is a collagenous compartment composed predominantly of type I collagen. Importantly, the mineralization of this collagenous compartment proceeds after that of the afibrillar interface region [47]. Fully differentiated osteoblasts are responsible for the formation of the collagen compartment, and they move backward from the progressive mineralization front. Sometimes, they are surrounded by mineralized tissue during this backward movement [22], and when this occurs, the osteoblast becomes an osteocyte within a bone cavity. This results in the formation of an immature woven bone that progresses appositionally from the implant surface to the edges of the bone to which it is attached, and this process is known as "contact osteogenesis" [48].

Bone formation can also occur in the opposite direction; i.e., it progresses from the bone surface to the implant, and this type of ossification is called "distance osteogenesis" [16, 48]. During implantation, osteocytes at the open bone margins die due to thermal necrosis, e.g., the opened bone surface where the screw is in contact with the pedicle screw. This extends to a depth of 100–500 μm in the bone, and the resulting dead tissue is destroyed by osteoblasts [47, 49].

Differentiating osteoblasts migrate to the surface of the destroyed bone and produce a knitted bone by apposition that extends from the cut bone surface and surrounds the implant surface. Thus, bone formation occurs in two opposite directions, i.e., contact osteogenesis toward the implant, and restoration from the implant on the surface of the bone tissue adjacent to the implant, i.e., distance osteogenesis. Moreover, it has been reported that contact osteogenesis occurs 30% faster than distance osteogenesis [29, 47], with both resulting in the formation of an immature woven bone around the implant.

Importantly, this provides secondary stabilization after the surgeon anchors the implant into the patient's bone, and therefore, there is a transition from primary stabilization caused by the friction of the implant in the host bone to secondary stabilization caused by the formation of woven bone around the implant [50], and primary stabilization is reduced. Over time, the host bone in direct contact with the implant dies and is reabsorbed by osteoclasts, and if the surface topography of the implant permits contact osteogenesis, secondary stability of the implant may result from bone attachment. If the surface topography of the implant is three-dimensionally complex, with pores and undercuts, it can become intertwined with the implant surface, resulting in bone bonding. If the implant surface does not have a suitable topography, the bone only grows toward the implant through distant osteogenesis, and bone attachment may not be achieved [48].

21.7 Implant Surface Design and Osteointegration

The success of a metal implant depends on the rate of bone–implant healing and the resulting mechanical strength of the bone–implant interface. Both of these parameters can be improved through surface modification of the implant. The two most commonly used methods to improve implant surface are (1) porous coating on the implant surface and (2) plasma spray coating of metals or ceramics on the implant surface (Fig. 21.4).

A single- or multilayer porous coating on Co-Cr-Mo or titanium alloy implants involves heating the implant to high temperatures for long periods of time to create a porous coating; however, high temperatures can change the mechanical properties of the implant and reduce metal strength. Bone growth into the pores of the coating stabilizes the implant within the bone but weakens the strength of the implant. Hence, for optimum bone growth, the size of the pores should be greater than 100 μm [51].

Plasma spray involves superheating titanium or ceramic powder and spraying the resulting

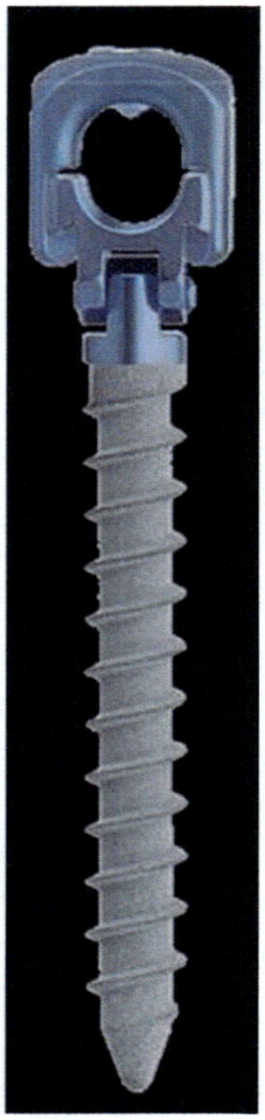

Fig. 21.4 A screw for spinal implantation, with a plasma-sprayed coating of hydroxyapatite

plasma onto the surface of a titanium alloy implant, which then solidifies rapidly and forms a deposit on the surface, which confers an irregular surface topography that can allow bone attachment at the implant surface [52].

The plasma spray process is commonly used to coat implants with hydroxyapatite, but the deposition occurring on the implant surface is actually a mixture of different calcium phosphate phases, e.g., hydroxyapatite tricalcium phosphate, tetracalcium phosphate, and amorphous calcium phosphate, because of the loss of normal stoichiometry upon overheating [53]. Therefore, hydroxyapatite-sprayed implants should aptly be named coated implants, i.e., predominantly calcium phosphate–coated implants. Both titanium and hydroxyapatite plasma–sprayed coatings rely on bone attachment for implant fixation within the host bone; hence, the strength of the final bone fixation is essentially the same with both coatings. However, hydroxyapatite plasma–sprayed implants appear to have faster peri-implant healing than titanium-sprayed implants, probably due to enhanced osteoconductivity secondary to chemical factors (e.g., an increase in peri-implant concentrations of Ca^{2+} and PO_4^{3-}) but more so due to the enhanced topography properties of the calcium phosphate coating (e.g., enhanced platelet activation) [54]. Remodeling of the bone that is in contact with the implant surface continues throughout the life of the implant and may allow greater contact between the implant and the bone over time.

21.8 Late Remodeling of the Bone–Implant Interface

The desired outcome is lamellar bone formation around the implant. However, woven bone forms first and rapidly and consists of randomly arrayed and loosely packed collagen fibers of varying sizes. In contrast, collagen fibers of the lamellar bone developing on the woven bone are arranged in thicker bundles and have a regular shape along the developing bone lamella, making the lamellar bone mechanically stronger than the woven bone [55].

However, this may not always be the case. Normally, formation and destruction of the bone are balanced, but maintenance of this balance requires some load on it, e.g., the daily activities of a healthy person, such as walking and running. However, in some cases, if the implant removes the load on the bone, osteoclastic activity overtakes osteoblastic activity, and the bone weakens. This is the stress-shielding mechanism that causes bone loss after the placement of an implant that is harder than the bone [53].

21.9 The Logic of Two-Stage Surgery

The rationale behind two-stage surgery lies in the failure of the surgery performed using instruments and the subsequent chronic instability due to the poor quality of the bone in elderly patients and the hypermobility of the unstable segment. For an implant to function properly, the stability of the primary implant must be exceptional, and the implant–bone compatibility must be harmonious in the presence of primary instability. However, while providing primary stabilization of a functional segment of the instrument where the neutral zone is too wide, excessive mobility in the functional segment will cause excessive load on the instrument. After the establishment of primary stability, osteoblastic activity due to excessive mobility in the bone–implant distance will lead to destruction by osteoclastic activity and the formation of fibrous tissue in the bone–joint distance. Eventually, the screw will loosen, and instrument failure will occur. As this is also true for long instrumentation, in patients with poor bone quality, screws loosen due to the effects of additional shear forces on the screws at the proximal and distal ends, resulting in instrument failure.

Poor quality of the bone is another important factor that prevents strong primary stability, and therefore, in diseases such as osteoporosis, rheumatoid arthritis, or ankylosing spondylitis, long instruments are designed to reduce the load per screw and prevent screw loosening due to poor bone quality.

The union of the screw to the bone and the healing of the broken bone occur concurrently, and according to Wolff's law, some load must be placed on the fracture ends or the graft for the broken bone to heal. As explained in detail above, this also applies to screws, but the load on the screw should not impair primary stability. If primary stability cannot be adequately achieved, it will result in pseudoarthrosis and instrument failure in fusion and screw loosening and instrument failure in dynamic stabilizations.

Screws are the most basic structures of construction, and in two-stage surgery, when the screws are first inserted, we easily pass the stage of accepting the implant from the bone to eliminate the load on the screws. The remodeling phase in the broken bone occurs between days 21 and 35 after surgery and lasts for months or even years [56]. As remodeling time increases, secondary stability gradually becomes stronger, and despite changing designs in knee and hip prostheses that are directly loaded, the patient is allowed to walk normally after an average of 12 weeks. This time can be used for pedicular screws that are not directly loaded, and second-stage surgery can be performed between 16–20 weeks, depending on the bone quality of the patient. Additionally, at this stage, the rods on the screws that are solidly fused to the bone can also be affixed.

Both surgeries can be performed with spinal anesthesia if the patient does not have any problems. This is a great advantage for patients with additional medical problems.

21.10 Patient Selection

Two-stage surgery should be especially considered in osteoporotic patients with a T-score below −1.5 or in patients with additional medical problems. Two-stage surgery can be used for single- or multilevel chronic instability. Broad-based contained or non-contained disc herniations, painful black discs, degenerative spondylolisthesis, lumbar stenosis, foraminal stenosis, lateral recess syndrome, and adult scoliotic or kyphotic deformities are the main pathologies in which chronic instability occurs.

In patients with good bone quality, if there is a medical problem that poses a risk in general anesthesia, two-stage surgery can be performed.

21.11 Surgical Technique

In dynamic system surgeries in our department, the Safinaz polyaxial dynamic hinged screw system (Medicon AS, Turkey), the Orthrus system (TıpSan), and the DYNESYS® spinal stabilization device (Zimmer Inc., Warsaw, IN), which are two-headed dynamic screws, are used.

The DYNESYS® system was described by Dubois in 1994 [57]. The system consists of pedicle screws and the polyester cord Sulene–polyethylene terephthalate (PET) that connects them. In addition, the Sulene–polycarbonate urethane (PCU) cylindrical spacers used in this system prevent excessive compression. In flexion, movement is controlled by tension on the band; in extension, spacers allow a limited amount of extension. Compared with other pure band-like systems, such as Graff ligaments, the spacer provides protection against compression at the posterior annulus and preserves the foramen volume, while also providing symmetrical load distribution. This prevents nerve root compression within the foramen under compressive loading.

The Orthrus system is made up of screws with two screwheads, each of which is designed to be individually fitted with a rod, and both heads can move on a hinge. The screw has up and down movement but not rotational movement. Each bass serves for one movement segment. It is designed for multilevel instabilities. For example, when three motion segments are stabilized, the inner heads act to stabilize one segment, and the outer heads act to stabilize the other segment. The screwheads are attached to each other with polyetheretherketone (PEEK) rods (Fig. 21.5).

In short-level stabilizations, a Safinaz screw with a polyaxial head is used, together with a PEEK rod. Safinaz screws have motion in all directions, even when the screw is tightened and its rotation is limited.

The patient is given a spinal anesthetic and placed in the prone position. After the surgical area is cleaned and the surgical field is draped sterilely. Screws may be placed by making several small skin incisions, through which the screws are inserted percutaneously using a C-arm or neuronavigation (Fig. 21.6).

Alternatively, scars from multiple incisions may be avoided by making a single midline incision and then inserting the screws through small incisions in the fascia. The most important element of the first stage of the surgery is the placement of screws such that pairs of screwheads face each other at exactly equivalent positions on either side and are at the same height. If screw placement is not precise, the attachment of the rods in the second surgery will be problematic, and this cannot be corrected during the second stage.

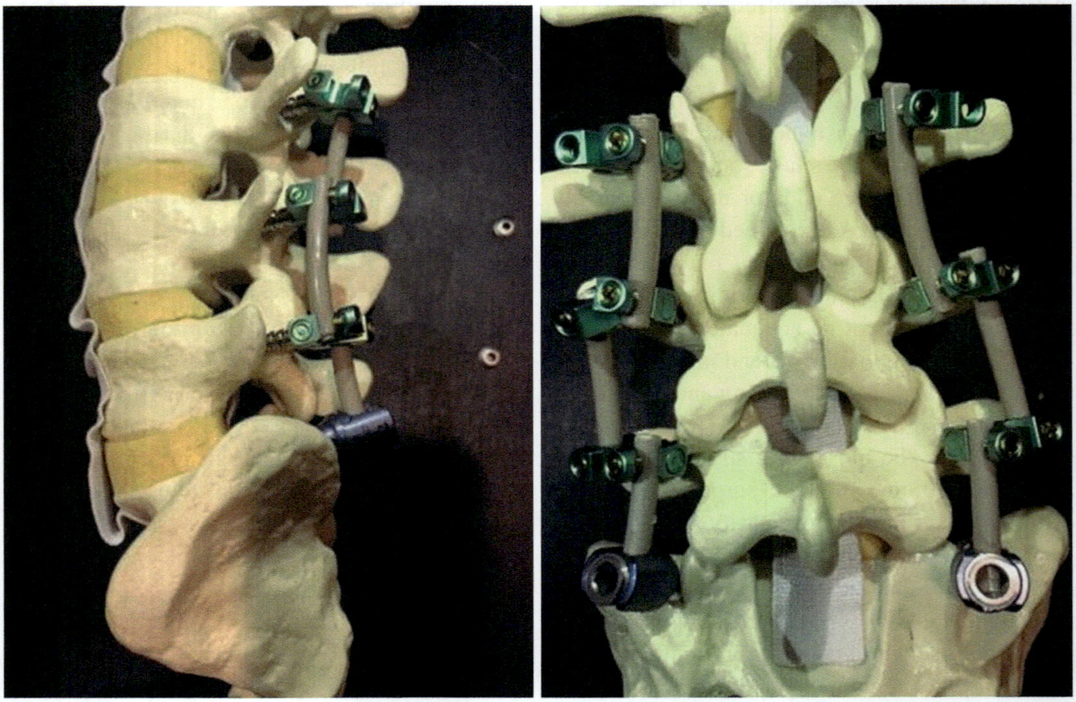

Fig. 21.5 The Orthrus dynamic spinal stabilization system. The heads of hinged dynamic screws are divided into two. The two halves of a screw are placed opposite one another at each relevant level of the spine. Once connected to a rod, each screw is then responsible for stabilizing the moving segments

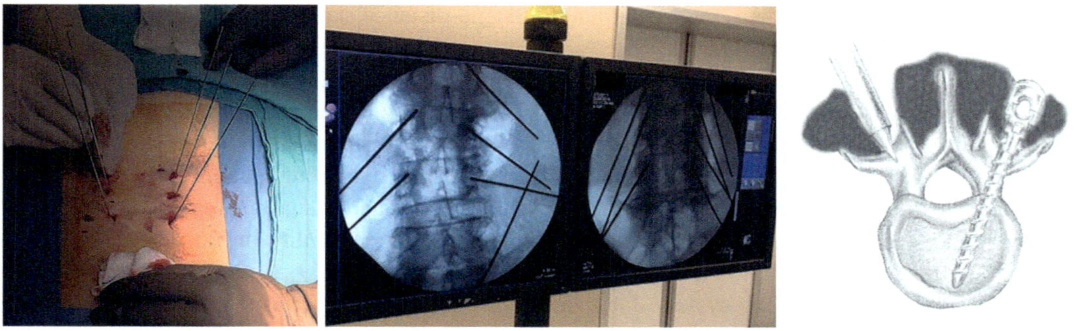

Fig. 21.6 Surgical placement of spinal screws. Small incisions are made in the skin over the intended placement point for each screwhead, and the screws are placed percutaneously. To avoid many incision scars, small incisions can be made over the fascia via a single midline incision

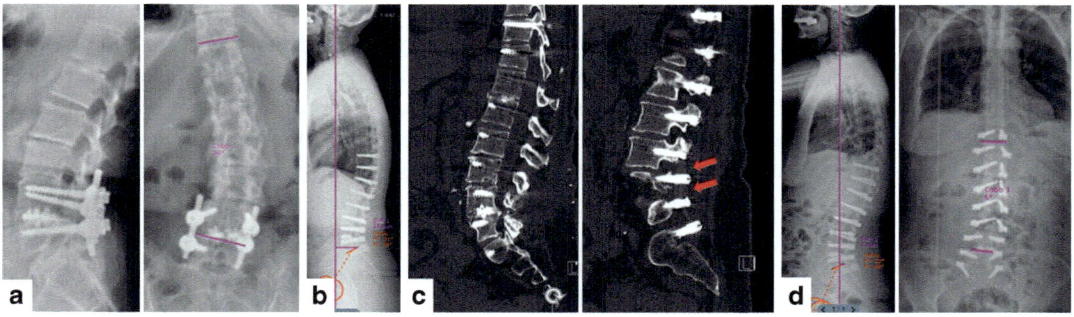

Fig. 21.7 Two-stage surgery for scoliotic and kyphotic deformities resulting from L3–4 disc degeneration in a patient with poor bone density. (**a**) L4–5 interbody fusion surgery was performed on a patient with severe lower back pain resulting from L4–5 disc degeneration. Ten years after the operation, the patient's lower back pain recurred. The adjacent L3–4 segment was found to have degenerated. Radiographs of the patient's spine revealed scoliotic and kyphotic deformities beginning in the L3–4 region. (**b**) The patient's T-score was found to be −2, indicating very poor bone density. Therefore, two-stage T10–S1 surgery was deemed the best option. In the first stage, spinal screws were placed. (**c**) A temporary rod was also placed during the first stage to prevent disc herniation or progression of the deformity to the adjacent segment. (**d**) The second stage was performed 4 months later. In the second operation, the temporary rods were replaced with DYNESYS® rods, with the patient in a normal position. Postoperatively, the patient's deformities improved significantly, and his spinopelvic parameters returned to healthy, functional levels

At this stage, if there is a narrow canal, a level with root irritation, or there is compression in the nerve root due to foraminal stenosis, this segment can be stabilized by decompressing, sometimes unilaterally or bilaterally, because it is unthinkable for the patient to spend the waiting period painfully. When using this method, the number of screws being loosened is limited if there is at least some loosening (Fig. 21.7). If the long segment is to be stabilized, bilateral temporary stabilization can also be applied only to the decompressed segment (Fig. 21.7).

If there are no clinical issues resulting from compression, decompression should be left to the second surgery. Patients can be discharged on the same day or 1 or 2 days after surgery.

The second stage is usually the weighted stage of the surgery. Patients are evaluated with CT after a minimum of 16–20 weeks of surgery. After it is determined that the osteointegration of screws is completed, patients are taken to the second surgery. At this stage, a midline incision is made, and only the required segments are stripped subperiosteally from the midline and decompressed. Then, the screws are found with the Wiltse paraspinal approach, and the rods are attached.

It is necessary to restore the impaired lumbar lordosis in patients. In order to bring the forward-slipped sagittal vertical axis back to the sacrum, the patient is placed in a lordotic position on the table and controlled with a C-arm in patients with a flat back deformity. If necessary, the iliac long-segment dynamic system stabilization is performed to ensure the continuity of the lordotic position [58].

21.12 Clinical Evaluation

Ten male and 13 female adult patients were included in this single-center retrospective study conducted between 2018 and 2021. The mean age of the patients was 65.6 years. T-scores were checked for all patients aged over 50, regardless of their gender, and two-stage surgery was recommended in patients with a T score of -1.5 and above.

Our average follow-up rates of patients 30 months. We did not have any complaints in the single-distance stabilization group. In the patient group with multilevel instability, the screw system was removed due to the development of metal allergy in one patient, and one patient was followed up with superficial wound infection, and in the remaining patient group, both the radiological and visual analog scale (VAS) and the Oswestry Disability Index scores returned to reasonable levels [59].

In the scoliotic deformity group, dynamic stabilization had serious advantages for the patients. First of all, the development of the deformity is stopped with a simple instrumentation system. Although the other advantage is not as much as in rigid systems, some improvement is possible. They are mobile deformities in their indications, and they are not used in advanced, rigid deformities. Two-stage surgery was applied to the patient with sagittal deformity. There was a significant improvement in the VAS and Oswestry results of the patients, and there was a significant improvement in the sagittal vertical axis, depending on the degree of mobilization of the radiological deformity (Fig. 21.8).

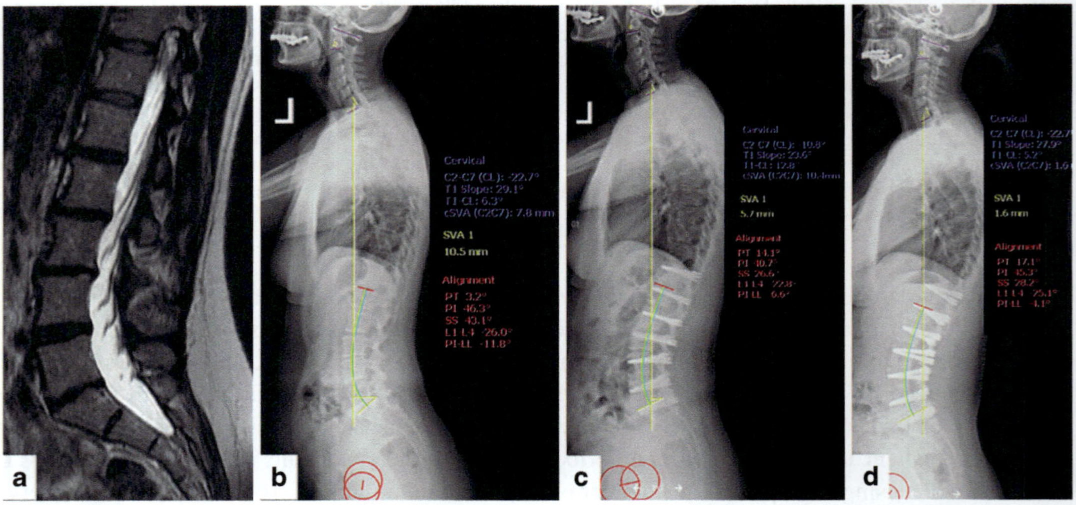

Fig. 21.8 Two-stage surgery for multilevel degenerative disc disease. A 46-year-old female patient presented with pain when standing or walking. (**a**) Magnetic resonance imaging of the T2 sections of the patient's spine showed multilevel degenerative disc disease. (**b**) The patient's sagittal vertical axis was forward-shifted, and sagittal imbalance was detected. (**c**) A spine X-ray taken 4 months after the screws were placed. At this point, it was established that the patient was able to maintain her balance using her muscles. (**d**) After the rods were placed, the sagittal parameters of the spine returned to healthy, functional levels

Patients treated for spinal degeneration are usually aware that treatment cannot return their radiological parameters to a pre-degeneration level, but it is important to discuss possible outcomes with them and establish realistic surgical goals that are acceptable to the patient. The recency with which we began using two-stage surgery with dynamic instability systems has limited our patient follow-up periods. While none of our patients have experienced any hardware problems in the 2 years after surgery, longer follow-up is needed to ensure the safety and efficacy of the approach.

21.13 Conclusion

In conclusion, two-stage surgery should be considered for patients who are of advanced age and/or have one or more comorbidities. The two-stage approach significantly reduces the incidence of surgical complications and can be performed using spinal anesthesia, eliminating the risks inherent in general anesthesia. Hospital stays are short, and the process is more cost-effective than a single major surgery.

References

1. Kirkaldy-Willis WH, Farfan HF. Instability of the lumbar spine. Clin Orthop Relat Res. 1982;165:110–23.
2. Manchikanti L, Singh V, Pampati V. Evaluation of the relative contributions of various structures in chronic low back pain. Pain Physician. 2001;4(4):308–16.
3. He L, Hu X, Tang Y, et al. Efficacy of coblation annuloplasty in discogenic low back pain: a prospective observational study. Medicine (Baltimore). 2015;94(19):e846. https://doi.org/10.1097/MD.0000000000000846.
4. Allegri M, Montella S, Salici F, et al. Mechanisms of low back pain: a guide for diagnosis and therapy. F1000Res. 2016;5:F1000 Faculty Rev-1530. Published 2016 Jun 28. https://doi.org/10.12688/f1000research.8105.2.
5. Yang KH, King AI. Mechanism of facet load transmission as a hypothesis for low-back pain. Spine. 1984;9(6):557–65. https://doi.org/10.1097/00007632-198409000-00005. PMID: 6238423.
6. DePalma MJ, Ketchum JM, Saullo T. What is the source of chronic low back pain and does age play a role? Pain Med. 2011;12(2):224–33. https://doi.org/10.1111/j.1526-4637.2010.01045.x.
7. Cavanaugh JM, Lu Y, Chen C, et al. Pain generation in lumbar and cervical facet joints. J Bone Joint Surg Am. 2006;88(Suppl 2):63–70.
8. Lettin AW. Diagnosis and treatment of lumbar instability. J Bone Joint Surg Br. 1967;49(3):520–9.
9. Morgan FP, King T. Primary instability of lumbar vertebrae as a common cause of low back pain. J Bone Joint Surg Br. 1957;39-B(1):6–22. https://doi.org/10.1302/0301-620X.39B1.6.
10. Macnab I. The traction spur. An indicator of segmental instability. J Bone Joint Surg Am. 1971;53(4):663–70.
11. Graf H. Lumbar instability: surgical treatment without fusion. Rachis. 1992;412:123–37.
12. Farfan HF, Gracovetsky S. The nature of instability. Spine (Phila Pa 1976). 1984;9(7):714–9. https://doi.org/10.1097/00007632-198410000-00011.
13. Pope MH, Panjabi M. Biomechanical definitions of spinal instability. Spine (Phila Pa 1976). 1985;10(3):255–6. https://doi.org/10.1097/00007632-198504000-00013.
14. Paris SV. Physical signs of instability. Spine (Phila Pa 1976). 1985;10(3):277–9. https://doi.org/10.1097/00007632-198504000-00016.
15. Benzel EC. The anatomic basis of spinal instability. In: Clinical neurosurgery. Baltimore: Williams and Wilkins; 1993. p. 224–41.
16. Kuzyk PR, Schemitsch EH. The basic science of peri-implant bone healing. Indian J Orthop. 2011;45(2):108–15. https://doi.org/10.4103/0019-5413.77129.
17. Davies JE. Bone bonding at natural and biomaterial surfaces. Biomaterials. 2007;28(34):5058–67. https://doi.org/10.1016/j.biomaterials.2007.07.049.
18. Cameron HU, Pilliar RM, MacNab I. The effect of movement on the bonding of porous metal to bone. J Biomed Mater Res. 1973;7(4):301–11. https://doi.org/10.1002/jbm.820070404.
19. Franchi M, Fini M, Martini D, Orsini E, Leonardi L, Ruggeri A, Giavaresi G, Ottani V. Biological fixation of endosseous implants. Micron. 2005;36(7–8):665–71. https://doi.org/10.1016/j.micron.2005.05.010.
20. Cullinane DM, Fredrick A, Eisenberg SR, Pacicca D, Elman MV, Lee C, Salisbury K, Gerstenfeld LC, Einhorn TA. Induction of a neoarthrosis by precisely controlled motion in an experimental mid-femoral defect. J Orthop Res. 2002;20(3):579–86. https://doi.org/10.1016/S0736-0266(01)00131-0.
21. Gerstenfeld LC, Cullinane DM, Barnes GL, Graves DT, Einhorn TA. Fracture healing as a post-natal developmental process: molecular, spatial, and temporal aspects of its regulation. J Cell Biochem. 2003;88(5):873–84. https://doi.org/10.1002/jcb.10435.
22. Marco F, Milena F, Gianluca G, Vittoria O. Peri-implant osteogenesis in health and osteoporosis. Micron. 2005;36(7–8):630–44. https://doi.org/10.1016/j.micron.2005.07.008.

23. Pilliar RM, Lee JM, Maniatopoulos C. Observations on the effect of movement on bone ingrowth into porous-surfaced implants. Clin Orthop Relat Res. 1986;208:108–13.
24. Goodman S, Aspenberg P. Effects of mechanical stimulation on the differentiation of hard tissues. Biomaterials. 1993;14(8):563–9. https://doi.org/10.1016/0142-9612(93)90171-w.
25. Futami T, Fujii N, Ohnishi H, Taguchi N, Kusakari H, Ohshima H, Maeda T. Tissue response to titanium implants in the rat maxilla: ultrastructural and histochemical observations of the bone-titanium interface. J Periodontol. 2000;71(2):287–98. https://doi.org/10.1902/jop.2000.71.2.287.
26. Ratner BD. New ideas in biomaterials science--a path to engineered biomaterials. J Biomed Mater Res. 1993;27(7):837–50. https://doi.org/10.1002/jbm.820270702.
27. Kanagaraja S, Lundström I, Nygren H, Tengvall P. Platelet binding and protein adsorption to titanium and gold after short time exposure to heparinized plasma and whole blood. Biomaterials. 1996;17(23):2225–32. https://doi.org/10.1016/0142-9612(95)00311-8.
28. Hanson SR. Blood coagulation and blood-material interations. In: Ratner RD, Hoffman A, Schoen F, Lemons J, editors. Biomaterials science. 2nd ed. San Diego: Academic Press; 2005. p. 332–8.
29. Davies JE, Hosseini MM, Hosseini MM. Histodynamics of endosseous wound healing. In: Davies JE, editor. Bone engineering. Toronto: EM Squared Inc; 2000. p. 1–14.
30. Anderson JM. Blood inflammation, wound healing and foreign body response. In: Ratner RD, Hoffman A, Schoen F, Lemons J, editors. Biomaterials science. 2nd ed. San Diego: Academic Press; 2005. p. 296–304.
31. Spisani S, Giuliani AL, Cavalletti T, Zaccarini M, Milani L, Gavioli R, Traniello S. Modulation of neutrophil functions by activated platelet release factors. Inflammation. 1992;16(2):147–58. https://doi.org/10.1007/BF00918954.
32. Ammon C, Kreutz M, Rehli M, Krause SW, Andreesen R. Platelets induce monocyte differentiation in serum-free coculture. J Leukoc Biol. 1998;63(4):469–76. https://doi.org/10.1002/jlb.63.4.469.
33. Tang Y, Wu X, Lei W, Pang L, Wan C, Shi Z, Zhao L, Nagy TR, Peng X, Hu J, Feng X, Van Hul W, Wan M, Cao X. TGF-beta1-induced migration of bone mesenchymal stem cells couples bone resorption with formation. Nat Med. 2009;15(7):757–65. https://doi.org/10.1038/nm.1979.
34. Gorbet MB, Sefton MV. Biomaterial-associated thrombosis: roles of coagulation factors, complement, platelets and leukocytes. Biomaterials. 2004;25(26):5681–703. https://doi.org/10.1016/j.biomaterials.2004.01.023.
35. Einhorn TA. The science of fracture healing. J Orthop Trauma. 2005;19(10 Suppl):S4–6. https://doi.org/10.1097/00005131-200511101-00002.
36. De Long WG Jr, Einhorn TA, Koval K, McKee M, Smith W, Sanders R, Watson T. Bone grafts and bone graft substitutes in orthopaedic trauma surgery. A critical analysis. J Bone Joint Surg Am. 2007;89(3):649–58. https://doi.org/10.2106/JBJS.F.00465.
37. Sumner DR, Turner TM, Purchio AF, Gombotz WR, Urban RM, Galante JO. Enhancement of bone ingrowth by transforming growth factor-beta. J Bone Joint Surg Am. 1995;77(8):1135–47. https://doi.org/10.2106/00004623-199508000-00001.
38. Lin M, Overgaard S, Glerup H, Søballe K, Bünger C. Transforming growth factor-beta1 adsorbed to tricalciumphosphate coated implants increases peri-implant bone remodeling. Biomaterials. 2001;22(3):189–93. https://doi.org/10.1016/s0142-9612(00)00165-4.
39. Liu Y, Huse RO, de Groot K, Buser D, Hunziker EB. Delivery mode and efficacy of BMP-2 in association with implants. J Dent Res. 2007;86(1):84–9. https://doi.org/10.1177/154405910708600114.
40. Park J, Lutz R, Felszeghy E, Wiltfang J, Nkenke E, Neukam FW, Schlegel KA. The effect on bone regeneration of a liposomal vector to deliver BMP-2 gene to bone grafts in peri-implant bone defects. Biomaterials. 2007;28(17):2772–82. https://doi.org/10.1016/j.biomaterials.2007.02.009.
41. Carmeliet P. Mechanisms of angiogenesis and arteriogenesis. Nat Med. 2000;6(4):389–95. https://doi.org/10.1038/74651.
42. Ferrara N, Davis-Smyth T. The biology of vascular endothelial growth factor. Endocr Rev. 1997;18(1):4–25. https://doi.org/10.1210/edrv.18.1.0287.
43. Fischbach C, Mooney DJ, et al. Polymeric systems for bioinspired delivery of angiogenic molecules. In: Abe A, Albertsson A, Duncan R, Dusek K, de Jeu W, Joanny J, editors. Advances in polymer science, vol. 203. Berlin, Heidelberg: Springer; 2006. p. 191–221.
44. Gerstenfeld LC, Cho TJ, Kon T, Aizawa T, Cruceta J, Graves BD, Einhorn TA. Impaired intramembranous bone formation during bone repair in the absence of tumor necrosis factor-alpha signaling. Cells Tissues Organs. 2001;169(3):285–94. https://doi.org/10.1159/000047893.
45. Crisan M, Yap S, Casteilla L, Chen CW, Corselli M, Park TS, Andriolo G, Sun B, Zheng B, Zhang L, Norotte C, Teng PN, Traas J, Schugar R, Deasy BM, Badylak S, Buhring HJ, Giacobino JP, Lazzari L, Huard J, Péault B. A perivascular origin for mesenchymal stem cells in multiple human organs. Cell Stem Cell. 2008;3(3):301–13. https://doi.org/10.1016/j.stem.2008.07.003.
46. Gruber R, Karreth F, Kandler B, Fuerst G, Rot A, Fischer MB, Watzek G. Platelet-released supernatants increase migration and proliferation, and decrease osteogenic differentiation of bone marrow-derived mesenchymal progenitor cells under in vitro conditions. Platelets. 2004;15(1):29–35. https://doi.org/10.1080/09537100310001643999.

47. Puleo DA, Nanci A. Understanding and controlling the bone-implant interface. Biomaterials. 1999;20(23–24):2311–21. https://doi.org/10.1016/s0142-9612(99)00160-x.
48. Davies JE. Understanding peri-implant endosseous healing. J Dent Educ. 2003;67(8):932–49.
49. Listgarten MA. Soft and hard tissue response to endosseous dental implants. Anat Rec. 1996;245(2):410–25. https://doi.org/10.1002/(SICI)1097-0185(199606)245:2<410::AID--AR20>3.0.CO;2-R.
50. Raghavendra S, Wood MC, Taylor TD. Early wound healing around endosseous implants: a review of the literature. Int J Oral Maxillofac Implants. 2005;20(3):425–31.
51. Pilliar RM. Cementless implant fixation–toward improved reliability. Orthop Clin North Am. 2005;36(1):113–9. https://doi.org/10.1016/j.ocl.2004.08.001.
52. Edwards JT, Brunski JB, Higuchi HW. Mechanical and morphologic investigation of the tensile strength of a bone-hydroxyapatite interface. J Biomed Mater Res. 1997;36(4):454–68. https://doi.org/10.1002/(sici)1097-4636(19970915)36:4<454::aid-jbm3>3.0.co;2-d.
53. Glassman AH, Bobyn JD, Tanzer M. New femoral designs: do they influence stress shielding? Clin Orthop Relat Res. 2006;453:64–74. https://doi.org/10.1097/01.blo.0000246541.41951.20.
54. Kikuchi L, Park JY, Victor C, Davies JE. Platelet interactions with calcium-phosphate-coated surfaces. Biomaterials. 2005;26(26):5285–95. https://doi.org/10.1016/j.biomaterials.2005.01.009.
55. Currey JD. The many adaptations of bone. J Biomech. 2003;36(10):1487–95. https://doi.org/10.1016/s0021-9290(03)00124-6.
56. Einhorn TA, Gerstenfeld LC. Fracture healing: mechanisms and interventions. Nat Rev Rheumatol. 2015;11(1):45–54. https://doi.org/10.1038/nrrheum.2014.164.
57. Dubois G, De Germay B, Schaerer NS, Fennema P. Dynamic neutralization: a new concept for restabilization of the spine. In: Szpalski M, Gunzburg R, Pope MH, editors. Lumbar segmental instability. Philadelphia: Lippincott Williams & Wilkins; 1999. p. 233–24.
58. Özer AF, Aydın AL, Hekimoğlu M, Çerezci Ö, Başak AT, Ates O, Oktenoglu T, Sasani M. Should iliac wing screws be included in long segment dynamic stabilization? Cureus. 2021;13:e13543.
59. Özer AF, Başak AT, Özbek MA, Hekimoğlu M, Aydın AL, Ateş Ö, Günerbüyük C, Akgül T, Sasani M, Öktenoğlu T. Lumbar dynamic stabilization with 2-stage surgery: early results. Int J Spine Surg. 2022:8306. https://doi.org/10.14444/8306.

Vertebral Body Tethering

22

Turgut Akgul and Murat Korkmaz

The reported incidence rate for adolescent idiopathic scoliosis (AIS) is 1–3%, without etiological acknowledgment. Dickson et al. theorized that AIS's development and progression were due to an imbalance in sagittal alignment. On the basis of this data, it was thought that thoracal lordosis resulted in rotational instability, causing the spine to rotate and laterally translate, creating three-dimensional (3D) scoliotic deformity [1].

Progression of this deformity has been described as a vicious cycle in which constant pathologic pressure inhibits the endochondral longitudinal growth of the posterior aspect of the spine. At the same time, reduced compression accelerates the growth of the anterior aspect of the spine. Two scientists described this phenomenon, and this theory is known as the Hueter–Volkmann effect. According to this theory, longitudinal growth is decelerated at the compression side and accelerated at the distraction level [2]. If the scoliotic deformity is greater than >20 Cobb angle, the apex vertebral body becomes asymmetrical due to unbalanced forces focused on the vertebral body [3].

T. Akgul (✉) · M. Korkmaz
Faculty of Medicine, Department of Orthopaedics and Traumatology, Koç University Hospital Spine Center, Istanbul, Turkey
e-mail: takgul@kuh.ku.edu.tr

Conservative or growth-friendly treatments attempt to balance or reverse the compression and distraction forces' effect on the vertebra. The growth-friendly method, which is the growing rod, is based on the distraction method performed by the surgeon at reported time intervals. On the other hand, the anterior approach with apical instrumentation is based on compression at the convex side and distraction at the concave side indirectly with longitudinal growing (Fig. 22.1). The first reported data with this type of surgery was published with anterior vertebral body stapling. However, the reported results varied due to nonstandard patient selection [4, 5]. Although the overall results reported in the literature are promising, this treatment option has yet to be popularized. Newton et al. performed anterolateral instrumentation with a flexible, ultrahigh-molecular-weight polyethylene ribbon combination in an immature porcine model in 2008 [6]. The results showed that anterolateral flexible tethering has a high chance of controlling forces that can deform the vertebra. They conclude that dynamic anterolateral instrumentation is safe and beneficial in treating scoliosis. The latest clinical study by Crawford et al. showed that anterolateral tethering reverses a vicious cycle, according to the Hueter–Volkmann theory, in patients with scoliotic deformity. Charles and colleagues reported that if the patients have scoliotic deformity with a curve degree between 21° and 30° at pubertal onset, the fusion rate would be 75%.

A. F. Özer et al. (eds.), *Dynamic Lumbar Spine Stabilization*,
https://doi.org/10.1007/978-3-032-12122-6_22

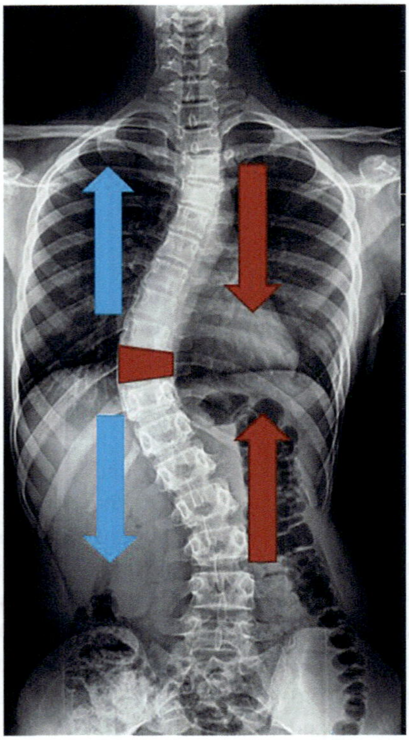

Fig. 22.1 The figures show distraction (blue arrows) and compression (red arrows) forces that act on the apical vertebra of deformity. The apical vertebral deformity occurred after the unbalanced action of the forces. The main idea of VBT is to create a compression force at the convex side and a distraction force at the concave side

This rate is higher in patients with a scoliotic deformity magnitude higher than 30° [7]. Fusion surgery is accepted as the gold standard for scoliosis surgery. Fusion is an irreversible procedure and has negative effects such as growth arrest, decreased range of motion (ROM), decreased spinal mobility, and adjacent disc degeneration [8]. Nowadays, to protect patients from fusion's side effects, the non-fusion method seems to be a better solution for scoliosis surgical treatment.

22.1 Indication

Amir Samdani introduced vertebral body tethering (VBT) in 2015 [9]. They reported their 1-year clinical results for their first 32 patients with immature adolescent idiopathic scoliosis. They emphasized that VBT is a safe and potentially effective treatment modality in the selected patient group. On the other hand, Crawford published the first case in the literature in 2010. The author emphasized that this procedure is safe and effective in growing children [10]. Samdani et al. reported that the indication for VBT is skeletally immature patients with idiopathic scoliosis and curves between 35° and 60°. In addition, the curves must demonstrate 50% flexibility, with 40 kyphosis (Fig. 22.2). Also, they recommended this surgery for children above 10 years of age due to the implant design and a rib hump prominence bigger than 20°. Several studies showed clinically and radiologically satisfactory results [9, 11].

Samdani recommended VBT indication for patients with thoracal or thoracolumbar scoliosis. Later, the authors reported lumbar curve tethering indication as a lumbar curve magnitude between 35° and 75° [11–14] (Fig. 22.3). Current FDA humanitarian device exemption (HDE) indications include skeletally immature patients with major Cobb angles of 30°–65° involving thoracic or lumbar curves for which bracing has failed or who are intolerant to brace wear. The main issue is the determination of the remaining growth potential for VBT. Authors agree that the Sanders skeletal maturity staging is better than the Risser sign. According to Alanay et al., follow-up curve behavior after VBT differs in patients with different Sanders stages. Sanders 2 patients experienced overcorrection more; thus, the timing and correction should be adjusted. Sanders 3, 4, and 5 patients displayed a lower risk of mechanical complications [15]. Trobishi et al. performed VBT surgery in all patients with Sanders 7 [11]. Also, the Sanders skeletal maturity staging is used to calculate the estimated correction ratio individually. Vertebral body tethering (VBT) is a motion-preserving method compared to fusion surgery. There are limited clinical studies focused on motion preservation. Pehlivanoğlu et al. showed that patients with VBT have a superior range of motion compared to patients in the posterior spinal fusion group [16]. Mathew et al.

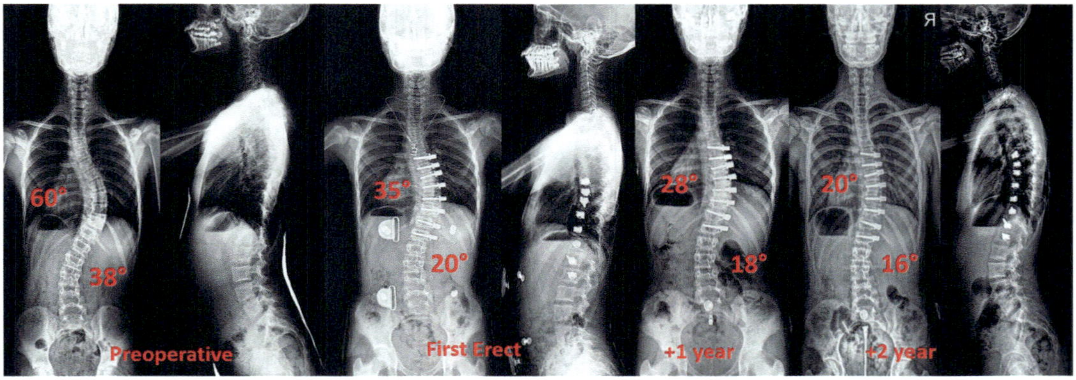

Fig. 22.2 The Lenke Type 1A AIS patient was treated with thoracal VBT

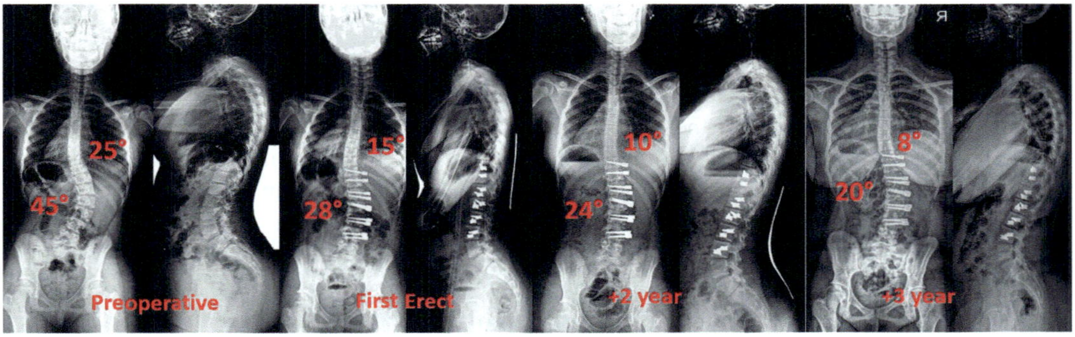

Fig. 22.3 The Lenke Type 5C AIS patient was treated with lumbar VBT with double tethering

reported the results after lumbar and thoracolumbar VBT with respect to patients' lumbar range of motion. According to this study, lumbar VBT resulted in preserved flexion and extension motion 1 year postoperatively [17]. Also, they noted some preserved coronal plane motion, but this was decreased compared with the preoperative values by ~50%. Buyuk et al. presented their patients' thoracal range of motion after thoracal VBT surgery. These patients maintained coronal (mean 7°) and sagittal (21°) arcs of motion at the 1-year follow-up, even though the coronal movement was significantly reduced from a preoperative value of 30° [18]. Human cadaver study performed by Nicolini et al. was designed to achieve the change in the range of motion at the thoracolumbar area (T10–L3). This biomechanical study showed similar results to clinical studies, as VBT techniques preserve the global ROM of the spine in flexion, extension, and axial rotation while reducing the ROM in lateral bending [19].

22.2 Surgical Technique

The VBT device is made up of two components. The tether component is a tubular construct with a uniform width, manufactured from Ultra-high-molecular-weight polyethylene (UHMWPE). It is anchored to a vertebral body component made of titanium alloy. Some of the authors suggest the usage of staple (Fig. 22.4).

Patients are induced under general anesthesia using a double-lumen endotracheal tube. Deflating the lung gives a better visualization and approach to the thoracal vertebral bodties. Patients are positioned in a lateral decubitus posi-

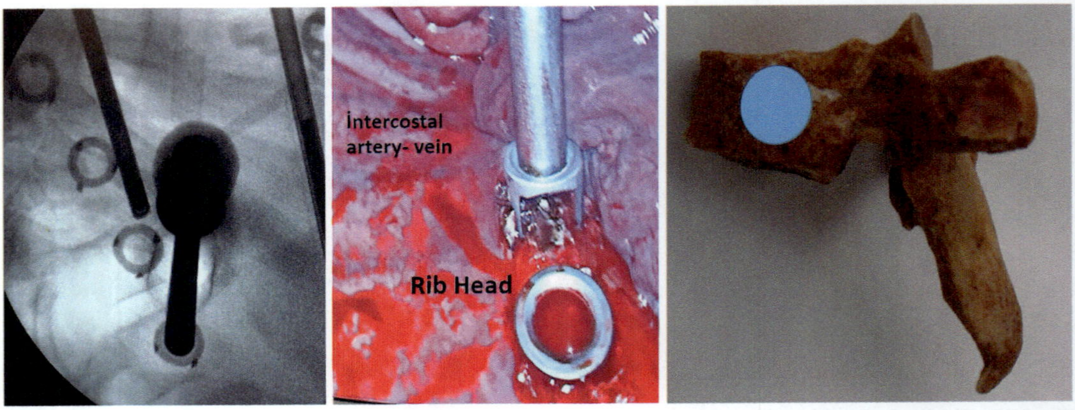

Fig. 22.4 The staple was positioned under a fluoroscopic view. The ideal position is the center of the vertebra corpus at the lateral area, just in front of the costal head for the thoracal area. The ideal position is the center of the vertebra corpus at the lateral area for the lumbar area

tion, with the convex side of the deformity facing upward. A soft gel roll supports the axilla area and the knee to protect against compression injury. Patients are stabilized with external support and tape. After the patient is positioned, the instrumentation level is checked with fluoroscopy with two positions: lateral and anterioposterior (AP) views. Thoracoscopic or mini-open thoracotomy can be chosen for exposure, and for lumbar exposure, the mini-open retroperitoneal approach is recommended. The first viewing portal is at the T5–T6 intercostal space along the anterior axillary line. Access to this first portal is usually done in a blind fashion, and the surgeon needs to be careful not to damage the lungs. Generally, a 10-mm, 45° scope is used during thoracoscopy. A second portal is made along the anterior axillary at the T8–T9 intercostal space through direct visualization using a thoracoscope. This portal facilitates dissection, instrument handling, and cable tensioning. The viewing portals are 1 cm in length. The instrumentation portals are 3 cm in length or long enough to pass the instruments (Fig. 22.5). Generally, five portals are enough for VBT surgery. With this approach, it is possible to reach the vertebral body from the T4 to the L2 vertebra corpus.

The pleura is dissected off 1 cm anteriorly from the rib head and vertebral junction, and the vertebral body is exposed to receive the instrumentation using electrocautery. The segmental vessels are dissected, exposed, and ligated using electrocautery. Due to the learning curve of thoracoscopy and setup requirements, mini-thoracotomy can be used for VBT. In mini-thoracotomy, a 5-cm, oblique incision, parallel to the ribs, is performed at the apex of deformity at the convex side. Due to the lack of reach proximally and distally for vertebral body instrumentation, extra instrumentation portals are performed at the proximal and distal sides, according to instrumentation level (Fig. 22.6). Determining the instrumentation level is suggested Cobb to Cobb and tether tensioned to bring the tilted discs into neutral alignment where possible. Instrumentation is performed under fluoroscopy view. The screw placement is anterior to the rib head, center at the thoracal vertebra in the lateral plane (Fig. 22.7), and parallel to the end plate in the coronal plane. All implanted screws can have either a unicortical or a bicortical purchase. The screw length will be measured after the vertebra is tapped. The positioned screw is either 6.0 or 6.5 mm in diameter. The screw length starts from 35 mm in the classic design. If a small screw is needed, the screw should be cut.

After all the screws are inserted, cable insertion and deformity correction are performed. Cable insertion is started at the proximal through the distal level. Segmental tensioning, transla-

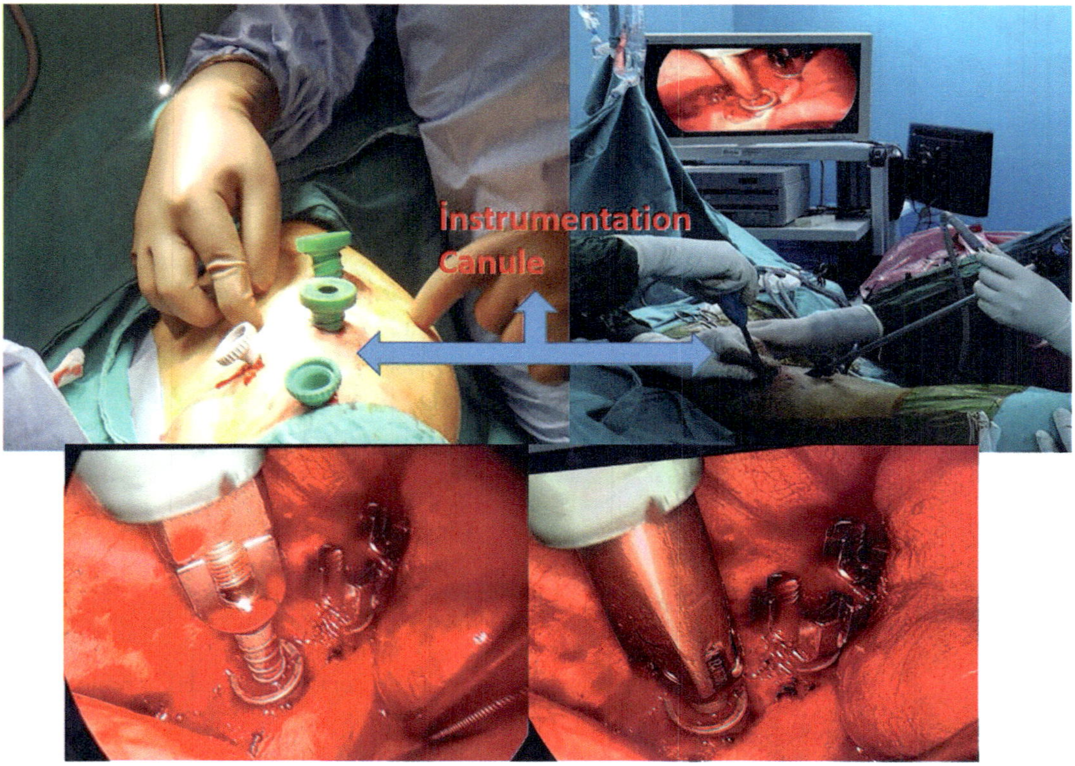

Fig. 22.5 The viewing portals are 1 cm in length and located anteriorly (white portal). The instrumentation portals are 3 cm long or long enough to pass the instruments and are located posteriorly (green portal). Generally, five portals are enough for VBT surgery. This approach makes it possible to reach from the T4 to the L2 vertebral bodies

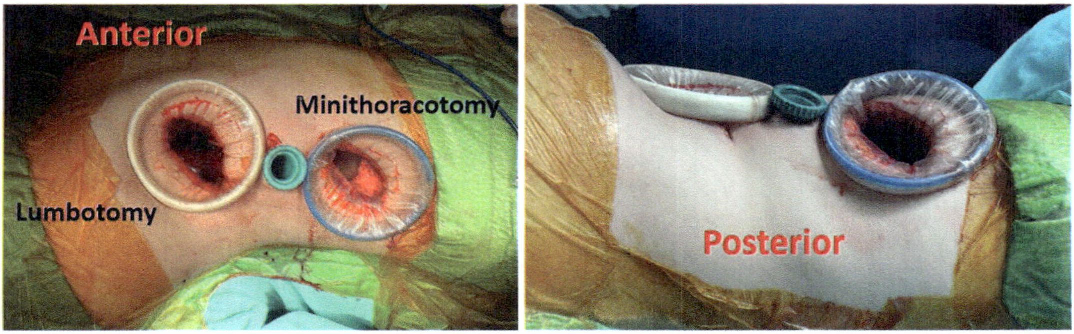

Fig. 22.6 Mini-thoracotomy and mini-lumbotomy could be performed for instrumentation

tion, and derotation are performed in each segment subsequently (Fig. 22.8). Tensioning is performed via a special external device or by grasping the cable with forceps and rotating the forceps at the base of the screw. Maximal tension is applied at the apex of deformity. In our practice, we tried to bring the end plates of the vertebra parallelly under fluoroscopy control for defor-

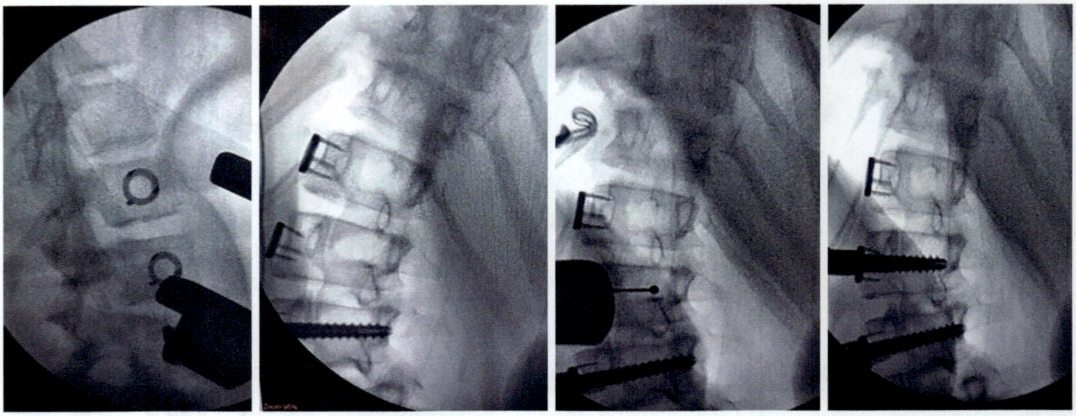

Fig. 22.7 The screw placement was performed under AP and lateral fluoroscopic views. At the lateral view, the screw entry point should be the center of the vertebral body, and the trajectory of the screw should be parallel to the disc space at the AP plane

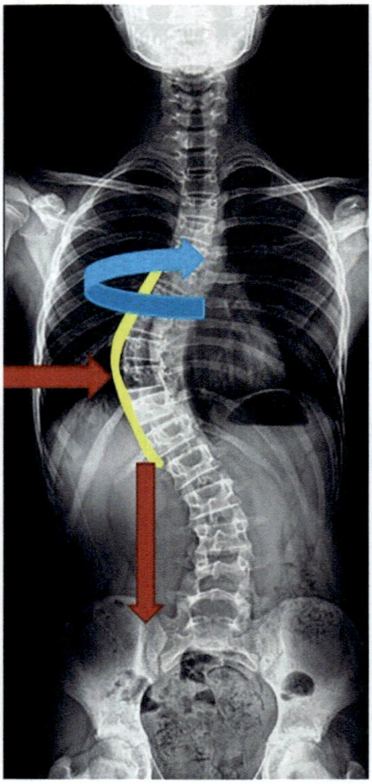

Fig. 22.8 The figure shows the correction maneuver. Segmental tensioning (red arrow), translation, and derotation (blue arrow) are performed in each segment subsequently, using a screwdriver and a tether (yellow) tensioning device

mity correction (Fig. 22.9). It was recommended that the cable should be left a minimum of 2–3 cm out of the instrumentation level.

Mini-lumbotomy can be used to reduce classical lumbotomy problems in cases that require long-level instrumentation in the lumbar region. This technique is similar to minimally invasive lateral access, although the incision line is oblique and longer than discectomies for this technique. In this technique, the segmental vessel should be coagulated or ligated (Fig. 22.6). The psoas muscle should be mobilized posteriorly to create a safe instrumentation area at the vertebral body laterally. It is recommended to use double screws and a row to decrease the row rupture rate. The acceptable position of the screw is at the middle of the corpus and just parallel to the disc space. The row tensioning is started at the proximal level to distally under fluoroscopy. The tensioning of the anterior or posterior row is chosen according to lumbar lordosis. A 28-French chest tube is inserted after controlling lung inflation and bleeding. The chest tube is removed when the drainage amount is below 50 cc daily. A daily chest X-ray is taken for hemo- and pneumothorax.

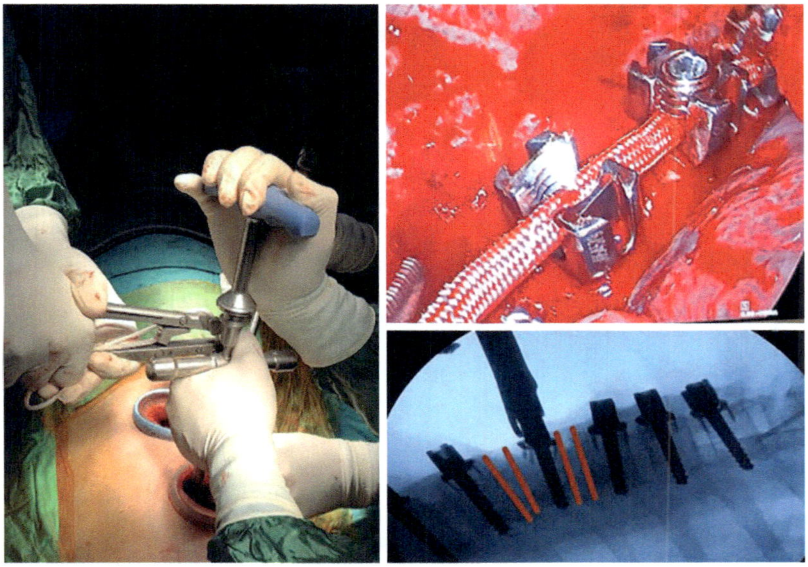

Fig. 22.9 In our daily practice, we tried to bring the end plates of the vertebra parallelly under fluoroscopy control for deformity correction, as shown in the figure

22.3 Complication

Complications were classified under three subgroups: perioperative, postoperative surgery-related, and tether-specific complications [20, 21].

Bleeding is the most common complication seen intraoperatively. Generally, it can occur due to inadequate segmental vessel dissection and coagulation. A formal thoracotomy can be performed to achieve adequate coagulation. Lung parenchyma damage is another rare complication. This complication should be treated with an expert thoracic surgeon for repair or follow-up. Chylothorax can be seen after VBT surgery. Dietary lipid intake restriction and prolonged thorax tube drainage are recommended to treat this complication. Atelectasis, hemothorax, and pneumothorax are reported complications after VBT surgery related to thorax surgery. Despite using navigation or fluoroscopy, screw malposition can be seen. If screw malposition has occurred, screw repositioning is recommended. cerebrospinal fluid (CSF) leakage after spinal canal penetration with screw malposition was reported in the literature [20, 21].

Tether-related complications are reported as overcorrection, tether breakage, and adding-on problem in patients with idiopathic scoliosis. This complication rate was reported at up to 41% [20]. Revision surgery suggested tethering revision or fusion surgery related to the complication. Tether breakage and overcorrection can be revised with tether revision or release (Fig. 22.10). Conversely, if the patient had an inadequate correction and adding on due to tethered breakage, then fusion surgery is recommended. A *tether breakage* was defined as a change of more than 5° in the angulation of two screws in the adjacent levels compared to previous images. It was reported that CT with 3D reconstruction has a high capability to show tether breakage. Alanay et al. reported tether breakage at 3% percent. However, other studies showed a higher breakage rate: 48% in Hoernschemeyer's study and 52% in Newton's work for thoracal VBT [15, 22, 23]. Vatkar et al. reported that overcorrection and mechanical complications were seen in 14.3% and 27.5% of cases, respectively.

Pulmonary complications, including atelectasis and pleural effusion, were seen in 9.7% of

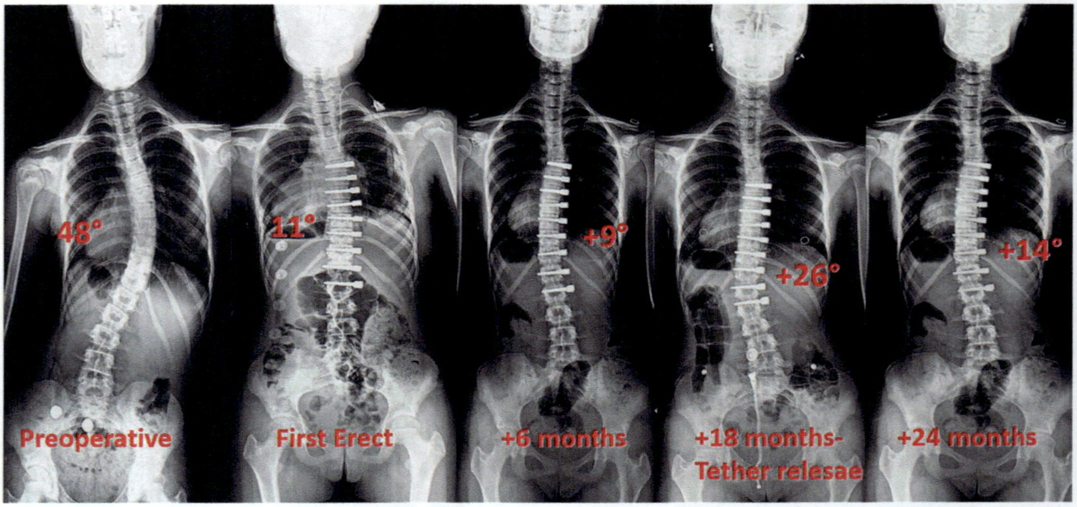

Fig. 22.10 The patient with scoliosis was treated with VBT. The overcorrection occurred at the time of follow-up. Tether release and physical therapy were performed for correction

patients. Tether revision was performed in 7.85% and revision to a spinal fusion in 7.88% [24].

Trobishi et al. reported tether breakage at 24% for single tether and 16% for double tether in patients with lumbar VBT. The revision rate for tethered breakage was reported at 10% by the same authors [12]. The latest reported data by the same team for VBT in the lumbar spine showed a 50% coronal curve correction 2 years postoperatively despite a tether breakage in 90% of patients. The revision for tether breakage was just for 2 out of 41 patients [25]. Boeyer et al. reported similar results regarding lumbar curve behavior after VBT. The success rate was 57%, regardless of the Lenke classification, and suspected tether breakage was observed in 16 of 28 consecutive patients [26].

Tether revision has risks of potential pulmonary complications due to scar tissue and adherence at the thorax. A surgical strategy for exposing the previous implants is a "back-to-front" dissection and exposure. This approach uses an ultrasonic dissector or a monopolar cautery to dissect from the posterior portion of the adherence or scar tissue adjacent to the lung parenchyma. This strategy allows anteriorly progressive lung mobilization, allowing exposure to the previous implants.

22.4 Results

"Clinical success" was defined a priori based on previously described criteria [21, 23]. Cases were considered a success if, at functional unit, they had not undergone (or were awaiting) fusion and their tethered curves were <35. The extensive data reported by Rushton et al. showed that the success rate according to clinical success criteria was 71% in 112 cases [27]. Patients with a smaller major Cobb angle and high flexibility had better results than others. This result is smaller than the first results reported by Samdani et al., with a 66% curve correction [11]. On the other hand, Newton et al. reported a high revision rate of 41% due to inappropriate patient selection [23]. Pioneers of VBT surgeries agreed that careful patient selection with appropriate Cobb angle is the key to successful results. In their latest paper, Samdani et al. reported that 80% of patients had curves of <30° at the most recent follow-up, where patients were followed up for an average of 55.2 ± 12.5 months [28]. Vatkar et al. reported the meta-analysis for VBT in the treatment of AIS. According to this paper, there was a significant correction of the main thoracic curve of scoliosis (mean preoperative Cobb angle of 48.5° and postoperative Cobb angle at the final

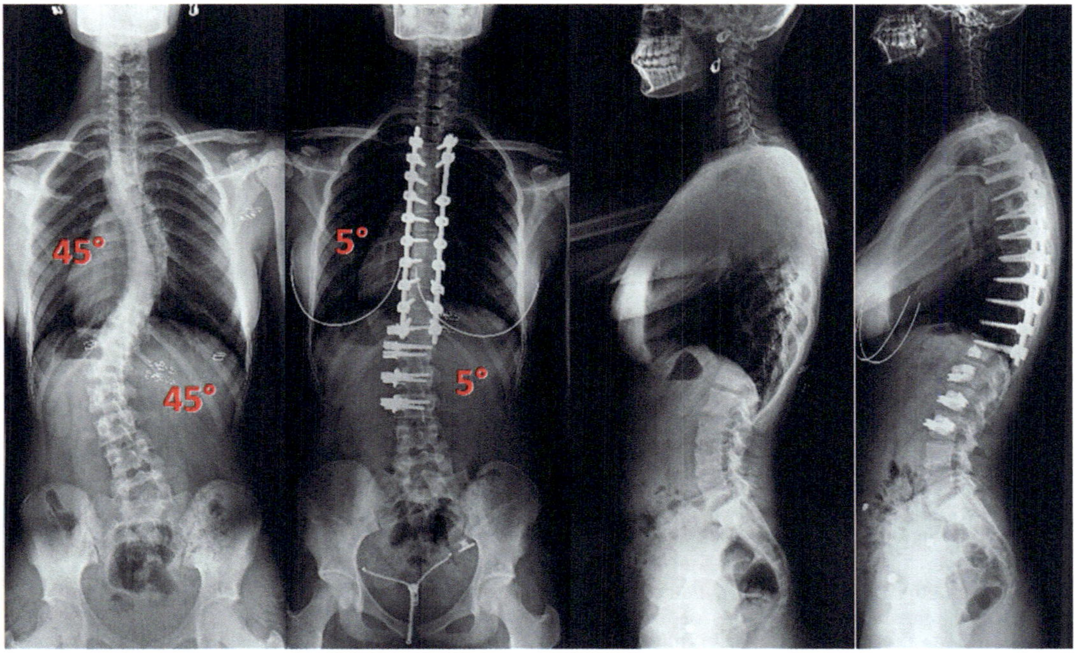

Fig. 22.11 In our daily practice, we use the hybrid system for AIS, which includes a selective thoracal fusion, with tethering for the lumbar area. A Lenke 6C patient was operated on with a hybrid system

follow-up of 20.1°, $P = 0.01$), with several complication rates.

It was well-known that VBT has a higher complication rate than fusion surgery, with a lower success rate in curve magnitude reduction [23, 24]. The studies showed that VBT successfully preserved spine motion [24].

Trobishi et al. defined clinical success criteria for lumbar VBT surgery. According to Trobishi et al., surgery was defined as "successful" when the lumbar curve measured <30 at the 1-year follow-up, "acceptable" for curves measuring 31–40, and "failed" for curves measuring >41. The overall success rate was 66%, and the acceptable was 26% in patients with lumbar VBT; on the other hand, the rate of failure was reported at 8% with lumbar VBT surgery [12]. The latest reported data by the same team for VBT in the lumbar spine showed a 50% coronal curve correction 2 years postoperatively despite a tether breakage in 90% of patients [25].

Instrumentation systems for Anterior Vertebral Body Growth Modulation (AVBGM) recently obtained approval from the FDA in 2019 for the vertebral body tethering system (Zimmer Biomet). This is a promising surgery for skeletally immature patients with scoliosis. The literature needs long-term follow-up and randomized controlled studies for VBT. In our daily practice, we use the hybrid system for AIS, which includes a selective thoracal fusion, with tethering for the lumbar area (Fig. 22.11). So far, the literature needs more data or publications about this hybrid model.

22.5 Conclusion

Vertebral body tethering (VBT) is a motion-preserving method using growth modulation against fusion surgery. Although the reported complication rate exceeds posterior spinal fusion (PSF), VBT surgery shows high radiological and clinical success in selected cases. The most important issue is selecting the appropriate patients for better results. Our knowledge about VBT changes with time and increases with the number of cases.

References

1. Dickson R, Lawton J, Archer I, et al. The pathogenesis of idiopathic scoliosis: biplanar spinal asymmetry. J Bone Joint Surg. 1984;66-B:8–15.
2. Arkin AM, Katz JF. The effects of pressure on epiphyseal growth. The mechanism of plasticity of growing bone. J Bone Joint Surg Am. 1956;38:1056–76.
3. Stokes IA, Spence H, Aronsson DD, Kilmer N. Mechanical modulation of vertebral body growth: implications for scoliosis progression. Spine. 1996;21(10):1162–7.
4. Betz RR, Kim J, D'Andrea LP, Mulcahey MJ, Balsara RK, Clements DH. An innovative technique of vertebral body stapling for the treatment of patients with adolescent idiopathic scoliosis: a feasibility, safety, and utility study. Spine. 2003;28(20):S255–65.
5. Betz RR, D'Andrea LP, Mulcahey MJ, Chafetz RS. Vertebral body stapling procedure for the treatment of scoliosis in the growing child. Clin Orthop Relat Res. 2005;434:55–60.
6. Newton PO, Upasani VV, Farnsworth CL, Oka R, Chambers RC, Dwek J, Kim JR, Perry A, Mahar AT. Spinal growth modulation with use of a tether in an immature porcine model. Spine (Phila Pa 1976). 2008;33(7):724–33.
7. Charles YP, Daures JP, de Rosa V, Diméglio A. Progression risk of idiopathic juvenile scoliosis during pubertal growth. Spine (Phila Pa 1976). 2006;31(17):1933–42.
8. Rinella A, Bridwell K, Kim Y, Rudzki J, Edwards C, Roh M, et al. Late complications of adult idiopathic scoliosis primary fusions to L4 and above: the effect of age and distal fusion level. Spine. 2004;29(3):318–25.
9. Samdani AF, Ames RJ, Kimball JS, Pahys JM, Grewal H, Pelletier GJ, Betz RR. Anterior vertebral body tethering for idiopathic scoliosis: two-year results. Spine. 2014;39(20):1688–93.
10. Crawford CH 3rd, Lenke LG. Growth modulation by means of anterior tethering resulting in progressive correction of juvenile idiopathic scoliosis: a case report. J Bone Joint Surg Am. 2010;92(1):202–9.
11. Samdani AF, Ames RJ, Kimball JS, Pahys JM, Grewal H, Pelletier GJ, Betz RR. Anterior vertebral body tethering for immature adolescent idiopathic scoliosis: one-year results on the first 32 patients. Eur Spine J. 2015;24(7):1533–9. Epub 2014 Dec 16.
12. Trobisch PD, Baroncini A. Preliminary outcomes after vertebral body tethering (VBT) for lumbar curves and subanalysis of a 1- versus 2-tether construct. Eur Spine J. 2021;30:3570–6.
13. Hoernschemeyer DG, Boeyer ME, Robertson ME, Loftis CM, Worley JR, Tweedy NM, Gupta SU, Duren DL, Holzhauser CM, Ramachandran VM. Anterior vertebral body tethering for adolescent scoliosis with growth remaining: a retrospective review of 2 to 5-year post-operative results. J Bone Joint Surg Am. 2020;102(13):1169–76.
14. Rushton PRP, Nasto L, Parent S, Turgeon I, Aldebeyan S, Miyanji F. Anterior vertebral body tethering for treatment of idiopathic scoliosis in the skeletally immature: results of 112 cases. Spine. 2021;46(21):1461–7.
15. Alanay A, Yucekul A, Abul K, Ergene G, Senay S, Ay B, Cebeci BO, Dikmen PY, Zulemyan T, Yavuz Y, Yilgor C. Thoracoscopic vertebral body tethering for adolescent idiopathic scoliosis: follow-up curve behavior according to sanders skeletal maturity staging. Spine. 2020. https://doi.org/10.1097/BRS.0000000000003643.
16. Pehlivanoglu T, Oltulu I, Erdag Y, Akturk UD, Korkmaz E, Yildirim E, Sarioglu E, Ofuoglu E, Aydogan M. Comparison of clinical and functional outcomes of vertebral body tethering to posterior spinal fusion in patients with adolescent idiopathic scoliosis and evaluation of quality of life: preliminary results. Spine Deform. 2021;9(4):1175–82.
17. Mathew SE, Milbrandt TA, Larson AN. Measurable lumbar motion remains 1 year after vertebral body tethering. J Pediatr Orthop. 2022;42(8):e861–7.
18. Buyuk AF, Milbrandt TA, Mathew SE, Larson AN. Measurable thoracic motion remains at 1 year following anterior vertebral body tethering, with sagittal motion greater than coronal motion. J Bone Joint Surg Am. 2021;103:2299–305. https://doi.org/10.2106/JBJS.20.01533.
19. Nicolini LF, Kobbe P, Seggewiß J, Greven J, Ribeiro M, Beckmann A, Da Paz S, Eschweiler J, Prescher A, Markert B, Stofel M, Hildebrand F, Trobisch PD. Motion preservation surgery for scoliosis with a vertebral body tethering system: a biomechanical study. Eur Spine J. 2022;31:1013–21.
20. Shin M, Arguelles GR, Cahill PJ, Flynn JM, Baldwin KD, Anari JB. Complications, reoperations, and mid-term outcomes following anterior vertebral body tethering versus posterior spinal fusion: a meta-analysis. JBJS Open Access. 2021;6(2):e21.00002.
21. Newton PO, Kluck DG, Saito W, Yaszay B, Bartley CE, Bastrom TP. Anterior spinal growth tethering for skeletally immature patients with scoliosis: a retrospective look two to four years post-operatively. J Bone Joint Surg Am. 2018;100(19):1691–7.
22. Hoernschemeyer DG, Boeyer ME, Robertson ME, et al. Anterior vertebral body tethering for adolescent scoliosis with growth remaining: a retrospective review of 2 to 5-year post-operative results. J Bone Joint Surg Am. 2020;102:1169–76.
23. Newton PO, Bartley CE, Bastrom TP, et al. Anterior spinal growth modulation in skeletally immature patients with idiopathic scoliosis: a comparison with posterior spinal fusion at 2 to 5 years post-operatively. J Bone Joint Surg Am. 2020;102:769–77.
24. Vatkar A, Najjar E, Patel M, Quraishi NA. Vertebral body tethering in adolescent idiopathic scoliosis with more than 2 years of follow-up- systematic review and meta-analysis. Eur Spine J. 2023. https://doi.org/10.1007/s00586-023-07724-2.

25. Trobisch PD, Castelein R, Da Paz S. Radiographic outcome after vertebral body tethering of the lumbar spine. Eur Spine J. 2023;32:1895–900.
26. Boeyer ME, Farid S, Wiesemann S, Hoernschemeyer DG. Outcomes of vertebral body tethering in the lumbar spine. Deform. 2023;11:909–18.
27. Rushton PRP, Nasto L, Parent S, Turgeon I, Aldebeyan S, Miyanji F. Anterior vertebral body tethering for treatment of idiopathic scoliosis in the skeletally immature: results of 112 cases. Spine (Phila Pa 1976). 2021;46(21):1461–7.
28. Samdani AF, Pahys JM, Ames RJ, Grewal H, Pelletier GJ, Hwang SW, Betz RR. Prospective follow-up report on anterior vertebral body tethering for idiopathic scoliosis: interim results from an FDA IDE study. J Bone Joint Surg Am. 2021;103(17):1611–9. https://doi.org/10.2106/JBJS.20.01503.

23 Reevaluation of Treatment in Lumbar Disc Surgery

Ali Fahir Özer and Erkan Kutlu Ekiz

23.1 Introduction

Since the publication of a landmark article by Mixter and Barr [1] 80 years ago, lumbar discectomy has become one of the most common spine surgeries worldwide. Nonetheless, it is still a controversial surgery due to several problems that have been encountered over time. Numerous articles have been published on lumbar disc herniation. The key aspects investigated in these studies are recurrence rates and evaluation of patient satisfaction. With the advances in knowledge and technology, several changes have been made in the surgical approach to improve these outcomes. In this article, we discuss the most important risk factors leading to the development of lumbar disc herniation and underline the key considerations that can help improve the chances of successful surgery in patients with disc herniation.

The first discectomy results pertained to the classical period. The subsequent introduction of the microscope in the field of lumbar disc surgery helped achieve better results compared to the classical approach. However, later studies found no significant difference in outcomes compared to the classical approach [2–4]. The same phenomenon now applies to endoscopic approaches. Despite the very good results obtained with endoscopic surgery, there is no robust evidence of its superiority over the microscopic approach. Most studies pertaining to endoscopic discectomy have concluded that, despite the better results of the endoscopic approach, there is a need for larger studies involving long-term follow-up to obtain more definitive evidence [5–8]. A meta-analysis of many studies reported identical success rates of classical discectomy, microdiscetomy, and endoscopic discectomy (79% success rate with all three approaches) [9].

In our opinion, the focus on overall recurrence rates and patient satisfaction evaluation in the contemporary literature is not particularly meaningful. This is because some underlying pathologies that play a role in the development of lumbar disc herniation, which we will discuss later, affect the recurrence rates and, thus, patient satisfaction. It would be more appropriate to assess satisfaction and recurrence rates specifically among groups of patients with these underlying pathologies. We believe that evaluating the groups separately will also inform changes in the treatment approach for these patients. A literature review published by Drazinn in 2016 found no consensus on the optimal approach after rediscectomy, and the same situation has persisted to date [10].

In this section, we will discuss the factors affecting the outcomes of lumbar disc herniation surgery and the appropriate treatment algorithms.

A. F. Özer (✉)
Department of Neurosurgery, Koc University School of Medicine, Istanbul, Turkey

E. K. Ekiz
Cam Sakura Hospital, Istanbul, Turkey

A. F. Özer et al. (eds.), *Dynamic Lumbar Spine Stabilization*,
https://doi.org/10.1007/978-3-032-12122-6_23

While lumbar disc herniation has long been considered a separate pathology compared to degenerative disc disease, it actually represents a variation of it. Under laboratory conditions, inducing herniation of a healthy disc necessitates a load of tens of Newtons [11, 12]. For most patients, the clinical picture of disc herniation develops gradually with much smaller loads. This is because the degenerative process is initiated much before the development of disc herniation. Initially, the nucleus pulposus starts to lose water, followed by bulging, resulting from decreasing intradiscal pressure, and the occurrence of tears in the annulus [13–18]. Almost all patients have a history of chronic lower back pain and acute painful attacks, which constitute the clinical picture of degenerative disc disease.

In the vast majority of cases, segmental instability resulting from disc deterioration due to a degenerative process is the main pathology underlying the development of disc herniation, as described by Panjabi [19]. For successful outcomes of lumbar disc surgery, the musculotendinous system of the patient is as important as the skill of the surgeon. The patient's musculature should also be strong enough to compensate for the discectomized segment. The main point we wish to reinforce here is that even if a discectomy is performed in a small area with a microscope or an endoscope, the muscular compartment of the patients should be able to compensate for the segment that is further deteriorated after discectomy. If not, recurrence and patient dissatisfaction due to pain are inevitable. Of note, disc surgery is a destructive surgery, and in order to reduce the possibility of recurrence, healthy tissue is removed during discectomy along with the damaged disc. In a significant proportion of patients, the leg pain is replaced by a serious lower back pain, leading to the continuation of patient dissatisfaction. Our overall recurrence rate was 15.42% in all patients. This result is consistent with the literature. However, what is the recurrence rate and satisfaction rate in the group of patients who are at a high risk of recurrence? The answer to this question is very important for appropriate patient evaluation and treatment decision-making.

23.2 Factors Affecting Recurrence

In this section, we review the important factors that affect recurrence in patients presenting with recurrent disc herniation after lumbar discectomy. These factors were identified using the ready-to-publish data of our own department [20].

The first factor that particularly draws our attention in these patients is the large rupture of the annulus. The mean rupture of the annulus is 13.31 mm, while the mean rupture of the annulus in patients with recurrence is 25.85 mm. Although many previous studies have investigated lower back pain and annular rupture, Carrage [21] stated the importance of disc herniation in the treatment/outcome relationship. This study identified a relationship between the size of the rupture in the annulus and recurrence, and only fragmentectomy was recommended for extruded fragments. The patient's complaint is important in cases with preserved integrity of the annulus but the presence of a large annular defect. It has been stated that if the patient does not have many complaints, not touching the disc is an important option. If a discectomy is to be performed, a subtotal discectomy has been recommended to reduce the rate of recurrence. In our recurrence cases, the annular rupture is approximately 2 cm (Fig. 23.1).

It should be noted that the surgeon may also contribute to enlarging the rupture while performing a discectomy. Other authors have also emphasized the importance of rupture in the annulus [22–26]. A key consideration is the choice between subtotal discectomy and limited discectomy. Carrage [21] recommended fragmentectomy and limited discectomy for patients with a small annulus defect or an undetectable annulus defect and an extruded fragment. We fully support this approach. However, subtotal discectomy was recommended for patients with a large defect in the annulus in order to reduce the recurrence rate. Subtotal discectomy has been commonly performed for the same reason, and when patients were treated in this way, the concepts of instability were not as well-known as at present [27]. However, after subtotal discectomy,

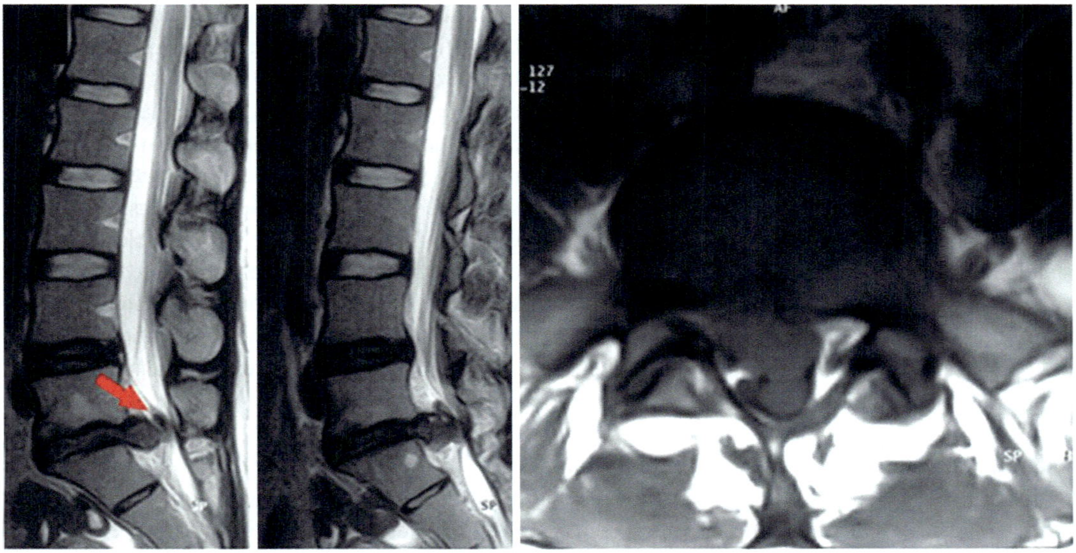

Fig. 23.1 There is a direct correlation between the size of the rupture in the annulus and the recurrence of disc herniation

some patients developed instability leading to severe lower back pain. In this emerging situation, it was argued that instead of removing the entire disc, only the fragment should be removed, and the intact disc tissue should not be touched [28, 29]. Naturally, recurrence rates are higher after limited discectomy, but the lack of consensus between limited discectomy and subtotal discectomy is an ongoing debate even today.

In the prospective randomized study by Barth et al. [30], limited discectomy was performed in 40 patients, and subtotal discectomy was performed in 38 patients. The patients were followed up for 2 years. At the end of the follow-up, there was no significant between-group difference with respect to the recurrence rate (12.5% in the limited discectomy group and 10.5% in the subtotal discectomy group). However, many retrospective studies comparing these two techniques have reported contradictory results. In one study, limited discectomy was associated with a lower recurrence rate [31], while another study found a recurrence rate of 21% after limited discectomy and 0% after subtotal discectomy [32].

McGirt et al. [33] performed a meta-analysis of 54 studies involving 13,359 lumbar discectomy cases to compare the two methods (6135 patients had undergone limited discectomy, while 7224 patients had undergone aggressive discectomy). The incidence of recurrent lower back pain or leg pain shortly after surgery was found to be similar in the two groups (mean: 14.5% for limited discectomy and 14.1% for aggressive discectomy). However, more than 2 years after surgery, the reported incidence of recurrent lower back pain or leg pain was 2.5 times lower after limited discectomy (11.6%) compared to that after aggressive discectomy (27.8%). In contrast, more than 2 years after surgery, the incidence of recurrent disc herniation after limited discectomy (7%) was higher than that after aggressive discectomy (3.5%).

On the premise that evidence from randomized studies is more robust and that meta-analyses provide a reliable synthesis of evidence from multiple studies, a question that needs to be answered is this: "Why we chose limited discectomy if aggressive discectomy reduces recurrence rates?" The answer to this question is important. After aggressive discectomy, there should be no deterioration in the function of the functional segment. Development of any instability in the functional segment that cannot be overcome with compensatory mechanisms is liable to cause recurrent disc herniation. If instability occurs immediately after surgery, the patient may emerge from anesthesia with instability, or the instability may develop later. The risk of development of recurrent disc herniation is directly proportional to the degree of instability. Even if there is no recurrence, abnormal motion in the functional segment may cause lower back pain. A patient may complain of low back pain immediately upon standing or feel pain after walking a few steps; some patients may even develop compensatory scoliosis. Therefore, the patient's quality of life may decrease after aggressive discectomy. If recurrent disc herniation is not detected in a patient with low back pain, spinal segment instability is often overlooked, misinterpreted as a secondary gain quest, and the symptoms are attributed to psychological causes. However, if a herniation is present, the patient's symptoms are assumed to be real, which is incorrect because the likelihood of these patients benefiting from rediscectomy surgery is reduced. The problem here is segmental instability. The operated motion segment cannot support the patient's torso, and abnormal movements within the segment cause low back pain. This condition may or may not be accompanied by a herniated disc. In this case, the cause of the pain is uncompensated segmental instability, and the correct approach is to stabilize the segment.

An intervertebral disc affected by Modic degeneration is characterized by impaired metabolism, resulting in a state of chronic starvation [34–38]. This results in Modic degeneration via two modes. In the first, the disc develops internal disruption, progresses to Modic type III stage, and shows spontaneous impairment of mobilization due to calcification. In the other mode, the disc height is high and cannot tolerate the developing Modic degeneration. The impaired structural integrity of the disc results in herniation. Discectomy performed on such a disc usually ends with reherniation. Studies have shown that Modic types I and II are painful [39–42]. When a discectomy is performed on a herniated disc with Modic degeneration, it is very difficult for the chronically starved disc to preserve the integrity of the functional unit. The unrecoverable disc increases the segmental instability in the functional unit and causes reherniation from the discectomy defect in the annulus. In our patient series, 12 patients had Modic degeneration with a large defect in the annulus. In five of these patients, there was no motion in the lower segment due to sacralization. When we consider the contribution of each factor to recurrence, the recurrence rate in this group of patients is much higher than the general average. In our own series, this rate is 78%. These findings suggest that the overall recurrence rate in an unselected cohort of patients who have undergone discectomy is not very meaningful in the context of underlying factors. It is undeniable that the development of Modic degeneration not only increases degeneration in the disc but also facilitates the formation of the defect in the annulus (Fig. 23.2).

On review of our patient series, seven patients showed no motion in the functional unit under the disc where herniation developed due to sacralization, spontaneous fusion, or other causes. Biomechanical studies have shown that the loss of motion in the functional unit due to sacralization or another reason causes hypermobility in the upper segment. Accordingly, it is

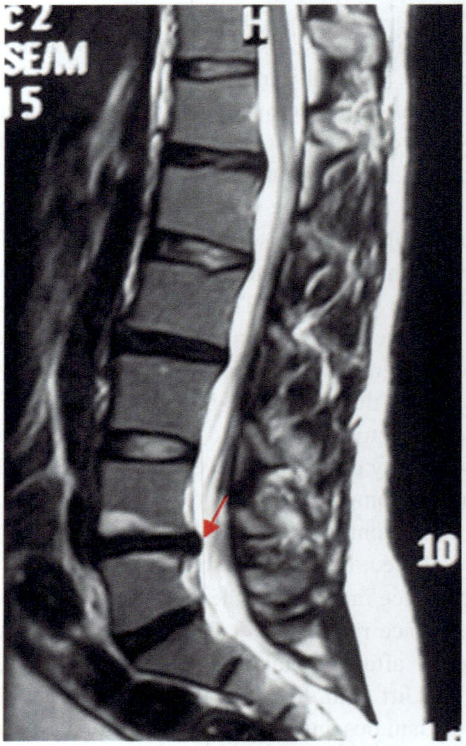

Fig. 23.2 Modic degeneration and disc herniation

known that intradiscal pressure increases as a result of increased stress in the upper disc. Whether degeneration in an upper segment is due to natural aging or increased disc pressure and hypermobility has been contested in the literature. On the other hand, another fact is that the immobile segment also causes stress on the facet joints above. It is inevitable that these persistent changes in the functional unit above the immobile segment will cause degeneration and, ultimately, hypermobility. The hypermobility and degeneration cascade of the disc is an important factor leading to the development of disc herniation. Even if a simple discectomy is performed, because discectomy is a destructive surgery, the continuation of the hypermobility and degeneration cascade after discectomy is liable to lead to reherniation (Fig. 23.3).

Failure of the muscle compartment to control the abnormal movement in the functional unit is liable to lead to recurrence in these patients [43–54]. However, it is important to note that hypermobility may not always be associated with instability. Gymnasts do not experience any pain during their maneuvers, although the spine is extremely mobile. Therefore, in this article, we are referring to hypermobility that develops as a result of abnormal motion caused by the functional unit due to structural failure [55].

Finally, it is necessary to talk about muscles. Although muscles are known to be major contributors to spinal stabilization, there is no method for the quantitative evaluation of their contribution. Indirect information about paraspinal muscles can be obtained by visual examination of MR sections, based on the assessment of the color, amount, and volume of fatty degeneration. The examination of 29 patients with recurrence in our series revealed an age-related decrease in muscle volume and enlarged fat areas in some of the muscle bundles. Thus, it is plausible that the preexisting age-related deterioration of muscle quality may lead to the emergence of a suitable environment for recurrence in advanced age because of the gradual age-related deactivation of the most important natural protection system that provides segmental stability (Fig. 23.4).

Ultimately, there must be practical conclusions to be drawn from this knowledge. Regardless of the method used for lumbar disc surgery, surgical treatment methods should be reconsidered, especially in patients with the above risk factors. Rediscectomy can be considered in a limited number of patients. Simple discectomy can be considered if there is remnant disc material abutting the nerve root in a patient in whom there is no residual material in the disc space and the distance between the vertebrae has

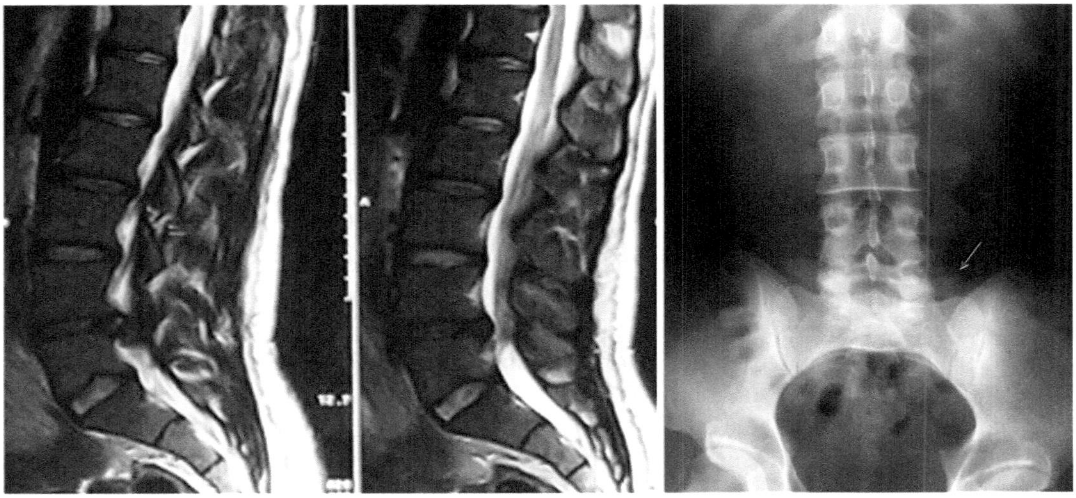

Fig. 23.3 Development of herniation in the disc above the sacralized segment is a common condition

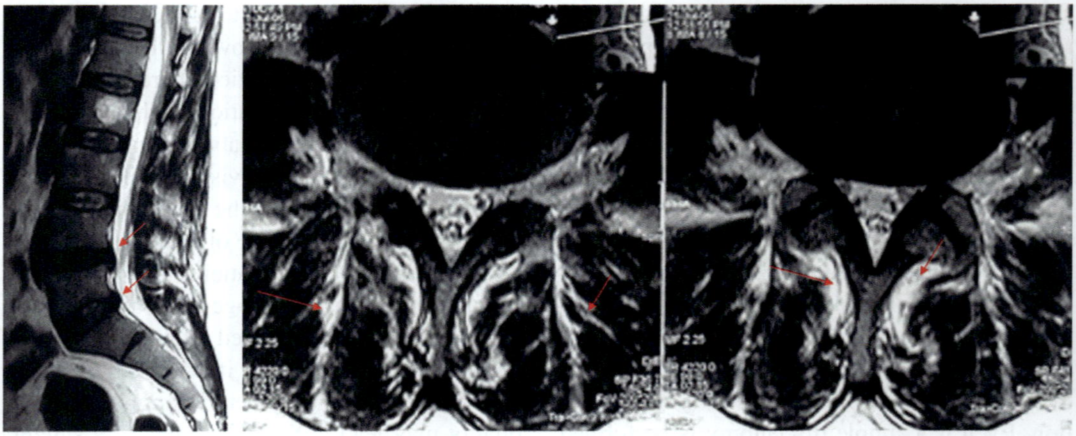

Fig. 23.4 MRI examination of a 63-year-old man showing enlarged areas of adipose tissue between the muscle tissue, whose volume has begun to decrease and color has begun to lighten. Wide-based disc herniation developed in the L4–5 and L5–S1 discs. Adele's compensation began to deteriorate

disappeared. Stabilization may not be considered in this motion segment, which has lost its mobility, and rediscectomy may be considered as an option in such cases. Successive discectomies following a simple discectomy have been shown to increase the complication rate, without any tangible beneficial effects [56–59]. Therefore, fusion surgery has become a widely used option in the United States for repeat surgery [56].

In patients with the abovementioned risks, stabilization can be considered even in the first surgery after discussing the high probability of recurrence with the patient. This is because the beneficial effects of surgery decrease with each discectomy operation, along with a concomitant increase in complication rates. Here, the following question will arise. Should we perform fusion right after discectomy? Fusion at the time of the first surgery for a simple discectomy is indeed an option that should be considered. However, fusion is not without its own ill effects. Indeed, fusion prepares the ground for adjacent segment disease. If there are signs of degeneration in the adjacent segment also, this probability is much higher [60, 61]. In order to reduce the risks, there is an increasing interest in the use of minimally invasive methods for fusion surgery. However, Singh [62] reported a 7% pseudoarthrosis rate in a cohort of 573 patients in whom it was used together with rhBMP-2. Again, if the disc height is >10 mm before the operation, there is an increased risk of pseudoarthrosis. In addition, angulated discs with a higher anterior disc height than posterior are more likely to develop pseudoarthrosis [63–65].

In addition, many other factors need to be considered, such as age, osteoporosis, obesity, and nicotine use. It should be noted that after the development of pseudoarthrosis, revision surgery has to be a larger surgery than the primary surgery. Therefore, rediscectomy is easier for surgeons but is often not the best cure for the patient. Therefore, treatment decision-making after post-discectomy recurrence is a large gray area. One can perform a simple discectomy surgery, but there is a high possibility of recurrence due to the reasons explained above; however, if one performs fusion after a simple discectomy, it will generally be considered overtreatment. This dilemma is experienced by many surgeons. Therefore, a simple discectomy is one of the most problematic surgeries in spine surgery when its results are taken into account.

From this perspective, pedicular dynamic systems are the surgical methods that are likely to fill this gap. Studies have shown acceptable outcomes of single-level dynamic stabilization. The procedure is relatively easy to perform in high-risk patient groups [66–74]. In patients with the abovementioned risk factors, it should be performed together with the primary surgery. The complication rates of this approach cannot be directly compared with fusion surgery because any revision is much easier than fusion surgery.

Lumbar disc surgery has continued to be a key challenge for spinal surgeons. In this article, we emphasized the fact that global recurrence rates are not particularly helpful in guiding the choice of surgical approach. The recurrence rates should be evaluated taking cognizance of the underlying risk factors for recurrence. This would require an in-depth evaluation of individual cases. In addition, we emphasize that simple soft stabilization systems can play an important role in solving the problem.

The conclusion we will draw here is that the main pathology underlying the development of disc herniation is segmental instability, which may occur with disc deterioration [19, 75, 76]. It may occur before surgery, but in most of the cases, it may develop after surgery. This is not so rare. If there is no instability in the patient after the discectomy operation, the surgeon and the patient are lucky; however, if there is instability, a rediscectomy should be followed by a second rediscectomy and then followed by fusion surgery. The next step that can pass through this cascade is the stabilization of the defective functional unit with a dynamic system. In particular, dynamic stabilization without deteriorating the structure of the disc is important in terms of maintaining motion (Fig. 23.5) [77].

In the setting of advanced disc degeneration, aside from maintaining motion, the segment to

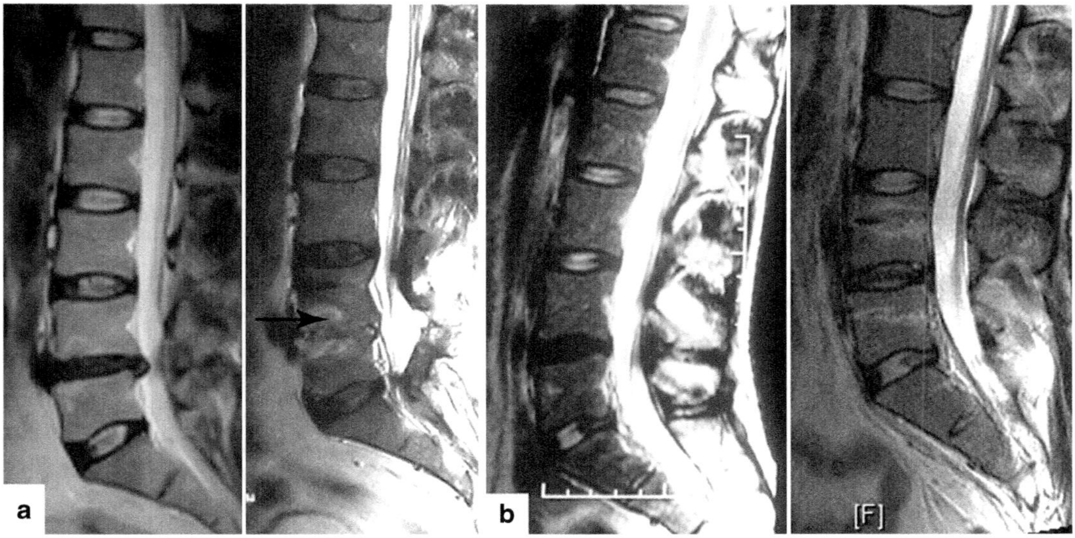

Fig. 23.5 (**a**) The first patient has an upper cartilage end plate Schmorl's nodule in the disc. Although the disc appears more hydrated compared to the second patient, it rapidly fused after discectomy. (**b**) In the second patient, the disc, which was more degenerate than in the first patient, was rehydrated

which the discectomy is made will go into fusion and will give a result equivalent to fusion.

References

1. Mixter WJ, Barr JS. Rupture of the intervertebral disc with involvement of the spinal canal. N Engl J Med. 1934;211:210–5.
2. Porchet F, Bartanusz V, Kleinstueck FS, Lattig F, Jeszenszky D, Grob D, Mannion AF. Microdiscectomy compared with standard discectomy: an old problem revisited with new outcome measures within the framework of a spine surgical registry. Eur Spine J. 2009;18 Suppl 3(Suppl 3):360–6. https://doi.org/10.1007/s00586-009-0917-9.
3. Rasouli MR, Rahimi-Movaghar V, Shokraneh F, Moradi-Lakeh M, Chou R. Minimally invasive discectomy versus microdiscectomy/open discectomy for symptomatic lumbar disc herniation. Cochrane Database Syst Rev. 2014;(9):CD010328. https://doi.org/10.1002/14651858.CD010328.pub2.
4. Türeyen K. One-level one-sided lumbar disc surgery with and without microscopic assistance: 1-year outcome in 114 consecutive patients. J Neurosurg. 2003;99(3 Suppl):247–50. https://doi.org/10.3171/spi.2003.99.3.0247.
5. Barber SM, Nakhla J, Konakondla S, Fridley JS, Oyelese AA, Gokaslan ZL, Telfeian AE. Outcomes of endoscopic discectomy compared with open microdiscectomy and tubular microdiscectomy for lumbar disc herniations: a meta-analysis. J Neurosurg Spine. 2019:1–14. https://doi.org/10.3171/2019.6.SPINE19532.
6. Katayama Y, Matsuyama Y, Yoshihara H, Sakai Y, Nakamura H, Nakashima S, Ito Z, Ishiguro N. Comparison of surgical outcomes between macro discectomy and micro discectomy for lumbar disc herniation: a prospective randomized study with surgery performed by the same spine surgeon. J Spinal Disord Tech. 2006;19(5):344–7. https://doi.org/10.1097/01.bsd.0000211201.93125.1c.
7. Meyer G, Rocha IDDA, Cristante AF, Marcon RM, Coutinho TP, Torelli AG, Petersen PA, Letaif OB, Filho TEPDEB. Percutaneous endoscopic lumbar discectomy versus microdiscectomy for the treatment of lumbar disc herniation: pain, disability, and complication rate-a randomized clinical trial. Int J Spine Surg. 2020;14(1):72–8. https://doi.org/10.14444/7010.
8. Kim M, Lee S, Kim HS, Park S, Shim SY, Lim DJ. A comparison of percutaneous endoscopic lumbar discectomy and open lumbar microdiscectomy for lumbar disc herniation in the korean: a meta-analysis. Biomed Res Int. 2018;2018:9073460. https://doi.org/10.1155/2018/9073460.
9. Dohrmann GJ, Mansour N. Long-term results of various operations for lumbar disc herniation: analysis of over 39,000 patients. Med Princ Pract. 2015;24(3):285–90. https://doi.org/10.1159/000375499.
10. Drazin D, Ugiliweneza B, Al-Khouja L, Yang D, Johnson P, Kim T, Boakye M. Treatment of recurrent disc herniation: a systematic review. Cureus. 2016;8(5):e622. https://doi.org/10.7759/cureus.622.
11. Adams MA, Hutton WC, Stott JR. The resistance to flexion of the lumbar intervertebral joint. Spine (Phila Pa 1976). 1980;5(3):245–53. https://doi.org/10.1097/00007632-198005000-00007.
12. Oktenoglu T, Ece K. Biomechanics of lumbar spine and lumbar disc; lomber degenerative disc disease and dynamic stabilisation. In: Ozer AF, Cosar M, editors. . Turkey: Intertip Publishing House; 2016. p. 23–37.
13. Adams MA, Roughley PJ. What is intervertebral disc degeneration, and what causes it? Spine (Phila Pa 1976). 2006;31(18):2151–61. https://doi.org/10.1097/01.brs.0000231761.73859.2c.
14. Abbott RD, Purmessur D, Monsey RD, Brigstock DR, Laudier DM, Iatridis JC. Degenerative grade affects the responses of human nucleus pulposus cells to link-N, CTGF, and TGFβ3. J Spinal Disord Tech. 2013;26(3):E86–94. https://doi.org/10.1097/BSD.0b013e31826e0ca4.
15. Chan WC, Sze KL, Samartzis D, Leung VY, Chan D. Structure and biology of the intervertebral disk in health and disease. Orthop Clin North Am. 2011;42(4):447–64, vii. https://doi.org/10.1016/j.ocl.2011.07.012.
16. Le Maitre CL, Freemont AJ, Hoyland JA. Accelerated cellular senescence in degenerate intervertebral discs: a possible role in the pathogenesis of intervertebral disc degeneration. Arthritis Res Ther. 2007;9(3):R45. https://doi.org/10.1186/ar2198.
17. Peng B, Wu W, Hou S, Li P, Zhang C, Yang Y. The pathogenesis of discogenic low back pain. J Bone Joint Surg Br. 2005;87(1):62–7.
18. Pfirrmann CW, Metzdorf A, Zanetti M, Hodler J, Boos N. Magnetic resonance classification of lumbar intervertebral disc degeneration. Spine (Phila Pa 1976). 2001;26(17):1873–8. https://doi.org/10.1097/00007632-200109010-00011.
19. Panjabi MM. The stabilizing system of the spine. Part II. Neutral zone and instability hypothesis. J Spinal Disord. 1992;5(4):390–6. https://doi.org/10.1097/00002517-199212000-00002.
20. Karadağ MK, Akıncı AT, Başak AT, Hekimoğlu M, Yıldırım H, Akyoldaş G, Aydın AL, Ateş Ö, Öktenoğlu T, Sasani M, Akgün MY, Günerbüyük C, Özer AF. Preoperative magnetic resonance imaging abnormalities predictive of lumbar herniation recurrence after surgical repair. World Neurosurg. 2022;165:e750–6.
21. Carragee EJ, Han MY, Suen PW, Kim D. Clinical outcomes after lumbar discectomy for sciatica: the effects of fragment type and anular competence. J Bone Joint Surg Am. 2003;85(1):102–8.

22. Tenny S, Gillis CC. Annular disc tear. [Updated 2021 Aug 11]. In: StatPearls [Internet]. Treasure Island (FL): StatPearls Publishing; 2021.
23. Ma XL. A new pathological classification of lumbar disc protrusion and its clinical significance. Orthop Surg. 2015;7(1):1–12. https://doi.org/10.1111/os.12152.
24. Parker SL, Mendenhall SK, Godil SS, Sivasubramanian P, Cahill K, Ziewacz J, McGirt MJ. Incidence of low back pain after lumbar discectomy for herniated disc and its effect on patient-reported outcomes. Clin Orthop Relat Res. 2015;473(6):1988–99. https://doi.org/10.1007/s11999-015-4193-1.
25. Bailey A, Araghi A, Blumenthal S, Huffmon GV, Anular Repair Clinical Study Group. Prospective, multicenter, randomized, controlled study of anular repair in lumbar discectomy: two-year follow-up. Spine (Phila Pa 1976). 2013;38(14):1161–9. https://doi.org/10.1097/BRS.0b013e31828b2e2f.
26. Wera GD, Marcus RE, Ghanayem AJ, Bohlman HH. Failure within one year following subtotal lumbar discectomy. J Bone Joint Surg Am. 2008;90(1):10–5. https://doi.org/10.2106/JBJS.F.01569.
27. O'Connele JE. Protrusions of the lumbar intervertebral discs, a clinical review based on five hundred cases treated by excision of the protrusion. J Bone Joint Surg Br. 1951;33-B(1):8–30. https://doi.org/10.1302/0301-620X.33B1.8.
28. Williams RW. Microlumbar discectomy: a conservative surgical approach to the virgin herniated lumbar disc. Spine (Phila Pa 1976). 1978;3(2):175–82.
29. Spengler DM. Lumbar discectomy. Results with limited disc excision and selective foraminotomy. Spine (Phila Pa 1976). 1982;7(6):604–7.
30. Barth M, Weiss C, Thomé C. Two-year outcome after lumbar microdiscectomy versus microscopic sequestrectomy: part 1: evaluation of clinical outcome. Spine (Phila Pa 1976). 2008;33(3):265–72. https://doi.org/10.1097/BRS.0b013e318162018c.
31. Rogers LA. Experience with limited versus extensive disc removal in patients undergoing microsurgical operations for ruptured lumbar discs. Neurosurgery. 1988;22(1 Pt 1):82–5. https://doi.org/10.1227/00006123-198801010-00013.
32. Faulhauer K, Manicke C. Fragment excision versus conventional disc removal in the microsurgical treatment of herniated lumbar disc. Acta Neurochir. 1995;133(3–4):107–11. https://doi.org/10.1007/BF01420059.
33. McGirt MJ, Ambrossi GL, Datoo G, Sciubba DM, Witham TF, Wolinsky JP, Gokaslan ZL, Bydon A. Recurrent disc herniation and long-term back pain after primary lumbar discectomy: review of outcomes reported for limited versus aggressive disc removal. Neurosurgery. 2009;64(2):338–44. https://doi.org/10.1227/01.NEU.0000337574.58662.E2.
34. Modic MT, Steinberg PM, Ross JS, Masaryk TJ, Carter JR. Degenerative disk disease: assessment of changes in vertebral body marrow with MR imaging. Radiology. 1988;166(1 Pt 1):193–9. https://doi.org/10.1148/radiology.166.1.3336678.
35. Carragee EJ, Spinnickie AO, Alamin TF, Paragioudakis S. A prospective controlled study of limited versus subtotal posterior discectomy: short-term outcomes in patients with herniated lumbar intervertebral discs and large posterior anular defect. Spine (Phila Pa 1976). 2006;31(6):653–7. https://doi.org/10.1097/01.brs.0000203714.76250.68.
36. Han C, Ma X, Ma J, et al. Distribution characteristics of Modic changes of lumbar endplate and its relationship with low back pain. Zhongguo Xiu Fu Chong Jian Wai Ke Za Zhi. 2009;23:1409–12. (in Chinese).
37. Hutton MJ, Bayer JH, Powell JM. Modic vertebral body changes: the natural history as assessed by consecutive magnetic resonance imaging. Spine (Phila Pa 1976). 2011;36(26):2304–7. https://doi.org/10.1097/BRS.0b013e31821604b6.
38. Ma XL, Ma JX, Wang T, Tian P, Han C. Possible role of autoimmune reaction in Modic Type I changes. Med Hypotheses. 2011;76(5):692–4. https://doi.org/10.1016/j.mehy.2011.01.035.
39. Eser O, Gomleksiz C, Sasani M, Oktenoglu T, Aydin AL, Ataker Y, Suzer T, Ozer AF. Dynamic stabilisation in the treatment of degenerative disc disease with modic changes. Adv Orthop. 2013;2013:806267. https://doi.org/10.1155/2013/806267.
40. Laustsen AF, Bech-Azeddine R. Do Modic changes have an impact on clinical outcome in lumbar spine surgery? A systematic literature review. Eur Spine J. 2016;25(11):3735–45. https://doi.org/10.1007/s00586-016-4609-y.
41. Shahmohammadi MR, Behrouzian S. Effect of preoperative modic change in the outcome of patients with low back pain following posterior spinal fusion or laminectomy. Asian J Neurosurg. 2019;14(2):432–5. https://doi.org/10.4103/ajns.AJNS_41_18.
42. Rahme R, Moussa R. The modic vertebral endplate and marrow changes: pathologic significance and relation to low back pain and segmental instability of the lumbar spine. AJNR Am J Neuroradiol. 2008;29(5):838–42. https://doi.org/10.3174/ajnr.A0925.
43. Ha KY, Schendel MJ, Lewis JL, Ogilvie JW. Effect of immobilization and configuration on lumbar adjacent-segment biomechanics. J Spinal Disord. 1993;6(2):99–105.
44. Ohtonari T, Kitagawa T, Ota T, Nishihara N. Preliminary results on radiological hypermobility at upper adjacent disc level in posterior lumbar interbody fusion compared to advanced dynamic stabilization. Neurol Med Chir (Tokyo). 2020;60(8):375–82. https://doi.org/10.2176/nmc.oa.2019-0255.
45. Cakir B, Carazzo C, Schmidt R, Mattes T, Reichel H, Käfer W. Adjacent segment mobility after rigid and semirigid instrumentation of the lumbar spine. Spine (Phila Pa 1976). 2009;34(12):1287–91. https://doi.org/10.1097/BRS.0b013e3181a136ab.

46. Bastian L, Lange U, Knop C, Tusch G, Blauth M. Evaluation of the mobility of adjacent segments after posterior thoracolumbar fixation: a biomechanical study. Eur Spine J. 2001;10(4):295–300. https://doi.org/10.1007/s005860100278.
47. Chow DH, Luk KD, Evans JH, Leong JC. Effects of short anterior lumbar interbody fusion on biomechanics of neighboring unfused segments. Spine (Phila Pa 1976). 1996;21(5):549–55. https://doi.org/10.1097/00007632-199603010-00004.
48. Esses SI, Doherty BJ, Crawford MJ, Dreyzin V. Kinematic evaluation of lumbar fusion techniques. Spine (Phila Pa 1976). 1996;21(6):676–84. https://doi.org/10.1097/00007632-199603150-00003.
49. Saavedra-Pozo FM, Deusdara RA, Benzel EC. Adjacent segment disease perspective and review of the literature. Ochsner J. 2014;14(1):78–83.
50. Lau KKL, Samartzis D, To NSC, Harada GK, An HS, Wong AYL. Demographic, surgical, and radiographic risk factors for symptomatic adjacent segment disease after lumbar fusion: a systematic review and meta-analysis. J Bone Joint Surg Am. 2021;103(15):1438–50. https://doi.org/10.2106/JBJS.20.00408.
51. Hekimoğlu M, Başak A, Yılmaz A, Yıldırım H, Aydın AL, Karadag K, Özer AF. Adjacent segment disease (ASD) in incidental segmental fused vertebra and comparison with the effect of stabilization systems on ASD. Cureus. 2021;13(10):e18647. https://doi.org/10.7759/cureus.18647.
52. Penta M, Sandhu A, Fraser RD. Magnetic resonance imaging assessment of disc degeneration 10 years after anterior lumbar interbody fusion. Spine (Phila Pa 1976). 1995;20(6):743–7. https://doi.org/10.1097/00007632-199503150-00018.
53. Etebar S, Cahill DW. Risk factors for adjacent-segment failure following lumbar fixation with rigid instrumentation for degenerative instability. J Neurosurg. 1999;90(2 Suppl):163–9. https://doi.org/10.3171/spi.1999.90.2.0163.
54. Hilibrand AS, Robbins M. Adjacent segment degeneration and adjacent segment disease: the consequences of spinal fusion? Spine J. 2004;4(6 Suppl):190S–4S. https://doi.org/10.1016/j.spinee.2004.07.007.
55. Paris SV. Physical signs of instability. Spine (Phila Pa 1976). 1985;10(3):277–9. https://doi.org/10.1097/00007632-198504000-00016.
56. Lubelski D, Senol N, Silverstein MP, Alvin MD, Benzel EC, Mroz TE, Schlenk R. Quality of life outcomes after revision lumbar discectomy. J Neurosurg Spine. 2015;22(2):173–8. https://doi.org/10.3171/2014.10.SPINE14359.
57. Patel N, Pople IK, Cummins BH. Revisional lumbar microdiscectomy: an analysis of operative findings and clinical outcome. Br J Neurosurg. 1995;9(6):733–7. https://doi.org/10.1080/02688699550040684.
58. Papadopoulos EC, Girardi FP, Sandhu HS, Sama AA, Parvataneni HK, O'Leary PF, Cammisa FP Jr. Outcome of revision discectomies following recurrent lumbar disc herniation. Spine (Phila Pa 1976). 2006;31(13):1473–6. https://doi.org/10.1097/01.brs.0000219872.43318.7a.
59. O'Sullivan MG, Connolly AE, Buckley TF. Recurrent lumbar disc protrusion. Br J Neurosurg. 1990;4(4):319–25. https://doi.org/10.3109/02688699008992741.
60. Wang H, Ma L, Yang D, Wang T, Liu S, Yang S, Ding W. Incidence and risk factors of adjacent segment disease following posterior decompression and instrumented fusion for degenerative lumbar disorders. Medicine (Baltimore). 2017;96(5):e6032. https://doi.org/10.1097/MD.0000000000006032.
61. Wang T, Ding W. Risk factors for adjacent segment degeneration after posterior lumbar fusion surgery in treatment for degenerative lumbar disorders: a meta-analysis. J Orthop Surg Res. 2020;15(1):582. https://doi.org/10.1186/s13018-020-02032-7.
62. Singh K, Nandyala SV, Marquez-Lara A, Cha TD, Khan SN, Fineberg SJ, Pelton MA. Clinical sequelae after rhBMP-2 use in a minimally invasive transforaminal lumbar interbody fusion. Spine J. 2013;13(9):1118–25. https://doi.org/10.1016/j.spinee.2013.07.028.
63. Sato S, Yagi M, Machida M, Yasuda A, Konomi T, Miyake A, Fujiyoshi K, Kaneko S, Takemitsu M, Machida M, Yato Y, Asazuma T. Reoperation rate and risk factors of elective spinal surgery for degenerative spondylolisthesis: minimum 5-year follow-up. Spine J. 2015;15(7):1536–44. https://doi.org/10.1016/j.spinee.2015.02.009.
64. Lee YP, Sclafani J, Garfin SR. Lumbar pseudarthrosis: diagnosis and treatment. Semin Spine Surg. 2011;23:275–81.
65. Emami A, Faloon M, Sahai N, Dunn CJ, Issa K, Thibaudeau D, Sinha K, Hwang KS. Risk factors for pseudarthrosis in minimally-invasive transforaminal lumbar interbody fusion. Asian Spine J. 2018;12(5):830–8. https://doi.org/10.31616/asj.2018.12.5.830.
66. Ozer AF, Oktenoglu T, Egemen E, Sasani M, Yilmaz A, Erbulut DU, Yaman O, Suzer T. Lumbar single-level dynamic stabilization with semi-rigid and full dynamic systems: a retrospective clinical and radiological analysis of 71 patients. Clin Orthop Surg. 2017;9(3):310–6. https://doi.org/10.4055/cios.2017.9.3.310.
67. Oktenoglu T, Erbulut DU, Kiapour A, Ozer AF, Lazoglu I, Kaner T, Sasani M, Goel VK. Pedicle screw-based posterior dynamic stabilisation of the lumbar spine: in vitro cadaver investigation and a finite element study. Comput Methods Biomech Biomed Engin. 2015;18(11):1252–61. https://doi.org/10.1080/10255842.2014.890187.
68. Erbulut DU, Zafarparandeh I, Ozer AF, Goel VK. Biomechanics of posterior dynamic stabilization systems. Adv Orthop. 2013;2013:451956. https://doi.org/10.1155/2013/451956.
69. Kaner T, Sasani M, Oktenoglu T, Aydin AL, Ozer AF. Minimum two-year follow-up of cases with recurrent disc herniation treated with microdiscectomy and

posterior dynamic transpedicular stabilisation. Open Orthop J. 2010;4:120–5. https://doi.org/10.2174/1874325001004010120.
70. Kaner T, Sasani M, Oktenoglu T, Cosar M, Ozer AF. Clinical outcomes after posterior dynamic transpedicular stabilization with limited lumbar discectomy: Carragee classification system for lumbar disc herniations. SAS J. 2010;4(3):92–7. https://doi.org/10.1016/j.esas.2010.06.001.
71. Ammerman J, Watters WC, Inzana JA, Carragee G, Groff MW. Closing the treatment gap for lumbar disc herniation patients with large annular defects: a systematic review of techniques and outcomes in this high-risk population. Cureus. 2019;11(5):e4613. https://doi.org/10.7759/cureus.4613.
72. Liao Z, Chen W, Wang Z, Wei H. Clinical study of a new transpedicular nonfusion posterior dynamic stabilization system for treating herniated lumbar intervertebral disks. Neurosurg Q. 2015;25(3):427–31. https://doi.org/10.1097/WNQ.0000000000000182.
73. Huo X, Hu C, Zhang Y, Yang S, Yang D, Ding W. Curative effects of Dynesys dynamic stabilization system for lumbar intervertebral disc herniation. Int J Clin Exp Med. 2017;10(11):15459–64.
74. Ozer AF, Suzer T, Cezayirli P, Erbulut D. Evaluating lumbar disc herniation and other motion segment pathologies from the window of dynamic stabilization systems. J Spine Neurosurg. 2014;2. https://doi.org/10.4172/2325-9701.S2-001.
75. Panjabi MM. The stabilizing system of the spine. Part I. Function, dysfunction, adaptation, and enhancement. J Spinal Disord. 1992;5(4):383–9; discussion 397. https://doi.org/10.1097/00002517-199212000-00001.
76. Pope MH, Panjabi M. Biomechanical definitions of spinal instability. Spine (Phila Pa 1976). 1985;10(3):255–6. https://doi.org/10.1097/00007632-198504000-00013.
77. Yilmaz A, Senturk S, Sasani M, Oktenoglu T, Yaman O, Yildirim H, Suzer T, Ozer AF. Disc rehydration after dynamic stabilization: a report of 59 cases. Asian Spine J. 2017;11(3):348–55. https://doi.org/10.4184/asj.2017.11.3.348.

Reevaluation of the Treatment of Chronic Degenerative Spine Disease

24

Ali Fahir Özer and Utku Özgen

24.1 Introduction

As discussed in the previous chapters, the key to success in spine surgery lies in either avoiding the creation of an unstable spine during the operation or, if such a concern arises, stabilizing the spine to successfully conclude the surgery. The challenge lies in determining how this should be executed. Examining the history of spinal stabilization reveals a predominant focus on trauma. Despite the coexistence of open and closed methods in the historical development process, closed methods have consistently taken precedence over open surgery. The primary objective is to protect the spinal cord, which is at risk of being crushed or compressed during trauma. In the context of open surgery, no measures are taken to ensure the continuity of the spine. Thus, closed methods are more advantageous. This is because allowing healing without damaging the spinal cord and ensuring the continuity of the fractured spine parts could enable the patient to stand up. If we briefly review these methods, the first treatment ever applied was traction. Traction, which has been employed since ancient times, involves restoring the alignment of the spine and waiting for the fractured spine to stabilize and return to its normal anatomy before discontinuing the treatment. Edwin Smith Papyrus (4000 BC) and, later, Hippocrates (470–410 BC) suggested using traction for the treatment of spine injuries. Şerafeddin Sabuncuoğlu (1386–1470) first utilized traction in Anatolia. Sir Geoffrey Jefferson (1886–1961) developed the Halter traction. Sir Reginald Watson-Jones (1902–1972) used two tables for traction in the prone position. W. Gayle Crutchfield (1900–1972) developed the first skeletal traction in 1933, and Vernon Nickel developed the halo traction in 1955 [1–7]. These treatment methods were mostly applied for traumatic injuries.

In 1911, two surgeons, Dr. Albee and Dr. Hibbs [8, 9], independently performed the first spinal fusion surgery to prevent deformities in patients with tuberculosis. Subsequently, fusion surgery would become the sole treatment method for spinal instabilities. It remains an indispensable option because of the enhanced clinical results with instrumentation [10]. During this significant development, information regarding the anatomy and mechanics of the spine was gradually emerging.

The detection and treatment of lumbar disc herniation, a significantly important condition in the population that leads to nerve root compression, were pioneered by Mixter and Barr in 1933.

A. F. Özer (✉)
Department of Neurosurgery, Koc University School of Medicine, Istanbul, Turkey

U. Özgen
Department of Neurosurgery, American Hospital, Istanbul, Turkey
e-mail: utkuo@amerikanhastanesi.org

A. F. Özer et al. (eds.), *Dynamic Lumbar Spine Stabilization*,
https://doi.org/10.1007/978-3-032-12122-6_24

Although substantial progress has been made, it would be premature to assert that the challenges associated with this condition have been entirely resolved [11]. These two developments are pivotal in the history of spine, as they mark the emergence of two distinct treatment concepts for pathologies other than trauma.

One treatment approach entails decompression and fusion with instrumentation to ensure spinal continuity, which is described as stabilization. The other approach advocates performing surgery through the smallest possible incision, causing minimal anatomical disruption, and directly decompressing the affected nerve. The rationale behind this is that minimal anatomical damage does not compromise stabilization, which would require additional stabilization procedures. Surgical microscopes were introduced to reinforce the latter approach [12]. Subsequently, endoscopy was incorporated, further minimizing the surgical field.

The progress of spinal surgery has been significantly influenced by developments in related fields. William Conrad Roentgen pioneered the use of X-rays for imaging. Dr. Jean A. Sicard introduced myelography. Dr. Kunt Lindblom introduced discography in 1948, Dr. William Oldendorf introduced computerized tomography (CT), and Dr. Raymond V. Damadian (1977) and Dr. A Reid (1980) introduced magnetic resonance (MR) technology. These technological advancements have provided crucial insights to surgeons regarding the nature of the issues they may encounter preoperatively. In particular, CT and MR technologies offer detailed information regarding the pathology and mechanisms of spinal injuries. MR, which provides detailed information regarding soft tissues, has been particularly beneficial for ensuring the accuracy of surgeries. Another significant development in the understanding of spinal pathologies is attributed to the advancements in laboratory and computer technologies [13–15]. The emergence of mechanical systems capable of achieving high speeds and precision measurement devices and the use of cadaver and human-like models in laboratories have led to a better understanding of pathologies, particularly those arising due to trauma, in real life. Consequently, in addition to understanding the spinal anatomy, its kinematics became more comprehensible. Thus, concepts of stability and instability in a spine with an elastic structure, particularly in trauma studies, started to emerge. What is instability? What are its boundaries? What defines a stable spine? The answers to these questions would significantly impact the evolution of spinal surgery. Because of advancements in computer technology, the finite element method allowed the transfer of spinal biological characteristics to a computer. The subsequent simulations conducted in the computer environment aimed to comprehend the mechanisms of pathologies observed in real life. The effectiveness and durability of instruments designed for use on the spine were tested in computer simulations before being used in laboratories, which reduced laboratory usage, was time-saving, and was cost-effective.

These developments have contributed significantly to the advancements in spinal surgery, leading to the development of new instrumentation techniques for effective spinal stabilization. Instrumentation was, in fact, a method that had been previously tested. Some believed that, instead of waiting for traction to produce results in spinal injuries, some interventions were necessary. Hadra [16] attempted spinal fixation with a wire in 1891, which was subsequently attempted by Toumey [17] in 1943. In 1944, King [18] performed the first facet screw fixation. In 1953, Wenger used the first anterior distraction device. Although it ended in failure, it was a significant experimental effort. In 1962, building on years of accumulated knowledge, Dr. Harrington developed a rod system for stabilizing the posterior column, which was subsequently named after him [19, 20].

The current stabilization methods, such as the transpedicular screw and rod system, which address the shortcomings of Harrington's system, were developed by Dr. Cotrel and Dr. Dubousset [21]. The screw and plate system was constructed by Dr. Roy-Camille [22, 23]. Dwyer developed the first anterior system in 1969, which paved the way for anterior instrumentation in spinal surgery [24]. Zielke improved the technology in anterior systems in 1976 [25]. Kaneda used the first anterior plate and double rod system in 1991 [26]. Routine placement of metal supports between vertebral bodies to ensure continuity was first introduced by Rezaian in 1983 [27, 28].

Currently, the chances of success of any surgical intervention are minimal if spinal continuity and stability are not maintained. In traumatic pathologies, where continuity is suddenly disrupted, or in degenerative disorders, where continuity gradually deteriorates, ensuring continuity at the site of disruption is the key to ensuring treatment success. A current literature review reveals that the reduction in surgical field size has not necessarily translated into positive outcomes. For instance, in the case of microsurgery for lumbar disc herniation, there is no clear superiority of the results over those of open surgery [29–33]. Even when endoscopic discectomy was first attempted via the transforaminal route, some studies demonstrated poor outcomes. Translaminar endoscopic discectomy does not demonstrate clear superiority over microdiscectomy for lumbar disc herniation in terms of recurrence rates [34–36]. In contrast, endoscopic fusion surgeries performed using the biportal technique are quite popular today. Our intention is not to discredit endoscopy. It is undoubtedly a superior technology in cases where segmental instability is unlikely to develop, such as in a fragmentectomy for a minimally torn annulus. However, its superiority cannot be generalized for all disc herniations.

Taking a general look at this history, what do we observe? The solution proposed by Albee and Hibbs for spinal continuity was fusion surgery. Remarkable developments in spinal stabilization, screw and rod technology, and agents that promote ossification are all centered around fusion surgery. There have been two significant rebellions against spinal fusion surgery. The first is the concept of a dynamic rod for simple stabilization, and the second involves disc prostheses aimed at preserving motion. Thus, the concept of "stabilizing while in motion" for the spine has emerged.

After years of addressing complications through new designs, the team led by Dr. Katrine Butner Janz introduced the CHARITE disc prosthesis for the first time in spinal surgeries in 1988 [37]. Subsequently, the accumulation of extensive experience and knowledge has led to the creation of numerous cervical and lumbar disc prosthesis models. Developments in cervical disc prostheses continue to gain momentum. In the lumbar region, because of the challenges in usage, long-term results not being superior to those of classical fusion surgery, and difficulties in resolving complications, progress in the development of prostheses has stalled. Over time, there will undoubtedly be further developments.

Systems that dynamically stabilize the spine from the back have also been considered. The creator of the concept of the posterior dynamic stabilization system was Dr. Henry Graf in 1991. He created a tension band using the Graf ligament on the posterior screws [38]. The second significant step in the dynamic pedicle system was the development of the dynamic screw concept by von Strempel in 1999. We believe that this has been one of the most important advances in dynamic systems and has provided a new perspective on fusion surgery. Dynamic systems, such as total disc replacements, were developed not to preserve motion but to provide stabilization for simple instabilities. Current dynamic rod systems and dynamic screw systems were not designed for preserving motion. However, for example, when used in the treatment of lumbar disc herniation at the onset of degeneration, the system can preserve motion. This situation is more realistic when the two systems are used together.

24.2 Pathologies That Are Treated with the Dynamic Pedicle System

Because lumbar disc herniation has been discussed separately in this book, it will not be discussed in this section.

24.2.1 Degenerative Spondylolisthesis

Degenerative spondylolisthesis arises from the degeneration of a motion segment, and unlike in isthmic spondylolisthesis, there is no congenital defect in the isthmus. Often, patients may not have any clinical symptoms, especially young patients in whom the muscle compartment is sufficient. Thus, patients are often unaware of it. The diagnosis is often incidentally made, following routine/random examinations. In individuals with ongoing muscle compartment support, the slow progression of degeneration in the disc and annulus, involvement of the facet joints, and spontaneous fusion allow individuals to overcome this condition without noticing it or developing significant symptoms. Clinical symptoms appear when the destabilized motion segment is no longer stabilized by compensatory mechanisms.

Clinical symptoms of degenerative spondylolisthesis manifest in the following three ways: disruption of alignment, compression of the nerve roots in the foramen, and development of spinal stenosis. All three may be present in a single patient.

Pain in a mobile segment, where one vertebra slides forward over another, is caused by stretching structures containing painful nerve endings, such as the annulus, capsular ligaments, and anterior and posterior ligaments. This is a mechanical pain caused by the damaged structures. A second cause of pain is when the nerve root exiting the foramen becomes compressed between the pedicle of the displaced upper vertebra and the underlying ruptured disc, causing nerve root pain. (Fig. 24.1).

This condition is crucial, and if central canal stenosis also exists, it can easily be overlooked. In such cases, opening the central canal alone does not relieve the patient's symptoms. The foramen will also need to be decompressed. The third source of pain is the arcus vertebra, which forms the back of the sliding upper vertebra. By advancing forward within the spinal canal and involving the dura mater, it causes a narrowing of the entire diameter of the spinal canal between the rear upper part of the lower vertebra and the deteriorated disc, leading to spinal canal stenosis. These patients develop the classic neurogenic claudication symptoms, and over time, their ability to stand and walk decreases (Fig. 24.2).

Based on the classical treatment methods, if spontaneous fusion has developed and there is no significant foraminal or central canal narrowing, then no intervention is required. These patients are usually asymptomatic. If spontaneous fusion has developed and it is associated with foraminal or central canal stenosis, there is no need for fusion or instrumentation. A foraminal and/or central canal decompression alone is sufficient. However, when opening up the foramen, it is not sufficient to remove only the facet joints that make up the rear wall of the foramen because the nerve root is compressed between the pedicle and the lower vertebra. It is essential to significantly widen the foramen by removing the calcified disc and either all (pediculectomy) or a portion of (partial pediculectomy) the upper pedicle (Fig. 24.3).

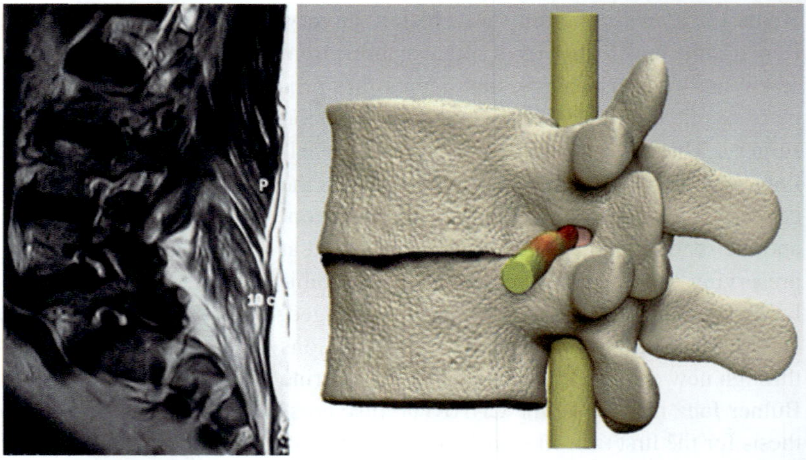

Fig. 24.1 Due to spondylolisthesis, the nerve roots get compressed between the pedicle of the upper vertebra and the disc below it, resulting in radicular symptoms

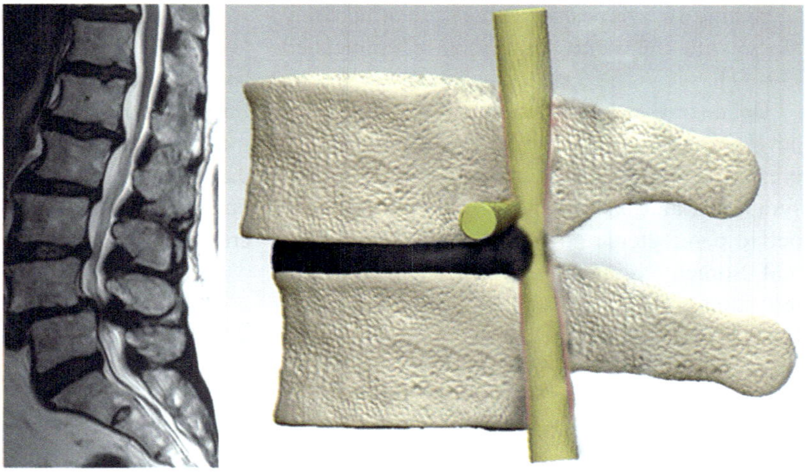

Fig. 24.2 Spinal canal stenosis caused by degenerative spondylolisthesis

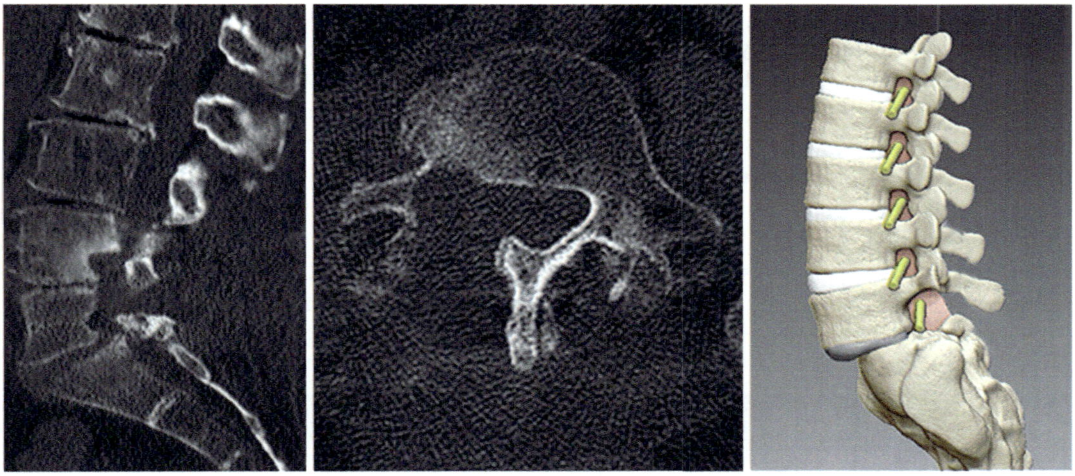

Fig. 24.3 If spontaneous fusion has developed in the mobile segment, instrumentation is not necessary. By removing a portion or all of the pedicle to create a new foramen, a comfortable space can be created for the passage of the nerve root

If osteophytes are present, they should also be excised. For the central canal, we routinely perform a unilateral decompression, which is usually sufficient for patients suffering from this condition. Because the spontaneous fusion develops in the anterior column, instrumentation and fusion are not necessary. In most cases, these patients do not demonstrate deterioration in the spinopelvic parameters, which is seen in some patients with isthmic spondylolisthesis. Therefore, decompression alone is generally adequate for the treatment of patients with spontaneous fusion.

If there is segmental movement in patients with degenerative spondylolisthesis, decompression alone is not sufficient; surgical stabilization is required. The classical approach is to place a cage with an autologous bone graft to elevate the disc space, especially if there is foraminal stenosis. This increases the disc height, expands the foraminal space, and restores the alignment to normal. If there is no foraminal stenosis and the pain is due to abnormal movements at the mobile segment, the segment will require stabilization to relieve the symptoms. In patients where there is a coexisting central canal stenosis, laminectomy along with the same surgery is recommended [39–41].

Degenerative spondylolisthesis is a slowly developing minor instability. Patients usually present to the doctor because of root irritation symptoms and back pain. In most patients, the pelvic parameters and sagittal balance are normal. Some patients may have a scoliotic deformity that does not disrupt the coronal balance. In these patients, providing decompression and stabilizing the unstable segment is sufficient. In worst-case scenarios, if pseudoarthrosis or infection develops after placing an interbody cage in a patient with a disrupted posterior tension band, the entire system may need to be dismantled. Furthermore, after the complication has resolved, a fusion surgery or even a larger one may need to be performed. A procedure that stabilizes the unstable segment with a simple system after decompression is sufficient to keep the patient erect without disrupting the normal or compensatory spinal alignment, walking ability, and mobility capacity. Using a dynamic system to support the mobile segment is usually sufficient (Fig. 24.4).

The likelihood of screw loosening in a single-level system is 4% at any age [42]. If the patient has advanced osteoporosis, surgery can be performed in two stages. These patients present to the doctor ambulating without pain and leave in the same condition with the same spine. It is sufficient to resolve the existing pathology without creating a new spine.

24.2.2 Lumbar Canal Stenosis

Degenerative lumbar canal stenosis is another chronic instability pathology. It is a progressive disease that affects all mobile spinal segments. Relative instability initiated by the degeneration of the intervertebral discs leads to hypermobility of vertebral segments, resulting in increased pressure on the posterior facet joints. This leads to narrowing of the intervertebral disc space, increased extension angle, and hypertrophy of the facet joints. As degeneration progresses slowly, the joints ankylose. The joint hypertrophy results in localized ankylosis. In addition, calcification or thickening of the yellow ligament is a significant mechanism involved in ste-

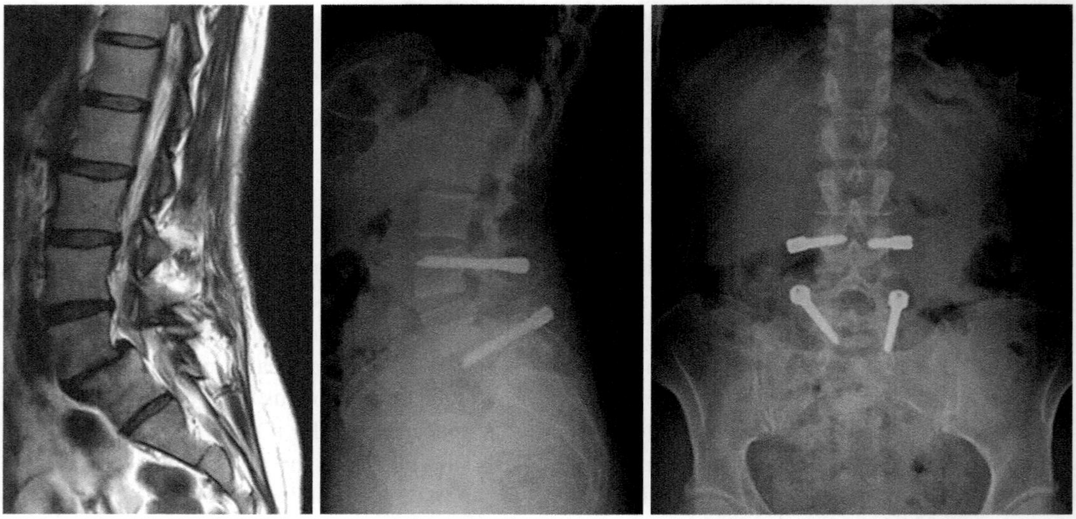

Fig. 24.4 In patients without balance issues, stabilization of the mobile segment with a dynamic system is sufficient. Due to sliding, the screwheads can come in contact with each other; i.e., a screw placed on L5 can be positioned on L4. Because the system is mobile, there is no significant loss of function in the patient's movements at the lumbar region

nosis. Joint tropism also contributes to the development of degenerative lumbar canal stenosis. It causes narrowing of the spinal canal and compression of the nerve roots, resulting in intermittent neurogenic claudication due to the obstruction of the epidural venous circulation and increased vascular pressure. Although minor trauma or work-related repetitive stimuli may not significantly contribute to the development of such narrowing, they can worsen the symptoms of an existing stenosis. No symptoms are felt while at rest. Symptoms develop when walking or standing for the following reasons. As the condition progresses, the metabolic rate of the nerve roots simultaneously increases, with lower extremity movement. However, the increased blood flow cannot keep up with the worsening condition. The cauda equina nerve roots provide energy for metabolism from the arteries on the surface of the nerve roots and from the cerebrospinal fluid by diffusion. In lumbar canal stenosis, increased pressure on the nerve roots in the spinal canal can lead to neural ischemia and impaired nerve conduction. Symptoms can also occur because of venous obstruction and may contribute to the development of lumbar canal stenosis that spans two or more segments. If nerve roots are damaged, central sensitization in pain perception may occur, which leads to chronic pain [43–45].

Degenerative lumbar canal stenosis primarily progresses because of the degenerative process of vertebral joints and the yellow ligament [45, 46]. Imaging studies may reveal advanced spondyloarthrosis in such patients. These abnormal findings can be found bilaterally but are most commonly seen between L4 and L5, followed by between L5 and the sacrum and between L3 and L4 [47]. Additionally, disc herniation and spondylolisthesis can acutely exacerbate the clinical symptoms related to this type of stenosis. Spondylolisthesis and degenerative spondyloarthropathy rarely cause stenosis in young patients. However, these degenerative changes can lead to lateral recess or foraminal stenosis in patients aged >50 years. After the primary surgical procedure for lumbar canal stenosis, stenosis can often recur. Several studies have evaluated the rates of reoperation after different surgical procedures for lumbar canal stenosis. However, there is still a dilemma regarding surgical procedures, accompanying comorbidities, and reoperation rates. Reoperation rates for lumbar stenosis surgery generally vary between 5% and 23% [48–53]. A meta-analysis identified that the following factors contribute to reoperation: smoking, type of surgical procedure performed, decompression without fusion, length of the postoperative period, patient's age, and the presence of comorbidities, such as diabetes mellitus [54].

In degenerative conditions, while the anatomy slowly deteriorates, the repair system also gets activated to immobilize the deteriorating structure. Whether the spine system is mobile or not can be determined using dynamic graphs. For structures that have deteriorated but not lost their mobility, even a unilateral approach with bilateral decompression can make the patient's spine more mobile and unstable than it was preoperatively. Although these patients do not lose their ability to walk postoperatively, axial pain may replace the neurogenic claudication. Over time, complications such as spondylolisthesis or restenosis are commonly encountered, which require a secondary surgery that is more challenging [55].

If there is no significant preoperative spinal instability, a unilateral approach with bilateral decompression, as described by Young [56], is an ideal approach because it minimizes the anatomical damage. No instrumentation is required in such cases. Canal stenosis itself is a slowly progressing impairment of stability, which can be managed due to the development of compensatory mechanisms. Although patients may undergo this surgery, they inevitably develop a more unstable spine postoperatively. If the muscle system is still active and the facet joints have ankylosed due to age, the patient will be satisfied with this surgery. However, if their instability cannot be compensated, then complications such as restenosis and instability may occur. Therefore, we believe that instrumentation with dynamic systems is necessary for mobile spinal canal stenosis. The classical approach involves rigid stabilization in addition to interbody fusion. This approach has been used for several years in patients with lumbar canal stenosis, and the undesirable results have been extensively discussed. For elderly patients with comorbidities, dynamic system stabilization is sufficient. Because the mobile segment is compromised even if a unilateral approach is used, although not as obvious as in a laminectomy, the approach can destabilize the segment, resulting in restenosis. Alternatively, a fusion operation, which is currently popular, can be recommended. The biggest issue in older patients is the rapid degeneration of the adjacent segment. Reportedly, there is no difference in the clinical outcomes between patients with stable restenosis and those with fusion after lumbar decompression surgery [57]. However, providing physiological support ensures a more guaranteed result. Dynamic systems provide this physiological support. Despite the possibility of screw loosening, a single-stage surgery can be performed in patients with good bone quality, and a two-stage surgery can be considered for patients with poor bone quality. This is a physiological surgery; the spine is preserved with very little damage, which is essential if the instrumentation system has to be removed for any reason. This is not possible after fusion surgery or after a simple discectomy. Thus, we believe that stabilization with a dynamic system provides sufficient support in these patients [58–60].

If the bone quality is not good, a two-staged procedure is suitable. If there are neurological or root irritation symptoms, screws are placed in the first stage, necessary decompression is performed at the symptomatic areas, and a short unilateral temporary rod is placed. There is a risk of one screw loosening following this stage. In the second stage, if the rods are placed and a screw has loosened, it is skipped or replaced with a thicker screw (Fig. 24.5).

The two-stage procedure allows a more delicate and softer stabilization [61]. Although these patients may still develop adjacent segment disease, incorporating the affected segment into the system is a simpler procedure.

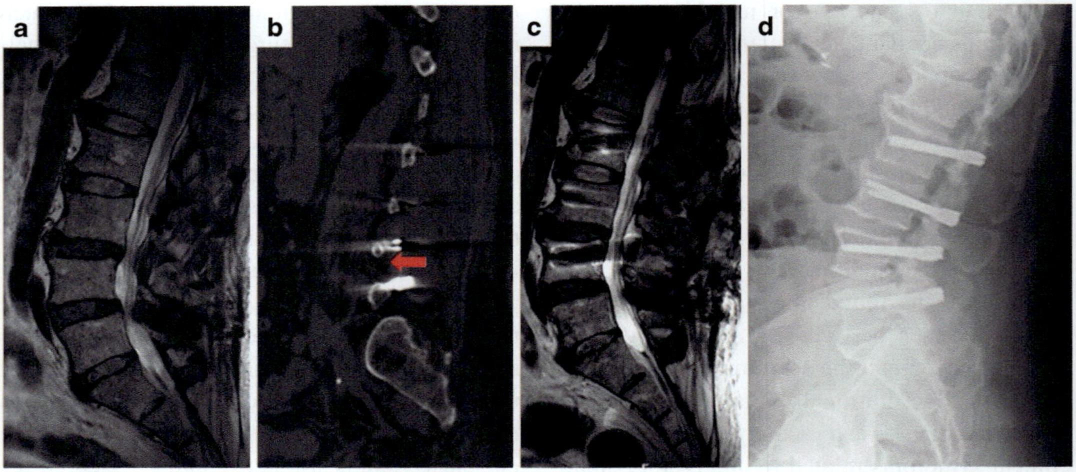

Fig. 24.5 A 58-year-old male, who had been previously operated for cervical canal stenosis, presented with paraparesis and a spastic gait. He complained of claudication pain for the past 5 months. (**a**) Magnetic resonance imaging (MRI) revealed canal stenosis at the L4–L5 and L3–L4 levels, without vascular problems. A two-stage surgery was planned. (**b**) In the first stage, a unilateral temporary rod was placed at the narrowest level of the L4–L5 mobile segment (red arrow). (**c**) The patient's MRI at the 4th postoperative month revealed a relaxed canal. (**d**) In the second stage, the temporary rod was removed, and all screws were connected with rods (the DYNESYS®. system)

24.2.3 Painful Black Disc

Painful black disc is a significant cause of lumbar pain. Age-related degeneration in the disc is a normal process. However, degeneration of one disc earlier than the others is abnormal and causes a painful condition when the structure of the other discs is normal. MR imaging (MRI) is the best diagnostic tool for this condition (Fig. 24.6).

In this condition, the pain mechanism is not the root compression but the annular tears [62–65]. When the disc's resistance is reduced, the patient can become locked and immobile with a slightly higher load than normal. The onset of pain can sometimes be triggered by a violent sneeze or even by bending over the sink to wash the face. Patients are often bent over and maintain that position due to severe muscle spasms. The MRIs of such patients may not highlight annular tears; a discography may be required to identify the tears [66].

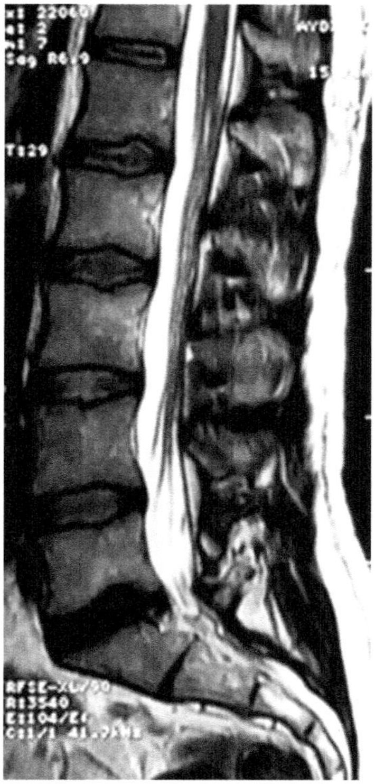

Fig. 24.6 It is abnormal for one of the discs to undergo degeneration earlier than the others. It causes a painful condition if the structure of all the other discs is normal. Magnetic resonance imaging is the best diagnostic tool

Muscle spasm is actually a reflex response to prevent the torn annular leaflets from moving and causing pain. Attempting to resolve the spasm is ineffective. The pain decreases after the connective tissue in the annulus is repaired, following which the spasm resolves spontaneously. During this period, a combination of anti-inflammatory and analgesic drugs should be administered, and rest is essential. Sometimes, all the discs may appear normal on an MRI. In such cases, discography is significantly important (Fig. 24.7) [66].

The classical approach for a painful black disc involves interbody fusion and rigid instrumentation for stabilization. However, in the majority of these patients, the disc is in the early stages of degeneration based on Pfirrmann's criteria [67]. Thus, we are sacrificing a relatively healthy disc for an annular tear. If an early-stage dynamic stabilization is performed and the load is bypassed through the dynamic system, the disc can recover over time [68–70]. If stabilized using a dynamic system with a movable rod and a movable screw, the movement at the mobile segment is preserved [71–74]. In most young patients, dynamic system stabilization is a much easier and more effective method, and the likelihood of screw loosening is very low [42]. For patients with compromised bone quality, which generally constitutes older adults, performing a two-staged surgery is a more reliable approach.

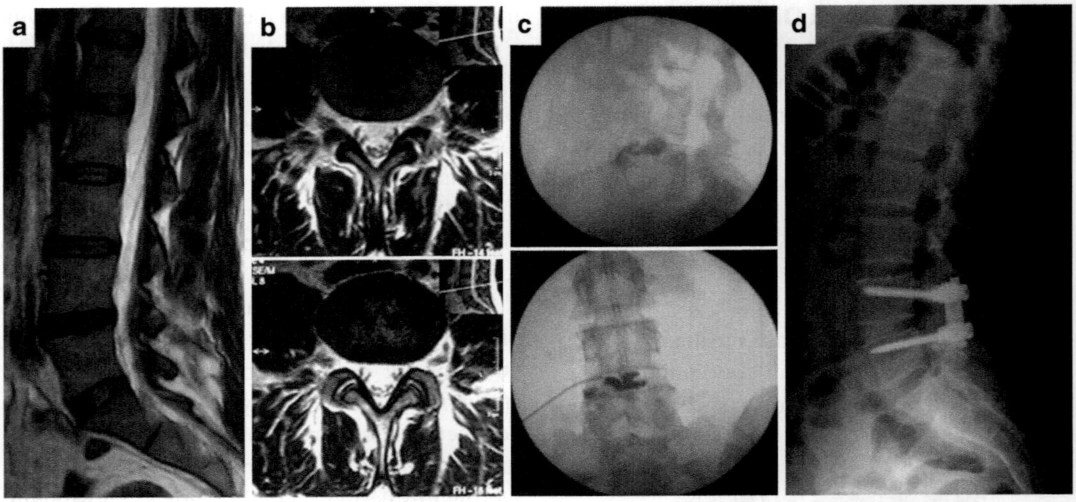

Fig. 24.7 A 56-year-old female patient suddenly developed lower back pain while lifting a heavy load 2 years ago. The pain gradually improved over 10 days, and the patient was able to stand up. However, in the following months, she continued to experience episodes of lower back pain every 2 months. Currently, even the slightest movement causes pain and stiffness in her lower back. The patient underwent multiple physical therapy sessions and pain management approaches. However, the symptoms were not relieved. Eventually, considering a psychiatric component, she was referred to a psychiatrist. (**a**, **b**) MRI revealed a healthy L5–S1 disc and a partially degenerated (Pfirrmann Grade 1) L4–L5 disc. The discs above the L4–L5 disc also appeared to be healthy. (**c**) Discography revealed a full-thickness tear in the anterior annulus of the L4–L5 disc, with the contrast material leaking out. The pain provocation test was also positive. (**d**) Dynamic stabilization (the Cosmic system) was performed at the L4–L5 level, resulting in the complete resolution of her symptoms. MRI: magnetic resonance imaging

24.2.4 Modic Degeneration with Pain

Modic degeneration is a specific degenerative process of the disc for which the cause remains unknown [75]. It progresses through three stages. In the first stage, there is edema in the cartilage end plates. Because the nutrition of the disc relies on diffusion from the cartilage end plates, the nutrition starts to deteriorate. Spontaneous resolution has been reported at this stage [76]. The edema appears hypointense on T1-weighted MR images and hyperintense on T2-weighted MR images in the adjacent upper and lower cartilage end plates. In the second stage, edema gives way to the accumulation of fatty tissue, which further compromises the nutrition of the disc. Disc herniation is prominent in this stage, and there is a higher likelihood of recurrence after a simple discectomy. If the pathology involves a segment with sacralization, the recurrence rate is 78.6% [77]. The fatty infiltration appears hyperintense on T1- and T2-weighted MR images in the adjacent upper and lower cartilage end plates. In the third stage, the fatty tissue is replaced by calcium, and these areas appear sclerotic. Because the annulus is also calcified, the disc does not move and decreases in height. This stage marks the resolution of the condition and appears hypointense on T1- and T2-weighted MR images. The first two stages of Modic degeneration are reportedly painful, which can sometimes significantly affect the patient's quality of life. If the condition progresses to the third stage, with the patient experiencing the painful process, the pain eventually disappears. In some cases, the condition progresses in this manner, resulting in the spontaneous collapse of the disc. In patients experiencing pain, the classical approach involves insertion of interbody cages with graft and rigid stabilization. Performing a surgical procedure using a dynamic system in the first stage allows the resolution of the symptoms with a simple sta-

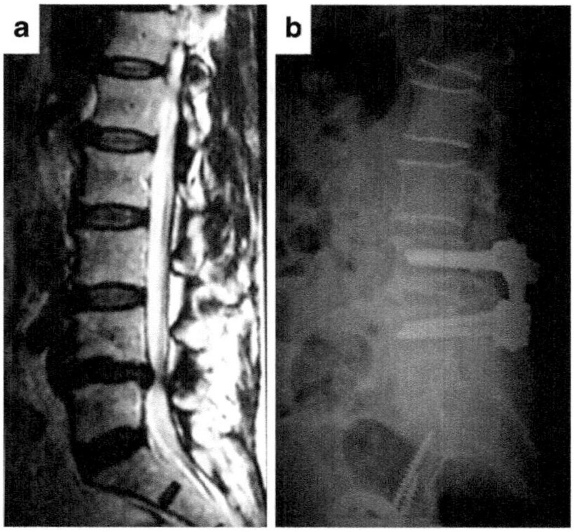

Fig. 24.8 A 48-year-old male had been experiencing frequent and disabling lower back pain for the past 6 months. He had become fearful of any movement. (**a**) MRI revealed a progressive disc herniation, with Modic degeneration at the L4–L5 level. (**b**) After dynamic stabilization of the L4–L5 level (the Safinaz system), the patient's symptoms resolved

bilization and even preservation of the disc mobility. In patients with poor bone quality or comorbid medical conditions, a two-stage surgery may be necessary. In these patients, performing a dynamic stabilization in the first stage has proven to be a sufficient solution for the patients' painful condition (Fig. 24.8) [61].

After stabilization, the development of fusion or preservation of disc movement depends on the level of disc degeneration [68].

24.2.5 Foraminal Stenosis

Foraminal stenosis can develop due to various reasons, and its treatment is distinctive [78]. Before addressing the foraminal stenosis, it is essential to examine the anatomy and pathology of the foramen.

The foramen begins with the lateral recess. The lateral recess, known as the "entry zone," starts at the medial border of the superior articular process and extends to the medial border of the pedicle. In this region, the nerve roots exit the dura and proceed to the foramen while in contact with the lateral recess. The boundaries of the lateral recess comprise the vertebral pedicle on the lateral side, the superior articular process of the facet joint on the dorsal side, the intervertebral disc and posterior ligaments on the anterior side, and the spinal canal on the medial side. The main causes of stenosis at the entry zone are a posteriorly herniated intervertebral disc and hypertrophic osteoarthritis of the posterior joints, leading to osteoporosis-induced facet tropism and superior articular process thickening. Narrowing of the lateral recess causes compression of the nerve root as it enters the foramen.

The "mid-zone" refers to the foraminal region located in front of the midsection (pars) of the vertebra. Its boundaries include the lateral recess medially, the vertebral body and intervertebral disc anteriorly, the pars and intertransverse ligaments posteriorly, and the pedicle surface and foramen continuation laterally. Narrowing in this area occurs because of the thickening of defective partial fibrocartilaginous tissue or the formation of osteophytes. Thickening of the yellow ligament can sometimes cause narrowing up to the neural foramen. Osteophyte formation under the pars defect is also associated with narrowing in the "mid-zone" (Fig. 24.9).

In spondylolisthesis and degenerative scoliosis, rotational malalignment of the vertebral body or asymmetric narrowing of the intervertebral disc can cause one vertebral pedicle to be relatively lower than the others. This can lead to nerve root compression at this level [43, 78, 79].

The "exit zone" is a teardrop-shaped area created by the intervertebral foramen, and the neural foramen lies between the lower part of the upper vertebral pedicle and the upper part of the lower vertebral pedicle. It is limited posteriorly by the lower pars. Its boundaries are formed by the inferior articular process of the upper vertebra and the superior articular process of the lower vertebra posteriorly and the posterior surface of the vertebral body and the intervertebral disc anteriorly. The dorsal root ganglia and ventral motor roots cover approximately 30% of this area. In this region, the nerve roots within the dura begin to wrap around the epineurium. Here, the nerve roots can be compressed because of a far-lateral disc herniation, spondylolisthesis-related sublux-

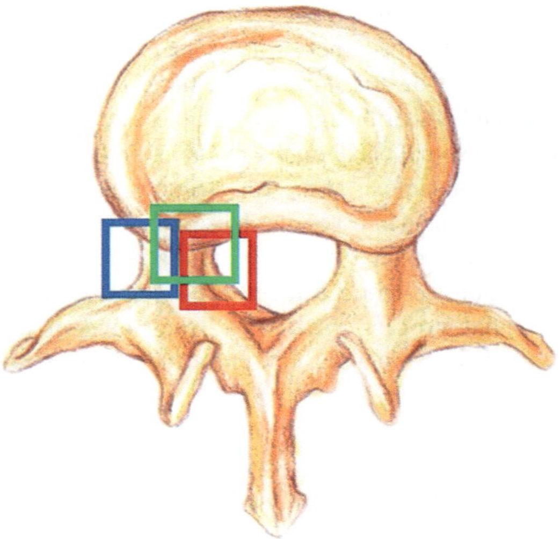

Fig. 24.9 Zone 1 (red square) is where the nerve root passes laterally and enters the foramen. Here, it can be compressed in the following two ways: (i) The facet joint can undergo osteoporosis-related facet tropism and collapse toward the vertebral body, causing nerve root compression between the facet joint and the vertebral body, or (ii) the nerve root can be compressed due to disc herniation. In some patients, both mechanisms can occur simultaneously. The most significant issue in Zone 2 (green square) is the compromised facet joint, which can cause narrowing of this part of the foramen and compression of the nerve root. Occasionally, osteophytes in this area can push the nerve root backward, causing compression at the undersurface of the facet joint. The most significant pathology causing foraminal stenosis in Zone 3 (blue square) is a far-lateral disc herniation

ation, or facet joint arthritis. The most common cause of nerve root compression in this region is degenerative spine arthritis [78, 80].

Two key points are important to note. First, if stenosis has occurred in a mobile segment that has undergone spontaneous fusion, decompression is sufficient, and instrumentation for stabilization is not necessary. Second, if spondylolisthesis has undergone spontaneous fusion, it is necessary to create a new foramen via a partial pediculectomy. This entails removal of the posterior wall of the facet joint, including the inferior and superior joint surfaces, as well as the calcified disc, lateral recess, and part of the pedicle. This procedure is required because the root is compressed between the upper pedicle and the lower vertebral body, and removal of the posterior wall of the facet joint alone is not sufficient [81, 82] (Fig. 24.10).

If there is movement in the foramen and the spondylolisthesis is bilateral, as discussed in the section on degenerative spondylolisthesis, it is necessary to use a bilateral dynamic system and perform a partial facetectomy along the posterior facet wall. In addition, reducing the disc size by coagulating the annulus and creating a space for the nerve root to pass through is essential. In such patients, the upper screw needs to be placed at the level of the L4 vertebra because the screwheads

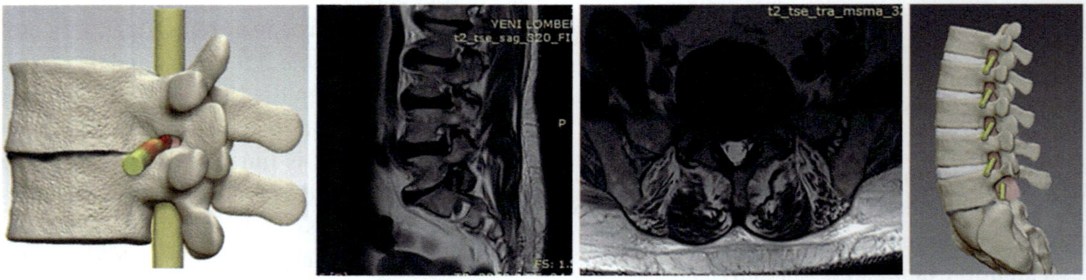

Fig. 24.10 If a disc collapses and causes nerve root compression between two pedicles, a partial pediculectomy should be performed at the upper pedicle level

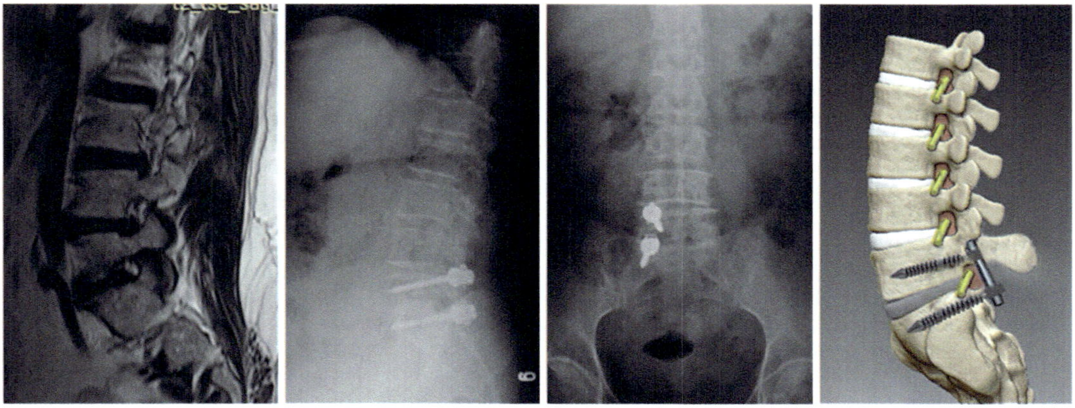

Fig. 24.11 If the nerve root in the foramen is compressed by a herniated disc or a degenerated facet joint, the compression can be relieved by performing a discectomy or removing the damaged facet joint, respectively. Unilateral dynamic stabilization is sufficient in such a case to replace the removed facet joint

at the L5 and S1 levels will sit on top of each other due to spondylolisthesis.

If the stenosis is unilateral, the procedure can be performed on the symptomatic side. Furthermore, instrumentation on that side alone is sufficient. If foraminal stenosis has occurred not due to slippage but due to the deterioration of the facet joints, then removal of the posterior wall of the facet joint, including the inferior and superior protrusions, is sufficient. Furthermore, a dynamic system can be applied on this side alone (Fig. 24.11).

In rare cases, if the disc collapses and the nerve root is compressed between the two pedicles, a partial pediculectomy should be performed at the level of the upper pedicle (Fig. 24.10) [83, 84].

References

1. van Middendorp JJ, Sanchez GM, Burridge AL. The Edwin Smith papyrus: a clinical reappraisal of the oldest known document on spinal injuries. Eur Spine J. 2010;19(11):1815–23.
2. Silver JR. History of the treatment of spinal injuries. Postgrad Med J. 2005;81(952):108–14.
3. Knoeller SM, Seifried C. Historical perspective: history of spinal surgery. Spine (Phila Pa 1976). 2000;25(21):2838–43.
4. Walker CT, Kakarla UK, Chang SW, Sonntag VKH. History and advances in spinal neurosurgery. J Neurosurg Spine. 2019;31(6):775–85.
5. Canale DJ. Milestones leading to the development of spinal surgery in the late 19th century. Henry Ford Hosp Med J. 1977;25(3):131–44.
6. Khoo LT, Ozer AF, Cosar M, Asgarzadie F. History of minimally invasive spine surgery In: Khoo LT, Ozer AF, editors. Minimally invasive procedures in spine surgery. İzmir: Intertıp Yayınevi; 2015. ISBN: 978-605-50004-08-8.
7. Lifshutz J, Colohan A. A brief history of therapy for traumatic spinal cord injury. Neurosurg Focus. 2004;16(1):E5.
8. Hibbs RA. An operation for progressive spinal deformities: a preliminary report of three cases from the service of the orthopaedic hospital. 1911. Clin Orthop Relat Res. 2007;460:17–20.
9. Albee FH. Transplantation of a portion of the tibia into the spine for Pott's disease. JAMA. 1911;57:885–6.
10. Virk S, Qureshi S, Sandhu H. History of spinal fusion: where we came from and where we are going. HSS J. 2020;16(2):137–42.
11. Mixter WJ, Barr JS. Rupture of the intervertebral disc with involvement of the spinal canal N Engl J Med. 1934;211:210–5.
12. Yasargil MG. Microsurgical operation for herniated disc. In: Wullenweber R, Brock M, Hamer J, Klinger M, Spoerri O, editors. Advances in neurosurgery. Berlin: Springer-Verlag; 1977. p. 81.
13. Hesselink JR. Spine imaging: history, achievements, remaining frontiers. AJR Am J Roentgenol. 1988;150(6):1223–9.
14. Harada GK, Siyaji ZK, Younis S, Louie PK, Samartzis D, An HS. Imaging in spine surgery: current concepts and future directions. Spine Surg Relat Res. 2019;4(2):99–110.
15. Nimsky C, Carl B. Historical, current, and future intraoperative imaging modalities. Neurosurg Clin N Am. 2017;28(4):453–64.

16. Hadra BE. Wiring of the vertebrae as a means of immobilization in fracture and Potts' disease. 1891. Clin Orthop Relat Res. 2007;460:11–3.
17. Tourney J. Internal fixation in fusion of the lumbosacral joint. Lahey Clin Bull. 1943;3:188–91.
18. King D. Internal fixation for lumbosacral fusion. J Bone Joint Surg Am. 1948;30:560–78.
19. Harrington PR, Tullos HS. Reduction of severe spondylolisthesis in children. South Med J. 1969;62(1):1–7.
20. Harrington PR, Dickson JH. Spinal instrumentation in the treatment of severe progressive spondylolisthesis. Clin Orthop Relat Res. 1976;117:157–63.
21. Cotrel Y, Dubousset J, Guillaumat M. New universal instrumentation in spinal surgery. Clin Orthop Relat Res. 1988;227:10–23.
22. Roy-Camille R, Roy-Camille M. Demeulenaere C. Ostéosynthèse du rachis dorsal, lombaire et lombo-sacré par plaques métalliques vissées dans les pédicules vertébraux et les apophyses articulaires [Osteosynthesis of dorsal, lumbar, and lumbosacral spine with metallic plates screwed into vertebral pedicles and articular apophyses]. Presse Med (1893). 1970;78(32):1447–8. French.
23. Roy-Camille R, Saillant G, Berteaux D, Salgado V. Osteosynthesis of thoraco-lumbar spine fractures with metal plates screwed through the vertebral pedicles. Reconstr Surg Traumatol. 1976;15:2–16.
24. Dwyer AF, Newton NC, Sherwood AA. An anterior approach to scoliosis. A preliminary report. Clin Orthop. 1969;62:192–202.
25. Zielke K, Stunkat R, Beaujean F. Ventrale derotations spondylodesis. Arch Orthop Unfallchir. 1976;85:257–77.
26. Kaneda K, Shono Y, Satoh S, Abumi K. New anterior instrumentation for the management of thoracolumbar and lumbar scoliosis. Application of the Kaneda two-rod system. Spine. 1996;21:1250–61.
27. Rezaian SM, Dombrowski ET, Ghista DN. Spinal fixator for the management of spinal injury (the mechanical rationale). Eng Med. 1983;12(2):95–7.
28. Matur AV, Mejia-Munne JC, Plummer ZJ, Cheng JS, Prestigiacomo CJ. The history of anterior and lateral approaches to the lumbar spine. World Neurosurg. 2020;144:213–21.
29. Daneyemez M, Sali A, Kahraman S, Beduk A, Seber N. Outcome analyses in 1072 surgically treated lumbar disc herniations. Minim Invasive Neurosurg. 1999;42:63–8.
30. Gibson JN, Grant IC, Wadell G. The Cocharane review of surgery for lumbar disc prolapse and degenerative lumbar spondylosis. Spine. 1999;24:1820–32.
31. Katayama Y, Matsuyama Y, Yoshihara H, et al. Comparison of surgical outcomes between macro discectomy and micro discectomy for lumbar disc herniation: a prospective randomized study with surgery performed by the same spine surgeon. J Spinal Disord Tech. 2006;19(5):344–7.
32. Tureyen K. One-level one-sided lumbar disc surgery with and without microscopic assistance: 1-year outcome in 114 consecutive patients. J Neurosurg Spine. 2003;99:247–50.
33. Porchet F, Bartanusz V, Kleinstueck F, et al. Microdiscectomy compared with standard discectomy: an old problem revisited with new outcome measures within the framework of a spine surgical registry. Eur Spine J. 2009;18(Suppl 3):360–6.
34. Lee SH, Chung SE, Ahn Y, Kim TH, Park JY, Shin SW. Comparative radiologic evaluation of percutaneous endoscopic lumbar discectomy and open microdiscectomy: a matched cohort analysis. Mt Sinai J Med. 2006;73(5):795–801.
35. Anichini G. Lumbar endoscopic microdiscectomy: where are we now? An updated literature review focused on clinical outcome, complications, and rate of recurrence. Biomed Res Int. 2015;238:1–14.
36. Kim M, Lee S, Kim HS, Park S, Shim SY, Lim DJ. A comparison of percutaneous endoscopic lumbar discectomy and open lumbar microdiscectomy for lumbar disc herniation in the Korean: a meta-analysis. Biomed Res Int. 2018;2018:9073460.
37. Buttner Janz K, Schellnack K, Zippel H. Biomechanics of the SB Charité lumbar intervertebral disc endoprosthesis. Int Orthop. 1989;13:173–6.
38. Graff H. Lumbar instability surgical treatment without fusion: soft system stabilisation. J Turk Spinal Surg. 1991;2:132–40.
39. Takahashi T, Hanakita J, Minami M, Kitahama Y, Kuraishi K, Watanabe M, Takeshima Y, Uesaka T. Clinical outcomes and adverse events following transforaminal interbody fusion for lumbar degenerative spondylolisthesis in elderly patients. Neurol Med Chir (Tokyo). 2011;51(12):829–35.
40. Oliveira L, Marchi L, Coutinho E, Pimenta L. A radiographic assessment of the ability of the extreme lateral interbody fusion procedure to indirectly decompress the neural elements. Spine (Phila Pa 1976). 2010;35(26 Suppl):S331–7.
41. Sato J, Ohtori S, Orita S, et al. Radiographic evaluation of indirect decompression of mini-open anterior retroperitoneal lumbar interbody fusion: oblique lateral interbody fusion for degenerated lumbar spondylolisthesis. Eur Spine J. 2017;26(3):671–8.
42. Ozer AF, Oktenoglu T, Egemen E, Sasani M, Yilmaz A, Erbulut DU, Yaman O, Suzer T. Lumbar single-level dynamic stabilization with semi-rigid and full dynamic systems: a retrospective clinical and radiological analysis of 71 patients. Clin Orthop Surg. 2017;9(3):310–6.
43. Lee CK, Rauschning W, Glenn W. Lateral lumbar spinal canal stenosis: classification, pathologic anatomy and surgical decompression. Spine (Phila Pa 1976). 1988;13:313–20.
44. Abbas J, Peled N, Hershkovitz I, Hamoud K. Facet tropism and orientation: risk factors for degenerative lumbar spinal stenosis. Biomed Res Int. 2020;2020:2453503.
45. Lee BH, Moon SH, Suk KS, Kim HS, Yang JH, Lee HM. Lumbar spinal stenosis: pathophysiology and

treatment principle: a narrative review. Asian Spine J. 2020;14(5):682–93.
46. Chiba D, Tsuda E, Wada K, et al. Lumbar spondylosis, lumbar spinal stenosis, knee pain, back muscle strength are associated with the locomotive syndrome: rural population study in Japan. J Orthop Sci. 2016;21:366–72.
47. Lee SY, Kim TH, Oh JK, Lee SJ, Park MS. Lumbar stenosis: a recent update by review of literature. Asian Spine J. 2015;9:818–28.
48. Jansson KA, Németh G, Granath F, Blomqvist P. Spinal stenosis re-operation rate in Sweden is 11% at 10 years – a national analysis of 9,664 operations. Eur Spine J. 2005;14:659–63.
49. Hansraj KK, Cammisa FP Jr, O'Leary PF, Crockett HC, Fras CI, Cohen MS, Dorey FJ. Decompressive surgery for typical lumbar spinal stenosis. Clin Orthop Relat Res. 2001;384:10–7.
50. Herno A, Airaksinen O, Saari T. Long term results of surgical treatment of lumbar spinal stenosis. Spine (Phila Pa 1976). 1993;18:1471–4.
51. Jönsson B, Annertz M, Sjöberg C, Strömqvist B. A prospective and consecutive study of surgically treated lumbar spinal stenosis. Part II: five-year followup by an independent observer. Spine (Phila Pa 1976). 1997;22:2938–44.
52. Hee HT, Wong HK. The long term results of surgical treatment for spinal stenosis in the elderly. Singapore Med J. 2003;44:175–80.
53. Oertel MF, Ryang YM, Korinth MC, Gilsbach JM, Rohde V. Long term results of microsurgical treatment of lumbar spinal stenosis by unilateral laminotomy for bilateral decompression. Neurosurgery. 2006;59:1264–9.
54. Goel SA, Modi HN. Reoperations following lumbar spinal canal stenosis. Indian J Orthop. 2018;52(6):578–83.
55. Shimauchi-Ohtaki H, Minami M, Takahashi T, Kanematsu R, Honda F, Hanakita J. Lumbar canal stenosis caused by marked bone overgrowth after decompression surgery. Case Rep Orthop. 2022;2022:9462399.
56. Young S, Veerapen R, O'Laoire SA. Relief of lumbar canal stenosis using multilevel subarticular fenestrations as an alternative to wide laminectomy: preliminary report. Neurosurgery. 1988;23(5):628–33.
57. Miyahara J, Yoshida Y, Nishizawa M, et al. Treatment of restenosis after lumbar decompression surgery: decompression versus decompression and fusion. J Neurosurg Spine. 2022;36(6):892–9.
58. Kaner T, Sasani M, Oktenoglu T, Aydin AL, Ozer AF. Clinical outcomes of degenerative lumbar spinal stenosis treated with lumbar decompression and the cosmic "semi-rigid" posterior system. SAS J. 2010;4(4):99–106.
59. Maleci A, Sambale RD, Schiavone M, Lamp F, Özer F, von Strempel A. Nonfusion stabilization of the degenerative lumbar spine. J Neurosurg Spine. 2011;15(2):151–8.
60. Kaner T, Ozer AF. Dynamic stabilization for challenging lumbar degenerative diseases of the spine: a review of the literature. Adv Orthop. 2013;2013:753470.
61. Özer AF, Başak AT, Özbek MA, et al. Lumbar dynamic stabilization with 2-stage surgery: early results. Int J Spine Surg. 2022;16(4):638–45.
62. Saifuddin A, Mitchell R, Taylor BA. Extradural inflammation associated with annular tears: demonstration with gadolinium-enhanced lumbar spine MRI. Eur Spine J. 1999;8(1):34–9.
63. Brinjikji W, Diehn FE, Jarvik JG, Carr CM, Kallmes DF, Murad MH, Luetmer PH. MRI findings of disc degeneration are more prevalent in adults with low back pain than in asymptomatic controls: a systematic review and meta-analysis. AJNR Am J Neuroradiol. 2015;36(12):2394–9.
64. Lagerstrand K, Hebelka H, Brisby H. Identification of potentially painful disc fissures in magnetic resonance images using machine-learning modelling. Eur Spine J. 2022;31(8):1992–9.
65. Sharifi S, Bulstra SK, Grijpma DW, Kuijer R. Treatment of the degenerated intervertebral disc; closure, repair and regeneration of the annulus fibrosus. J Tissue Eng Regen Med. 2015;9(10):1120–32.
66. Ozer AF, Oktenoglu T, Sasani M, Kaner T, Ercelen O, Canbulat N. Unusual cause of acute low-back pain: sudden annulus fibrosus rupture. Orthop Rev (Pavia). 2012;4(2):e22.
67. Pfirrmann CW, Metzdorf A, Zanetti M, Hodler J, Boos N. Magnetic resonance classification of lumbar intervertebral disc degeneration. Spine (Phila Pa 1976). 2001;26:1873–8.
68. Yilmaz A, Senturk S, Sasani M, Oktenoglu T, Yaman O, Yildirim H, Suzer T, Ozer AF. Disc rehydration after dynamic stabilization: a report of 59 cases. Asian Spine J. 2017;11(3):348–55.
69. Wang W, Huang W, Yu X, Wang L, Xu X. Lumbar disc rehydration after dynamic stabilization: a systematic review. Medicine (Baltimore). 2023;102(15):e33163.
70. Cho BY, Murovic J, Park KW, Park J. Lumbar disc rehydration postimplantation of a posterior dynamic stabilization system. J Neurosurg Spine. 2010;13(5):576–80.
71. Oktenoglu T, Erbulut DU, Kiapour A, Ozer AF, Lazoglu I, Kaner T, Sasani M, Goel VK. Pedicle screw-based posterior dynamic stabilisation of the lumbar spine: in vitro cadaver investigation and a finite element study. Comput Methods Biomech Biomed Engin. 2015;18(11):1252–61. https://doi.org/10.1080/10255842.2014.890187.
72. Erbulut DU, Kiapour A, Oktenoglu T, Ozer AF, Goel VK. A computational biomechanical investigation of posterior dynamic instrumentation: combination of dynamic rod and hinged (dynamic) screw. J Biomech Eng. 2014;136(5):051007.
73. Kaner T, Sasani M, Oktenoglu T, Cosar M, Ozer AF. Utilizing dynamic rods with dynamic screws in the surgical treatment of chronic instability: a prospective clinical study. Turk Neurosurg. 2009;19(4):319–26.

74. Ozer AF, Crawford NR, Sasani M, Oktenoglu T, Bozkus H, Kaner T, Aydin S. Dynamic lumbar pedicle screw-rod stabilization: two-year follow-up and comparison with fusion. Open Orthop J. 2010;4:137–41.
75. Modic MT, Steinberg PM, Ross JS, Masaryk TJ, Carter JR. Degenerative disk disease: assessment of changes in vertebral body marrow with MR imaging. Radiology. 1988;166(1 Pt 1):193–9. https://doi.org/10.1148/radiology.166.1.3336678.
76. Shan Z, Fan S, Xie Q, Suyou L, Liu J, Wang C, Zhao F. Spontaneous resorption of lumbar disc herniation is less likely when modic changes are present. Spine (Phila Pa 1976). 2014;39(9):736–44.
77. Karadağ MK, Akıncı AT, Başak AT, Hekimoğlu M, Yıldırım H, Akyoldaş G, Aydın AL, Ateş Ö, Öktenoğlu T, Sasani M, Akgün MY, Günerbüyük C, Özer AF. Preoperative magnetic resonance imaging abnormalities predictive of lumbar herniation recurrence after surgical repair. World Neurosurg. 2022;165:e750–6.
78. Özer AF, Akyoldaş G, Çevik OM, Aydın AL, Hekimoğlu M, Sasani M, Öktenoğlu T, Çerezci Ö, Süzer T. Lumbar foraminal stenosis classification that guides surgical treatment. Int J Spine Surg. 2022;16(4):666–73.
79. Kjaer P, Leboeuf-Yde C, Korsholm L, Sorensen JS, Bendix T. Magnetic resonance imaging and low back pain in adults: a diagnostic imaging study of 40-year-old men and women. Spine (Phila Pa 1976). 2005;30:1173–80.
80. Jensen RK, Jensen TS, Koes B, Hartvigsen J. Prevalence of lumbar spinal stenosis in general and clinical populations: a systematic review and meta-analysis. Eur Spine J. 2020;29:2143–63.
81. Akgun MY, Toklu S, Gunerbuyuk C, Ates O, Aydin AL, Baran O, Oktenoglu T, Sasani M, Ozer AF. Foraminoplasty with partial pediculectomy in degenerative spondylolisthesis cases with nerve compression. World Neurosurg. 2023;172:e532–9.
82. Ozer AF, Suzer T, Sasani M, Oktenoglu T, Egemen E. Enlargement of neural foramina and dynamic stabilization in spondylolisthesis without restoring the alignment: technical note. Korean J Spine. 2016;13(1):37–9.
83. Bozkus H, Sasani M, Oktenoglu T, Aydin AL, Ozer AF. Unilateral dynamic stabilization for unilateral lumbar spinal pathologies; a new surgical concept. Turk Neurosurg. 2012;22(6):718–23.
84. Ozer AF, Suzer T, Sasani M, Oktenoglu T, Cezayirli P, Marandi HJ, Erbulut DU. Simple facet joint repair with dynamic pedicular system: technical note and case series. J Craniovertebr Junction Spine. 2015;6(2):65–8.

Rehabilitation After Lumbar Transpedicular Dynamic Stabilization Surgery

25

Nazan Canbulat, Yaprak Ataker, and Tunç Öktenoğlu

25.1 Introduction

Developing a standardized postoperative rehabilitation plan is essential because of the growing trend of dynamic lumbar spine stabilization surgery. There are currently no uniform standards for the rehabilitation of patients after dynamic lumbar spine stabilization surgery. A structured, well-planned postoperative rehabilitation program can result in significant improvements in the parameters of pain and quality of life and does not increase the risk of postoperative complications. Successful management of the patient after dynamic lumbar stabilization surgery is often dependent on the specific surgical intervention, as well as the appropriately planned and executed rehabilitation. All patients who have undergone spinal surgery do not progress in their rehabilitation at the same rate. Clinicians must consider anatomy and biomechanics, underlying pathophysiology, mechanobiology of collagen tissue healing, and the specific surgical intervention to appropriately adjust the postoperative course of rehabilitation for each patient. Exercise programs considering both the core area and the full kinetic chain are important.

Patient education, accurate information about the postoperative course, and information about limitations as well as pain management seem to have an important role in the final outcome of the operation. Ideally, these procedures should be performed preoperatively or repeatedly from the first postoperative day following lumbar spine surgery. There are studies that showed that greater levels of fear of movement were related to greater levels of lower back disability following lumbar spine surgery. It is recommended to address the fear of movement in prehabilitation/rehabilitation pre- or postsurgically to improve health outcomes for patients who undergo lumbar spine surgery [1].

Different types of depressive symptoms are associated with poor outcomes after lumbar spine surgery. This was observed in pain intensity, functional disability, and response to pain medication. It would be important to evaluate depression pre- and postoperatively. Offering a tailored rehabilitation program to patients with depression should be considered [2].

The purpose of this chapter is to make recommendations for the postoperative rehabilitation after dynamic lumbar stabilization surgery regarding mobilization, weight bearing, and return to full activities of daily living. These recommendations are based on current evidence and experience in our institution [3].

N. Canbulat (✉) · Y. Ataker
Koç University School of Medicine, Department of Physical Medicine and Rehabilitation, Istanbul, Turkey
e-mail: YaprakA@amerikanhastanesi.org

T. Öktenoğlu
Department of Neurosurgery, Koç University School of Medicine, Istanbul, Turkey

A. F. Özer et al. (eds.), *Dynamic Lumbar Spine Stabilization*,
https://doi.org/10.1007/978-3-032-12122-6_25

A rehabilitation plan following dynamic lumbar stabilization surgery should be formulated on the basis of basic sciences. The goals of the surgery are the decompression of the neural tissue, restoration of the vertebral alignment, and stabilization. Planning the phases of the rehabilitation program following transpedicular dynamic stabilization depends on the biology of implant osseointegration and the mechanobiology of collagen tissue healing.

In the first part, we will discuss the importance of osseointegration and the phases of collagen tissue healing in determining the rehabilitation plan following transpedicular dynamic lumbar stabilization. In the second part, we will discuss the rationale of the exercise programs after dynamic lumbar stabilization surgery. Exercise programs after surgery of the spine begin with the goal of improving the alignment and posture. Lumbar stabilization and core strengthening exercises that strengthen the muscles supporting the spine will be discussed. The concept of neutral zone and elastic zone is important in spinal rehabilitation. Active, passive, and neural control subsystems of the spinal stabilization system work together in the kinetic chain rehabilitation approach, which focuses on rehabilitating the entire neuromuscular system, integrating multiple body segments into the exercise.

25.2 Important Factors in Planning the Phases of the Rehabilitation Program Following Transpedicular Dynamic Stabilization

All patients who have undergone spinal surgery do not progress in their rehabilitation at the same rate. There are many important factors that affect the functional outcome. These factors are age, level of activity, duration of symptom, smoking, surgical technique, presence of other spinal pathologies, medications, systemic diseases, tissue quality and muscle atrophy, sagittal balance problems, the presence of segmental instability, the degree of annular tear, and the presence of transitional vertebrae.

Rehabilitation protocols are based on basic principles but should always be tailored according to the patient. The biology of implant osseointegration and healing timelines of the collagen tissue are the two main factors in determining the phases of the rehabilitation programs.

25.2.1 Biology of Implant Osseointegration and Healing Timelines of the Collagen Tissue

The degeneration of the intervertebral disk, which is the primary stabilizer of the spine, causes segmental instability. The degenerated segment cannot carry the body weight. Segmental instability resulting from disk degeneration is the source of the pain occurring with the movement of the spine. The symptoms of degenerative disk disease most commonly start between 30 and 50 years of age. This is the period of life during which challenging work and sports activities are performed. Age-related degenerative changes affecting the intervertebral disks, vertebrae, facet joints, and ligaments cause entrapment of the spinal nerves and spinal nerve roots. When the resulting pain due to degenerative disk disease, spinal stenosis, and degenerative spondylolisthesis cannot be controlled by conservative treatment, surgery can be considered.

Until recently, spinal fusion surgery has been preferred as the gold standard for controlling the pain related to the instability of a degenerated spinal segment. The aim of fusion surgery is to control the pain by eliminating the motion on the painful segment. However, the outcomes of spinal fusion are still controversial. Normal spinal biomechanics cannot be achieved following fusion surgery [4–7].

The philosophy of dynamic instrumentation surgery is just opposite to that of spinal fusion surgery. The purpose of fusion surgery is to eliminate motion. On the other hand, the aims of dynamic instrumentation systems are to control the spinal segmental motion, stop the pathological motion, neutralize the excessive load, prevent the progressive deformity, protect the function, and allow controlled movement at the affected segment. According to the Pfirrmann criteria, it is possible to preserve motion in patients stabilized with the dynamic system in the early phases of degeneration. In the late phases, the dynamic system brings the motion segment to fusion in a controlled manner, but the patient spends this period painlessly as the impaired motion segment is stabilized [8].

These systems are indicated in cases of painful degenerative disk disease, symptomatic lumbar stenosis, chronic lumbar pain due to facet syndrome and discogenic pain, recurrent disk herniation, degenerative spondylolisthesis, iatrogenic instability, and adjacent segment disease after fusion surgery [9–11].

Rehabilitation planning after lumbar transpedicular dynamic stabilization should be based on the biology of implant osseointegration. The rehabilitation specialist should be aware of the osseointegration process, which is an important determinant of the rehabilitation plan.

Osseointegration refers to the direct structural and functional connections between the living bone and the surface of a load-carrying implant. An implant is considered osseointegrated when there is no movement between the implant and the bone with which it has direct contact [12] (Fig. 25.1).

There is a tissue response to the implant and peri-implant bone formation (osteogenesis) that starts on the first day after implant fixation. Peri-implant trabecular bone formation begins 10–14 days after surgery. At 3 months after implantation, woven and lamellar bone formation is observed around the titanium implant. Maturation (remodeling) of the bone around the implant may take up to 1 year [13].

Various factors may enhance or inhibit osseointegration. Factors enhancing osseointegration include implant-related factors such as the design of the implant or chemical composition, implant surface coatings, status of the host bone and intrinsic healing potential, mechanical stability of the implant, adjuvant treatments like bone grafting or osteogenic biological coatings, biophysical stimulation, and pharmacological agents like simvastatin and bisphosphonates.

Factors inhibiting osseointegration include excessive implant mobility and micromotion, inappropriate porosity of the porous coating of the implant, radiation therapy, and pharmacological agents like cyclosporin A, methotrexate, warfarin, low-molecular-weight heparins, and nonsteroidal anti-inflammatory drugs, especially selective Cyclooxygenase-2 (COX2) inhibitors. There are also patient-related factors inhibiting osseointegration, such as osteoporosis, rheumatoid arthritis, advanced age, nutritional deficiency, smoking, and renal insufficiency [12].

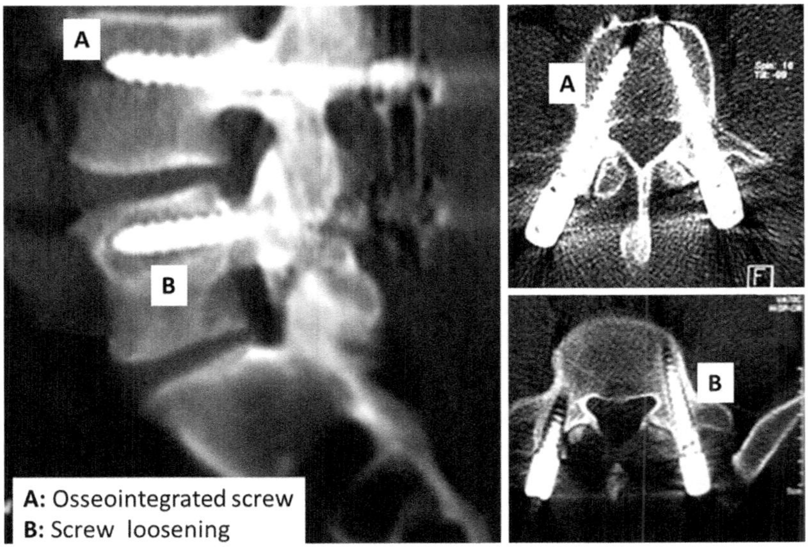

Fig. 25.1 (a) Osseointegrated screw. (b) Screw loosening

The osseointegration process is important, and if aggressive rehabilitation is performed before osseointegration is complete, loosening of the implant may result. Bone strength is also important for stability. Controlled movement is necessary and stimulates new bone formation. It has been shown that dynamic loads, rather than static loads; short-term mechanical loads; and the response of bone cells to these loads are important determinants of the bone adaptation process [14].

Another important aspect in planning the rehabilitation program after dynamic lumbar stabilization surgery is the healing timeline of the collagen tissue. Collagen tissue healing is primarily divided into three phases. The inflammatory phase, the proliferative phase, and the remodeling (maturation) phase. The inflammatory phase occurs during the first 7 days, when platelets from blood plasma enter to initiate clot formation. The inflammatory phase gradually transforms into the proliferative phase, which occurs 2–3 weeks after surgery. Fibroblasts initially produce type III collagen, which is arranged irregularly in the absence of cross-linking. The maturation, or remodeling, phase begins around week 3 after surgery, and scar tissue organizes. Immature type III collagen is replaced by mature type I collagen during this phase, and the type I collagen aligns along tensile forces. The collagen is continually remodeled until permanent repair tissue is formed. There is variation during the maturation phase. Studies suggest that collagen healing takes 12–16 weeks to 1 year to reach the final tensile strength [15, 16].

From the point of view of the mechanobiology of collagen tissue healing, excessive movement in a region that has recently undergone surgery damages collagen tissue healing. Complete removal of load is also harmful to normal healing. Controlled loading can enhance healing in most settings; however, a fine balance must be reached between loads that are too low, like immobilization, and loads that are too high, leading to damage [17].

Considering the stages of the osseointegration process and the time intervals of collagen tissue healing, the rehabilitation program after transpedicular dynamic stabilization is divided into five main phases.

The first phase is the "preoperative evaluation phase." This is followed by the postoperative phases. The second phase is named the "active rest phase" and is composed of the first six postoperative weeks. In this period, it is important to teach the correct posture (Fig. 25.2a, b) to the patient, and the avoidance of excessive movements is emphasized.

The third phase is the "minimum movement phase," which is the period between the 6th and the 12th postoperative weeks. During this period, pelvic tilt exercise (Fig. 25.3) is started, and general body exercises such as swimming and walking are recommended in pain-free limits.

The fourth phase is named the "dynamic phase" and is the period between the 12th postoperative week and the 6th postoperative month. In this period, dynamic lumbar stabilization exercises are initiated in consultation with the surgical team (Figs. 25.4 and 25.5).

The fifth phase is the "back to sports" phase, which starts after the sixth postoperative month. Patients are allowed to participate in low-resistance and high-repetition sport activities. Contact sports are allowed, but the risks of falling and impact are explained to the patients (Table 25.1).

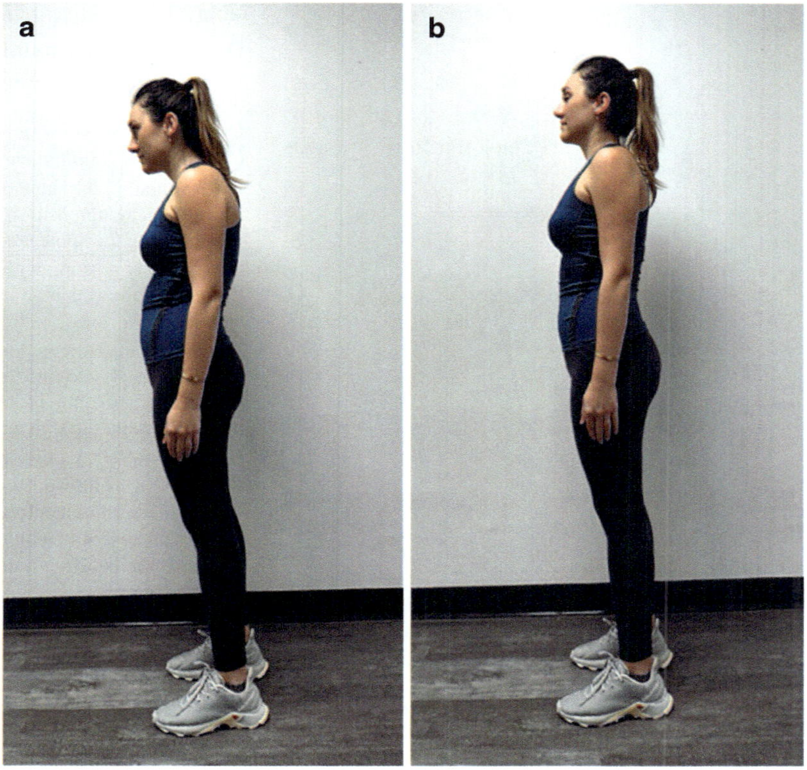

Fig. 25.2 (**a**) Incorrect posture. (**b**) Correct posture

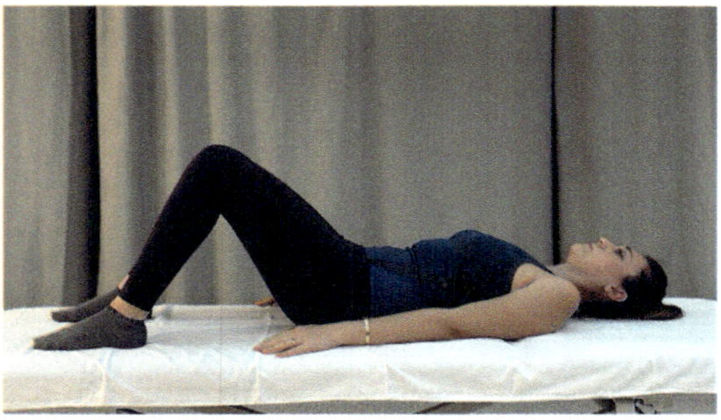

Fig. 25.3 Pelvic tilt exercise

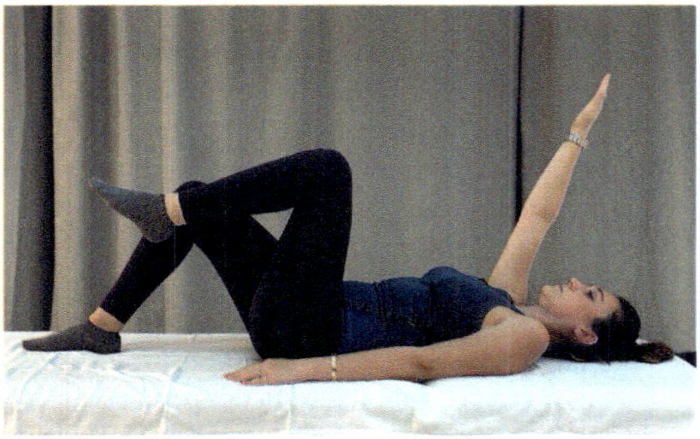

Fig. 25.4 Dynamic lumbar stabilization exercise: core strengthening exercise with arms and legs

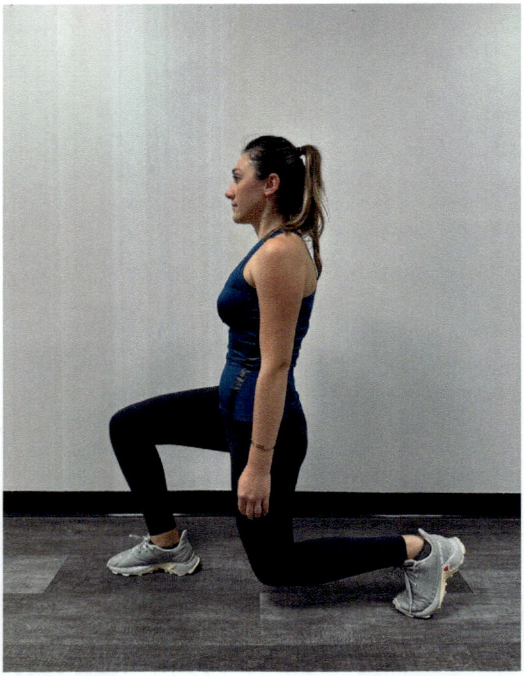

Fig. 25.5 Dynamic lumbar stabilization exercise: step forward (lunge)

Table 25.2 Principles of lumbar care

Do not sit in the same position for more than 30 min. Change your position, stand up, walk for 3–5 s, and sit down again
Do not sit on very low or very soft seats
Chairs with a good lumbar support should be preferred
Do not stand in the same position for more than 30 min; changing position and redistributing the weight along the spine are important
Correct body posture, with the shoulders retracted, should be followed at all times, especially in the sitting and working position
The lying and sleeping position should be comfortable and painless. Try to find the least painful and most comfortable position. Lying on one's side with a pillow between the legs may help
Do not carry heavy objects. Instead of carrying 20 kg at once, carry 2 kg ten times
While lifting an object from the floor, squatting is correct, instead of bending from the lumbar spine
The object to be lifted should be kept close to the body while lifting
Any sport, activity, or exercise aggravating the back pain should be stopped
While driving, the seat should be adjusted in a proper position, with the back straight

Table 25.1 Rehabilitation protocol after transpedicular dynamic stabilization

Phase 1: Preoperative evaluation phase
The patients are informed about the surgery and the period after posterior dynamic instrumentation
Lumbar protection principles are explained (Table 25.2)
Phase 2: Active rest phase (0–6 weeks)
On the first postoperative day, the patient is mobilized
The correct posture is taught (Fig. 25.2a, b)
Patients are informed about pain-aggravating movements. Prolonged sitting (more than 30 min), standing in the same position (more than 30 min), lumbar twisting, lumbar hyperflexion, hyperextension, and lifting heavy objects should be avoided
Phase 3: Minimum movement phase (6–12 weeks)
Pelvic tilt exercises are started in this period (Fig. 25.3)
Swimming and walking are allowed in pain-free limits. The duration and frequency of walking are determined according to the patient's tolerance
Phase 4: Dynamic phase (12 weeks to 6 months)
Dynamic lumbar stabilization exercises are initiated in this phase
The first group of these exercises is done in the supine position by moving only the upper and lower extremities while doing pelvic tilt (Fig. 25.4)
Dynamic lumbar stabilization exercises in the standing position are also added to the program (Fig. 25.5)
Dynamic lumbar stabilization exercises are gradually advanced according to the patient's tolerance (Figs. 25.6 and 25.7)
In these weeks, it is especially important to avoid rotational movements of the lumbar spine
Swimming and walking are continued in pain-free limits
Phase 5: Back to sports phase (after the 6th month)
In this phase, return to sports is planned
Sport-specific exercises are started
Special precautions are taken according to the preferred sports activity, and the training program is individualized

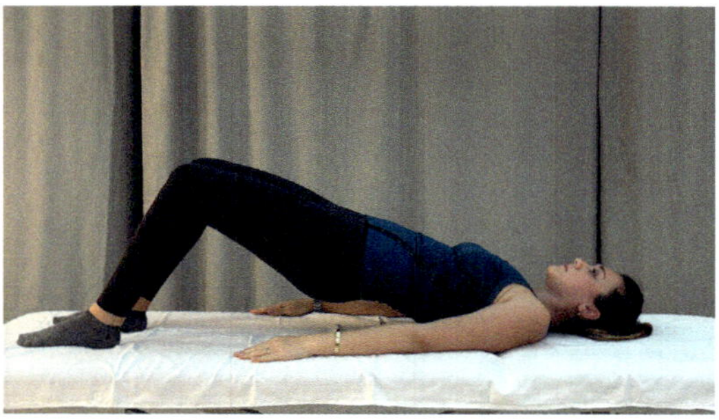

Fig. 25.6 Dynamic lumbar stabilization exercise: bridge exercise

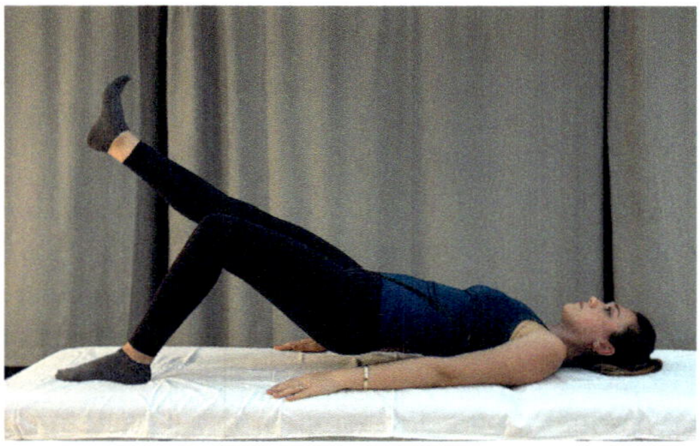

Fig. 25.7 Dynamic lumbar stabilization exercise: leg extension in bridge position

25.3 Rationale of Exercise Programs After Spinal Surgery

25.3.1 Why Exercise? Which Exercise?

25.3.1.1 Developing a Muscle Brace Around the Spine Through Exercise

The stabilization system of the spine, defined by Panjabi, consists of three subsystems. These are the passive subsystem, the active subsystem, and the neural control subsystem.

The passive subsystem is composed of the vertebrae, disks, and ligaments. The active subsystem is composed of all muscles and tendons surrounding the spinal column that can apply forces to the spinal column. The neural control subsystem is composed of the nerves and the central nervous system. The neural control subsystem monitors the various transducer signals

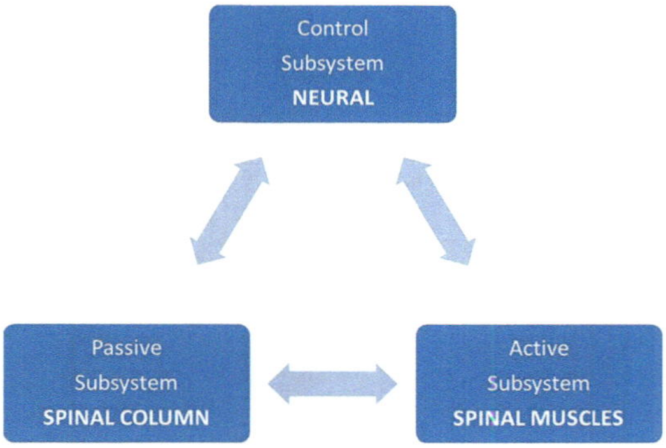

Fig. 25.8 Stabilization system of the spine

and directs the active subsystem to provide the needed stability. The passive, active, and neural control subsystems are functionally interdependent. The dysfunction of a component of any one of the subsystems may lead to immediate compensation response from other subsystems, resulting in normal function. When the dysfunction of a component of any one of the subsystems results in a long-term adaptation response, there is normal function of the spine but with altered spinal stabilization. The failure of one of the subsystems to be compensated by the other subsystems and the collapse of the whole system results in instability and lower back pain [18] (Fig. 25.8).

The most important subsystem that can be strengthened with exercise is the active subsystem, formed by the muscles surrounding the spine. Spinal stability can be increased with exercise programs that create tension in the muscles around the spine. The active subsystem informs the neural control subsystem about the position and movements of the spine. The rationale of exercise programs is to develop dynamic stability in the spine by creating a muscle brace around the spine.

Panjabi stated that the total physiological range of motion has two components, which he called the neutral and elastic zones. Neutral zone movement is the physiological intervertebral movement of the spine against the minimal resistance exerted by the passive subsystem.

Neutral zone movement is the movement of the most stable part of the spine segment, and the movement is performed with minimal resistance.

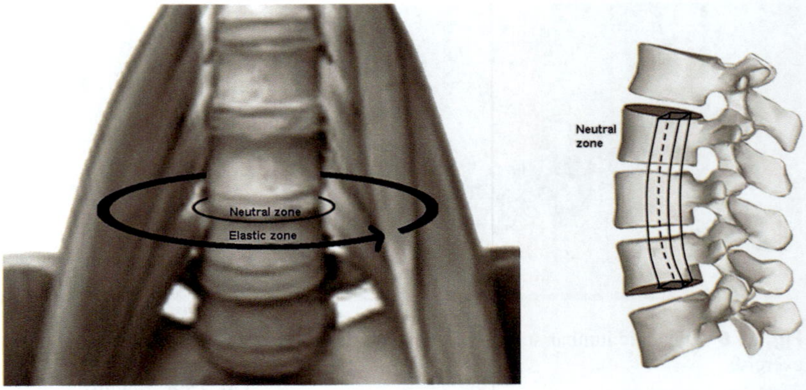

Fig. 25.9 Neutral and elastic zones

The neutral zone is clinically important and is a measure of spinal stability. In case of any damage to the spine or weakening of the muscles around the spine, there is neutral zone expansion, resulting in spinal instability and lower back problems. The neutral zone can be reduced by osteophyte formation, surgical fixation/fusion, or muscle-strengthening exercises. The elastic zone is the part of the physiological intervertebral movement that can be measured from around the neutral zone to the physiological limits. There is maximal resistance to spinal movement in the elastic zone. Here, the spine moves against resistance, and the resistance against movement is created by the joints (Fig. 25.9).

The logic and purpose of exercise programs is to keep the neutral zone within physiological limits.

25.4 Core Stabilization Exercises and Kinetic Chain Exercises

The main purpose of the exercise programs applied after spine surgery is to strengthen the area called the "core," formed by the deep muscles that stabilize the spine in the lumbopelvic junction. Thus, spine control is provided during dynamic movements of body parts. Key muscles to condition are the multifidus, transversus abdominus, internal oblique, paraspinal, and pelvic floor muscles.

Core stability is critically important for load balance and load transfer across the spine, pelvis, and the entire kinetic chain.

According to the kinetic chain model, the body consists of interdependent segments. Body parts often move in a proximal-to-distal sequence to elicit a desired movement in the distal segment [19, 20].

Normal motor development takes place from the proximal to the distal direction, and the body acts as a dynamic unit. Proximal stability (core control) is important, and movement in one part of the body facilitates movement in the adjacent segment. The kinetic chain model explains the contribution of the whole body to the activity rather than the movement in a single segment in sportive activities.

The stability of the core area and the motor control of this stability are essential for initiating functional arm and leg movements. It has been shown that trunk muscles contract before upper extremity and lower extremity movements [21, 22].

Core stabilization exercises mainly focus on strengthening the multifidus and transversus abdominus muscle groups. Multifidus is an important lumbar extensor and stabilizer. The lumbopelvic junction of the body creates a muscular support, which plays an important role in transferring the load from the upper to the lower part of the body. This role is maintained during standing, sitting, walking, and other body move-

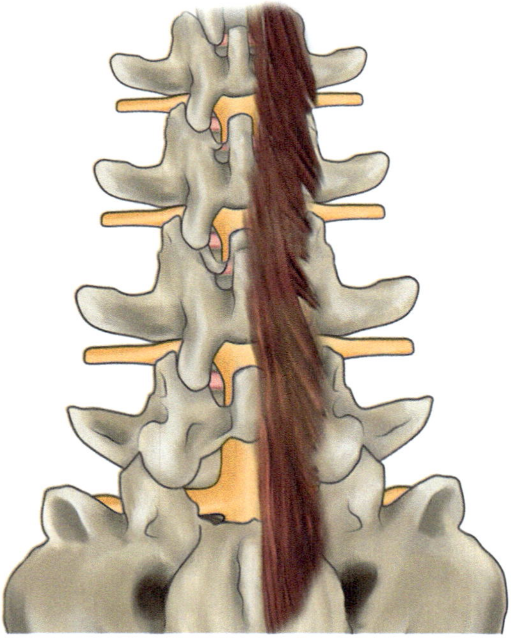

Fig. 25.10 The multifidus muscle

ments and while carrying objects. The multifidus muscle has deep and superficial fibers and segmental innervation. The deep fibers of the multifidus have a role in lumbar stabilization, and the superficial fibers have a role in maintaining lumbar lordosis during spinal movements (Fig. 25.10).

Multifidus dysfunction plays an important role in the recurrence of subacute pain and chronic lower back pain. Particular attention should be given to the multifidus muscle for stabilizing the lumbopelvic area [23]. Transversus abdominus muscles, in conjunction with external oblique muscles and internal oblique muscles, through the thoracolumbar fascia, play a role in the stabilization of the spine. Abdominal, gluteal, hip girdle, paraspinal, and other muscles work together to provide spinal stability.

The purpose of rehabilitation is to strengthen the stabilizing muscles of the spine and increase neuromuscular control. Although the aim in the rehabilitation program after spinal surgery seems to be to strengthen the isolated muscle groups, the main goal is to strengthen multiple muscle groups and motor patterns by means of anatomical connections. Not only the lumbar region but also the junction of the hip, spine, and shoulder girdle should be worked together. Exercises such as walking and swimming, which work many muscles of the body at the same time, should be included in the rehabilitation program. The entire kinetic chain should be included in the rehabilitation process. Therefore, exercise programs should involve strengthening of the core muscles, lower back muscles, abdominal muscles, and the whole kinetic chain [24].

Exercises enhancing neuromuscular control are proprioceptive exercises, plyometric exercises combining strength and velocity, work- and sport-specific exercises, agility exercises, and progressive strengthening and functional training exercises. All of them start with proximal stabilization and integrate the whole kinetic chain into the program.

25.5 Importance of a Multidisciplinary Approach for Enhanced Recovery After Surgery

The treatment of patients who have undergone spinal surgery needs a multidisciplinary approach. Close communication and collaboration between the surgeon, pain specialist, rehabilitation team, and the patient are crucially important for the best functional outcome (Fig. 25.11).

According to a recent study about the clinical application of enhanced recovery after surgery

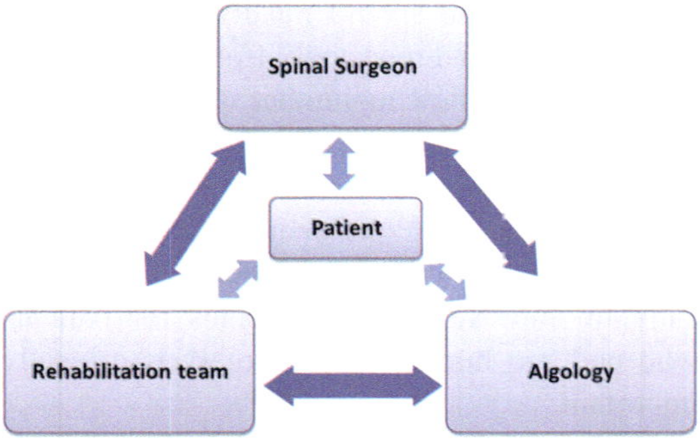

Fig. 25.11 Patient-centered multidisciplinary care

(ERAS) in lumbar disk herniation patients undergoing dynamic stabilization and discectomy, intraoperative blood loss, operation time, ambulation time, and the length of hospital stay were all lower in the ERAS group than in the control group. Results showed that the enhanced recovery after surgery (ERAS) protocol designed was feasible for patients undergoing dynamic lumbar stabilization and discectomy, with significantly improved perioperative outcomes [25].

ERAS protocols involve a multidisciplinary approach and start with a preoperative optimization of the patient during patient selection for spine surgery. Patients who are medically optimized before a major spine surgery demonstrate improvements in self-reported satisfaction scores, decreased postoperative complications, and decreased length of hospital stay. The ERAS protocol underlines several patient-specific, modifiable risk factors that could be targets for improvement before surgery: blood glucose control, smoking cessation, weight loss, osteoporosis treatment, opioid dependence, and the treatment of comorbid mental health disorders. Smoking is a strong risk factor for pseudarthrosis after spinal fusion. Uncontrolled diabetes mellitus is a strong risk factor for postoperative surgical site infection, poor wound healing, and pseudarthrosis after spinal surgery. Obesity is correlated with surgical site infection, poor wound healing, and pseudarthrosis after spinal surgery. Depression is correlated with poor patient satisfaction scores, regardless of whether the technical goals of surgery were achieved.

Patient education, accurate information about the postoperative course, activity limitations, and pain management should ideally be performed preoperatively and repeatedly from the first postoperative day following lumbar spine surgery.

Fear of movement is related to greater levels of lower back disability following lumbar spine surgery. Addressing the fear of movement in prehabilitation/rehabilitation pre- or postsurgically to improve health outcomes for patients who undergo lumbar spine surgery is critically important.

Early mobilization, immediate activation of the lower limb muscles within hours after surgery, and standing up within 24 h should be ensured. Physical exercise and limb pneumatic pump applications are valuable for improving microcirculation and preventing deep vein thrombosis.

The good outcomes can be achieved by a combination of very careful and restrictive patient selection, surgical technique, and a well-planned, patient-specific rehabilitation program.

References

1. Kemani MK, Hägg O, Jakobsson M, Lundberg M. Fear of movement is related to low back disability during a two-year period in patients who have undergone elective lumbar spine surgery. World Neurosurg. 2020;137:e416–24.
2. Järvimäki V, Kautiainen H, Haanpää M, Koponen H, Spalding M, Alahuhta S, Vakkala M. Depressive symptoms are associated with poor outcome for lumbar spine surgery. Scand J Pain. 2016;12:13–7.
3. Canbulat N, Oktenoglu T, Ataker Y, Sasani M, Ercelen O, Cerezci O, Suzer T, Ozer AF. A rehabilitation protocol for patients with lumbar degenerative disc disease treated with posterior transpedicular dynamic stabilization. Turk Neurosurg. 2017;27(3):426–35.
4. Hilibrand AS, Robbins M. Adjacent segment degeneration and adjacent segment disease: the consequences of spinal fusion? Spine J. 2004;4(6 Suppl):190S–4S.
5. Ishihara H, Kanamori M, Kawaguchi Y, Nakamura H, Kimura T. Adjacent segment disease after anterior cervical interbody fusion. Spine J. 2004;4(6):624–8.
6. Mayer HM, Korge A. Non-fusion technology in degenerative lumbar spinal disorders: facts, questions, challenges. Eur Spine J. 2002;11 Suppl 2(Suppl 2):S85–91.
7. Fritzell P, Hägg O, Wessberg P, Nordwall A, Swedish Lumbar Spine Study Group. 2001 Volvo Award Winner in Clinical Studies: lumbar fusion versus nonsurgical treatment for chronic low back pain: a multicenter randomized controlled trial from the Swedish Lumbar Spine Study Group. Spine (Phila Pa 1976). 2001;26(23):2521–32; discussion 2532–4.
8. Yilmaz A, Senturk S, Sasani M, Oktenoglu T, Yaman O, Yildirim H, Suzer T, Ozer AF. Disc rehydration after dynamic stabilization: a report of 59 cases. Asian Spine J. 2017;11(3):348–55.
9. Dooris AP, Goel VK, Grosland NM, Gilbertson LG, Wilder DG. Load-sharing between anterior and posterior elements in a lumbar motion segment implanted with an artificial disc. Spine (Phila Pa 1976). 2001;26(6):E122–9.
10. Hedman TP, Kostuik JP, Fernie GR, Hellier WG. Design of an intervertebral disc prosthesis. Spine (Phila Pa 1976). 1991;16(6 Suppl):S256–60.

11. Von Strempel A, Moosmann D, Stoss C, Martin A. Stabilization of the degenerated lumbar spine in the nonfusion technique with cosmic posterior dynamic system. WSJ. 2006;1:40–7.
12. Mavrogenis AF, Dimitriou R, Parvizi J, Babis GC. Biology of implant osseointegration. J Musculoskelet Neuronal Interact. 2009;9(2):61–71.
13. Roberts WE. Bone tissue interface. J Dent Educ. 1988;52(12):804–9.
14. Turner CH. Three rules for bone adaptation to mechanical stimuli. Bone. 1998;23(5):399–407.
15. Carpenter JE, Thomopoulos S, Flanagan CL, DeBano CM, Soslowsky LJ. Rotator cuff defect healing: a biomechanical and histologic analysis in an animal model. J Shoulder Elb Surg. 1998;7(6):599–605.
16. Guo S, Dipietro LA. Factors affecting wound healing. J Dent Res. 2010;89(3):219–29.
17. Killian ML, Cavinatto L, Galatz LM, Thomopoulos S. The role of mechanobiology in tendon healing. J Shoulder Elb Surg. 2012;21(2):228–37.
18. Panjabi MM. The stabilizing system of the spine. Part I. Function, dysfunction, adaptation, and enhancement. J Spinal Disord. 1992;5(4):383–9; discussion 397.
19. Feltner ME, Dapena J. Three-dimensional interactions in a two-segment kinetic chain, part I: general model. Int J Sport Biomech. 1989;5:403–19.
20. Putnam CA. Sequential motions of body segments in striking and throwing skills: description and explanations. J Biomech. 1993;26:125–35.
21. Cordo PJ, Nashner LM. Properties of postural adjustments associated with rapid arm movements. J Neurophysiol. 1982;47:287–302.
22. Zattara M, Bouisset S. Posturo-kinetic organisation during the early phase of voluntary upper limb movement. 1. Normal subjects. J Neurol Neurosurg Psychiatry. 1988;51(7):956–65.
23. Akuthota V, Ferreiro A, Moore T, Fredericson M. Core stability exercise principles. Curr Sports Med Rep. 2008;7(1):39–44.
24. Bonetti F, Curti S, Mattioli S, Mugnai R, Vanti C, Violante FS, Pillastrini P. Effectiveness of a 'Global Postural Reeducation' program for persistent Low Back Pain: a non-randomised controlled trial. BMC Musculoskelet Disord. 2010;11(1):285.
25. Zhang H, Wang Z, Li K. Clinical application of enhanced recovery after surgery in lumbar disk herniation patients undergoing dynamic stabilization and discectomy. J Back Musculoskelet Rehabil. 2022;35(1):47–53.

26 Emerging Biological Treatments for Intervertebral Disc Degeneration Disease: A Regenerative Medicine Perspective

Nesrin Ercelen, Esmer Zeynep Duru Badakal, and Gizem Boyraz

26.1 Introduction

Intervertebral disc degeneration disease (IVDD) is one of the most common causes of lower back pain, significantly reducing individuals' quality of life and placing a substantial economic burden on global healthcare systems. Lower back pain, one of the most prevalent musculoskeletal problems worldwide, affects more than 70% of the population at some point in their lives [1]. Progressive disc degeneration leads not only to mechanical instability [2] but also to pathological processes such as inflammation, sensitization of nerve endings, and nerve root compression [3]. Although traditional treatment methods—including physical therapy, pain management, anti-inflammatory drugs, epidural injections, and surgical interventions in advanced cases—provide symptomatic relief, they generally fail to reverse the underlying degenerative process [4].

N. Ercelen (✉)
Uskudar University Faculty of Medicine, Department of Medical Genetics, Biotechnology Application and Research Center (BİYOTEKMER), Istanbul, Turkey

Geneis Genetic System Solutions, Istanbul, Turkey
e-mail: nesrin.ercelen@uskudar.edu.tr

E. Z. D. Badakal · G. Boyraz
Geneis Genetic System Solutions, Istanbul, Turkey
e-mail: ndal@ku.edu.tr

In recent years, regenerative medicine technics like biological therapies have emerged as a promising research area for alleviating symptoms and promoting tissue regeneration in intervertebral disc diseases. Cellular therapies, growth factors, genetic engineering techniques, and tissue engineering approaches hold potential to restore disc tissue homeostasis and slow down progressive degeneration [4].

This section will address the basic characteristics of disc biology, the molecular and cellular foundations of degeneration, and biological treatment alternatives, providing a multidisciplinary perspective on the current status and future directions.

26.2 Biology of the Disc and Degenerative Mechanisms

26.2.1 Structural Characteristics of the Intervertebral Disc

The intervertebral disc is an avascular structure that provides spinal flexibility and mechanical stability, playing essential roles in load bearing and shock absorption. It consists of three main components: the nucleus pulposus (NP), the annulus fibrosus (AF), and the cartilaginous end

A. F. Özer et al. (eds.), *Dynamic Lumbar Spine Stabilization*,
https://doi.org/10.1007/978-3-032-12122-6_26

plates (CEPs) [4]. The NP is located at the center of the disc and is a gel-like structure with high water content. It primarily contains proteoglycans such as aggrecan and type II collagen, enabling it to absorb axial loads [5]. Surrounding the NP, the AF is composed of concentric lamellae rich in type I and type II collagen, providing resistance against tensile and torsional forces [6]. The CEPs, which separate the disc from the vertebral bodies, are hyaline-like structures that play a key role in the nutrient transport between the vertebrae and the disc tissue [4]. Due to its avascular nature, the disc is metabolically vulnerable. Nutrients and metabolites can only reach the disc cells via diffusion, so any disruption in this transport system or any impairment of cellular metabolism can trigger degenerative changes [5].

26.2.2 Degenerative Processes and Molecular Mechanisms

Intervertebral disc degeneration is a multifactorial and progressive condition marked by the loss of tissue homeostasis. It involves interconnected cellular and molecular mechanisms, including senescence, inflammation, oxidative stress, matrix degradation, and immune dysregulation. At the cellular level, nucleus pulposus cells exhibit increased senescence and apoptosis, leading to reduced extracellular matrix (ECM) production and altered cytokine profiles. These aged cells secrete pro-inflammatory mediators and fail to maintain tissue homeostasis, thereby contributing to structural decline [2]. Mitochondrial dysfunction and the accumulation of reactive oxygen species (ROS) exacerbate this decline by inducing oxidative DNA damage, promoting cell death, and accelerating degenerative cascades [7]. On a structural level, degeneration is characterized by the loss of key ECM components such as aggrecan and type II collagen, which results in decreased hydration, disc height reduction, and impaired shock absorption. Concurrently, there is a compensatory increase in fibrotic type I collagen, which stiffens the disc and reduces its biomechanical flexibility [8]. Inflammatory cytokines—particularly interleukin-1β (IL-1β) and tumor necrosis factor–alpha (TNF-α)—are upregulated in degenerating discs. These cytokines stimulate the expression of catabolic enzymes, including matrix metalloproteinases (MMP-3 and MMP-13) and aggrecanases (ADAMTS-5), accelerating ECM breakdown and disrupting tissue integrity [5].

As disc degeneration progresses, structural disruptions in the annulus fibrosus may expose normally sequestered NP components to the immune system. This breach can activate macrophage infiltration and T-cell responses, triggering chronic inflammation and amplifying tissue degradation. Such immune-mediated processes further contribute to nerve sensitization and discogenic pain [6].

26.3 Risk Factors and Etiopathogenic Mechanisms Underlying Intervertebral Disc Degeneration

Intervertebral disc degeneration disease is a complex, multifactorial condition influenced by genetic, biochemical, structural, and immunological components. In recent years, there has been a growing emphasis on the roles of genetic predisposition; collagen matrix integrity, particularly type II collagen; and autoimmune-inflammatory processes in the onset and progression of IVDD.

26.3.1 Genetic Susceptibility and Molecular Markers

Recent meta-analyses have confirmed a substantial heritable component in IVDD, estimating that up to 60–80% of susceptibility is genetically determined. Among the most studied genes are those encoding for collagen, particularly COL1A1, COL11A1, and COL9A2/9A3, which are involved in maintaining extracellular matrix integrity and biomechanical function. A comprehensive meta-analysis by Xie et al. (2021) demonstrated a significant association between the COL1A1 Sp1 (+1245G>T) polymorphism and the increased risk of IVDD, particularly in Caucasian populations [9]. Similarly, the COL11A1 C4603T variant was linked to a higher susceptibility to disc degeneration due to its involvement in ECM remodeling and structural resilience. These polymorphisms affect collagen fiber formation and increase the tissue's vulnerability to mechanical and inflammatory stress [9]. Other gene variants implicated in IVDD include those coding for aggrecan, matrix metalloproteinases, IL-1β, and the vitamin D receptor, all of which participate in ECM metabolism and inflammation regulation [10].

26.3.2 Type II Collagen and Structural Vulnerability

Type II collagen, encoded by the COL2A1 gene, is the principal structural protein of the nucleus pulposus and the inner annulus fibrosus. It provides compressive strength and elasticity, crucial for load distribution in the spine. Mutations or polymorphisms in COL2A1 can lead to weakened fibril organization, decreased hydration, and altered osmotic balance, thereby promoting early fibrotic changes and disc collapse. In degenerated discs, the loss of type II collagen is typically accompanied by an increased expression of type I collagen, which creates a stiffer, fibrotic ECM, less capable of absorbing mechanical loads. This imbalance not only reduces the functional capacity but also facilitates microstructural damage, such as annular tears and nucleus extrusion [2].

26.3.3 Autoinflammatory and Immune-Mediated Mechanisms

In addition to structural deterioration, IVDD involves a significant immunological component. The intervertebral disc is considered an immune-privileged site; however, degeneration disrupts this status by exposing normally sequestered disc antigens, such as type II collagen and aggrecan, to immune surveillance. This can trigger autoimmune responses, including T-cell activation and macrophage infiltration [10, 11]. Recent studies have demonstrated increased levels of pro-inflammatory cytokines such as TNF-α, IL-1β, IL-6, and IL-17 in degenerated discs. These cytokines contribute to ECM degradation by upregulating catabolic enzymes such as MMPs and ADAMTS while simultaneously promoting apoptosis and inhibiting regeneration. In particular, NLRP3 inflammasome activation has been identified as a key pathway in disc inflammation and cell pyroptosis, linking innate immunity to disc tissue breakdown [12, 13]. Macrophage polarization also plays a role in disease trajectory. While M1 macrophages promote inflammation through nitric oxide and TNF-α release, M2 macrophages exhibit anti-inflammatory properties and may aid in tissue repair. An imbalance in M1/M2 phenotypes contributes to chronic inflammation within the disc microenvironment [11].

26.4 Conventional and Palliative Therapuetic Approaches in Intervertebral Disc Degeneration

Intervertebral disc degeneration disease is typically managed with conventional therapies that are largely palliative in nature. These treatments aim to reduce pain and maintain functionality rather than directly modify the degenerative process. Interventions primarily focus on symptom control through pharmacological agents, physical rehabilitation, and interventional or surgical techniques. Nonsteroidal anti-inflammatory drugs (NSAIDs), such as ibuprofen and naproxen, are commonly prescribed to alleviate inflammation and pain, though their prolonged use is associated with gastrointestinal, renal, and cardiovascular side effects [14]. For patients experiencing muscle spasms or radiculopathy, muscle relaxants, gabapentinoids, or serotonin-norepinephrine reuptake inhibitors (SNRIs) may be added. Short-term corticosteroid use may be considered during acute exacerbations, but long-term administration is generally discouraged due to systemic risks [15].

Non-pharmacological treatments, such as physical therapy and exercise programs, form the cornerstone of conservative management. Therapeutic exercises—including core stabilization, lumbar extension movements (e.g., the McKenzie method), and aerobic conditioning—have been shown to improve spinal mobility, reduce pain intensity, and enhance the overall functional status. Manual therapy and postural retraining may further complement these strategies [16]. However, while beneficial for symptom relief, these approaches do not directly influence disc cell biology or promote structural regeneration.

Interventional pain procedures are reserved for patients with persistent symptoms. Epidural steroid injections (ESIs), which involve the delivery of corticosteroids and local anesthetics into the epidural space, are widely used for managing radicular pain due to nerve root inflammation. Similarly, facet joint injections and medial branch blocks may relieve axial back pain originating from degenerative facet arthropathy. Although effective in selected cases, the relief is usually temporary, and repeated procedures increase the risk of complications such as infection, dural puncture, and tissue fibrosis [17]. When conservative measures fail to provide adequate relief—typically after 6–12 months—surgical intervention may also be considered.

In conclusion, conventional treatment approaches in IVDD focus on managing symptoms and maintaining functional capacity but fall short in reversing the underlying degenerative cascade. These treatments cannot restore the extracellular matrix integrity, prevent cellular senescence, or modulate inflammatory pathways inherent to disc pathology. Moreover, the long-term use of analgesics—especially opioids—carries serious risks such as dependency, tolerance, and systemic side effects [18]. Thus, while traditional therapies remain indispensable for symptomatic relief, the growing demand for regenerative and biologically targeted therapies has drawn significant attention. In this context, recent clinical studies on the intradiscal delivery of biological agents report promising results.

26.5 Biological Treatment Approaches

Intervertebral disc degeneration disease is not merely a result of mechanical deterioration; it also involves a complex interplay of inflammatory, cellular, and molecular processes. Therefore, biological treatment strategies targeting the etiopathogenesis of the disease have gained significant attention in recent years. The primary objective of biological therapies is to preserve the native disc structure, promote regeneration, and halt or slow down the degenerative cascade. Among the methods developed within this scope are growth factors, mesenchymal stem cells (MSCs), exosomes, gene therapies, and tissue engineering–based biomaterials. This section focuses on evaluating biological treatment approaches, particularly MSC- and exosome-based strategies.

26.5.1 Mesenchymal Stem Cells (MSCs)

Mesenchymal stem cells have emerged as one of the most extensively studied cell types in the biological treatment of IVDD due to their anti-inflammatory, immunomodulatory, and tissue regenerative (Table 26.1) properties. These cells can be isolated from various sources, including the bone marrow (BM-MSCs), the adipose tissue (AD-MSCs), and the umbilical cord (UC-MSCs), and are known for their ability to remain functional even in hypoxic and inflammatory microenvironments. The therapeutic effect of MSCs is attributed not only to their differentiation capacity but also to their ability to regulate inflammation and immune responses through the secretion of paracrine factors [19, 20].

These properties suggest that MSCs could be effective not only in local tissue repair but also in systemic inflammatory conditions. For instance, their potential was demonstrated in severe forms of COVID-19, where cytokine storms played a critical role in disease severity. In two recent

Table 26.1 Recent clinical trials investigating MSC-based therapies for intervertebral disc degeneration disease

Study/registry ID	Year	Intervention	Phase/status	Key outcomes
NCT04759105	2023	Autologous BM-MSC intradiscal injection	Phase IIb—Completed	VAS, ODI, MRI (Pfirrmann), disc height
Mesoblast Rexlemestrocel-L (FDA RMAT)	2021	Allogeneic MPC intradiscal injection	Phase III—Recruiting	Pain, disability, safety
RESPINE—NCT03737461	Ongoing	Allogeneic BM-MSC intradiscal injection	Phase III—Active, not recruiting	VAS, ODI, MRI disc hydration

studies—a meta-analysis by Qu et al. (2022) and a clinical report by Ercelen et al. (2021), respectively—UC-MSC treatment was shown to significantly reduce the levels of inflammatory cytokines such as IL-6 and TNF-α, improve oxygenation, and enhance clinical outcomes. These findings indicate that the ability of MSCs to modulate systemic inflammation could also be beneficial in chronic inflammatory conditions such as IVDD [21, 22].

MSCs exert multifaceted therapeutic effects on degenerated discs. They suppress the expression of pro-inflammatory cytokines (e.g., IL-1β and TNF-α), enhance the synthesis of matrix proteins such as type II collagen and aggrecan, and support extracellular matrix remodeling. Moreover, MSCs prevent apoptosis by modulating intracellular signaling pathways like the Bcl-2/Bax ratio and promote the survival of nucleus pulposus cells. Immunologically, they induce the polarization of macrophages from the M1 (pro-inflammatory) phenotype to the M2 (anti-inflammatory) phenotype, thereby contributing to immune regulation [5, 23].

These biological mechanisms have been supported by several clinical studies. Yoshikawa et al. (2010) conducted a pilot study in two patients with severely degenerated intervertebral discs and applied autologous BM-MSCs, combined with collagen sponges, into the disc space after a partial laminotomy. After 2 years, both patients experienced significant pain relief, and T2-weighted MRIs revealed a high signal intensity within the treated discs, indicating improved NP hydration [24]. Following this, Orozco et al. (2011) performed direct intradiscal MSC injections in ten patients with chronic lower back pain. Pain and disability scores significantly improved within 3 months and were sustained at the 6- and 12-month follow-ups [25]. In a larger clinical trial, Pettine et al. (2015) treated 26 patients with moderate-to-severe discogenic pain using autologous bone marrow concentrate (BMC). The results showed statistically significant improvements in functional scores (ODI) and MRI-based degeneration scores at 3, 6, and 12 months. Importantly, patients whose aspirates contained more than 2000 colony-forming unit-fibroblasts (CFU-F) per mL experienced significantly better clinical outcomes compared to those with fewer than 2000 CFU-Fs/mL [26].

Despite these promising outcomes, MSC-based therapies face some limitations. The avascular nature of the disc poses a challenge for transplanted cell survival. Additionally, maintaining MSC phenotypic stability remains difficult, and risks such as tumorigenicity or immune reactions, although rare, cannot be completely ruled out. The lack of standardized protocols concerning dosage, cell sourcing, and application procedures also hampers the widespread clinical adoption of MSC therapy [27, 28].

26.5.2 Exosomes

A significant portion of the therapeutic efficacy attributed to mesenchymal stem cells is now known to be mediated not through the cells themselves but through paracrine signaling molecules, particularly exosomes [19]. Exosomes are extracellular vesicles ranging from 30 to 150 nm in diameter, encapsulated by a lipid bilayer and capable of modulating the behavior of target cells via their cargo of miRNAs, mRNAs, proteins, and lipids. Exosomes derived from MSCs have been demonstrated to exert anti-inflammatory effects, reduce cellular apoptosis, promote ECM synthesis, and modulate oxidative stress in various preclinical models [5, 29].

In an in vitro study, Bhujel et al. (2022) reported that exosomes derived from mesenchymal stem cells cultured under hypoxic conditions suppressed pro-inflammatory cytokines such as IL-1β and TNF-α, modulated the Bcl-2/Bax ratio, and promoted the expression of aggrecan, type II collagen, and anabolic genes such as *COL2A1* and *ACAN* in IL-1β-stimulated nucleus pulposus cells [5]. Zhao et al. (2024) emphasized both ECM-protective and anti-inflammatory roles of MSC-derived exosomes in a model of IVDD. Their findings highlighted the exosomes' ability to suppress inflammatory pathways linked to endoplasmic reticulum stress and mitochondrial dysfunction [29].

Exosome-based therapies offer distinct advantages over cell-based approaches. Their cell-free nature reduces the risk of immunogenicity, they are easier to store and transport, and they demonstrate higher stability in hypoxic environments such as the intervertebral disc. However, challenges remain, including the need for optimized carrier systems to enhance bioavailability, a lack of standardized dosing and administration protocols, and limited long-term clinical data [5, 29].

In summary, exosomes represent a promising class of biological agents in the treatment of IVDD due to their safety profile, practicality, and immunological advantages. Current evidence suggests that exosomes, either alone or in combination with stem cell therapies, may support regenerative processes, particularly in the early stages of degeneration.

26.5.3 Other Biological Therapies: Peptides (Growth Factors and Cytokines), Gene Therapies, and Biomaterial-Based Tissue Engineering

Although MSCs and exosomes have been the primary focus in biological treatment approaches, several other regenerative strategies have garnered attention in recent years. Among these are growth factors, gene therapies, and biomaterial-based tissue engineering [30, 31]. Growth factors and cytokines are critical peptides that regulate the proliferation, differentiation, and ECM synthesis of disc cells. In degenerated discs, the decline or dysfunction of these molecules contributes to the loss of regenerative potential. Exogenous administration of factors such as TGF-β, GDF-5, BMP-7, IGF-1, and IL-1Ra has been shown to enhance ECM synthesis and reduce inflammation [23, 30, 32]. However, due to their short half-life, it is recommended that they be delivered using carrier systems for sustained therapeutic effects.

Gene therapy aims to promote ECM synthesis or suppress inflammation through long-term protein expression by delivering specific genes to disc cells. Preclinical studies targeting genes like SOX9, TIMP-1, TGF-β, and IL-1Ra have demonstrated potential in slowing degenerative processes. Gene delivery via viral (adenoviral and lentiviral) and nonviral (plasmid and nanoparticle) vectors enables prolonged production of therapeutic proteins within the disc. Nevertheless, concerns about immunogenicity and the lack of long-term safety data remain significant limitations for clinical application [23, 30].

Tissue engineering– and biomaterial-based therapies aim to reconstruct the biomechanical integrity of the disc while providing a supportive microenvironment for cell survival and function. These strategies are often combined with cells or growth factors. Hydrogels (such as alginate, hyaluronic acid, and PEG) can be injected into the disc to support regeneration in the nucleus pulposus region. Scaffolds enhance three-dimensional cell adhesion and direct differentiation, while nanoparticles can serve as delivery systems for genes and therapeutic agents. Notably, silk-elastin-based hydrogel products have been reported to improve disc height and reduce pain scores [31]. In addition, pioneering data have demonstrated the successful transplantation of fresh donor-derived intervertebral disc allografts in human patients [33]. Although these methods remain in preclinical or early clinical stages, they offer promising cell-free biological alternatives for intervertebral disc regeneration.

26.5.4 Emerging Delivery Strategies for Biologic Therapies in Intervertebral Disc Degeneration

As regenerative therapies continue to advance, the method of administering biological products is becoming increasingly critical to therapeutic success. Among these, intradiscal injection (Figs. 26.1, 26.2, and 26.3) remains the most extensively studied approach for local delivery. Under fluoroscopic guidance, agents such as mesenchymal stem cells, platelet-rich plasma (PRP), or hydrogels are directly injected into the nucleus pulposus, allowing for precise targeting of the affected tissue while minimizing systemic exposure. Clinical studies have reported promising outcomes, including significant improvements in pain and functional scores, as well as increased disc hydration [25, 26]. However, the avascular and acidic microenvironment of the degenerated disc presents substantial challenges in terms of cell retention, distribution, and long-term viability.

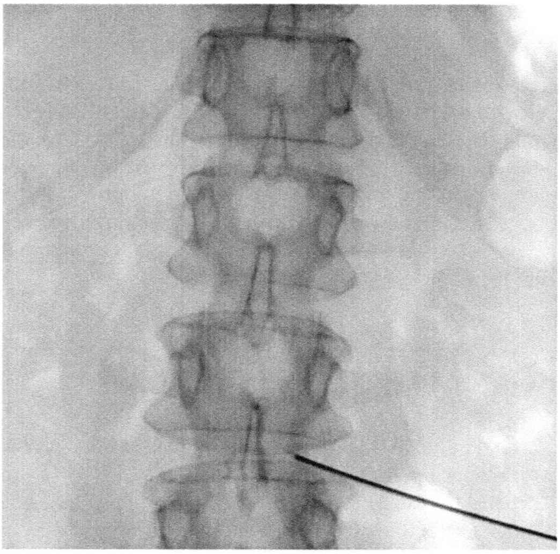

Fig. 26.1 Fluoroscopic lateral view of the targeted disc level. (Courtesy of Prof. Dr. Ömür Erçelen. All rights reserved)

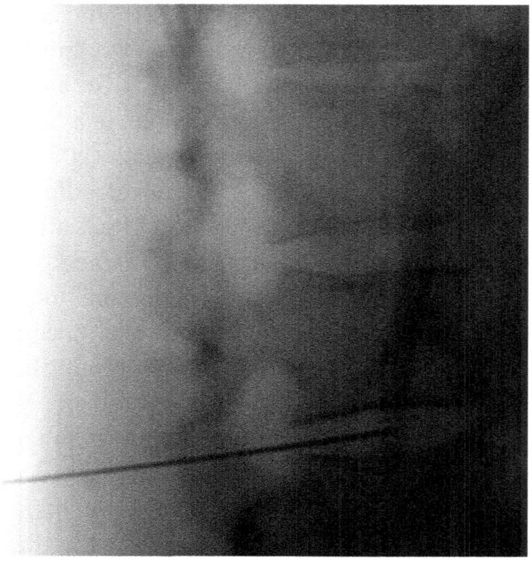

Fig. 26.2 Anteroposterior view showing the central needle placement. (Courtesy of Prof. Dr. Ömür Erçelen. All rights reserved)

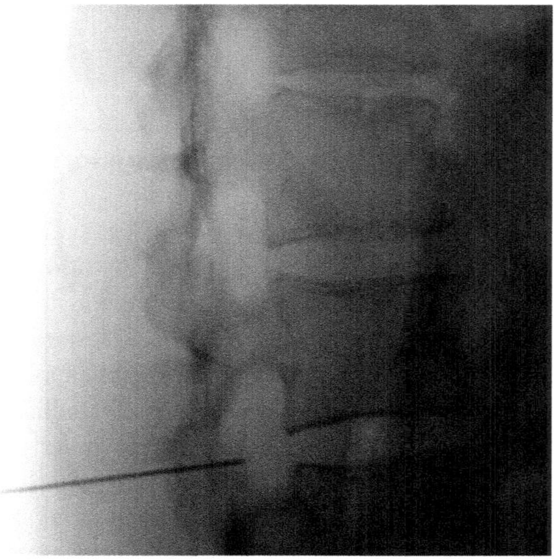

Fig. 26.3 Oblique view confirming the correct intradiscal positioning under fluoroscopy. (Courtesy of Prof. Dr. Ömür Erçelen. All rights reserved)

Intravenous (IV) infusion, while lacking direct targeting capability, offers systemic immunomodulatory effects. This route has been successfully employed in treating inflammatory conditions such as COVID-19 using MSC- and exosome-based therapies. Benefits observed include the suppression of systemic inflammation, attenuation of cytokine storms, and improvement in oxygenation [21, 22]. In addition, preclinical evidence suggests that IV-administered MSCs may exhibit neuroprotective and anti-inflammatory effects. For example, in a rat model of sciatic nerve injury, Miyano et al. (2022) demonstrated that IV administration of adipose tissue– and umbilical cord–derived MSCs alleviated pain, suppressed inflammatory markers (ATF-3 and Iba-1), and reversed demyelination [19]. Although these findings were not specific to intervertebral disc tissue, they highlight the systemic immunoregulatory potential of MSCs, which may provide indirect support in inflammatory or multifocal degenerative processes. Despite these promising developments, both delivery routes still lack adequate standardization regarding dosing, timing, formulation, and carrier systems. Therefore, well-designed prospective clinical trials are urgently needed to determine the most effective and safe application strategies tailored to the pathophysiology of disc degeneration.

26.6 Discussion and Conclusion

Intervertebral disc degeneration disease remains a highly prevalent and progressive condition that imposes a substantial burden on individual well-being and public health systems. Despite the widespread use of conventional treatments, current therapeutic strategies are largely palliative and insufficient to halt or reverse the underlying degenerative cascade. This therapeutic gap has catalyzed interest in biological treatments and new-generation biotechnological approaches, which aim to promote tissue regeneration and restore disc homeostasis rather than merely alleviate symptoms.

Mesenchymal stem cells and MSC-derived exosomes are among the most studied candidates in regenerative disc therapy. Both demonstrate anti-inflammatory, antiapoptotic, and matrix-restorative properties, supported by increasing preclinical and clinical data. Other strategies, such as growth factors, gene transfer systems, and biomaterial-assisted delivery platforms, further expand the therapeutic landscape. These approaches not only support extracellular matrix synthesis and cell survival but also facilitate structural restoration of the disc.

However, several critical limitations must be addressed before these therapies can be widely adopted. The harsh avascular and acidic environment of the degenerated disc impairs the survival and function of transplanted cells or molecules. Moreover, no consensus currently exists on optimal dosing, delivery methods, or product bioavailability, which hinders the reproducibility and standardization of biological interventions across clinical settings.

In this context, well-designed, large-scale prospective studies are urgently needed to evaluate the safety, efficacy, optimal dosage, and biodistribution of biological products. These studies should aim to establish standardized protocols and guide regulatory pathways for clinical application.

In conclusion, regenerative medicine paves the way for innovative biological and biotechnology-driven therapy strategies that hold great promise for IVDD. While still evolving, these approaches exhibit the potential to move beyond symptom control and toward true regenerative repair. With continued interdisciplinary research and clinical validation, they may soon form the foundation of next-generation spine care.

Acknowledgments We would like to express our sincere gratitude to Prof. Dr. Ali Fahir Özer and Prof. Dr. Ömür Erçelen for their valuable contributions to the development of this chapter. The fluoroscopic images included in the manuscript were kindly provided by Prof. Dr. Ömür Erçelen from his personal archive, and we deeply appreciate his generosity in granting permission for their use.

References

1. Andersson GB. Epidemiological features of chronic low-back pain. Lancet. 1999;354(9178):581–5.
2. Feng C, Liu H, Yang M, Zhang Y, Huang B, Zhou Y. Disc cell senescence in intervertebral disc degeneration: causes and molecular pathways. Cell Cycle. 2016;15(13):1674–84.
3. Molinos M, Almeida CR, Caldeira J, Cunha C, Gonçalves RM, Barbosa MA. Inflammation in inter-

vertebral disc degeneration and regeneration. J R Soc Interface. 2015;12(104):20141191.

4. Pennicooke B, Moriguchi Y, Hussain I, Bonssar L, Härtl R. Biological treatment approaches for degenerative disc disease: a review of clinical trials and future directions. Cureus [Internet]. 2016 [cited 2025 Jul 10]. Available from: http://www.cureus.com/articles/4056-biological-treatment-approaches-for-degenerative-disc-disease-a-review-of-clinical-trials-and-future-directions.
5. Bhujel B, Shin HE, Choi DJ, Han I. Mesenchymal stem cell-derived exosomes and intervertebral disc regeneration: review. Int J Mol Sci. 2022;23(13):7306.
6. Lu L, Xu A, Gao F, Tian C, Wang H, Zhang J, et al. Mesenchymal stem cell-derived exosomes as a novel strategy for the treatment of intervertebral disc degeneration. Front Cell Dev Biol. 2022;9:770510.
7. Chen X, Zhang A, Zhao K, Gao H, Shi P, Chen Y, et al. The role of oxidative stress in intervertebral disc degeneration: mechanisms and therapeutic implications. Ageing Res Rev. 2024;98:102323.
8. Li ZP, Li H, Ruan YH, Wang P, Zhu MT, Fu WP, et al. Stem cell therapy for intervertebral disc degeneration: clinical progress with exosomes and gene vectors. World J Stem Cells. 2025;17(4):102945.
9. Xie G, Liang C, Yu H, Zhang Q. Association between polymorphisms of collagen genes and susceptibility to intervertebral disc degeneration: a meta-analysis. J Orthop Surg Res. 2021;16(1):616.
10. Munir S, Rade M, Määttä JH, Freidin MB, Williams FMK. Intervertebral disc biology: genetic basis of disc degeneration. Curr Mol Biol Rep. 2018;4(4):143–50.
11. Ren Q, Chen L, Ma Y, Huang Y, Wang S. Immune microenvironment in intervertebral disc degeneration: pathophysiology and therapeutic potential. Front Immunol [Internet]. 2025 [cited 2025 Jul 10];16. Available from: https://www.frontiersin.org/journals/immunology/articles/10.3389/fimmu.2025.1563635/full.
12. Chao-yang G, Peng C, Hai-hong Z. Roles of NLRP3 inflammasome in intervertebral disc degeneration. Osteoarthr Cartil. 2021;29(6):793–801.
13. Suyama K, Sakai D, Watanabe M. The role of IL-17-mediated inflammatory processes in the pathogenesis of intervertebral disc degeneration and herniation: a comprehensive review. Front Cell Dev Biol. 2022;10:857164.
14. Qaseem A, Wilt TJ, McLean RM, Forciea MA, for the Clinical Guidelines Committee of the American College of Physicians*. Noninvasive treatments for acute, subacute, and chronic low back pain: a clinical practice guideline from the American College of Physicians. Ann Intern Med. 2017;166(7):514–30.
15. Deyo RA, Mirza SK, Turner JA, Martin BI. Overtreating chronic back pain: time to back off? J Am Board Fam Med. 2009;22(1):62–8.
16. Foster NE, Anema JR, Cherkin D, Chou R, Cohen SP, Gross DP, et al. Prevention and treatment of low back pain: evidence, challenges, and promising directions. Lancet. 2018;391(10137):2368–83.
17. Manchikanti L, Abdi S, Atluri S, Benyamin RM, Boswell MV, Buenaventura RM, et al. An update of comprehensive evidence-based guidelines for interventional techniques in chronic spinal pain. Part II: guidance and recommendations. Pain Physician. 2013;16(2 Suppl):S49–283.
18. Petzke F, Klose P, Welsch P, Sommer C, Häuser W. Opioids for chronic low back pain: an updated systematic review and meta-analysis of efficacy, tolerability and safety in randomized placebo-controlled studies of at least 4 weeks of double-blind duration. Eur J Pain. 2020;24(3):497–517.
19. Miyano K, Ikehata M, Ohshima K, Yoshida Y, Nose Y, Yoshihara S-I, et al. Intravenous administration of human mesenchymal stem cells derived from adipose tissue and umbilical cord improves neuropathic pain via suppression of neuronal damage and anti-inflammatory actions in rats. Minami M, editor. PLoS One. 2022;17(2):e0262892.
20. Ercelen N, Karasu N, Kahyaoglu B, Cerezci O, Akduman RC, Ercelen D, et al. Clinical experience: outcomes of mesenchymal stem cell transplantation in five stroke patients. Front Med. 2023;10:1051831.
21. Qu W, Wang Z, Engelberg-Cook E, Yan D, Siddik AB, Bu G, et al. Efficacy and safety of MSC cell therapies for hospitalized patients with COVID-19: a systematic review and meta-analysis. Stem Cells Transl Med. 2022;11(7):688–703.
22. Ercelen NO, Pekkoc-Uyanik KC, Alpaydin N, Gulay GR, Simsek M. Clinical experience on umbilical cord mesenchymal stem cell treatment in 210 severe and critical COVID-19 cases in Turkey. Stem Cell Rev Rep. 2021;17(5):1917–25.
23. Jin Y, Wu O, Chen Z, Chen L, Zhang K, Chen Q, et al. Exploring extracellular vesicles as novel therapeutic agents for intervertebral disc degeneration: delivery, applications, and mechanisms. Stem Cell Res Ther [Internet]. 2025 [cited 2025 Jul 10];16(1). Available from: https://stemcellres.biomedcentral.com/articles/10.1186/s13287-025-04299-1.
24. Yoshikawa T, Ueda Y, Miyazaki K, Koizumi M, Takakura Y. Disc regeneration therapy using marrow mesenchymal cell transplantation: a report of two case studies. Spine. 2010;35(11):E475–80.
25. Orozco L, Soler R, Morera C, Alberca M, Sánchez A, García-Sancho J. Intervertebral disc repair by autologous mesenchymal bone marrow cells: a pilot study. Transplantation. 2011;92(7):822–8.
26. Pettine KA, Murphy MB, Suzuki RK, Sand TT. Percutaneous injection of autologous bone marrow concentrate cells significantly reduces lumbar discogenic pain through 12 months. Stem Cells. 2015;33(1):146–56.
27. Tan F, Li X, Wang Z, Li J, Shahzad K, Zheng J. Clinical applications of stem cell-derived exosomes. Signal Transduct Target Ther. 2024;9(1):17.
28. Hamdan H, Hashmi SK, Lazarus H, Gale RP, Qu W, El Fakih R. Promising role for mesenchymal stromal cells in coronavirus infectious disease-19 (COVID-

19)-related severe acute respiratory syndrome? Blood Rev. 2021;46:100742.
29. Zhao Y, Dong H, Xia Q, Wang Y, Zhu L, Hu Z, et al. A new strategy for intervertebral disc regeneration: the synergistic potential of mesenchymal stem cells and their extracellular vesicles with hydrogel scaffolds. Biomed Pharmacother. 2024;172:116238.
30. Masuda K. Biological repair of the degenerated intervertebral disc by the injection of growth factors. Eur Spine J. 2008;17(S4):441–51.
31. Berlemann U, Schwarzenbach O. An injectable nucleus replacement as an adjunct to microdiscectomy: 2 year follow-up in a pilot clinical study. Eur Spine J. 2009;18(11):1706–12.
32. Krut Z, Pelled G, Gazit D, Gazit Z. Stem cells and exosomes: new therapies for intervertebral disc degeneration. Cells. 2021;10(9):2241.
33. Ruan D, He Q, Ding Y, Hou L, Li J, Luk KD. Intervertebral disc transplantation in the treatment of degenerative spine disease: a preliminary study. Lancet. 2007;369(9566):993–9.

From Rigidity to Flexibility: Where Is Spinal Surgery Evolving?

27

Ali Fahir Özer, Mehmet Yiğit Akgün, Tunç Öktenoğlu, and Özkan Ateş

27.1 Introduction

To accurately assess the current state and future trajectory of spinal surgery, it is essential to first present an objective overview of its historical development and present-day practices. The foundational principles of decompression and stabilization—both critical to successful surgical outcomes—should be examined through a historical lens, with particular attention to how these approaches have evolved, both independently and in combination.

Within this framework, the development of surgical strategies for spinal trauma and tumors will also be reviewed where relevant.

27.2 Spinal Decompression: Historical Development and Surgical Milestones

Spinal decompression is a surgical intervention performed in response to structural deterioration within a motion segment, often due to degenerative processes that result in neural compression. This condition typically arises when the structural integrity of the intervertebral disc is compromised, leading to the protrusion of annulus fibrosus or nucleus pulposus components, which in turn exert pressure on adjacent neural structures.

Historically, the evolution of spinal surgery has been closely linked to advances in antisepsis and anesthesia. Following Joseph Lister's introduction of antiseptic principles [1], spinal procedures began to be conducted under aseptic conditions with the aid of general anesthesia from the 1840s onward, significantly improving the safety and efficacy of such operations. Notably, in the fourth century, Caelius Aurelianus described intervertebral disc spaces and recognized that sciatica could manifest at any age [2–5].

Paulus of Aegina [6] proposed that surgically removing fractured bone fragments could benefit patients with spinal cord paralysis secondary to vertebral fractures, although the success of his interventions remains undocumented. In the fifth century, the Turkish physician Sabuncuoğlu advocated for cauterization in cases of sciatica unresponsive to analgesics [7].

The correlation between radicular pain and the sciatic nerve was established by Domenico Cotugno in his 1764 monograph, leading to the designation of this clinical entity as "Cotugno's disease" [8]. In 1857, Virchow described disc

A. F. Özer (✉) · T. Öktenoğlu
Department of Neurosurgery, Koc University School of Medicine, Istanbul, Turkey

M. Y. Akgün · Ö. Ateş
Department of Neurosurgery, Koc University Hospital, Spine Center, Istanbul, Turkey
e-mail: makgun@kuh.ku.edu.tr; oates@kuh.ku.edu.tr

A. F. Özer et al. (eds.), *Dynamic Lumbar Spine Stabilization*,
https://doi.org/10.1007/978-3-032-12122-6_27

herniation pathologies [9, 10], and a year later, Luschka provided more detailed morphological descriptions, albeit without associating them with clinical syndromes [11]. During this period, the refinement of the clinical definition of sciatica laid the groundwork for considering disc pathology as surgically treatable.

In 1864, Ernest Lasègue introduced the straight leg raise test, marking a pivotal advancement in the clinical diagnosis of sciatica [2, 4]. Subsequently, in 1908, Fedor Krause performed the first discectomy under the guidance of Hermann Oppenheim. Postoperatively, the patient's symptoms resolved entirely; although the excised tissue was initially misidentified as a tumor, it was later confirmed to be intervertebral disc material [12, 13].

Alfred Taylor conducted the first unilateral laminectomy on a cadaver in 1909, while Victor Horsley had previously achieved the first spinal tumor resection in 1887 [14, 15]. These early successes contributed to the broader adoption of laminectomy for various indications, including trauma, infections, and congenital anomalies. In 1929, Walter Dandy identified free cartilage fragments within the epidural space, later understood to be sequestered disc material resulting from trauma [16].

A major milestone occurred in 1932 when Mixter and Barr performed the first surgery specifically diagnosed as a "ruptured intervertebral disc," achieving complete symptomatic resolution [17]. Collaboration with pathologist Kubik confirmed that the excised mass was indeed disc tissue [18, 19]. By 1934, surgical intervention had become increasingly accepted as a viable treatment for disc herniation. Love's 1938 description of the intralaminar and extradural discectomy technique provided the foundation for modern lumbar disc surgery [5, 7, 20, 21].

By the 1940s, the term "nucleus pulposus herniation" had gained currency. However, the contemporary term "lumbar disc herniation," which encompasses both the nucleus and annulus components, is now considered more accurate [22]. In 1967, Yaşargil pioneered the use of an operating microscope in spinal surgery, and in 1977, Caspar introduced a microdiscectomy technique utilizing smaller incisions with microscopic assistance [23].

During the 1980s, aggressive surgical intervention was often advocated for patients presenting with acute symptoms [24–26]. However, randomized controlled trials by Weber [27] and Hakelius [28] demonstrated that conservative treatment yielded comparable long-term outcomes. Although surgery resulted in earlier symptom relief, both groups had similar outcomes after a decade. McCulloch [29] argued that surgical intervention offered only marginally superior results compared to the natural progression of the disease. These findings reinforced the case for conservative management among many clinicians.

Histopathological studies in the 1990s revealed that herniated disc material could be resorbed through macrophage-mediated phagocytosis following inflammation [24]. In 1947, Inman and Saunders identified pain-conducting nerve fibers within the annulus fibrosus [30], and subsequent studies confirmed that nociceptive transmission occurs via the sinuvertebral nerve [31].

Murphey [32] popularized the concept of segmental immobilization for alleviating mechanical back pain. This marked the emergence of spinal stabilization as a core surgical objective, leading to the increasing use of fusion procedures in conjunction with decompression [33]. The notion that mechanical instability was a significant pain generator, and that its surgical correction could provide relief, gained widespread acceptance [15].

Advances in imaging during the 1980s allowed for the classification of disc herniations into subtypes such as anterior and posterolateral. The diagnosis of far-lateral herniations became more straightforward, and Wiltse described a lateral surgical approach for such cases [34–36]. Due to the limited success of surgery for midline herniations, these were often excluded from surgical consideration [31, 37]. In later classifications, the size of the annular defect emerged as a key predictor of recurrence risk [38].

Early radical discectomy techniques involving extensive removal of the nucleus pulposus and cartilaginous endplates were associated with increased risk of nerve root injury and long-term mechanical instability. This led to chronic postoperative pain in many cases. In response, Williams and his colleagues advocated for a more conservative approach, removing only sequestered fragments. Subsequent studies confirmed that this limited technique did not significantly increase the rate of recurrence [1, 25, 39–41].

27.3 The Role of Fusion in Lumbar Disc Herniation

The utility of spinal fusion in the treatment of lumbar disc herniation (LDH) has been a subject of ongoing debate for decades. In 1947, Barr [42] reported superior outcomes in patients undergoing decompression with fusion compared to those treated with discectomy alone. However, these initial findings were later reevaluated, and Barr himself subsequently retracted his earlier stance, asserting that "fusion does not significantly enhance surgical outcomes and may instead increase complication rates" [18, 43]. By 1988, several authors concluded that fusion was "entirely unnecessary" in the treatment of LDH [31].

Nonetheless, in specific subgroups predisposed to postoperative instability—such as patients with spondylolisthesis—discectomy alone often yielded suboptimal results [44–46]. Consequently, fusion has gained broader acceptance, particularly in the context of recurrent disc herniation. While some authors advocate for fusion following a second recurrence, others support repeated discectomy as the preferred approach [47, 48].

In a 1988 study, Vaughan et al. compared discectomy alone versus discectomy with concomitant fusion in a cohort of 85 patients [49]. After a mean follow-up of 7.3 years, the non-fusion group demonstrated a significantly higher incidence of chronic low back pain. Patient satisfaction was markedly higher in the fusion group (85%) compared to the discectomy group (39%). Furthermore, the reoperation rate was substantially lower in the fusion group (3%) than in the non-fusion group (13.5%). These findings suggest that fusion may offer mechanical stabilization in addition to neural decompression.

Supporting these results, Samartzis et al. [50] reported a 5-year reoperation rate of approximately 3% in patients treated with fusion, in contrast to 13–14% in those who underwent discectomy alone. Patel et al. also emphasized the superior satisfaction rates among fusion patients, with 85% expressing satisfaction, compared to 39% in the discectomy group [51].

The increasing recognition of axial low back pain as a component of disc pathology has led to a growing preference for fusion in these patients. Concurrently, the development of various interbody fusion cages and disc arthroplasty systems has expanded surgical options and clinical applications [7].

Recent randomized controlled trials indexed in MEDLINE indicate that surgical treatment offers short-term symptomatic improvement in patients with lumbar disc herniation and spinal stenosis. However, the long-term benefits appear to diminish over time. For non-radicular low back pain associated with diffuse degenerative changes, fusion has not demonstrated superiority over intensive rehabilitation, though it may offer modest advantages over decompression alone [52].

27.4 Microsurgery for Lumbar Disc Herniation

A central trend in the surgical management of lumbar disc herniation has been the minimization of iatrogenic soft tissue damage. To this end, specialized retractor systems have been developed to facilitate deep access through minimal skin incisions. This approach aims to reduce surgical morbidity and preserve paraspinal muscle integrity.

Foley and Smith were among the first to describe the use of tubular retractor systems in microendoscopic discectomy, laying the groundwork for modern minimally invasive techniques [53]. Lebl [54] further emphasized the role of such instruments in minimizing tissue trauma and reducing overall morbidity.

By the 1990s, the use of tubular retractors had significantly decreased incision length, paraspinal muscle injury, and the formation of dead space [55]. The concept of lumbar microdiscectomy was initially introduced by Yaşargil in 1967 with the use of an operating microscope, and the technique was systematically documented in 1977 [56]. In 1979, Williams [41] published a series involving 534 patients, reporting favorable outcomes using a microscope-assisted approach that emphasized fragmentectomy—specifically, the excision of only sequestered disc fragments.

In the 1990s, John McCulloch [29] refined and popularized the microdiscectomy technique, which has since been widely recognized as the "gold standard" by many spinal surgeons [57]. Advances in illumination, magnification, and retractor systems have enabled the performance of highly effective surgeries through minimal incisions. Improvements in anesthesia techniques, especially the adoption of epidural anesthesia, have further contributed to reduced hospital stays, with many procedures now performed in outpatient settings [58–62].

While extended bed rest was once standard postoperative practice, studies in the 1990s by Carragee et al. challenged this paradigm, demonstrating that prolonged immobilization did not enhance outcomes or reduce recurrence rates [63, 64]. These findings underscored the importance of early mobilization in postoperative recovery.

In 1977, Salenius and Laurent reported that 56% of 886 patients who underwent discectomy experienced favorable outcomes, with 63% returning to their previous occupations [65]. Comparative results from Caspar et al. in a cohort of 418 patients revealed that those undergoing microdiscectomy experienced less intraoperative bleeding, fewer complications, shorter hospital stays, and a more rapid return to work [66].

Silvers [67], in a 1988 analysis of 540 patients, demonstrated that microdiscectomy offered advantages in terms of both clinical efficacy and cost-effectiveness. Recovery times and return-to-work intervals were notably shorter in the microdiscectomy group. However, Tullberg et al. [68] conducted a randomized trial suggesting that the use of an operating microscope did not significantly influence recovery time or intraoperative blood loss. While several studies support the role of microsurgery in accelerating early recovery, long-term outcome differences remain minimal [69–71].

27.5 Evolution of Minimally Invasive Techniques and Endoscopic Spine Surgery

The principle "less tissue disruption leads to improved outcomes" has served as a primary driver in the development of minimally invasive spinal surgical techniques. During the early phases of this evolution, the concept of segmental instability had not yet gained widespread clinical traction, and biomechanical models such as column theories were still in their developmental stages. In 1968, Wiltse et al. laid the groundwork for tissue-sparing surgical approaches by describing a technique that minimized damage to the paraspinal musculature, thereby reinforcing the paradigm that minimal invasiveness correlates with better postoperative outcomes [72]. Similarly, the microendoscopic discectomy technique introduced by Foley and Smith further exemplified the shift toward soft tissue preservation through technological innovation [53].

Although Knutsson first defined the concept of segmental instability in 1944 [73], it had not yet been integrated into standard clinical practice during this formative period. In the 1970s, Japanese surgeon Hijikata expanded upon the posterolateral approach used in diagnostic discography, developing a procedure termed "percutaneous nucleotomy" under fluoroscopic guidance [74]. This method involved aspirating disc material via cannulated instruments introduced through the annulus. At the time, it was postulated that reducing intradiscal pressure might prevent herniation and alleviate symptoms. However, subsequent advances in the understanding of spinal biomechanics revealed that this assumption failed to address the more complex issues of segmental stability and instability.

In the 1980s, Parviz Kambin achieved access to central disc herniations via a transforaminal approach, supplementing existing techniques for foraminal and extraforaminal discs [75–78]. This led to the identification of the anatomical "Kambin triangle," a safe working zone for percutaneous endoscopic procedures. Building upon this, Hal Mathews [79] and Tony Yeung [80, 81] developed alternative routes, including lateral transforaminal and interlaminar approaches, which enabled the effective removal of both lateral and more centrally located herniations.

Choi et al. introduced continuous saline irrigation, often referred to as "underwater dissection," which enhanced intraoperative visualization while reducing bleeding and infection risk [82]. This technique significantly improved surgical field clarity and procedural safety, contributing to increased success rates and reduced recurrence in endoscopic spinal surgery. Hoogland et al. further reported that the transforaminal endoscopic approach achieved favorable clinical outcomes, including low recurrence rates, owing to its minimally invasive advantages [83].

The adoption of endoscopic spinal techniques has been particularly rapid in Asia, where major innovations in surgical instrumentation and technique have emerged. In the early 2000s, German surgeon Sebastian Rutten [84–86] adapted endoscopic systems to interlaminar access routes, helping popularize their use in Western surgical practice. Subsequently, biportal endoscopic techniques were developed, allowing surgeries traditionally performed via microscopy to be conducted using endoscopy as well [82].

Park and colleagues demonstrated the clinical efficacy of unilateral biportal lumbar interbody fusion (ULIF) when compared to posterior lumbar interbody fusion (PLIF), validating biportal techniques in contemporary practice [87]. Chung's biportal endoscopic fusion procedures exemplify the early stages of robotic integration, while Zhang and Li's series on robot-assisted unilateral biportal endoscopic lumbar interbody fusion (UBE-LIF) illustrated the successful application of the Tianji robotic system in conjunction with biportal methods [88, 89]. These developments signal the likely expansion of robotic assistance in endoscopic spine surgery in the near future.

Today, complex spinal procedures can be performed using biportal endoscopy, and the distinctions between monoportal and biportal techniques continue to be explored and debated [90–92]. In the thoracic spine, endoscopic approaches evolved independently through the efforts of Mack and Regan [93, 94], as well as Rosenthal [95]. Thoracoscopy is now widely employed in the management of thoracic disc herniation and other intrathoracic spinal pathologies [96–101].

27.6 Historical Development of Spinal Instrumentation

Since antiquity, spinal interventions have largely relied on external methods such as traction and orthotic bracing for stabilization. The inception of modern spinal instrumentation, however, dates back to 1891, when Hadra pioneered internal stabilization by wrapping silver wire around the spinous processes to manage spinal fractures and instability [102]. This marked the first known use of internal fixation for spinal pathology.

In 1908, Lang expanded on Hadra's technique by introducing internal stabilization with steel wires and cables, particularly for spinal deformities such as kyphosis secondary to tuberculosis. This cabling method is considered one of the earliest systematic attempts at internal fixation and was shown to offer significantly improved outcomes and shorter recovery times compared to external immobilization with braces or casts [103]. A 2019 review on the historical development of spinal neurosurgery reaffirmed the clinical benefits of these early internal counter-stabilization techniques [104].

In 1911, Albee [105] and Hibbs [106] introduced the principles of posterolateral arthrodesis.

Hibbs' technique involved excision of the spinous processes, decortication of the lamina and facet joints, and fusion using autologous bone grafts. For decades, wiring remained the mainstay of posterior spinal fixation. In 1943, Tourney [107] introduced the concept of facet screw fixation to enhance fusion stability, which was later refined by King [108]. Nevertheless, the prevailing view at the time held that instrumentation alone was insufficient; successful outcomes required fusion (arthrodesis) as the central component of surgical intervention.

In 1944, Briggs and Milligan [109] introduced interbody fusion by placing grafts between the posterior lumbar vertebrae, laying the foundation for modern intervertebral arthrodesis. A major advancement came in the 1950s with Harrington's development of the first segmental instrumentation system using stainless steel rods and hooks, initially designed for scoliosis treatment [110]. This system was subsequently adapted for use in thoracolumbar trauma and other spinal pathologies [110–113]. However, the absence of concomitant fusion in the early applications revealed significant limitations in achieving lasting spinal stability, thereby underscoring the necessity of combining instrumentation with arthrodesis.

In 1959, Boucher [114] introduced the pedicle screw, revolutionizing posterior fixation techniques. Harrington and Tullos [115] later advanced and popularized its clinical application. This innovation was further refined by Magerl [116], and by Dick and colleagues [117, 118], who developed biomechanically optimized systems that enhanced segmental control and load distribution.

In parallel, Roy-Camille and Robert Judet pioneered anterior cervical plating by affixing plates to the lateral masses, a technique that was later adapted for the thoracolumbar spine. Despite his pivotal contributions, Roy-Camille remains underappreciated in the historical narrative of spinal instrumentation development.

Further innovation came in 1982 when Steffee [119] introduced a segmental spinal plate fixation system, which allowed for more rigid segmental stabilization. In 1986, Luque [112] enhanced spinal alignment in both the coronal and sagittal planes using sublaminar wire and rod constructs, enabling effective correction through a posterior-only approach. Notably, these methods did not address anterior column support unless combined with pedicle screw technology. This conceptual shift contributed to the emergence of the "universal clamp system" and paved the way for dynamic screw systems designed to partially engage the anterior column.

In 1987, Cotrel and Dubousset [120] developed a rod-based system designed for scoliosis correction. Their innovation involved pre-contoured rods that could be anchored to the spine using either hooks or pedicle screws, thereby creating a modular and adaptable system suitable for a wide range of spinal deformities. Despite certain limitations, this system played a seminal role in the advancement of deformity surgery and catalyzed the development of more ergonomic and versatile instrumentation platforms used today.

27.7 The Role of Imaging and Technological Innovation in the Advancement of Spinal Surgery

The most transformative advancements in spinal surgery over the past century have undeniably been driven by the evolution of imaging technologies. Following the introduction of radiographic imaging, the use of contrast-enhanced myelography emerged in the early twentieth century, facilitating visualization of the spinal canal and neural structures [121, 122].

The subsequent invention of computed tomography (CT) in 1972 and magnetic resonance imaging (MRI) in 1974 revolutionized spinal diagnostics, enabling detailed assessment of bony and soft tissue structures. These modalities rapidly supplanted myelography as routine diagnostic tools, which became reserved for select cases requiring dynamic or adjunctive evaluation. Beyond enhancing diagnostic precision, the development of CT and MRI also enabled histopathological differentiation of spinal lesions, improving surgical planning and prognostication.

Intraoperative imaging advancements have further refined surgical precision. Mobile fluoroscopy units and intraoperative CT now allow for real-time guidance during procedures such as pedicle screw insertion, reducing the risk of misplacement, particularly in anatomically complex regions such as the craniocervical junction. These innovations have significantly enhanced the safety and efficacy of spinal instrumentation.

A pivotal advancement in this domain has been the introduction of spinal navigation systems. These technologies reduce ionizing radiation exposure to both surgical teams and patients while improving the accuracy of hardware placement. In a landmark 2000 study, Rampersaud et al. [123] demonstrated that the use of navigated pedicle screw placement significantly minimized radiation exposure for the surgical team compared to conventional fluoroscopy. Building on this, Tabaraee et al. [124] in 2018 reported that navigation systems not only enhanced screw placement accuracy in minimally invasive transforaminal lumbar interbody fusion (TLIF) procedures but also significantly reduced radiation doses. Similarly, Sroka et al. [125] in 2019 affirmed that navigated spinal instrumentation decreases both patient and surgeon radiation exposure while maintaining high accuracy in screw positioning.

More recently, the integration of artificial intelligence and robotics into spinal navigation has marked a new frontier. Robotic systems such as Mazor X (Medtronic) and ExcelsiusGPS represent early but significant steps toward fully automated and intelligent surgical guidance. Although robotic spinal surgery remains in its developmental stages, emerging evidence supports its safety, feasibility, and clinical benefit.

As these technologies continue to evolve, it is widely anticipated that robotic navigation systems will become an integral component of standard spinal surgical practice, playing a central role in improving procedural accuracy and safety [126].

27.8 Spinal Stability and Instability: Biomechanical Principles and Evolving Surgical Strategies

27.8.1 Spinal Biomechanics and Stability Concepts

Spinal stability is a fundamental physiological requirement that ensures protection of the spinal cord and nerve roots while preserving the structural integrity of the spinal column. Although a variety of biomechanical and clinical definitions have been proposed, no universally accepted definition of spinal stability currently exists.

The spine's osseous structures, intervertebral discs, and ligaments act as biomechanical transducers, housing mechanoreceptors that provide proprioceptive feedback to the central nervous system. This feedback modulates muscle tone, reflex responses, and segmental coordination. Disruption to any of these structural or regulatory components can result in spinal instability of varying degrees.

White et al. [127] define clinical spinal stability as "the ability of the spine under physiological loads to limit patterns of displacement so as not to damage or irritate the spinal cord or nerve roots, cause deformity, or result in incapacitating pain." Similarly, the American Academy of Orthopaedic Surgeons characterizes stability as "the capacity to preserve structural integrity and maintain physiological range of motion during movement" [128]. According to White and Panjabi [129], spinal instability refers to the "loss of the spine's ability to maintain displacement patterns within normal limits under physiological loads."

The Functional Spinal Unit (FSU), composed of two adjacent vertebrae and the intervening disc and ligaments, facilitates motion in six degrees of freedom—three translational and three rotational axes. In addition to these primary movements, the FSU exhibits complex coupled motions. Instability may manifest either through excessive motion (quantitative) or through abnormal motion patterns (qualitative) [130].

The severity and clinical presentation of instability are influenced by the dominant lesion's location within the motion segment. Given the spine's inherently three-dimensional kinematics, instability frequently affects multiple planes of motion, necessitating multi-axial evaluation during surgical planning [131]. For instance, in the cervical spine, axial rotation and lateral flexion commonly occur in tandem due to the orientation of the facet joints and paraspinal musculature [132].

The physiological range of spinal motion is classically divided into two phases: the neutral zone (NZ) and the elastic zone (EZ) [133]. The NZ is a region of minimal resistance where passive structures are lax, allowing increased motion. In contrast, the EZ exhibits progressively increasing resistance, providing a stabilizing effect that limits excessive motion.

27.8.2 Column Theories and Models of Instability

Several theoretical frameworks have been proposed to conceptualize spinal stability. Holdsworth's [134] two-column model divides the spine into anterior and posterior elements, asserting that instability primarily results from disruption of the anterior column. In 1983, Denis [135] proposed the three-column model, which introduced the concept of a middle column (posterior half of the vertebral body, disc, and posterior longitudinal ligament). According to this model, injury to the middle column denotes instability. While this model has clinical utility in thoracolumbar trauma, it has been criticized for not incorporating neurologic status and for potentially leading to overtreatment in simple fractures.

Despite the emergence of more nuanced classification systems [136–139], the two- and three-column theories remain foundational tools in the assessment of instability.

27.8.3 Segmental Instability and Functional Classification

Panjabi [133, 140] advanced the understanding of spinal instability by introducing the neutral zone concept within the FSU. Increased motion in the NZ is indicative of segmental instability, often due to traumatic, degenerative, infectious, or neoplastic processes. Panjabi's model identifies three interacting subsystems: the passive (osteoligamentous), active (musculotendinous), and neural control systems. Instability arises when one subsystem fails and cannot be compensated by the others.

This model emphasizes the importance of rehabilitation and muscle strengthening to restore stability. Active therapeutic interventions have demonstrated superior outcomes compared to passive modalities in chronic low back pain [141–143]. Benzel's classification distinguishes between acute (discrete) and chronic (segmental movement dysfunction, glacial instability) forms of instability [144]. The central clinical dilemma remains: should decompression alone be performed, or should fusion be added?

27.9 Where We Stand?

27.9.1 Current Challenges and Future Directions

Advancements in endoscopic techniques, artificial intelligence-assisted navigation, and robotics have redefined the possibilities of spinal surgery [145, 146]. Despite these innovations, persistent challenges such as recurrent herniation and chronic axial pain remain. The prevailing belief that "the less invasive, the better" continues to guide surgical choices, often favoring fragmentectomy over subtotal discectomy due to reduced anatomical disruption.

Although minimally invasive and microsurgical approaches offer perioperative benefits—shorter hospitalization, faster mobilization, and quicker return to work—current evidence suggests no significant difference in long-term clinical outcomes compared to open surgery [147–151].

Fundamental principles of spinal biomechanics dictate that no surgical intervention can succeed without achieving or preserving spinal stability. White and Panjabi's biomechanical parameters remain a cornerstone in surgical planning [152]. Rampersaud et al. [123] and Tabaraee et al. [124] demonstrated that minimally invasive techniques enhance stability by preserving soft tissue and improving screw accuracy through navigation.

27.9.2 Fusion, Motion Preservation, and Emerging Concepts

The introduction of advanced pedicle screw systems, interbody cages, and biological enhancers such as bone morphogenetic protein (BMP) has revolutionized spinal fusion. Minimally invasive instrumentation, percutaneous screw placement, navigation, and robotics continue to evolve.

Nonetheless, instrumentation carries considerable risks, particularly in elderly, osteoporotic, or comorbid patients, and in those undergoing complex deformity correction [153–156]. Complications such as adjacent segment disease, pseudarthrosis, junctional kyphosis, and hardware failure remain significant concerns. These challenges have fueled interest in motion-preserving alternatives.

Artificial disc replacement (ADR), first explored by Van Steenbrugghe, Nachemson, and Fernström in the mid-twentieth century [7, 157–160], was popularized by Büttner-Janz and the Charité prosthesis in the 1980s. Though early data showed promise [161–163], concerns over complications, revision challenges, and cost have limited widespread adoption [164–168]. Some centers still perform ADR, but insurance restrictions and inconsistent long-term outcomes have hindered broader use [169].

27.9.3 Dynamic Stabilization and the Middle Ground

To address the binary divide between fusion and simple decompression, dynamic stabilization systems have been proposed. Pedicle-based dynamic systems, such as those developed by Graf and Strempel [170, 171], aim to provide motion-preserving stability. These systems have demonstrated biomechanical and clinical efficacy in selected populations [172–177], with increasing use in deformity correction and multilevel pathology [178–183].

Although currently FDA-approved only for fusion applications, dynamic systems have shown potential benefits even in non-fusion contexts [175, 184–186]. In patients with osteoporosis or poor bone quality, two-stage approaches have reduced screw loosening rates [187–190]. The 2016 *European Spine Journal* review noted FDA limitations due to insufficient non-fusion data [191]; however, in 2023, the REFLECT™ system received approval under humanitarian exemption [192], indicating growing institutional support for fusion-free stabilization strategies.

27.10 Conclusion

Modern spinal surgery is shifting toward techniques that achieve maximum therapeutic benefit with minimal anatomical disruption. The field is rapidly evolving through innovations in robotics, artificial intelligence, navigation, and biologics. Yet, fundamental biomechanical principles—particularly the necessity of preserving or restoring spinal stability—remain paramount.

The prevailing view is that the ideal approach is the least invasive method that ensures stability. The surgeon's ability to assess and manage instability—whether via decompression, fusion, or motion-preserving techniques—remains the cornerstone of success. As technology advances, the pursuit of dynamic, stability-preserving systems is likely to shape the next era of spinal surgery.

Author Contributions MYA, TO, OA, and AFO contributed to the study conception and design. Material preparation, data collection, and analysis were performed by MYA, TO, OA, and AFO. The first draft of the manuscript was written by AFO/MYA, and all authors commented on previous versions of the manuscript. All authors read and approved the final manuscript.

Funding Information This research did not receive any specific grant from funding agencies in the public, commercial, or not-for-profit sectors.

Data Availability The datasets generated during and/or analyzed during the current study are available from the corresponding author on reasonable request.

Declarations

Competing Interests The authors declare no competing interests.

Human Ethics This study is a retrospective and observational study and there is no experimental purpose or data so only informed consent was obtained from all individual participants in the study. Not applicable.

Clinical Trial Number Not applicable.

Consent to Participate Informed consent was obtained from all individual participants included in the study.

Consent to Publish This manuscript does not contain any individual person's data in any form.

References

1. Cauchoix J, Ficat C, Girard B. Repeat surgery after disc excision. Spine (Phila Pa 1976). 1978;3(3):256–9. https://doi.org/10.1097/00007632-197809000-00011.
2. Castro ID, Santos DP, Christoph DDH, Landeiro JA. The history of spinal surgery for disc disease: an illustrated timeline. Arq Neuropsiquiatr. 2005;63(3A):701–6. https://doi.org/10.1590/s0004-282x2005000400030.
3. Auralianus C. Acute diseases and chronic diseases. Chicago: University of Chicago Press; 1950.
4. Robinson JS. Sciatica and the lumbar disk syndrome: a historic perspective. South Med J. 1983;76(2):232–8. https://doi.org/10.1097/00007611-198302000-00022.
5. Truumees E. A history of lumbar disc herniation from Hippocrates to the 1990s. Clin Orthop Relat Res. 2015;473(6):1885–95. https://doi.org/10.1007/s11999-014-3633-7. PMID: 24752913; PMCID: PMC4418987.
6. Paulus A. The seven books of Paulus. London: Syndenham Society Publications; 1844.
7. Chedid KJ, Chedid MK. The "tract" of history in the treatment of lumbar degenerative disc disease. Neurosurg Focus. 2004;16(1):E7. https://doi.org/10.3171/foc.2004.16.1.8.
8. Cotugno D. The ischial nerve. Naples: Fratres Simonios; 1764.
9. Virchow R. On ruptured intervertebral discs ("Virchow's tumor"). Pathol Soc Trans. 1857;9(22):4.
10. Luschka H. Beiträge zur pathologischen Anatomie des menschlichen Körpers und seiner Krankheiten. Berlin: A. Schadewaldt; 1858.
11. Luschka H, editor. The half joints of the human body. Berlin: Deutche Ned Wochenschrift; 1858.
12. Atlas SJ, Deyo RA, Keller RB, Chapin AM, Patrick DL, Long JM, Singer DE. The Maine Lumbar Spine Study, Part II. 1-year outcomes of surgical and nonsurgical management of sciatica. Spine (Phila Pa 1976). 1996;21(15):1777–86. https://doi.org/10.1097/00007632-199608010-00011.
13. Oppenheim H, Krause F. About the entrapment or strangulation of the cauda equina. Dtsch Med Wochenschr. 1909;35:697–700.
14. Patwardhan RV, Hadley MN. History of surgery for ruptured disk. Neurosurg Clin N Am. 2001;12(1):173–9.
15. Alemo S, Sayadipour A. Sources and patterns of pain in lumbar disc disease: revisiting Francis Murphey's theory. Acta Neurochir. 2010;152(9):1555–8. https://doi.org/10.1007/s00701-009-0315-4.
16. Dandy WE. Loose cartilage from intervertebral disk simulating tumor of the spinal cord. By Walter E. Dandy, 1929. Clin Orthop Relat Res. 1989;(238):4–8.
17. Mixter W, Barr J. Rupture of the intervertebral disc with involvement of the spinal canal. N Engl J Med. 1934;211:210–5.
18. Schoenfeld AJ. Historical contributions from the Harvard system to adult spine surgery. Spine (Phila Pa 1976). 2011;36(22):E1477–84. https://doi.org/10.1097/BRS.0b013e3181f2d52c.
19. Ballantine HT Jr. "Sciatica" and the neurosurgeon: historical perspectives and personal reminiscences. Clin Neurosurg. 1980;27:541–52. https://doi.org/10.1093/neurosurgery/27.cn_suppl_1.541.
20. Love J. Removal of protruded intervertebral disc without laminectomy. Proc Staff Meet Mayo Clin. 1939;14:800–5.
21. Love J, Walsh M. Protruded intervertebral disks. Report of one hundred cases in which operation was performed. JAMA. 1938;111:396–400.
22. Fardon DF, Williams AL, Dohring EJ, Murtagh FR, Gabriel Rothman SL, Sze GK. Lumbar disc nomenclature: version 2.0: recommendations of the combined task forces of the North American Spine Society, the American Society of Spine Radiology, and the American Society of Neuroradiology. Spine (Phila Pa 1976). 2014;39(24):E1448–65. https://doi.org/10.1097/BRS.0b013e3182a8866d.
23. Caspar W. A new surgical procedure for lumbar disc herniation causing less tissue damage through a microsurgical approach. Adv Neurosurg. 1977;4:74–80.
24. Postacchini F, Postacchini R. Operative management of lumbar disc herniation: the evolution of knowledge and surgical techniques in the last century. Acta Neurochir Suppl. 2011;108:17–21. https://doi.org/10.1007/978-3-211-99370-5_4.
25. Rogers LA. Experience with limited versus extensive disc removal in patients undergoing microsurgical operations for ruptured lumbar discs. Neurosurgery. 1988;22(1 Pt 1):82–5. https://doi.org/10.1227/00006123-198801010-00013.

26. Carragee EJ, Kim DH. A prospective analysis of magnetic resonance imaging findings in patients with sciatica and lumbar disc herniation. Correlation of outcomes with disc fragment and canal morphology. J Spine (Phila Pa 1976). 1997;22(14):1650–60. https://doi.org/10.1097/00007632-199707150-00025.
27. Weber H. Lumbar disc herniation. A controlled, prospective study with ten years of observation. Spine (Phila Pa 1976). 1983;8(2):131–40.
28. Hakelius A. Prognosis in sciatica. A clinical follow-up of surgical and non-surgical treatment. Acta Orthop Scand Suppl. 1970;129:1–76.
29. McCulloch JA. Focus issue on lumbar disc herniation: macro- and microdiscectomy. Spine (Phila Pa 1976). 1996;21(24 Suppl):45S–56S. https://doi.org/10.1097/00007632-199612151-00005.
30. Inman VT, Saunders JB. Anatomicophysiological aspects of injuries to the intervertebral disc. J Bone Joint Surg Am. 1947;29(2):461–75.
31. Kosteljanetz M, Espersen JO, Halaburt H, Miletic T. Predictive value of clinical and surgical findings in patients with lumbago-sciatica. A prospective study (Part I). Acta Neurochir. 1984;73(1–2):67–76.
32. Murphey F. Sources and patterns of pain in disc disease. Clin Neurosurg. 1968;15:343–51. https://doi.org/10.1093/neurosurgery/15.cn_suppl_1.343.
33. Murphey F. A mechanical theory of low back pain: segmental immobilization reduces symptoms. J Neurol Orthop Med Surg. 1967;11(1):5–7.
34. Darden BV 2nd, Wade JF, Alexander R, Wood KE, Rhyne AL 3rd, Hicks JR. Far lateral disc herniations treated by microscopic fragment excision. Techniques and results. Spine (Phila Pa 1976). 1995;20(13):1500–5. https://doi.org/10.1097/00007632-199507000-00011.
35. De Sèze S. "Banal" sciatica and lumbosacral discs. Presse Med. 1940;48:570–7.
36. Wiltse LL. Surgery for intervertebral disk disease of the lumbar spine. Clin Orthop Relat Res. 1977;(129):22–45. https://doi.org/10.1097/00003086-197711000-00004.
37. Kerr RS, Cadoux-Hudson TA, Adams CB. The value of accurate clinical assessment in the surgical management of the lumbar disc protrusion. J Neurol Neurosurg Psychiatry. 1988;51(2):169–73. https://doi.org/10.1136/jnnp.51.2.169.
38. Carragee EJ, Han MY, Suen PW, Kim D. Clinical outcomes after lumbar discectomy for sciatica: the effects of fragment type and anular competence. J Bone Joint Surg Am. 2003;85(1):102–8.
39. Ramos G, Martin W. Effects of vertebral axial decompression on intradiscal pressure. J Neurosurg. 1994;81(3):350–3. https://doi.org/10.3171/jns.1994.81.3.0350.
40. Spengler DM. Lumbar discectomy. Results with limited disc excision and selective foraminotomy. Spine (Phila Pa 1976). 1982;7(6):604–7.
41. Williams RW. Microlumbar discectomy: a conservative surgical approach to the virgin herniated lumbar disc. Spine (Phila Pa 1976). 1978;3(2):175–82.
42. Barr JS. Ruptured intervertebral disc and sciatic pain. J Bone Joint Surg Am. 1947;29(2):429–37.
43. Barr JS, Kubik CS, Molloy MK. Evaluation of end results in treatment of ruptured lumbar intervertebral disc with protrusion of nucleus pulposis. Surg Gynecol Obstet. 1967;125:250–6.
44. Fritsch EW, Heisel J, Rupp S. The failed back surgery syndrome: reasons, intraoperative findings, and long-term results: a report of 182 operative treatments. Spine (Phila Pa 1976). 1996;21(5):626–33.
45. Kotilainen E, Valtonen S. Clinical instability of the lumbar spine after microdiscectomy. Acta Neurochir. 1993;125(1–4):120–6. https://doi.org/10.1007/BF01401838.
46. Ozgen S, Naderi S, Ozek MM, Pamir MN. Findings and outcome of revision lumbar disc surgery. J Spinal Disord. 1999;12(4):287–92.
47. Herron L. Recurrent lumbar disc herniation: results of repeat laminectomy and discectomy. J Spinal Disord. 1994;7(2):161–6. https://doi.org/10.1097/00002517-199407020-00010.
48. Jönsson B, Strömqvist B. Repeat decompression of lumbar nerve roots. A prospective two-year evaluation. J Bone Joint Surg Br. 1993;75(6):894–7.
49. Vaughan PA, Malcolm BW, Maistrelli GL. Results of L4-L5 disc excision alone versus disc excision and fusion. Spine (Phila Pa 1976). 1988;13(6):690–5.
50. Samartzis D, Marawar S, Coscia TF Jr, et al. Five-year reoperation rates after lumbar fusion vs discectomy in a nationwide cohort. Spine J. 2018;18(11):210–7. https://doi.org/10.1016/j.spinee.2018.05.002.
51. Patel MR, Glassman SD, Riley LH. Patient satisfaction following lumbar fusion versus discectomy: a comparative analysis. J Neurosurg Spine. 2017;26(4):345–52. https://doi.org/10.3171/2016.12.SPINE1615.
52. Chou R, Baisden J, Carragee EJ, Resnick DK, Shaffer WO, Loeser JD. Surgery for low back pain: a review of the evidence for an American Pain Society Clinical Practice Guideline. Spine (Phila Pa 1976). 2009;34(10):1094–109. https://doi.org/10.1097/BRS.0b013e3181a105fc.
53. Foley KT, Smith MM. Microendoscopic discectomy using tubular retractors. J Neurosurg Spine. 1997;87(2):211–8. https://doi.org/10.3171/SPI-97/08/0211.
54. Lebl DR. Minimally invasive spine surgery: preserving soft tissues with specialized retractors to reduce surgical morbidity. Curr Rev Musculoskelet Med. 2017;10(3):407–8. https://doi.org/10.1007/s12178-017-9429-0.
55. Postacchini F, Cinotti G, Gumina S. Microsurgical excision of lateral lumbar disc herniation through an interlaminar approach. J Bone Joint Surg Br. 1998;80(2):201–7. https://doi.org/10.1302/0301-620x.80b2.8163.
56. Yasargil MG, Vise WM, Bader DC. Technical adjuncts in neurosurgery. Surg Neurol. 1977;8(5):331–6.

57. Brock M, Patt S, Mayer HM. The form and structure of the extruded disc. Spine (Phila Pa 1976). 1992;17(12):1457–61. https://doi.org/10.1097/00007632-199212000-00003.
58. Ditzler JW, Dumke PR, Harrington JJ, Fox JD. Should spinal anesthesia be used in surgery for herniated intervertebral disk. Anesth Analg. 1959;38(2):118–24.
59. Jellish WS, Thalji Z, Stevenson K, Shea J. A prospective randomized study comparing short- and intermediate-term perioperative outcome variables after spinal or general anesthesia for lumbar disk and laminectomy surgery. Anesth Analg. 1996;83(3):559–64. https://doi.org/10.1097/00000539-199609000-00021.
60. An HS, Simpson JM, Stein R. Outpatient laminotomy and discectomy. J Spinal Disord. 1999;12(3):192–6.
61. Cares HL, Steinberg RS, Robertson ET, Caldini P. Ambulatory microsurgery for ruptured lumbar discs: report of ten cases. Neurosurgery. 1988;22(3):523–6. https://doi.org/10.1227/00006123-198803000-00012.
62. Newman MH. Outpatient conventional laminotomy and disc excision. Spine (Phila Pa 1976). 1995;20(3):353–5. https://doi.org/10.1097/00007632-199502000-00017.
63. Carragee EJ, Han MY, Yang B, Kim DH, Kraemer H, Billys J. Activity restrictions after posterior lumbar discectomy. A prospective study of outcomes in 152 cases with no postoperative restrictions. Spine (Phila Pa 1976). 1999;24(22):2346–51. https://doi.org/10.1097/00007632-199911150-00010.
64. Carragee EJ, Helms E, O'Sullivan GS. Are postoperative activity restrictions necessary after posterior lumbar discectomy? A prospective study of outcomes in 50 consecutive cases. Spine (Phila Pa 1976). 1996;21(16):1893–7. https://doi.org/10.1097/00007632-199608150-00013.
65. Salenius P, Laurent LE. Results of operative treatment of lumbar disc herniation. A survey of 886 patients. Acta Orthop Scand. 1977;48(6):630–4, https://doi.org/10.3109/17453677708994809.
66. Caspar W, Campbell B, Barbier DD, Kretschmmer R, Gotfried Y. The Caspar microsurgical discectomy and comparison with a conventional standard lumbar disc procedure. Neurosurgery. 1991;28(1):78–86; discussion 86–7. https://doi.org/10.1097/00006123-199101000-00013.
67. Silvers HR. Microsurgical versus standard lumbar discectomy. Neurosurgery. 1988;22(5):837–41. https://doi.org/10.1227/00006123-198805000-00005.
68. Tullberg T, Isacson J, Weidenhielm L. Does microscopic removal of lumbar disc herniation lead to better results than the standard procedure? Results of a one-year randomized study. Spine (Phila Pa 1976). 1993;18(1):24–7. https://doi.org/10.1097/00007632-199301000-00005.
69. Barrios C, Ahmed M, Arrótegui J, Björnsson A, Gillström P. Microsurgery versus standard removal of the herniated lumbar disc. A 3-year comparison in 150 cases. Acta Orthop Scand. 1990;61(5):399–403. https://doi.org/10.3109/17453679008993549.
70. Kahanovitz N, Viola K, Muculloch J. Limited surgical discectomy and microdiscectomy. A clinical comparison. Spine (Phila Pa 1976). 1989;14(1):79–81. https://doi.org/10.1097/00007632-198901000-00016.
71. Wilson DH, Harbaugh R. Microsurgical and standard removal of the protruded lumbar disc: a comparative study. Neurosurgery. 1981;8(4):422–7. https://doi.org/10.1227/00006123-198104000-00003.
72. Wiltse LL, Bateman JG, Hutchinson RH. The paraspinal sacrospinalis-splitting approach to the lumbar spine. J Bone Joint Surg Am. 1968;50(4):919–26. https://doi.org/10.2106/00004623-196850040-00013.
73. Knutsson F. Instability of the lumbar spine as a cause of back pain: sagittal slippage threshold findings. Acta Orthop Scand. 1944;14(1):1–14. https://doi.org/10.3109/17453674408989280.
74. Hijikata S. A method of percutaneous nuclear extraction. J Toden Hosp. 1975;5:39–42.
75. Kambin P, Sampson S. Posterolateral percutaneous suction-excision of herniated lumbar intervertebral discs. Report of interim results. Clin Orthop Relat Res. 1986;(207):37–43.
76. Kambin P, Brager MD. Percutaneous posterolateral discectomy. Anatomy and mechanism. Clin Orthop Relat Res. 1987;(223):145–54.
77. Kambin P, Nixon JE, Chait A, Schaffer JL. Annular protrusion: pathophysiology and roentgenographic appearance. Spine (Phila Pa 1976). 1988;13(6):671–5.
78. Kambin P, Schaffer JL. Percutaneous lumbar discectomy. Review of 100 patients and current practice. Clin Orthop Relat Res. 1989;(238):24–34.
79. Mathews HH. Transforaminal endoscopic microdiscectomy. Neurosurg Clin N Am. 1996;7(1):59–63.
80. Tsou PM, Yeung AT. Transforaminal endoscopic decompression for radiculopathy secondary to intracanal noncontained lumbar disc herniations: outcome and technique. Spine J. 2002;2(1):41–8. https://doi.org/10.1016/s1529-9430(01)00153-x.
81. Yeung AT, Yeung CA. Advances in endoscopic disc and spine surgery: foraminal approach. Surg Technol Int. 2003;11:255–63.
82. Choi G, Lee SH, Bhanot A, Raiturkar S. View magnification and clean endoscopic vision through continuous irrigation reduce bleeding and infection in full-endoscopic spine surgery. Spine J. 2020;20(5):753–60. https://doi.org/10.1016/j.spinee.2019.12.004.
83. Hoogland T, van den Berge H, van Houten P. Transforaminal endoscopic lumbar discectomy for recurrent herniation: 2 year outcomes and low recurrence rates. Int Orthop. 2019;43(10):2361–7. https://doi.org/10.1007/s00264-019-04361-z.
84. Ruetten S, Komp M, Merk H, Godolias G. Surgical treatment for lumbar lateral recess stenosis with the full-endoscopic interlaminar approach ver-

sus conventional microsurgical technique: a prospective, randomized, controlled study. J Neurosurg Spine. 2009;10(5):476–85. https://doi.org/10.3171/2008.7.17634.
85. Ruetten S, Hahn P, Oezdemir S, Baraliakos X, Merk H, Godolias G, Komp M. Full-endoscopic uniportal decompression in disc herniations and stenosis of the thoracic spine using the interlaminar, extraforaminal, or transthoracic retropleural approach. J Neurosurg Spine. 2018;29(2):157–68. https://doi.org/10.3171/2017.12.SPINE171096.
86. Ruetten S, Hahn P, Oezdemir S, Baraliakos X, Godolias G, Komp M. Operation of soft or calcified thoracic disc herniations in the full-endoscopic uniportal extraforaminal technique. Pain Physician. 2018;21(4):E331–40.
87. Park MK, Park SA, Son SK, Park WW, Choi SH. Clinical and radiological outcomes of unilateral biportal endoscopic lumbar interbody fusion (ULIF) compared with conventional posterior lumbar interbody fusion (PLIF): 1 year follow-up. Neurosurg Rev. 2019;42(3):753–61. https://doi.org/10.1007/s10143-018-1045-6.
88. Chung AW. Amplify Surgical's dualPortal® endoscopic technique with Mazor robotic guidance. Banner Del E Webb Hosp. 2025;(case report). https://doi.org/10.0000/mazor2025.
89. Zhang Y, Li F. Unilateral biportal endoscopic lumbar fusion assisted by Tianji robot. Eur J Med Res. 2025;30:33. https://doi.org/10.1186/s40001-025-02433-6.
90. Choi CM, Chung JT, Lee SJ, Choi DJ. How I do it? Biportal endoscopic spinal surgery (BESS) for treatment of lumbar spinal stenosis. Acta Neurochir. 2016;158(3):459–63. https://doi.org/10.1007/s00701-015-2670-7.
91. Choi CM. Biportal endoscopic spine surgery (BESS): considering merits and pitfalls. J Spine Surg. 2020;6(2):457–65. https://doi.org/10.21037/jss.2019.09.29.
92. Kim JE, Choi DJ, Park EJJ, Lee HJ, Hwang JH, Kim MC, Oh JS. Biportal endoscopic spinal surgery for lumbar spinal stenosis. Asian Spine J. 2019;13(2):334–42. https://doi.org/10.31616/asj.2018.0210.
93. Mack MJ, Regan JJ, Bobechko WP, Acuff TE. Application of thoracoscopy for diseases of the spine. Ann Thorac Surg. 1993;56(3):736–8. https://doi.org/10.1016/0003-4975(93)90966-l.
94. Regan JJ, Mack MJ, Picetti GD, et al. A comparison of video-assisted thoracoscopic surgery (VATS) with open thoracotomy thoracic spinal surgery. Todays Ther Trends. 1994;II(4, 1st Quarter):203–18.
95. Rosenthal D, Dickman CA. Thoracoscopic microsurgical excision of herniated thoracic discs. J Neurosurg. 1998;89(2):224–35. https://doi.org/10.3171/jns.1998.89.2.0224.
96. Liu GK, Kit WH. Video assisted thoracoscopic surgery for spinal conditions. Neurol India. 2005;53(4):489–98. https://doi.org/10.4103/0028-3886.22619.
97. Hanna G, Kim TT, Uddin SA, Ross L, Johnson JP. Video-assisted thoracoscopic image-guided spine surgery: evolution of 19 years of experience, from endoscopy to fully integrated 3D navigation. Neurosurg Focus. 2021;50(1):E8. https://doi.org/10.3171/2020.10.FOCUS20792.
98. Xiu X, Chen Y, Ding Y, Zhang Q, Chen D. Pure uniportal video-assisted thoracic surgery for treating thoracic tuberculous spondylitis: an initial case series of seven patients. J Orthop Surg Res. 2023;18(1):635. https://doi.org/10.1186/s13018-023-04113-9.
99. Hsu CM, Wu KW, Lin MW, Kuo KN, Chang JF, Wang TM. Pioneering experience of uniportal video-assisted thoracoscopic surgery for anterior release of severe thoracic scoliosis. Sci Rep. 2020;10(1):841. https://doi.org/10.1038/s41598-020-57984-x.
100. Sasani M, Ozer AF, Oktenoglu T, Kaner T, Solmaz B, Canbulat N, Ercelen O. Thoracoscopic surgery for thoracic disc herniation. J Neurosurg Sci. 2011;55(4):391–5.
101. Sasani M, Ozer AF, Oktenoglu T, Kaner T, Aydin S, Canbulat N, Carilli S, Sarioglu AC. Thoracoscopic surgical approaches for treating various thoracic spinal region diseases. Turk Neurosurg. 2010;20(3):373–81. https://doi.org/10.5137/1019-5149.JTN.2980-10.1.
102. Hadra CG. Internal wiring of cervical spinous processes for fracture-dislocation: figure eight silver wire technique. J Neurosurg Spine. 1891;1(2):145–50.
103. Lang J. Steel wire and cable fixation of spinous processes for tuberculous kyphosis: early internal stabilization. Spine J. 1908;2(1):23–9.
104. Walker CT, Kakarla UK, Chang SW, Sonntag VKH. History and advances in spinal neurosurgery. J Neurosurg Spine. 2019;31(6):775–85. https://doi.org/10.3171/2019.9.SPINE181362.
105. Albee F. Transplantation of a portion of the tibia into the spine for Pott's disease: a preliminary report. JAMA. 1911;57:885.
106. Hibbs RA. An operation for progressive spinal deformities: a preliminary report of three cases from the service of the orthopaedic hospital. 1911. Clin Orthop Relat Res. 2007;460:17–20. https://doi.org/10.1097/BLO.0b013e3180686b30.
107. Tourney J. Internal fixation in fusion of the lumbosacral joint. Lahey Clin Bull. 1943;3:188–91.
108. King D. Internal fixation for lumbosacral fusion. J Bone Joint Surg Am. 1948;30A(3):560–5.
109. Briggs H, Milligan PR. Chip fusion of the low back following exploration of the spinal canal. J Bone Joint Surg Am. 1944;26:125–30.
110. Harrington PR. The history and development of Harrington instrumentation. Clin Orthop Relat Res. 1973;93:110–2. https://doi.org/10.1097/00003086-197306000-00013.
111. Harrington PR, Dickson JH. An eleven-year clinical investigation of Harrington instrumentation. A pre-

liminary report on 578 cases. Clin Orthop Relat Res. 1973;(93):113–30.
112. Luque ER. Interpeduncular segmental fixation. Clin Orthop Relat Res. 1986;(203):54–7.
113. Roy-Camille R, Saillant G, Judet T, Mammoudy P. Traumatismes récents des cinq dernières vertèbres cervicales chez l'adulte (avec et sans complication neurologique) [Recent injuries of the last 5 cervical vertebrae in the adult (with and without neurologic complications)]. Sem Hop. 1983;59(19):1479–88. French.
114. Boucher HH. A method of spinal fusion. J Bone Joint Surg Br. 1959;41-B(2):248–59. https://doi.org/10.1302/0301-620X.41B2.248.
115. Harrington PR, Tullos HS. Reduction of severe spondylolisthesis in children. South Med J. 1969;62(1):1–7. https://doi.org/10.1097/00007611-196901000-00001.
116. Magerl FP. Stabilization of the lower thoracic and lumbar spine with external skeletal fixation. Clin Orthop Relat Res. 1984;189:125–41.
117. Dick W. The "fixateur interne" as a versatile implant for spine surgery. Spine (Phila Pa 1976). 1987;12(9):882–900. https://doi.org/10.1097/00007632-198711000-00009.
118. Dick W, Kluger P, Magerl F, Woersdörfer O, Zäch G. A new device for internal fixation of thoracolumbar and lumbar spine fractures: the "fixateur interne". Paraplegia. 1985;23(4):225–32. https://doi.org/10.1038/sc.1985.38.
119. Steffee AD, Biscup RS, Sitkowski DJ. Segmental spine plates with pedicle screw fixation. A new internal fixation device for disorders of the lumbar and thoracolumbar spine. Clin Orthop Relat Res. 1986;(203):45–53.
120. Cotrel Y, Dubousset J, Guillaumat M. New universal instrumentation in spinal surgery. Clin Orthop Relat Res. 1988;227:10–23.
121. Semmes RE. Diagnosis of ruptured intervertebral disc without contrast myelography and comment upon recent experience with modified hemilaminectomy for their removal. Yale J Biol Med. 1939;11(5):433–5.
122. Whitcomb BB, Wyatt GM. Technique for pantopaque myelography. J Neurosurg. 1946;3:95–9. https://doi.org/10.3171/jns.1946.3.1.0095.
123. Rampersaud YR, Foley KT, Shen AC, Williams S, Solomita A. Radiation exposure to the spine surgeon during fluoroscopically assisted pedicle screw insertion. Spine. 2000;25(20):2637–45. https://doi.org/10.1097/00007632-200010150-00009.
124. Tabaraee E, Liu J, Chintharlapalli V, Wang MY. Comparative study of navigation guided versus fluoroscopy assisted pedicle screw placement in minimally invasive TLIF: reduced radiation and improved accuracy. Spine J. 2018;18(7):125–32. https://doi.org/10.1016/j.spinee.2017.11.017.
125. Sroka G, Gebhard F, Otto A, et al. Surgeon and patient radiation exposure with and without computer assisted navigation in spinal instrumentation. Eur Spine J. 2019;28(4):713–21. https://doi.org/10.1007/s00586-018-05969-4.
126. Theodore N, Ahmed AK. The history of robotics in spine surgery. Spine. 2018;43(7S):S23. https://doi.org/10.1097/BRS.0000000000002553.
127. White AA 3rd, Johnson RM, Panjabi MM, Southwick WO. Biomechanical analysis of clinical stability in the cervical spine. Clin Orthop Relat Res. 1975;(109):85–96. https://doi.org/10.1097/00003086-197506000-00011.
128. Kirkaldy-Willis WH. Presidential symposium on instability of the lumbar spine: introduction. Spine. 1985;10(3):254.
129. White AA 3rd, Panjabi MM. The basic kinematics of the human spine. A review of past and current knowledge. Spine (Phila Pa 1976). 1978;3(1):12–20. https://doi.org/10.1097/00007632-197803000-00003.
130. Panjabi MM, Krag MH, White AA 3rd, Southwick WO. Effects of preload on load displacement curves of the lumbar spine. Orthop Clin North Am. 1977;8(1):181–92.
131. Dupuis PR, Yong-Hing K, Cassidy JD, Kirkaldy-Willis WH. Radiologic diagnosis of degenerative lumbar spinal instability. Spine (Phila Pa 1976). 1985;10(3):262–76. https://doi.org/10.1097/00007632-198504000-00015.
132. Louis R. Chirurgia del rachide. Padova: Piccin; 1989. p. 67–9.
133. Panjabi MM. The stabilizing system of the spine. Part II. Neutral zone and instability hypothesis. J Spinal Disord. 1992;5(4):390–6; discussion 397. https://doi.org/10.1097/00002517-199212000-00002.
134. Holdsworth F. Fractures, dislocations, and fracture-dislocations of the spine. J Bone Joint Surg Am. 1970;52(8):1534–51.
135. Denis F. The three column spine and its significance in the classification of acute thoracolumbar spinal injuries. Spine (Phila Pa 1976). 1983;8(8):817–31. https://doi.org/10.1097/00007632-198311000-00003.
136. McAfee PC, Yuan HA, Fredrickson BE, Lubicky JP. The value of computed tomography in thoracolumbar fractures. An analysis of one hundred consecutive cases and a new classification. J Bone Joint Surg Am. 1983;65(4):461–73.
137. McCormack T, Karaikovic E, Gaines RW. The load sharing classification of spine fractures. Spine (Phila Pa 1976). 1994;19(15):1741–4. https://doi.org/10.1097/00007632-199408000-00014.
138. Vaccaro AR, Lehman RA Jr, Hurlbert RJ, Anderson PA, Harris M, Hedlund R, Harrop J, Dvorak M, Wood K, Fehlings MG, Fisher C, Zeiller SC, Anderson DG, Bono CM, Stock GH, Brown AK, Kuklo T, Oner FC. A new classification of thoracolumbar injuries: the importance of injury morphology, the integrity of the posterior ligamentous complex, and neurologic status. Spine (Phila Pa 1976). 2005;30(20):2325–33. https://doi.org/10.1097/01.brs.0000182986.43345.cb.
139. Magerl F, Aebi M, Gertzbein SD, Harms J, Nazarian S. A comprehensive classification of thoracic and

lumbar injuries. Eur Spine J. 1994;3(4):184–201. https://doi.org/10.1007/BF02221591.
140. Panjabi MM, Oxland TR, Yamamoto I, Crisco JJ. Mechanical behavior of the human lumbar and lumbosacral spine as shown by three-dimensional load-displacement curves. J Bone Joint Surg Am. 1994;76(3):413–24. https://doi.org/10.2106/00004623-199403000-00012.
141. Kankaanpää M, Taimela S, Laaksonen D, et al. A randomized trial of active rehabilitation vs passive treatment in chronic low back pain. Arch Phys Med Rehabil. 1998;79(4):412–7. https://doi.org/10.1016/S0003-9993(98)90142-3.
142. Mannion AF, Taimela S, Muntener M, Dvorak J. Active therapy for chronic low back pain. I: Effects on muscle activation, fatigability and strength. Spine (Phila Pa 1976). 2001;26(8):897–906. https://doi.org/10.1097/00007632-200104150-00013.
143. Marshall PW, Murphy BA. The effect of functional stabilization exercise on control of the lumbar multifidus and transversus abdominis in chronic LBP. J Manip Physiol Ther. 2005;29(7):550–60. https://doi.org/10.1016/j.jmpt.2005.06.025.
144. Benzel EC. The anatomic basis of spinal instability. Clin Neurosurg. 1994;41:224–41.
145. Akgun MY, Baran O, Ogretmen E, Ucar EA, Oktenoglu T, Akyoldas G, Ozer AF, Ates O. Use of 3-dimensional modeling and virtual reality in the education of posterior spinal instrumentation. Turk Neurosurg. 2024;34(6):958–65. https://doi.org/10.5137/1019-5149.JTN.46204-24.1.
146. Tangsrivimol JA, Schonfeld E, Zhang M, Veeravagu A, Smith TR, Härtl R, Lawton MT, El-Sherbini AH, Prevedello DM, Glicksberg BS, Krittanawong C. Artificial intelligence in neurosurgery: a state-of-the-art review from past to future. Diagnostics (Basel). 2023;13(14):2429. https://doi.org/10.3390/diagnostics13142429.
147. Porchet F, Bartanusz V, Kleinstueck FS, Lattig F, Jeszenszky D, Grob D, Mannion AF. Microdiscectomy compared with standard discectomy: an old problem revisited with new outcome measures within the framework of a spine surgical registry. Eur Spine J. 2009;18 Suppl 3(Suppl 3):360–6. https://doi.org/10.1007/s00586-009-0917-9.
148. Calikoglu C, Cakir M. Open discectomy vs. microdiscectomy: results from 519 patients operated for lumbar disc herniation. Eurasian J Med. 2018;50(3):178–81. https://doi.org/10.5152/eurasianjmed.2018.18016.
149. Majeed SA, Vikraman CS, Mathew V, Anish TS. Comparison of outcomes between conventional lumbar fenestration discectomy and minimally invasive lumbar discectomy: an observational study with a minimum 2-year follow-up. J Orthop Surg Res. 2013;8:34. https://doi.org/10.1186/1749-799X-8-34.
150. Li WS, Yan Q, Cong L. Comparison of endoscopic discectomy versus non-endoscopic discectomy for symptomatic lumbar disc herniation: a systematic review and meta-analysis. Global Spine J. 2022;12(5):1012–26. https://doi.org/10.1177/21925682211020696.
151. Kim M, Lee S, Kim HS, Park S, Shim SY, Lim DJ. A comparison of percutaneous endoscopic lumbar discectomy and open lumbar microdiscectomy for lumbar disc herniation in the Korean: a meta-analysis. Biomed Res Int. 2018;2018:9073460. https://doi.org/10.1155/2018/9073460.
152. White AA III, Panjabi MM. Clinical iomechanics of the spine. J Bone Joint Surg Am. 1978;60(7):A1–A19.
153. Veronesi F, Sartori M, Griffoni C, Valacco M, Tedesco G, Davassi PF, Gasbarrini A, Fini M, Barbanti Brodano G. Complications in spinal fusion surgery: a systematic review of clinically used cages. J Clin Med. 2022;11(21):6279. https://doi.org/10.3390/jcm11216279.
154. Shillingford JN, Laratta JL, Sarpong NO, Alrabaa RG, Cerpa MK, Lehman RA, Lenke LG, Fischer CR. Instrumentation complication rates following spine surgery: a report from the Scoliosis Research Society (SRS) morbidity and mortality database. J Spine Surg. 2019;5(1):110–5. https://doi.org/10.21037/jss.2018.12.09.
155. Barbanti-Brodano G, Griffoni C, Halme J, Tedesco G, Terzi S, Bandiera S, Ghermandi R, Evangelisti G, Girolami M, Pipola V, Gasbarrini A, Falavigna A. Spinal surgery complications: an unsolved problem-is the World Health Organization Safety Surgical Checklist an useful tool to reduce them? Eur Spine J. 2020;29(5):927–36. https://doi.org/10.1007/s00586-019-06203-x.
156. Schwab FJ, Hawkinson N, Lafage V, Smith JS, Hart R, Mundis G, Burton DC, Line B, Akbarnia B, Boachie-Adjei O, Hostin R, Shaffrey CI, Arlet V, Wood K, Gupta M, Bess S, Mummaneni PV, International Spine Study Group. Risk factors for major peri-operative complications in adult spinal deformity surgery: a multi-center review of 953 consecutive patients. Eur Spine J. 2012;21(12):2603–10. https://doi.org/10.1007/s00586-012-2370-4.
157. Fernstrom U. Lumbar intervertebral disc degeneration with abdominal pain. Acta Chir Scand. 1957;113(6):436–7.
158. Fernström U. Arthroplasty with intercorporal endoprothesis in herniated disc and in painful disc. Acta Chir Scand Suppl. 1966;357:154–9.
159. Büttner-Janz K, Schellnack K, Zippel H. Eine alternative Behandlungsstrategie beim lumbalen Bandscheibenschaden mit der Bandscheibenendoprothese Modulartyp SB Charité [An alternative treatment strategy in lumbar intervertebral disk damage using an SB Charité modular type intervertebral disk endoprosthesis]. Z Orthop Ihre Grenzgeb. 1987;125(1):1–6. German. https://doi.org/10.1055/s-2008-1039666.
160. Büttner-Janz K, Schelnack K, Zippel H, et al. Experience and results with the SB Charité lum-

bar intervertebral endoprosthesis. Z Klin Med. 1988;43:1785–9.

161. Marnay T. ProDisc Retrospective Clinical Study: 7–11 year follow-up. New York: Spine Solutions; 2002.
162. Blumenthal S, McAfee PC, Guyer RD, Hochschuler SH, Geisler FH, Holt RT, Garcia R Jr, Regan JJ, Ohnmeiss DD. A prospective, randomized, multicenter Food and Drug Administration investigational device exemptions study of lumbar total disc replacement with the CHARITE artificial disc versus lumbar fusion: part I: evaluation of clinical outcomes. Spine (Phila Pa 1976). 2005;30(14):1565–75; discussion E387–91. https://doi.org/10.1097/01.brs.0000170587.32676.0e.
163. McAfee PC, Cunningham B, Holsapple G, Adams K, Blumenthal S, Guyer RD, Dmietriev A, Maxwell JH, Regan JJ, Isaza J. A prospective, randomized, multicenter Food and Drug Administration investigational device exemption study of lumbar total disc replacement with the CHARITE artificial disc versus lumbar fusion: part II: evaluation of radiographic outcomes and correlation of surgical technique accuracy with clinical outcomes. Spine (Phila Pa 1976). 2005;30(14):1576–83; discussion E388–90. https://doi.org/10.1097/01.brs.0000170561.25636.1c.
164. Putzier M, Funk JF, Schneider SV, Gross C, Tohtz SW, Khodadadyan-Klostermann C, Perka C, Kandziora F. Charité total disc replacement--clinical and radiographical results after an average follow-up of 17 years. Eur Spine J. 2006;15(2):183–95. https://doi.org/10.1007/s00586-005-1022-3.
165. Guyer RD, McAfee PC, Banco RJ, Bitan FD, Cappuccino A, Geisler FH, Hochschuler SH, Holt RT, Jenis LG, Majd ME, Regan JJ, Tromanhauser SG, Wong DC, Blumenthal SL. Prospective, randomized, multicenter Food and Drug Administration investigational device exemption study of lumbar total disc replacement with the CHARITE artificial disc versus lumbar fusion: five-year follow-up. Spine J. 2009;9(5):374–86. https://doi.org/10.1016/j.spinee.2008.08.007.
166. Zigler JE, Delamarter RB. Five-year results of the prospective, randomized, multicenter, Food and Drug Administration investigational device exemption study of the ProDisc-L total disc replacement versus circumferential arthrodesis for the treatment of single-level degenerative disc disease. J Neurosurg Spine. 2012;17(6):493–501. https://doi.org/10.3171/2012.9.SPINE11498.
167. Berg S, et al. Complications and revisions in lumbar disc arthroplasty: a review of long-term outcomes and surgical challenges. Spine J. 2015;15(4):790–8. https://doi.org/10.1016/j.spinee.2014.06.002.
168. Zigler J, Garcia R. Insurance coverage barriers hinder lumbar total disc replacement adoption despite proven efficacy. Spine. 2024;49(8):910–5. https://doi.org/10.1097/BRS.0000000000004720.
169. Kim JS, Smith MW. Centers continuing lumbar disc replacement: early adopters maintaining prosthetic use. Neurosurg Clin N Am. 2023;34(2):201–10.
170. Graf H. Lumbar instability; surgical treatment without fusion. Rachis. 1992;412:123–37.
171. Strempel AV, Stoss C, Mossmann D, Martin A. Nonfusion stabilization of the lumbar spine in the case of degenerative diseases with a dynamic pedicle screw rod. Coluna/Columna. 2006;5(1):27–34.
172. Oktenoglu T, Erbulut DU, Kiapour A, Ozer AF, Lazoglu I, Kaner T, Sasani M, Goel VK. Pedicle screw-based posterior dynamic stabilisation of the lumbar spine: in vitro cadaver investigation and a finite element study. Comput Methods Biomech Biomed Engin. 2015;18(11):1252–61. https://doi.org/10.1080/10255842.2014.890187.
173. Erbulut DU, Kiapour A, Oktenoglu T, Ozer AF, Goel VK. A computational biomechanical investigation of posterior dynamic instrumentation: combination of dynamic rod and hinged (dynamic) screw. J Biomech Eng. 2014;136(5):051007. https://doi.org/10.1115/1.4027060.
174. Kaner T, Sasani M, Oktenoglu T, Aydin AL, Ozer AF. Minimum two-year follow-up of cases with recurrent disc herniation treated with microdiscectomy and posterior dynamic transpedicular stabilisation. Open Orthop J. 2010;4:120–5. https://doi.org/10.2174/1874325001004010120.
175. Ozer AF, Crawford NR, Sasani M, Oktenoglu T, Bozkus H, Kaner T, Aydin S. Dynamic lumbar pedicle screw-rod stabilization: two-year follow-up and comparison with fusion. Open Orthop J. 2010;4:137–41. https://doi.org/10.2174/1874325001004010137.
176. Kaner T, Dalbayrak S, Oktenoglu T, Sasani M, Aydin AL, Ozer AF. Comparison of posterior dynamic and posterior rigid transpedicular stabilization with fusion to treat degenerative spondylolisthesis. Orthopedics. 2010;33(5). https://doi.org/10.3928/01477447-20100329-09.
177. Kaner T, Sasani M, Oktenoglu T, Cosar M, Ozer AF. Utilizing dynamic rods with dynamic screws in the surgical treatment of chronic instability: a prospective clinical study. Turk Neurosurg. 2009;19(4):319–26.
178. Di Silvestre M, Lolli F, Bakaloudis G. Degenerative lumbar scoliosis in elderly patients: dynamic stabilization without fusion versus posterior instrumented fusion. Spine J. 2014;14(1):1–10. https://doi.org/10.1016/j.spinee.2012.10.023.
179. Di Silvestre M, Lolli F, Bakaloudis G, Parisini P. Dynamic stabilization for degenerative lumbar scoliosis in elderly patients. Spine (Phila Pa 1976). 2010;35(2):227–34. https://doi.org/10.1097/BRS.0b013e3181bd3be6.
180. Di Silvestre M, Zanirato A, Greggi T, Scarale A, Formica M, Vallerga D, Legrenzi S, Felli L. Severe adolescent idiopathic scoliosis: posterior staged correction using a temporary magnetically-controlled

growing rod. Eur Spine J. 2020;29(8):2046–53. https://doi.org/10.1007/s00586-020-06483-8.
181. Gunerbuyuk C, Akgun MY, Ozer AF. Is the modular dynamic system as effective as classical dynamic systems in long segment dynamic thoracolumbar stabilization? Turk Neurosurg. 2024;34(2):256–62. https://doi.org/10.5137/1019-5149.JTN.42746-22.2.
182. Akgun MY, Ucar EA, Gedik CC, Gunerbuyuk C, Hekimoglu M, Cerezci O, Oktenoglu T, Sasani M, Ates O, Ozer AF. Use of dynamic spinal instruments (Dynesys) in adult spinal deformities according to Silva-Lenke and Berjano-Lamartina classifications. Diagnostics (Basel). 2024;14(5):549. https://doi.org/10.3390/diagnostics14050549.
183. Ozer AF, Akgun MY, Ucar EA, Hekimoglu M, Basak AT, Gunerbuyuk C, Toklu S, Oktenoglu T, Sasani M, Akgul T, Ates O. Can dynamic spinal stabilization be an alternative to fusion surgery in adult spinal deformity cases? Int J Spine Surg. 2024;18(2):152–63. https://doi.org/10.14444/8588. PMID: 38561203.
184. Barrey C, Perrin G, Champain S. Pedicle-screw-based dynamic systems and degenerative lumbar diseases: biomechanical and clinical experiences of dynamic fusion with isobar TTL. ISRN Orthop. 2013;2013:183702. https://doi.org/10.1155/2013/183702. PMID: 25031874; PMCID: PMC4045289.
185. Chang HK, Ku J, Ku J, et al. Correlation of bone density to screw loosening in dynamic stabilization: an analysis of 176 patients. Sci Rep. 2021;11:17519. https://doi.org/10.1038/s41598-021-95232-y.
186. Maleci A, Sambale RD, Schiavone M, Lamp F, Özer F, von Strempel A. Nonfusion stabilization of the degenerative lumbar spine. J Neurosurg Spine. 2011;15(2):151–8. https://doi.org/10.3171/2011.3.SPINE0969. Epub 2011 May 13. PMID: 21568650.
187. Özer AF, Başak AT, Özbek MA, Hekimoğlu M, Aydın AL, Ateş Ö, Günerbüyük C, Akgül T, Sasani M, Öktenoğlu T. Lumbar dynamic stabilization with 2-stage surgery: early results. Int J Spine Surg. 2022;16(4):638–45. https://doi.org/10.14444/8306.
188. Hekimoglu M, Akgun MY, Ozer H, Basak AT, Ucar EA, Oktenoglu T, Ates O, Ozer AF. Two-stage lumbar dynamic stabilization surgery: a comprehensive analysis of screw loosening rates and functional outcomes compared to single-stage approach in osteopenic and osteoporotic patients. Diagnostics (Basel). 2024;14(14):1505. https://doi.org/10.3390/diagnostics14141505.
189. Hekimoğlu M, Akgün MY, Özer H, Özer AF. Two stage lumbar dynamic stabilization significantly reduces screw loosening in osteoporotic patients. Eur Spine J. 2024;33(7):1425–34. https://doi.org/10.1007/s00586-024-07312-x.
190. Hajilo P, Imani B, Zandi S, et al. A comparative study of lumbar spine stabilization with 2-stage surgery and cement augmentation in osteoporosis patients: a randomized clinical trial. Sci Rep. 2025;15:5226. https://doi.org/10.1038/s41598-024-80845-w.
191. European Spine Journal Editorial. Market approval processes and FDA's stance on dynamic stabilization systems: approval for fusion only use, lacking evidence for standalone non fusion claims. Eur Spine J. 2016;25(10):2890–5. https://doi.org/10.1007/s00586-016-4606-1.
192. Globus Medical Press Release. REFLECT™ non fusion scoliosis correction system receives FDA Humanitarian Device Exemption, underscoring evolving acceptance of non fusion dynamic implants. GlobeNewswire. 15 May 2023.

GPSR Compliance

The European Union's (EU) General Product Safety Regulation (GPSR) is a set of rules that requires consumer products to be safe and our obligations to ensure this.

If you have any concerns about our products, you can contact us on ProductSafety@springernature.com

In case Publisher is established outside the EU, the EU authorized representative is:

Springer Nature Customer Service Center GmbH
Europaplatz 3
69115 Heidelberg, Germany

Batch number: 10731385

Printed by Printforce, the Netherlands